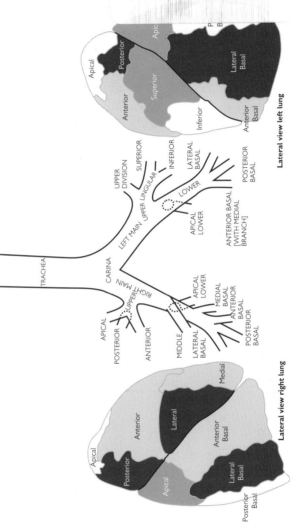

Lateral view left lung

TRACHEA

CARINA

LEFT MAIN

UPPER DIVISION

SUPERIOR

UPPER LINGULAR

INFERIOR

LATERAL BASAL

LOWER

APICAL LOWER

ANTERIOR BASAL [WITH MEDIAL BRANCH]

POSTERIOR BASAL

RIGHT MAIN

APICAL

POSTERIOR

ANTERIOR

UPPER

MIDDLE

LATERAL BASAL

APICAL LOWER

MEDIAL BASAL

ANTERIOR BASAL

POSTERIOR BASAL

Left lung (Lateral view left lung):
Apical · Posterior · Apical · Anterior · Superior · Inferior · Lateral Basal · Anterior Basal · P. B.

Lateral view right lung

Apical · Posterior · Anterior · Lateral · Apical · Medial · Anterior Basal · Lateral Basal · Posterior Basal

5/04/10

Index to emergency topics

Oxford American Handbook of
Pulmonary Medicine

Published and forthcoming Oxford American Handbooks

Oxford American Handbook of Clinical Medicine
Oxford American Handbook of Anesthesiology
Oxford American Handbook of Clinical Dentistry
Oxford American Handbook of Critical Care
Oxford American Handbook of Emergency Medicine
Oxford American Handbook of Nephrology and Hypertension
Oxford American Handbook of Obstetrics and Gynecology
Oxford American Handbook of Oncology
Oxford American Handbook of Otolaryngology
Oxford American Handbook of Pediatrics
Oxford American Handbook of Psychiatry
Oxford American Handbook of Pulmonary Medicine
Oxford American Handbook of Rheumatology
Oxford American Handbook of Surgery

Oxford American Handbook of **Pulmonary Medicine**

Kevin K. Brown, MD
Professor and Vice Chairman
Department of Medicine
National Jewish Health
Denver, Colorado

Teofilo Lee-Chiong, MD
Professor of Medicine
Head, Division of Sleep Medicine
Department of Medicine
National Jewish Health
University of Colorado
Denver School of Medicine
Denver, Colorado

with

Stephen Chapman
Grace Robinson
John Stradling
Sophie West

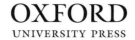

OXFORD
UNIVERSITY PRESS

OXFORD
UNIVERSITY PRESS

Oxford University Press, Inc., publishes works that further
Oxford University's objective of excellence
in research, scholarship, and education.

Oxford New York

Auckland Cape Town Dar es Salaam Hong Kong Karachi
Kuala Lumpur Madrid Melbourne Mexico City Nairobi
New Delhi Shanghai Taipei Toronto

With offices in

Argentina Austria Brazil Chile Czech Republic France Greece
Guatemala Hungary Italy Japan Poland Portugal Singapore
South Korea Switzerland Thailand Turkey Ukraine Vietnam

Copyright © 2009 by Oxford University Press, Inc.

Published by Oxford University Press, Inc.
198 Madison Avenue, New York, New York 10016

www.oup.com

Library of Congress Cataloging-in-Publication Data

Oxford American handbook of pulmonary medicine/edited by Kevin K. Brown,
Teofilo Lee-Chiong
p. ; cm.—(Oxford American handbooks)
Based on: Oxford handbook of respiratory medicine/Stephen Chapman ... [et al.], 2005.
ISBN 978-0-19-532956-8 (alk. paper)
1. Respiratory organs—Diseases—Handbooks, manuals, etc.
[DNLM: 1. Respiratory Tract Diseases—diagnosis—Handbooks.
2. Respiratory Tract Diseases—therapy—Handbooks. WF 39 O978 2008]
I. Title: Handbook of pulmonary medicine. II. Brown, Kevin K. III. Lee-Chiong, Teofilo
L, 1960. IV. Oxford handbook of pulmonary medicine. V. Series.
RC732.O95 2008
616.2—dc22   2007044658

9 8 7 6 5 4 3 2 1

Printed in China
on acid-free paper.

Preface

This handbook is designed to meet the needs of its various readers, from the pulmonary subspecialist who yearns to know "more about less," the pulmonary generalist who is required to know "something about every-thing," and the pulmonary trainee who wants to understand it all. To the busy clinician, this concise book can serve as an independent portable manual for the day-to-day management of patients with respiratory disorders as well as a complement to larger textbooks in the field. This book can be brought to the outpatient clinic, inpatient hospital ward, or intensive care unit, wherever patients are cared for.

We wish to express our sincere gratitude to the many contributors and colleagues, all of whom are major authorities on contemporary respiratory medicine, for the expert submissions and counsel they have generously provided us. We also thank the editorial board at Oxford University Press for their patience and unwavering enthusiasm for this project. We are especially indebted to Amy Hall at National Jewish Health, who almost single-handedly kept all the authors on schedule. Finally, we must gratefully acknowledge the support and encouragement given us by our families. To them we dedicate this book:

Kathleen A. Doyle, MD, MPH, Lily Clare Brown, and Mei Linn Brown

Dolores Grace Zamudio and Zoé Lee-Chiong.

Kevin K. Brown, MD

Teofilo Lee-Chiong, MD

Contents

Part I Clinical presentations—approaches to problems

Part II Clinical conditions

Part III Supportive care

Detailed contents

20 Viral respiratory infection 247

Contributors

John David Armstrong II, MD, MA [Phil]
Professor, Institute for Advanced BioMedical Imaging
National Jewish Health
Professor, Diagnostic Imaging and Division of Pulmonary Sciences & Critical Care Medicine
Faculty Associate, Center for Bioethics & Humanities
University of Colorado Denver School of Medicine
Denver, Colorado

David A. Badesch, MD
Professor of Medicine
Division of Pulmonary Sciences, Critical Care Medicine and Cardiology
Clinical Director, Pulmonary Hypertension Center
University of Colorado Denver School of Medicine
Denver, Colorado

Ronald Carlisle Balkissoon
Associate Professor of Medicine
National Jewish Health
Denver, Colorado

Robert Phillip Baughman, MD
Professor of Medicine
University of Cincinnati Medical Center
Cincinnati, Ohio

David A. Beuther, MD
Assistant Professor
Department of Medicine
Director of Medical Informatics
National Jewish Health
University of Colorado Denver School of Medicine
Denver, Colorado

Darren Boe, MD
Fellow
Division of Pulmonary Sciences and Critical Care Medicine,
University of Colorado Denver School of Medicine
Denver, Colorado

Kevin K. Brown, MD
Professor and Vice Chairman
Department of Medicine
National Jewish Health
Denver, Colorado

Todd M. Bull, MD
Associate Professor of Medicine
Pulmonary Hypertension Center
Division of Pulmonary Sciences and Critical Care Medicine
University of Colorado Denver School of Medicine
Denver, Colorado

Brendan J. Clark, MD
Fellow, Pulmonary and Critical Care Medicine
University of Colorado Denver School of Medicine
Denver, Colorado

Samay Dalal, MD
Instructor
Division of Pulmonary Sciences and Critical Care Medicine
University of Colorado Denver School of Medicine
Denver, Colorado

Charles S. Dela Cruz, MD, PhD
Senior Research Fellow
Pulmonary and Critical Care Medicine
Yale University School of Medicine
New Haven, Connecticut

Maxine E. Dexter, MD
University of Colorado Denver
School of Medicine
Denver, Colorado

Peter Doelken, MD
Associate Professor of Medicine
Director, Interventional Pleural Unit
Division of Pulmonary, Critical
Care, Allergy and Sleep Medicine
Medical University of South
Carolina Charleston,
South Carolina

Lior Dolgonos, MD
Fellow, Pulmonary and Critical
Care Medicine
University of Colorado Denver
School of Medicine
Denver, Colorado

James H. Ellis, Jr. MD
Clinical Professor of Medicine
and Pulmonary Disease
National Jewish Health
University of Colorado Denver
School of Medicine
Denver, Colorado

**Stephen K. Frankel, MD,
FCCP**
Associate Professor of Medicine,
Section Head, Critical Care &
Hospital Medicine
National Jewish Health
Associate Professor of Medicine,
Division of Pulmonary Sciences
and Critical Care Medicine
University of Colorado Denver
School of Medicine
Denver, Colorado

Adam L. Friedlander, MD
Instructor of Medicine
Division of Pulmonary Sciences
and Critical Care Medicine
University of Colorado Denver
School of Medicine
National Jewish Health
Denver, CO

**Mary Gilmartin, RN, RRT,
AE-C**
Principal Coordinator, NETT
Coordinator, COPD CRN
Nurse Specialist
National Jewish Health
Denver, Colorado

**E. Brigitte Gottschall, MD,
MSPH**
Assistant Professor of Medicine
National Jewish Health
Denver, Colorado

Brian Barkley Graham, MD
Fellow, Division of Pulmonary
Sciences and Critical Care Medicine
University of Colorado Denver
School of Medicine
Denver, Colorado

John J. Harrington, MD, MPH
Assistant Professor
National Jewish Health
Denver, Colorado

**Kristin B. Highland, MD,
MSCR**
Associate Professor of Medicine
Director, Pulmonary Hypertension
Program
Division of Pulmonary, Critical Care,
Allergy and Sleep Medicine
Division of Rheumatology and
Immunology
Medical University of South Carolina
Charleston, South Carolina

Stella E. Hines, MD
Fellow, Pulmonary Sciences and
Critical Care Medicine
Resident, Occupational and
Environmental Medicine
University of Colorado Denver
School of Medicine
Division of Environmental
and Occupational Health Sciences
National Jewish Health
Denver, Colorado

Katherine Hodgin, MD
Fellow
Division of Pulmonary Sciences
and Critical Care Medicine
University of Colorado Denver
School of Medicine
Denver, Colorado

Tristan J, Huie, MD
Fellow, Division of Pulmonary
Sciences and Critical Care
Medicine
University of Colorado Denver
School of Medicine
Denver, Colorado

Richard Stephen Irwin, MD
Professor of Medicine
University of Massachusetts
Medical School
Worcester, Massachusetts

Michael D. Iseman, MD
Professor of Medicine
National Jewish Health
Divisions of Pulmonary Sciences
and Critical Care Medicine and
Infectious Diseases
University of Colorado Denver
School of Medicine
Denver, Colorado

David A. Kaminsky, MD
Associate Professor of Medicine
Division of Pulmonary and Critical
Care Medicine
University of Vermont College of
Medicine
Burlington, Vermont

Mark Kearns, MD
Fellow, Division of Pulmonary
Sciences and Critical Care
Medicine
University of Colorado Denver
School of Medicine
Denver, Colorado

Ghulam Khaleeq, MD
Albert Einstein Medical Center
Philadelphia, Pennsylvania

Jeffrey S. Klein, MD
Soule and Tampas Green and Gold
Professor of Radiology
University of Vermont
College of Medicine
Fletcher Allen Health Care
Burlington, Vermont

Robert M. Kotloff, MD
Professor of Medicine
Chief, Section of Advanced Lung
Disease and Lung Transplantation
Hospital of the University
of Pennsylvania
Philadelphia, Pennsylvania

Heather R. LaChance, PhD
Assistant Professor of Medicine
National Jewish Health
Denver, Colorado

Esther L. Langmack, MD
Associate Professor of Medicine
National Jewish Health
Denver, Colorado

Pyng Lee, MD, FCCP
Senior Consultant
Department of Respiratory
and Critical Care Medicine
Singapore General Hospital
Singapore

Teofilo Lee-Chiong, MD
Professor of Medicine
Head, Division of Sleep Medicine
National Jewish Health
University of Colorado
Denver School of Medicine
Denver, Colorado

Mark E. Lund, MD, FCCP
Assistant Professor of Medicine
Drexel University College of Medicine
Philadelphia, Pennsylvania

J. Mark Madison, MD
Professor of Medicine and Physiology
Chief, Division of Pulmonary,
Allergy and Critical Care Medicine
University of Massachusetts Medical
School, Worcester, Massachusetts

Thomas L. Petty, MD
Professor of Medicine
University of Colorado Denver
School of Medicine
Denver, Colorado
Rush Presbyterian St. Luke's
Chicago, Illinois
Professor Emeritus
National Jewish Health
Denver, Colorado

Jason Phan, MD
Department of Radiology
University of Vermont College of
Medicine
Fletcher Allen Healthcare
Burlington, Vermont

Michael Risbano, MD, MA
Fellow, Division of Pulmonary
Sciences & Critical Care Medicine
University of Colorado Denver
School of Medicine
Denver, Colorado

Jay H. Ryu, MD
Professor of Medicine
Mayo Clinic College of Medicine
Consultant, Division of Pulmonary
and Critical Care Medicine
Director
Interstitial Lung Disease Clinic
Mayo Clinic
Rochester, Minnesota

Milene T. Saavedra, MD
Assistant Professor of Medicine
National Jewish Health
Denver, Colorado

Steven A. Sahn, MD
Professor of Medicine
Director, Division of Pulmonary,
Critical Care, Allergy and Sleep
Medicine
Medical University of South Carolina
Charleston, South Carolina

Barry Make, MD
Professor of Medicine
Co-Director, COPD Program
Director, Pulmonary
Rehabilitation and
Respiratory Care
National Jewish Health
Denver, Colorado

Richard A. Matthay, MD
Boehringer Ingelheim Professor of
Medicine
Associate Director, Pulmonary and
Critical Care Medicine Section
Department of Medicine
Yale University School of Medicine
New Haven, Connecticut

Marc Moss, MD
Roger S. Mitchell Professor of
Medicine
Head of Critical Care
Division of Pulmonary
Sciences and Critical Care
University of Colorado Denver
School of Medicine
Denver, Colorado

Ali I. Musani, MD, FCCP
Associate Professor of Medicine
Director,
Interventional Pulmonary
Program
Pulmonary Sciences and Critical
Care Medicine
University of Colorado Denver
School of Medicine
Denver, Colorado

Jerry A. Nick, MD
Associate Professor of Medicine
Director, Adult Cystic Fibrosis
Program
National Jewish Health
Denver, Colorado

George Samuel, MD, CM, MSc.
Assistant Professor
Division of Environmental and
Occupational Health Sciences
National Jewish Health
Denver, Colorado

Marvin I. Schwarz, MD
The James C. Campbell Professor of
Pulmonary Sciences and Critical
Care Medicine
Director, Fellowship Program
University of Colorado Denver
School of Medicine
Denver, Colorado

Amen Sergrew, MD
Fellow, Division of Pulmonary
Sciences and Critical Care
Medicine
University of Colorado Denver
School of Medicine
Denver, Colorado

**Om R. Sharma, MD, FRCP,
Master FCCP**
Professor of Medicine
Keck School of Medicine
Los Angeles, California

Daniel R. Smith, MD, FCCP
Assistant Professor of Medicine
National Jewish Health
Denver, Colorado

Jeff Swigris, DO, MS
Assistant Professor of Medicine
Autoimmune Lung Center and
Interstitial Lung Disease Program
National Jewish Health
Denver, Colorado

Masayoshi Takashima, MD
Program Director,
Bobby R. Alford Department of
Otolaryngology,
Head and Neck Surgery
Baylor College of Medicine
Houston, Texas

David R. Theil, MD
Medical Director,
Department of Anesthesiology
Rose Medical Center
Denver, Colorado

**Gregory Tino, MD, FCCP,
FACP**
Associate Professor of Medicine
Pulmonary, Allergy and Critical
Care Division
Chief, Pulmonary Clinical Service
Hospital of the University of
Pennsylvania
University of Pennsylvania School
of Medicine
Philadelphia, Pennsylvania

Frederick S. Wamboldt, MD
Professor of Medicine
Head, Division of Psychosocial
Medicine
National Jewish Health
Professor of Psychiatry
University of Colorado Denver
School of Medicine
Denver, Colorado

**Jennifer J. Weinberger, MS,
RN, ANP**
Division of Cardiology
Denver Health Medical Center
Denver, Colorado

**Howard D. Weinberger,
MD, FACC, FACP**
Professor of Medicine
Head, Division of Cardiology
National Jewish Health
Division of Cardiology
University of Colorado Denver
School of Medicine
Denver, Colorado

Carl W. White, MD
Professor of Pediatrics
National Jewish Health
University of Colorado Denver
School of Medicine
Denver, Colorado

Howard Yeong-Rung Li, MD
Fellow,
Division of Pulmonary Sciences and
Critical Care Medicine
University of Colorado Denver
School of Medicine
Denver, Colorado

Robert L. Young, MD, PhD
Assistant Professor of Medicine
National Jewish Health
Denver, Colorado

Jose P. Zevallos, MD
Bobby R. Alford Department of
Otolaryngology
Baylor College of Medicine
Houston, Texas

Symbols and abbreviations

A–a	alveolar to arterial gradient
ABC	airway, breathing, circulation
ABG	arterial blood gas
ABPA	allergic bronchopulmonary aspergillosis
ACCP	American College of Chest Physicians
ACE	angiotensin-converting enzyme
ACI	acute lung injury
ACTH	adrenocorticotrophic hormone
ADH	antidiuretic hormone
AECC	American–European Consensus Conference
AFB	acid-fast bacillus
AFP	α-fetoprotein
AG	anion gap
AHI	apnea–hypopnea index
AIA	aspirin-induced asthma
AIDS	acquired immune deficiency syndrome
AIP	acute interstitial pneumonia
ALI	acute lung injury
AML	acute myeloid leukemia
AMS	acute mountain sickness
ANA	antinuclear antibody
ANCA	antinuclear cytoplasmic antibody
ANP	atrial natriuretic peptide
AP	aortopulmonary
APACHE	acute physiology and chronic health evaluation (score)
APAP	automated positive airway pressure
APH	associated pulmonary hypertension
APTT	activated partial thromboplastin time
ARB	angiotensin II receptor blocker
ARDS	acute respiratory distress syndrome
ASV	adaptive servo ventilation
ATN	acute tubular necrosis
ATRA	all-*trans* retinoic acid
ATS	American Thoracic Society

AVM	arteriovenous malformation
BAC	bronchoalveolar carcinoma
BAL	bronchoalveolar lavage
BCG	bacille Calmette–Guérin
β-hCG	beta human chorionic gonadotrophin
bid	twice a day
BHR	bronchial hyperreactivity or hyperresponsiveness
BIPAP	bilevel positive airways pressure
BMD	bonemineral density
BMI	body mass index ($kg/meters^2$)
BMT	bone marrow transplantation
BNP	brain natriuretic peptide
BOOP	bronchiolitis obliterans organizing pneumonia
BP	blood pressure
BPAP	bilevel positive airway pressure
BPD	bronchopulmonary dysplasia
BTS	British Thoracic Society
CABG	coronary artery bypass graft
C-ANCA	cytoplasmic pattern of ANCA
CAP	community-acquired pneumonia
CBC	complete blood count
CBD	chronic beryllium disease
CCB	calcium channel blocker
CCHS	congenitally central hypoventilation syndrome
CF	cystic fibrosis
CFA	cryptogenic fibrosing alveolitis
CFRD	cystic fibrosis–related diabetes
CFT	complement fixation test
CFTR	cystic fibrosis transmembrane conductance regulator
CFU	colony-forming unit
CHART	continuous hyperfractionated accelerated radiotherapy
CHF	congestive heart failure
CI	contraindication
CLL	chronic lymphocytic leukemia
CMV	cytomegalovirus
CNS	central nervous system
CO	carbon monoxide
CO_2	carbon dioxide
COHb	carboxyhemoglobin

COP	cryptogenic organizing pneumonia
COPD	chronic obstructive pulmonary disease
CPAP	continuous positive airway pressure
CPK	creatine phosphokinase
CPT	chest physiotherapy
CRP	C-reactive protein
CRQ	Chronic Respiratory Questionnaire
CSA	central sleep apnea
CSF	cerebrospinal fluid
CSR	Cheyne–Stokes respiration
CT	computerized tomography
CTD	connective tissue disease
CTPA	computerized tomographic pulmonary angiogram
CTV	computed tomography venography
CURB	confusion, urea, respiration rate, blood pressure (score)
CVA	cardiovascular accident
CVD	cardiovascular disease
CVP	central venous pressure
CXR	chest radiograph
DAD	diffuse alveolar damage
DAH	diffuse alveolar hemorrhage
DEXA	dual energy X-ray absorptiometry
DFA	direct fluorescent-antibody
DIC	disseminated intravascular coagulation
DIF	direct immunofluorescence (test)
DIOS	distal intestinal obstructive syndrome
DIP	desquamative interstitial pneumonitis
DLCO	carbon monoxide diffusing capacity
DM	dermatomyositis
DOT	directly observed therapy
DPI	dry powder inhaler
DPLD	diffuse parenchymal lung disease
DPT	diffuse pleural thickening
DSA	digital subcutaneous angiography
dsDNA	double-stranded DNA
DST	drug susceptibility testing
DTH	delayed-type hypersensitivity
DVT	deep vein thrombosis
EBUS	endobroncheal ultrasound

EBV	Epstein–Barr virus
ECG	electrocardiogram
Echo	echocardiogram
ECMO	extracorporeal membrane oxygenation
ECOG	Eastern Cooperative Oncology Group
ED	emergency department
EEG	electroencephalogram
EGFR	epidermal growth factor receptor
EIA	enzyme immunoassay
EIB	exercise-induced bronchospasm
ELCAP	Early Lung Cancer Action Project
ELISA	enzyme-linked immunosorbent assay
EMG	electromyogram
ENA	extractable nuclear antigen
ENT	ear, nose, and throat
EOG	electrooculogram
EPAP	expiratory positive airways pressure
ESR	erythrocyte sedimentation rate
ESS	Epworth sleepiness scale/score
ETT	endotracheal tube
EUS	esophageal ultrasound
FBC	full blood count
FBG	fasting blood glucose
FDG-18	fluorodeoxyglucose
FeNO	inhaled nitric oxide
FEV_1	forced expiratory volume in 1 second
FFP	fresh frozen plasma
FiO_2	fractional inspired oxygen
FNA	fine needle aspirate
FOB	fibre optic bronchoscopy
FPAH	familial pulmonary arterial hypertension
FRC	functional residual capacity
FVC	forced vital capacity
g	gram
GBM	glomerular basement membrane
GERD	gastroesophageal reflux disease
GI	gastrointestinal
GM-CSF	granulocyte macrophage colony-stimulating factor
GU	genitourinary
H2	histamine receptors, type 2

HAART	highly active antiretroviral therapy
HACE	high-altitude cerebral edema
HADS	Hospital Anxiety and Depression Score
HAPE	high-altitude pulmonary edema
Hb	haemoglobin
HCG⁻	human chorionic gonadotrophin
HCO₃⁻	bicarbonate
HES	hypereosinphilic syndrome
HHT	hereditary hemorrhagic telangiectasia
HHV	human herpes virus
HIT	heparin-induced thrombocytopenia
HIV	human immunodeficiency virus
HLA	human leukocyte antigen
HP	hypersensitivity pneumonitis
HPA	hypothalamic–pituitary–adrenal (axis)
HPOA	hypertrophic pulmonary osteoarthropathy
HPS	hepatopulmonary syndrome
HRCT	high-resolution computerized tomography
HRT	hormone replacement therapy
HSV	herpes simplex virus
IA	invasive aspergillosis
IBD	inflammatory bowel disease
IBW	ideal body weight
ICS	inhaled corticosteroids
ICU	intensive care unit
IDSA	Infectious Diseases Society of America
IFA	indirect immunofluorescence assay
IgE	immunoglobulin E
IgG	immunoglobulin G
IgM	immunoglobulin M
IGRA	interferon-γ release assay
IIP	idiopathic interstitial pneumonia
ILD	interstitial lung disease
IM	intramuscular
INR	international normalized ratio
IPAH	idiopathic pulmonary arterial hypertension
IPAP	inspiratory positive airways pressure
IPF	idiopathic pulmonary fibrosis
IV	intravenous

IVC	inferior vena cava
IVIG	intravenous immunoglobulin
JVP	jugular venous pressure
KCO	carbon monoxide transfer factor
L	liter
LAM	lymphangioleiomyomatosis
LCH	Langerhans cell histiocytosis
LDH	lactate dehydrogenase
LFTs	liver function tests
LIP	lymphocytic or lymphoid interstitial pneumonia
LMA	laryngeal mask airway
LMWH	low-molecular-weight heparin
LRI	lower respiratory tract infection
LTOT	long-term oxygen therapy
LV	left ventricular
LVRS	lung volume reduction surgery
MAC	Mycobacterium avium complex
M, C, & S	microscopy, culture, and sensitivity
MDI	metered dose inhaler
MDR-TB	multidrug-resistant TB
MDT	multidisciplinary team
MEP	maximum expiratory pressure
mg	milligrams
MGUS	monoclonal gammopathy of uncertain significance
MHC	major histocompatibility complex
MI	myocardial infarction
min	minute
MIP	maximum inhibitory pressure
MND	motor neuron disease
MODS	multiple organ dysfunction syndrome
MPO	myeloperoxidase
MRA	magnetic resonance angiography
MRC	Medical Research Council
MRI	magnetic resonance imaging
MRSA	methicillin (or multiply) resistant Staphylococcus aureus
MTB	Mycobacterium tuberculosis
NAC	N-acetyl cysteine
NAEB	nonasthmatic eosinophil bronchitis
ng	nanograms

NGT	nasogastric tube
NIMV	noninvasive mechanical ventilation
NIPPV	noninvasive positive pressure ventilation
NIV	noninvasive ventilation
NNRTI	non-nucleoside reverse transcription inhibitor
NO	nitric oxide
NO_2	nitrogen dioxide
non-REM	non-rapid eye movement sleep
NPPE	negative pressure pulmonary edema
NPPV	noninvasive positive pressure ventilation
nREM	non-rapid eye movement sleep
NSAID	nonsteroidal anti-inflammatory drug
NSCLC	non-small cell lung cancer
NSIP	nonspecific interstitial pneumonia
NTM	nontuberculous mycobacteria
NYHA	New York Heart Association
OCP	oral contraceptive pill
od	once a day
OHS	obesity hypoventilation syndrome
OSA	obstructive sleep apnea
OSAHS	obstructive sleep apnea/hypopnea syndrome
OSAS	obstructive sleep apnea syndrome
OTC	over-the-counter (drugs)
PA	posteranterior; pulmonary artery
$PaCO_2$	arterial carbon dioxide tension
PAF	platelet-activating factor
PAH	pulmonary artery hypertension
pANCA	perinuclear pattern of ANCA
PaO_2	arterial oxygen tension
PAOP	pulmonary artery occlusion pressure
PAP	positive airway pressure; pulmonary artery pressure
PAS	para-aminosalicylic acid
PAVM	pulmonary arteriovenous malformation
PC_{20}	provocative concentration (of histamine or methacholine) causing a 20% fall in FEV_1
PCD	primary ciliary dyskinesia
PCO_2	carbon dioxide tension
PCP	*Pneumocystis carinii* (now *jiroveci*) pneumonia
PCR	polymerase chain reaction

PCT	procalcitonin
PCWP	pulmonary capillary wedge pressure
PE	pulmonary embolus
PEEP	positive end expiratory pressure
PEFR	peak expiratory flow rate
PEG	percutaneous endoscopic gastrostomy
PET	positron emission tomography
PFT	pulmonary function test
PFS-DQ	pulmonary Function Status–Dyspnea Questionnaire
PGD	primary graft dysfunction
PHT	pulmonary hypertension
PICC	peripherally inserted central catheter
PIOPED	Prospective Investigation of Pulmonary Embolism Diagnosis
PMF	progressive massive fibrosis
po	orally/by mouth
PO_2	oxygen tension
PPH	primary pulmonary hypertension
PPV	positive predictive value
PR3	proteinase 3
prn	as required
PSA	prostate-specific antigen
PSB	protected specimen brush
PSG	polysomnography
PSI	Pneumonia Severity Index
PT	prothrombin time
PTH	parathyroid hormone
PTLD	post-transplant lymphoproliferative disorder
PTT	partial thromboplastin time
PVR	pulmonary vascular resistance
qid	four times a day
RA	rheumatoid arthritis
RAD	right axis deviation
RADS	reactive airways dysfunction syndrome
RAST	radioallergosorbent test
RBBB	right bundle branch block
RB-ILD	respiratory bronchiolitis-associated interstitial lung disease
RCT	randomized controlled trial
REM	rapid eye movement sleep
RF	rheumatoid factor

RGM	rapidly growing mycobacteria
RHC	right heart catheterization
RML	right middle lobe
RNP	ribonuclear protein
RSV	respiratory syncytial virus
RTA	renal tubular acidosis
RT-PCR	reverse transcriptase polymerase chain reaction
RV	residual volume
RVH	right ventricular hypertrophy
RVSP	right ventricular systolic pressure
SABA	short-acting β-agonist
SaO_2	arterial oxygen saturation
SARS	severe acute respiratory syndrome
SBE	subacute bacterial endocarditis
SCLC	small cell lung cancer
SCL-70	scleroderma antibody (to topoisomerase 1)
SCUBA	self-contained underwater breathing apparatus
SE	side effect
SF-36	Short Form-36
SIADH	syndrome of inappropriate secretion of antidiuretic hormone
SIRS	systemic inflammatory response syndrome
SLE	systemic lupus erythematosus
SO_2	sulfur dioxide
SOB	shortness of breath
SVC	superior vena cava
SVCO	superior vena caval obstruction
TB	tuberculosis
TBB	transbronchial biopsy
TENS	transcutaneous electrical nerve stimulation
tid	three times a day
Th2	T-helper 2 cell
TIA	transient ischemic attack
TIPS	transjugular intrahepatic portosystemic shunt
TLC	total lung capacity
TLCO	total lung carbon monoxide transfer factor
TLTI	treatment of latent TB infection
TMP-SMX	trimethoprim-sulfamethoxazole
TNF	tumor necrosis factor
TPMT	thiopurine methyltransferase

TPN	total parenteral nutrition
TRALI	transfusion-related acute lung injury
TSH	thyroid-stimulating hormone
TST	tuberculin skin test
TTE	transthoracic echocardiogram
TTJV	transtracheal jet ventilation
UACS	upper airway cough syndrome
U & E	urea and electrolytes
UFH	unfractionated heparin
UIP	usual interstitial pneumonia
UNOS	United network for Organ Sharing
URT	upper respiratory tract
URTI	upper respiratory tract infection
V/Q	ventilation–perfusion ratio
VAP	ventilator-acquired pneumonia
VATS	video-assisted thoracoscopic surgery
VC	vital capacity
VCD	vocal cord dysfunction
VIP	vasoactive intestinal peptide
VKA	vitamin K antagonist
V/Q	ventilation–perfusion ratio
VTE	venous thromboembolism
VZV	varicella zoster virus
WBC	white blood cell count
WCC	white cell count
WHO	World Health Organisation
XDR-TB	extensive drug-resistant tuberculosis
XPTB	extrapulmonary tuberculosis
ZN	Ziehl–Neelson
6MWT	6-minute walk test

Part I

Clinical presentations: approaches to problems

Dyspnea

Clinical assessment and causes

Physiological mechanisms of dyspnea

Dyspnea refers to the sensation of labored breathing or shortness of breath. Its physiological mechanisms are poorly understood; possible afferent sources for the sensation include receptors in respiratory muscles, pulmonary juxtacapillary receptors, and chemoreceptors.

Clinical assessment

All patients with dyspnea need a thorough history and complete physical examination. Key points in this assessment include the following:

History

- *Characterization of dyspnea:* What was the rate of onset—acute, subacute, or chronic? Is it continuous or episodic? Box 1.1 lists the causes of dyspnea in groups based on rapidity of onset; please note that there is often variability and overlap.
- *Duration of dyspnea:* Patients often underestimate the duration of dyspnea or attribute it to inactivity, weight gain, or aging. Inquiring about exercise tolerance over a period of time is a useful way of assessing duration and progression.
- *Course of dyspnea:* Is it improving, stable, or worsening, and at what pace?
- *Severity of dyspnea:* Assess its impact and disability by asking about effects on lifestyle, work, and daily activities.
- *Specific features:* What provokes it? What, if anything, palliates it? Are other symptoms associated with it? Cough? Wheeze? Pain? Is there a relationship between its onset and time of day? Left ventricular failure may cause nocturnal dyspnea after a few hours of sleep; dyspnea from asthma is often accompanied by wheezing and may be brought on by exposure to environmental allergens or irritants, or it may occur later in the night or early morning.
- *Family, social, occupational history:* Most patients with asthma have a family history of atopy or asthma. What is the patient's occupation (present and past), and to what might they be exposed at work? Is dyspnea worse at work? What kinds of hobbies does the patient have? Might there be exposures in the home environment that would lead to dyspnea? What medications does the patient take? Has the patient taken any medications associated with parenchymal (e.g., chemotherapeutics), airways (e.g., beta blockers), or pulmonary vascular (e.g., anorexigens) disease? Has the patient smoked? Ever used illicit drugs? Are there pets at home?

Physical examination

- After a review of the vital signs and a global assessment of patient distress, the physical examination should focus on the cardiovascular and respiratory systems. However, signs in other systems can provide useful clues to the etiology of dyspnea.
- Observe the *pattern and rate of breathing*. Assess for signs of respiratory distress (e.g., rapid and shallow breathing, accessory muscle use, tripod position, intercostal retraction).
- Examine the *chest wall*. Is expansion symmetric? Asymmetric expansion suggests a unilateral problem. Is there full excursion of the chest with respiration? Hyperinflation often limits chest wall motion.
- *Percussion*: Dullness may suggest a pleural effusion. Hyperresonance suggests disorders associated with profound air-trapping.
- *Lung auscultation*: Are there abnormal sounds? Crackles? Wheeze? Rhonchi? Are they unilateral or bilateral? Upper zone or lower zone predominant?
- *Cardiovascular examination*: Is the jugular venous pulsation in the neck elevated with the patient 40°–45° recumbent? Is the point of maximum intensity over the left chest diffuse or focal? It should be about the size of a quarter—any larger suggests left ventricular abnormality. Is there a right ventricular lift or heave? Is there a murmur? Does the second heart sound split appropriately? Is the pulmonic component of the second heart sound louder than the aortic component? Is S3 or S4 audible?
- *Other clues*: Is there clubbing? Its presence suggests the possibility of long-standing pulmonary disease. Is there unilateral or bilateral lower extremity edema? Perform examination of the eyes, ears, nose, mouth, skin, joints, abdomen, and neurological systems to assess for signs of systemic disease and to gather more clues for the etiology of dyspnea.

Investigations

Initial investigations typically include resting oximetry, assessment of peak flow and spirometry, along with plain chest radiography and electrocardiography.

Further tests to order depend on clues from the history and physical examination. These might include full pulmonary function tests with measurement of lung volumes, flow-volume loop, and carbon monoxide diffusing capacity (DLCO); inspiratory and expiratory pressure measurement; an assessment of gas exchange (e.g., room air, resting arterial blood gas, exercise oximetry); maximum cardiopulmonary exercise test; bronchial provocation test (e.g., methacholine challenge); ventilation-perfusion scanning and computerized tomographic pulmonary angiogram (CTPA); transthoracic echocardiogram; blood tests (e.g., white blood cell count and differential, hemoglobin, cardiac enzymes, beta-natriuretic peptide, d-dimer); and several other possibilities as the scenario dictates.

Box 1.1 Causes of dyspnea grouped by speed of onset

Instantaneous
- Pneumothorax
- Pulmonary embolism
- Upper airway obstruction

Acute
- Cardiovascular disease (e.g., acute myocardial infarction, arrhythmia, aortic dissection)
- Obstructive airways disease (e.g., exacerbations of asthma or chronic obstructive pulmonary disease [COPD])
- Parenchymal process (e.g., infectious pneumonia, pulmonary edema, pulmonary hemorrhage, acute hypersensitivity pneumonitis)
- Metabolic acidosis
- Hyperventilation syndrome

Subacute (days)
- Many of the above, plus:
- Pleural effusion
- Lobar collapse
- Certain interstitial lung diseases
- Superior vena cava obstruction
- Pulmonary vasculitis

Chronic (months–years)
- Some of the above, plus:
- Airways diseases (e.g., asthma, COPD, bronchiectasis)
- Diffuse parenchymal disease
- Pulmonary vascular disease
- Hypoventilation (chest wall deformity, neuromuscular weakness, obesity)
- Anemia
- Thyrotoxicosis
- Deconditioning

Specific situations

Causes of dyspnea with possibility of a normal chest X-ray

- Airways disease (e.g. asthma, upper airways obstruction, bronchiolitis, COPD)
- Pulmonary vascular disease (e.g. acute or chronic pulmonary embolism, pulmonary hypertension, intrapulmonary shunt)
- Mild parenchymal disease (e.g. sarcoid, interstitial pneumonias)
- Infection—viral, pneumocystis
- Cardiac disease (e.g. angina, arrhythmia, valvular disease, intracardiac shunt)
- Neuromuscular weakness
- Metabolic acidosis
- Anemia
- Thyrotoxicosis
- Hyperventilation syndrome

Causes of episodic or intermittent dyspnea

- Asthma
- Pulmonary edema
- Angina
- Pulmonary embolism
- Hypersensitivity pneumonitis
- Hyperventilation syndrome

Distinguishing cardiac and respiratory causes of dyspnea

This is often challenging. Resting ECG is useful—in practice, a cardiac cause of dyspnea is unlikely in the setting of a completely normal electrocardiogram. Exercise electrocardiography, echocardiography, and cardiac catheterization may be required. Cardiopulmonary exercise testing can be helpful.

Chapter 2

Chronic cough
and normal chest X-ray

Etiology, clinical assessment, and treatment

Cough is the most common symptom that leads patients to seek medical attention. Although cough is often due to lung disease that is apparent on chest radiograph (CXR), it is a common clinical problem to have a patient with cough who has a normal or nearly normal CXR—a CXR that provides no clues to the etiology of the cough.

Cough is classified according to its duration: *acute cough* <3 weeks, *subacute cough* 3–8 weeks, and *chronic cough* >8 weeks. This chapter focuses on the diagnosis and management of chronic cough in immuno-competent adults who have a normal, or nearly normal, CXR.

An empirical integrative approach to diagnosis and treatment is rec-ommended. Therapy should be specifically directed at the underlying cause(s) of the chronic cough. Over the past three decades, specific antitussive therapy for chronic cough has led to a success rate in our seven published series that has averaged 95% (range 54%–100%).

Etiology

For non-cigarette-smoking patients who are not taking an angiotensin converting enzyme (ACE) inhibitor and who have a normal or nearly normal CXR, the most common causes of chronic cough are upper airway cough syndrome (UACS), asthma, nonasthmatic eosinophilic bronchitis (NAEB), and gastroesophageal reflux disease (GERD).

When evaluating a patient with chronic cough, it is important for the clinician to recognize that in at least 25% of such patients, there are multiple causes contributing to the cough simultaneously.

Clinical assessment

History

A history should be obtained, being certain to establish the following:

- Duration of cough. Chronic cough is cough persisting >8 weeks.
- Any recent (<2 months) history of a respiratory tract infection
- Active cigarette smoking or exposure to environmental irritants
- Current treatment with an ACE inhibitor
- Associated symptoms suggestive of asthma (dyspnea, wheezing), UACS (throat clearing, sensation of postnasal drip), and GERD (heartburn, dyspepsia)
- Prior history of respiratory disease(s)
- Whether cough is productive or not and the timing of cough (daytime or night time) are of little value diagnostically.

Physical examination

Physical examination is often not helpful in diagnosing the cause of chronic cough when the CXR is normal or nearly normal. Cobblestone appearance of the oropharynx mucosa can be an indication of GERD or an UACS; auscultation of the chest may reveal wheezing as a sign of asthma, crackles suggestive of cardiac dysfunction or occult interstitial lung disease, or rhonchi suggestive of unsuspected suppurative airway disease. Digital clubbing could indicate bronchiectasis or lung malignancy.

not detected on CXR. Neurological signs could indicate neuromuscular weakness, either focal or nonfocal, that predisposes to chronic aspiration.

Investigations

Investigations should begin by reviewing the CXR to be certain it is normal or nearly normal. If the CXR shows an abnormality, that finding should be pursued first as a potential cause of chronic cough.

Chronic bronchitis is one of the most common causes of chronic cough with a normal CXR. Therefore, if the patient is a cigarette smoker or exposed to other environmental irritants, that exposure should be eliminated before initiating extensive diagnostic testing. When chronic cough is due to cigarette-induced chronic bronchitis, cough improves in up to 94% of cases after abstinence from cigarettes for at least 4 weeks.

If the patient is taking an ACE inhibitor, that medication should be stopped, if possible, before undertaking diagnostic testing. ACE inhibitors commonly cause chronic cough, possibly in as many as 33% of patients treated with ACE inhibitors in hypertension trials.

If the CXR is normal or nearly normal and the patient is a nonsmoker who is not taking an ACE inhibitor, then an empirical integrative approach to diagnosis and treatment is recommended. Empirical therapy should be started (see Cause of chronic cough: UACS) and first directed at the most common causes of cough in the community in which the clinician practices. In the United States, empirical therapy focuses on UACS first because that diagnosis is the most common cause of chronic cough in adults in the United States. If the patient experiences resolution or partial resolution of cough in response to treatment, then UACS is considered to have been the cause, or a contributing cause, of cough.

If chronic cough has not completely resolved on empirical treatment for UACS, asthma should be considered next. Because bronchial provocation testing has a high negative predictive value, many clinicians begin a treatment trial for asthma only if this test is positive. However, if provocation testing is not available, empirical treatment for asthma is started and the effect on cough observed.

NAEB should be considered next. NAEB is characterized by sputum eosinophilia without bronchial hyperresponsiveness. The diagnosis is suspected by finding eosinophilia (>3% eosinophils of the nonsquamous cells present) in induced sputum samples. If this test is unavailable, patients should have a trial of inhaled corticosteroids. In most patients with NAEB, chronic cough will resolve within 4 weeks. A minority of patients require systemic corticosteroids.

Patients who do not respond completely to empirical therapy for UACS, asthma, or NAEB should next be evaluated for GERD as the underlying cause of cough. If gastrointestinal (GI) symptoms of GERD are prominent, the physician should institute therapy with an antireflux diet, lifestyle modifications, and a proton pump inhibitor. Prokinetic therapy may need to be added. If the patient does not have prominent GI symptoms of GERD, confirm the diagnosis with 24-hour esophageal pH monitoring before starting therapy. When this testing is not available, it is reasonable to begin an empirical trial of therapy for GERD without confirmatory testing.

For patients who have an inadequate response to empirical trials for the most common causes of chronic cough (see Box 2.1), further investigations off therapy may include methacholine challenge testing, sputum induction to assess for sputum eosinophilia, and 24-hour esophageal pH monitoring to assess for acid GERD, unless these studies have already been performed in conjunction with the empirical trials.

Additional studies to consider are endoscopic or videofluoroscopic evaluation for swallowing disorders, barium esophagogram, sinus imaging, high-resolution chest CT scan for interstitial lung disease and occult bronchiectasis, bronchoscopic evaluation for occult tumors and non-bronchiectatic suppurative airway disease, echocardiography for occult congestive heart failure, sputum for evaluation of tuberculosis depending on the clinical setting, and environmental and allergy assessments.

Cough should never be considered unexplained (previously referred to as idiopathic) until both common and uncommon causes of cough have been excluded. For patients with unexplained chronic cough a referral to a cough specialty clinic should be strongly considered.

Box 2.1 Causes of chronic cough with a normal CXR

Common

- Chronic bronchitis
- ACE inhibitor
- Upper airway cough syndrome (UACS) due to rhinosinus disease
- Asthma
- Nonasthmatic eosinophilic bronchitis (NAEB)
- Gastroesophageal reflux disease (GERD)

Less common

- Infectious processes (e.g., tuberculosis)
- Bronchiectasis
- Interstitial lung disease
- Airway foreign body
- Occult lung cancer not apparent on CXR
- Mediastinal pathology
- Left ventricular failure
- Esophageal pathology causing recurrent aspiration
- Bronchial-esophageal fistula
- Recurrent aspiration due to disorders of pharyngeal swallowing
- Inhaled medications
- Psychogenic (rare)
- Other (see *Chest* **129**(1 Suppl.):206S, 2006)

Causes of chronic cough: UACS

Upper airway cough syndrome (UACS) is the result of rhinosinus conditions that may cause cough by direct mechanical stimulation, irritation and inflammation of tissues in the pharynx and larynx, or a nasal cough reflex.

Typically, patients with UACS describe the sensation of fluid dripping down into their throats, nasal discharge, or the need to frequently clear their throats. Physical examination of the nasopharynx and oropharynx reveals mucoid or mucopurulent secretions or a cobblestone appearance of the mucosa.

Chronic cough may be the only symptom of UACS (so-called silent UACS). Therefore, the condition causing the cough can be definitively ascribed to UACS only when it responds to specific therapy for UACS.

Empirical therapy for UACS depends on the putative underlying rhinosinus condition and should begin with a trial of a first-generation antihistamine-decongestant unless contraindicated (e.g., because of benign prostatic hypertrophy, hypertension, or glaucoma). Intranasal ipratropium bromide may also be effective; the nonsedating antihistamines are not effective, however, unless the patient has allergic rhinitis or some other histamine-mediated rhinosinus condition.

If the patient experiences resolution or partial resolution of cough in response to treatment, then UACS is considered to have been the cause, or a contributing cause, of cough and the antihistamine-decongestant is continued. Noticeable improvement should occur within 2–4 days.

If the response to empirical therapy is only partial and the patient continues to have nasal symptoms suggestive of rhinosinus disease, the addition of a topical nasal steroid, nasal anticholinergic, or nasal antihistamine should be considered.

Persistent UACS symptoms despite topical therapy are an indication for sinus imaging, to look for evidence of occult sinusitis. The presence of air–fluid levels suggests that antibiotics for at least 3 weeks may be effective. Additionally, a decongestant nasal spray with an α-adrenergic agonist (e.g., oxymetazoline hydrochloride for a maximum of 5 days) may be of additional benefit.

If sinusitis fails to respond to treatment, a complete otolaryngologic evaluation is indicated. Measurement of serum immunoglobulin levels to assess for hypogammaglobulinemia, allergy testing, and an environmental assessment of home and workplace should also be considered.

Causes of chronic cough: asthma, NAEB

Asthma

Asthma should be suspected as the cause of chronic cough under any of three circumstances: (1) episodic wheezing and shortness of breath plus cough, and wheezing is heard on chest examination; (2) pulmonary function testing demonstrates reversible airflow obstruction, even in the absence of wheezing; or (3) methacholine inhalation challenge testing is positive in a patient with normal or near-normal results on routine spirometry, even in the absence of wheezing. It should be recognized, however, that chronic cough can be the sole presenting manifestation of asthma (i.e. cough-variant asthma).

Nonspecific pharmacologic bronchoprovocation challenge testing is extremely helpful in ruling out asthma as a possible cause of chronic cough because a negative methacholine challenge essentially rules out asthma as a cause of chronic cough. An exception is occupational asthma in its earliest stage. However, the methacholine challenge should become positive as the workplace exposure continues.

Asthma as the cause of chronic cough is confirmed only when the cough responds to specific therapy for asthma and the patient's subsequent clinical course is consistent with asthma. In this regard, the diagnosis of asthmatic cough is not made in any patient who has experienced an obvious respiratory tract infection within the previous 2 months, because cough and bronchial hyperresponsiveness can be transient and self-limited in this setting.

Empirical therapy for uncomplicated, cough-variant asthma is the same as treatment for asthma in general: inhaled β-adrenergic agonists and inhaled corticosteroids. On average, a chronic cough from asthma begins to improve after 6–7 days of treatment.

In select patients with a positive methacholine challenge test and a cough that persists despite therapy with inhaled medications, an oral leukotriene inhibitor may be successful. If cough still does not respond, it is reasonable to give a 5- to 10-day trial of oral corticosteroids (e.g., 40 mg/day of prednisone), provided the patient has no significant contraindications.

If properly used inhaled bronchodilators and inhaled corticosteroids do not decrease cough at least partially, either asthma is not the cause of the patient's cough or there is a concomitant condition making asthma difficult to control (e.g. sinusitis or GERD).

Nonasthmatic eosinophilic bronchitis (NAEB)

NAEB is characterized by sputum eosinophilia without bronchial hyper-responsiveness or other evidence of variable airflow obstruction. Although NAEB has been associated with occupational sensitizers and inhaled allergens, it also may occur spontaneously.

In patients with a negative bronchial provocation test, NAEB is suggested when examination of induced sputum shows eosinophilia (i.e., eosinophils constitute more than 3% of nonsquamous cells).

If the diagnosis is consistent with NAEB by sputum examination or if the test is unavailable, patients should have an empirical trial of inhaled corticosteroids. In most patients with NAEB, chronic cough resolves within 4 weeks of starting inhaled corticosteroids. A minority of patients may require a short course of oral corticosteroids.

For all patients with NAEB, the possibility of an occupation-related cause of NAEB should be considered and any relevant or suspected exposures eliminated.

Causes of chronic cough: GERD

Gastroesophageal reflux disease (GERD) appears to most commonly cause chronic cough by stimulating an esophageal-bronchial reflex in the mucosa of the distal esophagus. However, GERD can also stimulate cough by irritating the upper respiratory tract without aspiration (e.g. larynx/hypopharynx) or by irritating the lower respiratory tract during aspiration.

GERD should be suspected as the cause of chronic cough whenever a patient complains of frequent episodes of typical GI symptoms such as daily heartburn and regurgitation, especially when the chest radiograph or clinical picture suggests an aspiration syndrome. Alternatively, cough may be the only symptom of GERD ("silent" GERD).

In the absence of GI symptoms, chronic cough is most likely to be due to GERD if the patient is a nonsmoker, is not taking an ACE inhibitor, has a normal or near-normal chest radiograph, and asthma, UACS, and NAEB have been ruled out—92% of patients with silent GERD fit this clinical profile.

The use of 24-hour esophageal pH monitoring or 24-hour esophageal pH and impedance monitoring can help suggest that GERD is causing a cough. The latter test is preferable because it can assess non-acid as well as acid reflux disease. Correlation of cough and reflux events is possible when patients keep a symptom diary during the esophageal monitoring session. The monitoring session findings can be considered consistent with GERD as the cause of chronic cough when reflux events (acid or non-acid) appear to trigger cough, or when any reflux parameter falls out of the normal range.

Conventional diagnostic indices of GERD (e.g., percentage of time that pH is <4.0) that gastroenterologists use to diagnose reflux esophagitis can be misleadingly normal in patients with chronic cough from GERD. The test should be interpreted as normal only when conventional indices for acid reflux are within the normal range and no reflux-induced coughs are identified during the 24-hour monitoring study.

Confirmation of GERD as the cause of cough requires that the cough disappear when the patient starts antireflux therapy. Nevertheless, if treatment with proton pump inhibitors fails to eliminate cough in a patient who fits the clinical profile of GERD-induced chronic cough, GERD may nevertheless be causing the cough, albeit through a nonacid mechanism. Therefore, the term "acid reflux" can be misleading when describing chronic cough caused by GERD. Increasing evidence indicates that chronic cough can be caused by nonacid reflux as well as by acid reflux.

If a patient has prominent upper GI symptoms of GERD and chronic cough, the clinician should institute therapy with an antireflux diet, life-style modifications, and a proton pump inhibitor. If there is no response to this empirical therapy, a prokinetic agent should be added to the regimen.

If the patient does not have prominent GI symptoms, confirmation of the diagnosis of GERD should be obtained by 24-hour esophageal pH monitoring before starting therapy. However, because this testing may not be available and interpretation of these results can be controversial.

it is also reasonable to begin an empirical trial of therapy for GERD without confirmatory testing when the patient fits the clinical profile for cough from GERD.

Response to medical therapy is highly variable in cough from GERD, taking from less than 2 weeks to more than several months, and sometimes occurring only after a prokinetic agent is added. Some patients never respond to medical therapy.

When medical therapy appears to be failing, the clinician should review patient adherence and consider whether a comorbid disease (e.g., obstructive sleep apnea) or drugs used to treat a comorbid condition (e.g., progesterone, theophylline, nitrates, or calcium channel antagonists) may be exacerbating the patient's GERD. If cough still persists, perform 24-hour esophageal pH and impedance monitoring while the patient is receiving the most intensive medical therapy for GERD.

In selected cases, upper GI endoscopy or barium swallow testing may be indicated. On occasion, maximal medical therapy will fail to alter pathologic reflux, and such patients should be evaluated for reflux surgery.

Causes of chronic cough: chronic bronchitis, bronchiectasis, ACE inhibitors

Chronic bronchitis

Chronic bronchitis, especially from cigarette smoking, is one of the most common causes of chronic cough. However, although most smokers have a cough, they do not commonly seek medical attention for chronic cough.

Chronic bronchitis should be considered when one or more of the following three criteria are met: (1) the patient expectorates phlegm on most days during periods spanning at least 3 consecutive months, and such periods have occurred for more than 2 successive years; (2) alternative cough–phlegm syndromes such as UACS, asthma, and bronchiectasis have been ruled out; or (3) the patient has known exposure to dusts, fumes, or smoke.

Chronic bronchitis is confirmed as a cause of chronic cough when cough goes away after elimination of the respiratory irritant (e.g., cessation of cigarette smoking). In cases caused by cigarette smoking, chronic cough has improved in up to 94% of cases after abstinence from cigarettes for at least 4 weeks.

Bronchiectasis

Bronchiectasis should be suspected when cough is associated with expectoration of >30 mL of purulent sputum in 24 hours (i.e. bronchorrhea), with or without fever, hemoptysis, weight loss, and malaise; bronchorrhea is not specific for bronchiectasis.

Patients with chronic cough can have clinically unsuspected suppurative airway disease that may be detectable only with bronchoscopy. For this reason, a diagnosis of unexplained cough is not acceptable unless bronchoscopy has been performed.

CXR often suggests the diagnosis of bronchiectasis by revealing increased lung markings and increased size and loss of definition of segmental markings. When bronchiectasis is not apparent on CXR, but suspicion for this diagnosis remains high, high-resolution computerized tomography (HRCT) is the optimal method for further evaluation.

Cough from bronchiectasis has been successfully treated with theophylline or β_2-adrenergic agonists that increase mucociliary clearance, chest physiotherapy and postural drainage, and intermittent courses of antibiotics initially directed against *Haemophilus influenzae*, *Streptococcus pneumoniae*, and upper respiratory tract anaerobes.

If initial therapy is unsuccessful, antimicrobial coverage may need to be expanded depending on cultures to cover organisms such as facultative gram-negative enteric rods and *S. aureus*. Many clinicians extend antibiotic treatment for 3 weeks or longer.

ACE inhibitors

ACE inhibitors are a well-established cause of chronic cough. The pathogenesis may be related to bradykinin sensitization of afferent sensory nerves in the airways.

Although the reported frequency of cough associated with ACE inhibitors during hypertension trials has varied widely, from 0.2% to 33%, prospective studies have shown that ACE inhibitors account for 2% of chronic cough. Cough has been reported to appear within a few hours of taking a first dose in many patients, but it may not become apparent for weeks, months, or even longer.

ACE inhibitor–induced cough is diagnosed by stopping the drug and observing resolution of the cough.

Switching from one ACE inhibitor to another or decreasing the dose will usually not be beneficial in the elimination of chronic cough because cough is a class effect. When withdrawal of the ACE inhibitor is not a desirable option and the drug is being used to treat hypertension, an angiotensin II receptor blocker (ARB) may be substituted for the ACE inhibitor.

For patients in whom switching to an ARB is not an option, the clinician can add an agent to control the cough. Sodium cromoglycate, theophylline, sulindac, indomethacin, amlodipine, nifedipine, ferrous sulfate, aspirin in intermediate doses, and picotamide have all been suggested as potentially useful for controlling cough during continued ACE inhibitor administration.

Causes of chronic cough: miscellaneous

Miscellaneous conditions have usually comprised no more than 6% of the causes of chronic cough in prospective studies. The more frequently described miscellaneous causes are metastatic carcinoma; sarcoidosis; left ventricular failure; aspiration from a Zenker diverticulum or difficulty in swallowing; bronchogenic carcinoma; and tuberculosis, especially in underdeveloped countries and high-risk groups.

When the most common causes of chronic cough have been ruled out by testing and by failed empirical trials for UACS, asthma, NAEB, and GERD, other less common causes of chronic cough should be considered. Further testing in such patients may identify a disorder that is amenable to specific therapy.

Difficulty in swallowing from any cause may result in chronic cough because of recurrent aspiration of material into the airway. Recurrent aspiration is the cause in approximately 1% of patients presenting to a chronic-cough clinic. When pharyngeal dysfunction or aspiration is suspected, referral to a speech and language pathologist for video-fluoroscopic swallow evaluation or fiber-optic endoscopic evaluation of swallowing is appropriate.

Bronchogenic carcinoma is not a common cause of chronic cough, but should be included in the differential diagnosis because not all cases are evident on plain CXR. In addition, in long-term cigarette smokers, the new development of a chronic cough or a change in the character of an established cough should suggest bronchogenic carcinoma.

Chronic interstitial pneumonias (e.g., idiopathic pulmonary fibrosis) have not been reported as a common cause of chronic cough. In patients with interstitial lung disease who present with chronic cough, the interstitial lung disease is not necessarily causing the cough. One prospective study in patients with known interstitial lung disease found that 18 of 30 episodes of chronic cough were the result of other conditions, including UACS, asthma, GERD, bronchiectasis, and COPD exacerbation.

Although psychogenic cough, or habit cough, is sometimes reported to be relatively common, a full evaluation—which should include assessment for tic disorders—will typically reveal some other cause for the cough. Psychogenic cough is uncommon. There are no distinguishing clinical features and diagnostic tests for psychogenic cough—it is a diagnosis of exclusion.

Further information

Irwin RS (1997). Cough. In Irwin RS, Curley FJ, Grossman FR (Eds.), *Diagnosis and Treatment of Symptoms of the Respiratory Tract*, Armonk, NY: Futura Publishing.

Irwin RS, Baumann MH, Boulet LP, et al. (2006). Diagnosis and management of cough executive summary: ACCP evidence-based clinical practice guidelines. *Chest* **129**(1 Suppl.):1S.

Irwin, RS, Madison JM (2000). The diagnosis and treatment of cough. *N Engl J Med* **343**:1715.

Chest pain

Chest pain: overview

- Chest pain may originate from the cardiovascular, pulmonary, musculoskeletal, and/or gastrointestinal systems (see Fig. 3.1).
- The first priority is to identify and treat emergent and life-threatening causes such as acute myocardial infarction, aortic dissection, pulmonary embolism, and tension pneumothorax.
- Initial evaluation consists of focused history, physical examination, and appropriate diagnostic testing.

Chest pain characteristics

- *Quality:* Sharp, stabbing, pleuritic, pressure, tightness, heaviness, squeezing, burning
- *Severity:* 1 to 10 scale, severity at onset, time course to peak and pattern of change
- *Location and radiation:* Diffuse or localized, migratory, radiation patterns
- *Duration:* Time, constant or intermittent
- *Precipitating, exacerbating, or relieving factors:* Exercise, breathing, position
- *Associated symptoms:* Dyspnea, nausea/emesis, diaphoresis, nervousness/anxiety, sour brash/reflux, paresthesias

Physical examination

- *Vital signs:* Heart rate, respiratory rate, blood pressure, temperature
- *Pulmonary:* Air movement, breath sounds, fluid (interstitial, pleural), consolidation, rubs
- *Cardiovascular:* Murmurs, gallops, rubs, lifts/heaves, enlargement or displacement, pulses

Appropriate diagnostic testing

- *Oxygenation:* Saturation, arterial blood gas
- *ECG:* Ischemia, infarction, pericarditis, right heart strain
- *Chest X-ray:* Infiltrate, heart failure, vascular enlargement or distortion, pleural effusion, pneumothorax
- *Blood tests:* CBC (anemia, infection), metabolic panel

Additional specific testing for suspected pathology

- D-dimer: pulmonary embolus
- Troponin: myocardial infarction
- CT scan: pulmonary embolus, aortic dissection

Chest pain associated with pulmonary disease may originate from the pulmonary vasculature, lung parenchyma, or pleural tissue. Symptoms are primarily dyspnea and pleuritic pain localized to the site of pulmonary disease, and may be acute or chronic.

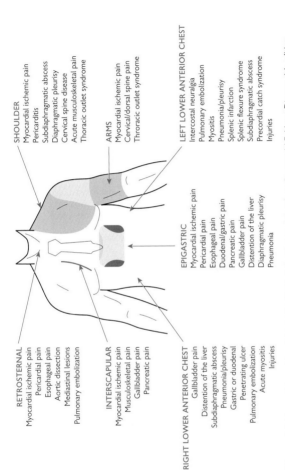

SHOULDER
Myocardial ischemic pain
Pericarditis
Subdiaphragmatic abscess
Diaphragmatic pleurisy
Cervical spine disease
Acute musculoskeletal pain
Thoracic outlet syndrome

ARMS
Myocardial ischemic pain
Cervical/dorsal spine pain
Throracic outlet syndrome

LEFT LOWER ANTERIOR CHEST
Intercostal neuralgia
Pulmonary embolization
Myositis
Pneumonia/pleurisy
Splenic infarction
Splenic flexure syndrome
Subdiaphragmatic abscess
Precordial catch syndrome
Injuries

EPIGASTRIC
Myocardial ischemic pain
Pericardial pain
Esophageal pain
Duodenal/gastric pain
Pancreatic pain
Gallbladder pain
Distention of the liver
Diaphragmatic pleurisy
Pneumonia

RIGHT LOWER ANTERIOR CHEST
Gallbladder pain
Distention of the liver
Subdiaphragmatic abscess
Pneumonia/pleurisy
Gastric or duodenal
Penetrating ulcer
Pulmonary embolization
Acute myositis
Injuries

INTERSCAPULAR
Myocardial ischemic pain
Musculoskeletal pain
Gallbladder pain
Pancreatic pain

RETROSTERNAL
Myocardial ischemic pain
Pericardial pain
Esophageal pain
Aortic dissection
Mediastinal lesions
Pulmonary embolization

Figure 3.1 Determining origin of chest pain. Reprinted with permission from Braunwald E: Heart Disease, 6th edition. Philadelphia: W.B. Saunders, 2001. Copyright Elsevier.

Acute chest pain

- *Acute myocardial infarction:* Cardiac risk factors; often described as pressure, squeezing, discomfort, rather than true pain; buildup in intensity; substernal, may radiate to neck, jaw, left shoulder or arm; duration usually longer than 20 minutes; worsened with activity; associated symptoms of dyspnea, nausea, diaphoresis
- *Aortic dissection:* Sudden onset, peak intensity at onset; often described as "tearing", or "knife like"; radiates through to back; may cause myocardial infarction or pericardial tamponade if extends to aortic root or into pericardial space
- *Acute pulmonary embolism:* Chest pain of sudden onset, often pleuritic; dyspnea; cough
- *Tension pneumothorax:* Sudden onset, pleuritic, progressive respiratory distress
- *Pulmonary infarction:* Usually days following pulmonary embolus
- *Pulmonary hypertension:* Symptoms related to underlying cause, dyspnea on exertion, decreased exercise tolerance; chest pain and syncope (both of which are often exertional)
- *Pneumonia:* Pleuritic pain over involved lung, fever, cough, productive sputum
- *Pneumothorax:* Sudden onset with peak intensity of pain at onset, dyspnea. Tension pneumothorax is a medical emergency and requires immediate decompression.
- *Tracheobronchitis:* Often burning mid-sternal pain
- *Pleuritis:* Usually viral, autoimmune (systemic lupus erythematosus, rheumatoid arthritis)
- *Esophageal:* May mimic myocardial ischemia; may be exertional

Chronic chest pain

- *Musculoskeletal*: Hours–days–weeks, often positional
- *Gastrointestinal*: May be similar to myocardial ischemic pain
- *Autoimmune diseases*: Systemic lupus erythematosus, rheumatoid arthritis
- *Cancer*: Lung, chest wall, pleural
- *Sarcoid*: Often with dyspnea, cough

Hemoptysis

Clinical assessment and causes

Hemoptysis is a common and nonspecific feature of many lung diseases. It can be a sign of significant underlying lung disease. In 5%–15% of cases, no cause will be found. An early assessment of the likely underlying cause needs to be made and investigated accordingly.

Diagnostic approach to hemoptysis

Small-volume hemoptysis (≤200 mL/day) is a commonly encountered problem in the outpatient department. It can usually be safely and efficiently investigated on an outpatient basis. Massive hemoptysis (>200–600 mL/day) is rare and usually encountered in trauma and in the emergency department, or in a hospitalized patient with known underlying lung disease. The approaches to small-volume and massive hemoptysis are different.

History

- Past history of lung disease?
- Document volume of blood and whether it is old (altered) or fresh (bright red).
- Time course (intermittent, constant)
- Is the bleeding from a nonpulmonary cause (upper airway, esophagus)? Is there a history of cirrhosis, alcoholism, nausea, or peptic ulcer disease?
- Anticoagulant or antiplatelet use?
- Presence of systemic features—associated infection, symptoms consistent with underlying malignancy, hematuria
- Smoking history
- Chest pain, edema, or history of thromboembolic disease

Examination

The examination may be normal. Look for signs of circulatory collapse. Signs of underlying lung disease, e.g., bronchiectasis, bronchial carcinoma, may be present. The usual differential diagnosis includes the disorders listed in Box 4.1.

Box 4.1 Differential diagnosis for hemoptysis

- Malignancy
- Bronchiectasis
- Acute or chronic bronchitis
- Tuberculosis/infection
- Pulmonary embolism
- Iatrogenic

Causes of hemoptysis

Common

- Bronchial tumor (benign, e.g., carcinoid, or malignant). Hemoptysis is a common presenting feature of bronchogenic malignancy, indicating endobronchial disease, which may be visible endoscopically.
- Bronchiectasis. Hemoptysis is a common feature of bronchiectasis, particularly during exacerbations. It can be a cause of massive hemoptysis, from dilated and abnormal bronchial artery branches that form around bronchiectatic cavities.
- Bronchitis (acute or chronic)
- Active tuberculosis. Hemoptysis occurs in cavitating and non-cavitating disease, active disease and inactive disease (bronchiectatic cavity, e.g., containing mycetoma).
- Pneumonia (especially pneumococcal)
- Lung abscess
- Pulmonary thromboembolic disease
- Warfarin with any of the above
- Iatrogenic, e.g., lung biopsy, bronchoscopy

Rare

- Vasculitides/alveolar hemorrhage syndromes, e.g., granulomatous small-vessel vasculitis, systemic lupus erythematosus (SLE), Goodpasture's syndrome
- Fungal, viral, or parasitic infections
- Fat embolism
- Arteriovenous malformation, e.g., in hereditary hemorrhagic telangiectasia (HHT) (see p. 629)
- Foreign body or broncholith (prior granulomatous disease infection)
- Severe pulmonary hypertension (PHT) (see p. 421)
- Mitral stenosis
- Congenital heart disease
- Aortic aneurysm
- Arteriobronchial fistula
- *Aspergillus*—invasive fungal disease (intracavity mycetoma) can be a cause of massive hemoptysis.
- Coagulopathy including disseminated intravascular coagulation
- Pulmonary endometriosis (catamenial hemoptysis)
- Pulmonary hemosiderosis

Investigations

The investigation of hemoptysis can often be carried out on an outpatient basis, but patients with significant bleeding or likely serious underlying cause should be admitted if there are concerns. Any patient with massive hemoptysis should be admitted to the ICU.

Beware of the apparently small bleed, which can itself be life threatening, or be a sentinel bleed with subsequent massive bleeding.

Outpatient investigations and management

First-line investigations

• *Blood tests*: CBC, PT/PTT, type and cross
• If vasculitis or autoimmunity suspected: antinuclear cytoplasmic anti-body (ANCA), anti-glomerular basement membrane (GBM), antinuclear antibody (ANA), and urinalysis
• *Sputum studies*: cytology, smears and cultures for bacteria, fungi, and acid-fast bacilli (AFB)
• CXR may show mass lesion, bronchiectasis, consolidation, or arterio-venous malformation (AVM)
• A *CT chest* should be done prior to bronchoscopy if possible, as prior knowledge of the site of abnormality leads to increased detection rates at bronchoscopy. Similarly, a definitive diagnosis, e.g. AVM, may be made from the CT, obviating the need for further investigations. CT may miss an airway abnormality, but bronchoscopy should not.
• *Bronchoscopy* to visualize airways and localize the site of bleeding. This may also be therapeutic, for example, if a bleeding tumor can be injected with vasoconstricting agent or a catheter inserted for tamponade (see Massive hemoptysis)
• *Transbronchial or surgical lung biopsies* if vasculitis is suspected

Second-line investigations

These are usually done if first-line investigations fail to demonstrate a cause.
• *CTPA or ventilation/perfusion (V/Q) scan* to exclude pulmonary embolism (PE)
• A *bronchial angiogram* can be both diagnostic and therapeutic. It is rare for the actual bleeding site to be identified; more often it is assumed from visualizing a mesh of dilated and tortuous vessels, e.g. around a bronchiectatic cavity. This is usually done during an episode of bleeding to maximize the chance of identifying the source.
• *Bronchial artery embolization* is a therapeutic approach to embolize the bleeding artery, usually with coils or
• *ENT evaluation* to evaluate the upper airway for the bleeding source.
• *Echocardiogram*: Moderate to severe PHT can cause hemoptysis, especially in a patient on anticoagulants.

Cryptogenic hemoptysis

In up to 15% of cases, despite appropriate investigations as outlined above, no cause for the hemoptysis can be found. This has a benign prognosis. Often the hemoptysis will resolve without treatment.

Management of massive hemoptysis

Massive hemoptysis (at least 200–600 mL blood in 24 hours) is a life-threatening emergency, with a mortality of up to 80%.

Massive hemoptysis is fortunately rare (1.5% of all hemoptysis cases). Investigations will follow treatment, which may be difficult, and is often unsuccessful. In some cases, active treatment may be inappropriate, and palliative treatment with oxygen and morphine may be warranted.

Airway protection and ventilation

Protection of the nonbleeding lung is vital to maintain adequate gas exchange. This may involve early endotracheal intubation and/or the patient lying in the lateral decubitus position with the bleeding side down (to prevent blood from flowing into the unaffected lung).

Selective intubation or intubation with a double lumen tube may be helpful in isolating the bleeding lung. If intubation is not needed or not appropriate, give high-flow oxygen.

Cardiovascular support

- Large-bore or central intravenous access
- CBC, PT/PTT, type and cross
- Fluid resuscitation and transfusion as necessary
- Reverse anticoagulants (vitamin K, fresh frozen plasma [FFP], etc.)
- Inotropes

Other treatment and investigations

- Nebulized or endobronchial epinephrine (5–10 mL of 1:10,000)
- CXR or chest CT (depending on stability of patient)
- Early bronchoscopy is diagnostic and therapeutic.
- Rigid bronchoscopy (with general anesthesia) is preferable. It may allow localization of the site of bleeding, and balloon tamponade with a Fogarty catheter.
- Bronchial artery embolization is the therapeutic approach to embolize a bleeding artery, usually with coils or glue.

Surgery: Resection of bleeding lobe (if all other measures have failed, there is adequate pulmonary reserve, and the patient is hemodynamically stable)

Unexplained respiratory failure

Causes

Definition

Acute respiratory failure is the inability of the respiratory system to provide either adequate oxygenation of the arterial blood or adequate elimination of carbon dioxide over the course of a few hours or days. Acute respiratory failure can be caused by lesions affecting several parts of the respiratory system including the airways, lung parenchyma, chest wall and respiratory muscles, and central nervous system processes involved in the control of breathing.

There are two physiological types of acute respiratory failure: hypoxic and ventilatory respiratory failure. *Acute hypoxic respiratory failure* is defined as a decrease in the delivery of oxygen from the atmosphere to the blood and, more specifically, as an arterial oxygen tension (PaO_2) of <60 mmHg with no impairment of ventilation. Although somewhat arbitrary, this value was selected on the basis of the beginning of the descent of the oxygen–hemoglobin dissociation curve at a PaO_2 of 60 mmHg.

Ventilatory (also known as hypercapneic or hypercarbic) *respiratory failure* is characterized by a rise in arterial carbon dioxide tension ($PaCO_2$) (>45 mmHg). These changes are associated with an acute respiratory acidosis. The prognostic significance and therapeutic implications of acute changes in $PaCO_2$ are clearly different from those of chronic hypercapnia associated with a renally compensated pH. Therefore, patients with $PaCO_2$ levels chronically elevated above 50 mmHg should not be considered to have acute ventilatory respiratory failure solely on the basis of their elevated $PaCO_2$.

Pathophysiology

The three most important causes of acute hypoxemic respiratory failure are alveolar hypoventilation, ventilation–perfusion (V/Q) mismatching, and intrapulmonary shunting. Pure alveolar hypoventilation is caused by neuromuscular or central nervous system dysfunction. The lung parenchyma is essentially normal. The hypoxemia occurs as a result of a continuous uptake of O_2 and the failure to eliminate CO_2. These patients will have a normal alveolar–arterial (A–a) gradient and a respiratory acidosis.

V/Q mismatching is the most common pathophysiological cause of acute hypoxemic respiratory failure. The degree of hypoxemia in patients with pure V/Q mismatching will improve in response to an increase in the fractional concentration of oxygen in the inspired air (F_iO_2). In contrast, patients with a pure intrapulmonary shunt will not improve their degree of hypoxemia in response to the inhalation of 100% oxygen.

The list below contains the most common and uncommon causes of acute respiratory failure. The conditions with asterisks (*) are those most commonly discovered when the cause is not immediately obvious.

Failure of respiratory drive

Brainstem abnormality
- Polio and post-polio syndrome* (exact mechanism unclear)
- Brainstem stroke

- Arnold–Chiari malformation—herniation of cerebellum into foramen magnum compressing the brainstem
- Syringobulbia—expansion of a fluid compartment in the middle of the spinal cord extending up into the medulla (can be associated with Arnold–Chiari malformation)
- Encephalitis
- Brainstem tumor
- Sarcoidosis
- Demyelinating disorders

Neurological suppression
- Sedative drugs*
- Metabolic alkalosis (hypokalemic alkalosis, diuretic-induced)

Respiratory pump failure

Neuromuscular (particularly if diaphragm is involved)
- Myopathies
  - Acid maltase deficiency (Pompe's); diaphragm paralysis commonly occurs early*
  - Duchenne muscular dystrophy
  - Myotonic dystrophy
  - Several other very rare myopathies
- Neuropathy
  - Motor neuron disease (MND), can affect diaphragm early*
  - Bilateral diaphragm paralysis, e.g., bilateral neuralgic amyotrophy, trauma*
  - Guillain–Barré syndrome*
  - Spinal muscular atrophy
  - High cord transection
- Neuromuscular junction abnormalities
  - Myasthenia gravis*
  - Eaton–Lambert syndrome
  - Anticholinesterase poisoning
- Mixed
  - Post-ICU ("critical care neuromuscular dysfunction"), post–muscle relaxant drugs*

Chest wall
- Obesity hypoventilation syndrome*
- Kyphoscoliosis*
- Post-thoracoplasty (usually "three stage," many ribs have caved in starting from the top down—done for tuberculosis prior to effective chemotherapy)
- Flail chest
- Pneumothorax/large effusion
- Severe ankylosing spondilitis

Airways obstruction/mixed
- Unrecognized COPD or severe asthma*
- Obstructive sleep apnea and associated COPD, obesity, or muscle weakness*
- Cystic fibrosis
- Laryngeal or tracheal stenosis.

Clinical presentation

Slow onset

When the PaO_2 rapidly falls below 40–50 mmHg, harmful effects may be observed in various organ systems. Patients may experience headache, somnolence, confusion, and convulsions. With more severe hypoxemia, permanent encephalopathy may occur. Cardiovascular sequelae from mild hypoxemia, including tachycardia and hypertension, may also develop. With severe hypoxemia, opposite effects may occur, such as bradycardia and hypotension.

Signs and symptoms of hypercapnia depend on not only the absolute levels of $PaCO_2$ but also the rate at which the level increases. Acute elevation in $PaCO_2$ to 80–90 mmHg may produce neurological symptoms including confusion, headaches, convulsions, and coma. A $PaCO_2$ level above 100 mmHg may be well tolerated if the hypercapnia develops slowly and acidemia is minimized by renal compensatory changes.

Triggers of respiratory failure

Sometimes the significance of these symptoms is missed and a relatively trivial respiratory tract infection can tip the balance. The increase in production of CO_2 may overwhelm the ability of the patient to properly ventilate and cause an acute respiratory acidosis that often requires mechanical ventilatory support with either noninvasive positive pressure ventilation (NIPPV) or endotracheal intubation with traditional mechanical ventilation. These patients are often difficult to wean and may present with recurrent ventilatory failure weeks after discharge.

Clinical assessment and management

History, examination, and investigations

History

A carefully taken history, particularly for symptoms of a subtle weakness prior to presentation, episode of shoulder pain (neuralgic amyotrophy), past history of polio, orthopnea (diaphragm weakness), drug history, or ascending paralysis may be helpful.

Examination

A careful neurological examination of a patient with acute hypercapnia may reveal agitation, coarse tremor, slurred speech, asterixis, and occasionally papilledema. These effects of hypercapnia on the central nervous system are fully reversible, in contrast to the potentially permanent neurological sequelae that are associated with acute hypoxemia. An elevated $PaCO_2$ is also associated with myocardial depression, arrhythmias, hyperkalemia, and gastrointestinal bleeding.

Blood gases taken breathing air (following >20 minutes off extra O_2)
- Supplemental oxygen required to maintain a minimum level of normoxia should not be removed to perform this investigation.
- Degree of CO_2 retention
- Presence of a base excess indicating chronicity of CO_2 retention
- Calculate A–a gradient to detect any V/Q mismatch.
- In pure hypoventilation there should be no significant A–a gradient, unless there is associated basal atelectasis from poor lung expansion and/or obesity.

Pulmonary function tests (p. 799)
- Presence of unexpected severe airways obstruction
- Reduction in vital capacity (VC) (neurological or chest wall)
- Further fall of VC on lying down—indicative of diaphragm paralysis
- The supine VC is most predictive of ventilatory failure; <1 liter indicates a high chance of this being the cause of the failure.
- Mouth pressures, sniff pressures, or transdiaphragmatic pressures are not much more helpful than VC, lying and standing.

Specific tests—for some of the conditions listed above:
- Electromyographic (EMG) studies: MND, myotonia
- Magnetic resonance imaging (MRI)—gadolinium enhanced: Arnold–Chiari malformation, brainstem lesion, syrinx
- Creatine phosphokinase (CPK): some myopathies
- Sleep study: rapid eye movement (REM) hypoxia, obstructive sleep apnea (OSA)
- Muscle biopsy: acid maltase deficiency (glycogen-containing vacuoles and low enzyme levels)

Management

Management of the underlying condition is paramount. NIPPV may also be tried when acute ventilatory failure is thought to be due to a rapidly reversible cause. Regardless of the indication for a trial of NIPPV, reassessment for signs of progressive respiratory failure or worsening mental status should be performed early and often, with rapid transition to endotracheal intubation if needed. In general, if the cause of acute ventilatory failure is not felt to be quickly reversible (within 24–48 hours), a trial of NIPPV should not be performed.

In cases of progressive chronic ventilatory failure due to an irreversible condition (such as muscular dystrophy), the decision will need to be made as to whether NIPPV is ethical and appropriate.

Lying down and sleeping with the ***whole bed tipped head up*** by about 20° improves ventilation in the presence of bilateral diaphragm paralysis. Just elevating the top half of the bed and leaving the patient's abdomen and legs horizontal does not work. The abdominal contents have to descend into the pelvis to effectively "offload" the diaphragm. This posture will also improve the ability to wean the patient from assisted ventilation.

Pleural effusion

Clinical assessment

Pleural effusion is a common presentation of a wide range of different diseases. The most common causes in the United Kingdom and United States are (in order) cardiac failure, pneumonia, malignancy, and pulmonary embolism.

The priority is to make a diagnosis and relieve symptoms with a minimum number of invasive procedures. Most patients do not require a chest drain and can be managed as outpatients. Procedures such as therapeutic thoracentesis may easily be performed as an outpatient.

Consider admission and chest drain insertion for the following:

- Patients with malignant effusions who are candidates for pleurodesis
- Empyema or parapneumonic effusion with purulent fluid or a pleural fluid pH <7.20 (the majority of these effusions are unlikely to resolve without drainage and antibiotics)
- Patients in distress with an acute massive effusion

Key steps in management of the patient with a pleural effusion are outlined below (see also abbreviated algorithm in the section "Diagnostic algorithm for the patient with a pleural effusion").

1. **History, examination, CXR** (PA and lateral)

2. Does the patient have heart failure? If so, this should be treated, with no need for pleural tap unless the patient has atypical features (such as very asymmetrical bilateral effusions, unilateral effusion, chest pain, or fever) or fails to respond within 3 days (cardiac failure effusions resolve following clearance of the pulmonary edema).

3. Thoracentesis ("pleural tap," or pleural fluid aspiration) may be diagnostic and/or therapeutic, depending on the volume of fluid removed. See pp. 770–771 for procedure details.

Diagnostic tap
- Note pleural fluid **appearance**.
- Send sample in sterile container to biochemistry for measurement of **protein** and **lactate dehydrogenase (LDH)**.
- Send a fresh, 20 mL sample in a sterile container to **cytology** for examination for malignant cells and differential cell count.
- Send samples in a sterile container and blood culture bottles to **microbiology** for Gram stain and microscopy, culture, and AFB stain and culture.
- Process nonpurulent, heparinized samples in arterial blood gas analyzer for **pH**.
- Consider measurement of cholesterol and triglycerides, hematocrit, glucose, and amylase, depending on the clinical circumstances.

If the patient is breathless he or she may benefit from removal of a larger volume of fluid (therapeutic tap, p. 771).

4. Is the pleural effusion a transudate or exudate? This information is helpful in narrowing the differential diagnosis. The effusion is exudative if:

Pleural fluid protein/serum protein ratio >0.50

Pleural fluid LDH is greater than two-thirds the upper limit of normal serum LDH

The criteria are very sensitive in the diagnosis of exudative effusions, although may occasionally falsely identify transudates as being exudates, e.g., patients treated for heart failure with diuretics may have protein ratios or LDH values in the exudative range.

5. Further investigations if the diagnosis remains unclear:
• Reconsider pulmonary embolism and tuberculosis
• Repeat pleural fluid cytology
• Further pleural fluid analysis, e.g., cholesterol, triglyceride, hematocrit, glucose, amylase, fungal stains
• CT chest with contrast (ideally scan prior to complete fluid drainage, to improve images of pleural surfaces; useful in distinguishing benign from malignant pleural disease, p. 328)
• Pleural tissue biopsy for histology and tuberculosis (TB) culture (ultrasound- or CT-guided, closed Abrams, or thoracoscopic biopsy. Image-guided biopsies are superior to Abrams for malignant disease; use Abrams biopsy only in cases when TB is suspected. Thoracoscopy is the gold standard—biopsies have sensitivity of 90% for malignancy—and allow therapeutic talc pleurodesis at the same time.)
• Consider thoracoscopy if there is persistent undiagnosed pleural effusion and malignancy is likely.

Bronchoscopy has no role in investigating undiagnosed effusions unless the patient has hemoptysis or a CXR or CT pulmonary abnormality is identified.

Further information

Holm KA, Antony VB (2001). Pleural effusions: the workup and treatment. *J Respir Dis* **22**:211–219.
Light RW (2002). Pleural effusion. *N Engl J Med* **346**:1971–1977.
Maskell NA, Butland RJA (2003). BTS guidelines for the investigation of a unilateral pleural effusion in adults. *Thorax* **58** (Suppl. II):ii8–ii17.

Diagnostic algorithm for the patient with a pleural effusion

1. **History, examination, CXR**
2. **Does the patient have heart failure**, with no atypical features (such as asymmetrical bilateral effusions, unilateral effusion, normal heart size on CXR, chest pain, fever)?

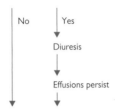

3. **Thoracentesis** (diagnostic +/- therapeutic)
   Pleural fluid analysis: Appearance, protein, LDH, cytology, microbiology, pH (triglyceride, hematocrit, glucose, amylase)
4. **Is the pleural effusion a transudate or exudate?**

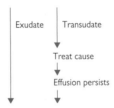

5. **Further investigations** if diagnosis remains unclear:
   - Reconsider pulmonary embolism and tuberculosis
   - Repeat pleural fluid cytology
   - Further pleural fluid analysis, e.g., cholesterol, triglyceride, hematocrit, glucose, amylase, fungal stains
   - CT chest with contrast
   - Pleural tissue biopsy for histology and TB culture (ultrasound- or CT-guided, closed Abrams, or thoracoscopic biopsy)
   - Consider thoracoscopy if there is persistent undiagnosed pleural effusion.

Transudative pleural effusions

Mechanisms involve either increased hydrostatic pressure or reduced osmotic pressure (due to hypoalbuminemia) in microvascular circulation.

Differential diagnosis
See Table 6.1.

Table 6.1 Differential diagnosis of transudative pleural effusions

Cause	Notes
Common	
Left ventricular failure	Investigate further if atypical features (very asymmetrical bilateral effusions, unilateral effusion, chest pain, fever); frequently complicated by pulmonary embolism (up to one-fifth of cases at autopsy)
Cirrhotic liver disease ("hepatic hydrothorax")	Clinical ascites usually but not invariably present; majority are right-sided; remove ascites and treat hypoalbuminemia (p. 574)
Pulmonary embolism	10%–20% are transudates (p. 342) from atelectasis
Peritoneal dialysis	Pleural fluid analysis resembles dialysis fluid, with protein <1 g/dL and glucose >300 mg/dL
Nephrotic syndrome	Usually bilateral; consider secondary pulmonary embolism if there are atypical features
Atelectasis	Common on ICU or postoperatively; usually small effusion, may be bilateral; rarely needs investigation
Less common	
Constrictive pericarditis	May be unilateral or bilateral
Hypothyroidism	May be transudate or exudate; pleural effusions occur most commonly in association with ascites, pericardial effusion, and cardiac failure, although may be an isolated finding
Meigs syndrome	Unilateral (often right-sided) or bilateral pleural effusions and ascites; occur in women with ovarian or other pelvic tumors; resolve following removal of tumor
Urinothorax	Effusion ipsilateral to obstructed kidney with retroperitoneal urine leak, resolves after treatment of obstruction; pleural fluid smells of urine, pH usually low; pleural fluid creatinine > serum creatinine is diagnostic
Malignancy	Up to 5% are transudates

Treatment of transudative effusions is directed at the underlying cause; consider further investigation if they fail to respond.

Exudative pleural effusions

Mechanisms involve an increase in capillary permeability and impaired pleural fluid resorption.

Differential diagnosis
See Table 6.2.

Table 6.2 Differential diagnosis of exudative pleural effusions

Cause	Notes and page references
Common	
Parapneumonic effusion	Occurs in 40%–57% of bacterial pneumonias; most common exudative effusion in young patients (p. 334)
Malignancy	Most common exudative effusion in patients >60 years (p. 330)
Pulmonary embolism	80%–90% are exudates (p. 342)
Rheumatoid arthritis	Typically low pleural fluid glucose, often <1.6 mmol/L (p. 342)
Mesothelioma	Pleural fluid cytological analysis has low sensitivity (pp. 352–3)
Less common	
Empyema	Frank pus in the pleural space; clinical features of infection, e.g., fever, sweats (p. 334)
Tuberculosis	Typically lymphocytic effusion; pleural fluid AFB smear positive in <10% of cases, culture positive in 25%, Abrams biopsy histology sensitivity 90% (p. 340)
Other infections	Very rare; include viral, parasitic, rickettsial, and fungal (e.g., aspergillus, histoplasma, coccidioidomycosis)
Hepatic, splenic, or subphrenic abscess	Sympathetic effusion with characteristics typical of uncomplicated parapneumonic effusion
Esophageal rupture	Initially sterile exudate, followed by empyema; pH <7.00, raised salivary amylase, often history of vomiting
Acute pancreatitis	Left-sided pleural fluid with elevated pancreatic amylase
SLE	Lupus erythematosus cells in fluid are diagnostic; may respond quickly to prednisolone

Table 6.2 (*Cont.*)

Cause	Notes and page references
Other autoimmune diseases	Churg–Strauss syndrome (intensely eosinophilic fluid), Sjögren's syndrome, scleroderma, dermatomyositis, Wegener's granulomatosis
Sarcoidosis	Effusions directly related to pleural sarcoid are uncommon (<2%)
Post–cardiac injury syndrome (Dressler's syndrome)	Pleural effusions common; may be blood-stained
Post–coronary artery bypass (CABG) surgery	Universally present within the first 30 days post-operatively (p. 343)
Radiotherapy	May cause small, unilateral effusions up to 6 months after treatment
Uremia	Effusions may develop in patients on chronic hemodialysis
Chylothorax	Presence of chylomicrons or pleural fluid triglyceride level >110 mg/dL (p. 50)
Benign asbestos-related pleural effusion	Over 50% of patient are asymptomatic with unilateral effusion on CXR
Drug-induced	Drugs include amiodarone, bromocriptine, methotrexate, phenytoin, and nitrofurantoin; see www.pneumotox.com for full list; effusions usually resolve following discontinuation of drug
Other, rare causes	Include yellow nail syndrome, amyloidosis, familial Mediterranean fever

Treatment

Treatment of exudates involves treatment of the underlying cause, as well as measures to improve breathlessness and remove pleural fluid, e.g., therapeutic thoracentesis (p. 771), intercostal drainage (p. 782), and pleurodesis (pp. 786–7).

Pleural fluid analysis 1

"Routine" pleural fluid analysis comprises assessment of the following:
• Pleural fluid appearance
• Biochemistry (protein, LDH, and glucose)
• Cytology (for malignant cells and differential cell count; ideally fresh 20 mL sample)
• Microbiology (Gram stain and microscopy, culture, and AFB stain and culture; inoculation of blood culture bottles with pleural fluid may increase yield)
• pH

Although considered routine, some of these investigations may be unnecessary and even misleading, depending on the clinical picture (e.g., microbiological analysis on patients suspected as having transudates).

Additional pleural fluid investigations such as measurement of cholesterol and triglycerides, hematocrit, and amylase may be helpful in certain clinical circumstances.

Appearance
See Table 6.3.

Table 6.3 Possible causes by appearance

Appearance	Possible causes
Bloody	Trauma, malignancy, pulmonary infarction, post-cardiac injury syndrome, pneumothorax (10%), benign asbestos-related pleural effusion, aortic dissection/rupture; defined as hemothorax if pleural fluid hematocrit >50% of peripheral blood hematocrit (p. 342)
Turbid or milky	Empyema, chylothorax, cholesterol effusion (clear supernatant after centrifuging favors empyema; cloudy after centrifuging suggests chylothorax or cholesterol effusion) (p. 50)
Putrid odor	Anaerobic empyema
Viscous	Mesothelioma
Food particles	Esophageal rupture
Urine odor	Urinothorax
Black	Aspergillus infection
Brown, "anchovy sauce"	Amebic liver abscess draining into pleural space

Differential cell count
See Table 6.4.

Table 6.4 Possible causes by differential cell count

Predominant cell type	Possible causes
Neutrophils	Any acute effusion, e.g., parapneumonic, pulmonary embolus
Mononuclear cells	Any chronic effusion, e.g., malignancy, tuberculosis
Lymphocytes	Tuberculosis, especially if over 80%; other causes include lymphoma, sarcoidosis, chronic rheumatoid pleurisy, late post-CABG, yellow nail syndrome, acute lung rejection
Eosinophils	Often unhelpful; associations include air or blood in pleural space (hemothorax, pulmonary infarct, pneumothorax), malignancy, infection (parapneumonic, fungal, parasitic), drug- and asbestos-induced effusions, Churg–Strauss syndrome or idiopathic
Mesothelial cells	Predominate in transudates; variable numbers in exudates, typically suppressed in inflammatory conditions, e.g., tuberculosis
Lupus erythematosus cells	Diagnostic of SLE

Pleural fluid analysis 2

Pleural fluid pH and glucose

Pleural fluid pH should be measured using an arterial blood pH analyzer. The sample should be appropriately heparinized—e.g., aspirate a few milliliters of pleural fluid into a preheparinized blood gas syringe. Frankly purulent samples do not need to be analyzed, as the pH value would not change management.

Normal pleural fluid pH is about 7.60. An abnormally low pH (<7.30) suggests pleural inflammation and is often associated with a low pleural fluid glucose (<3.3 mmol/L or pleural fluid/serum glucose ratio <0.50). The mechanism probably involves increased neutrophil phagocytosis and bacterial metabolism with increased glycolysis resulting in the accumulation of lactate and carbon dioxide.

Causes of low pH and low glucose effusions
- Parapneumonic effusion and empyema (pH <7.20 is indication for drainage of pleural space, as unlikely to resolve spontaneously)
- Rheumatoid pleuritis (glucose <1.7 mmol/L in 66% and <2.8 mmol/L in 80% of cases)
- Malignant pleural effusion (associated with advanced disease and poor survival, higher sensitivity of pleural fluid cytological analysis, and poorer response to pleurodesis)
- Tuberculous pleural effusion
- Esophageal rupture
- Lupus pleuritis.

Urinothorax is the only transudative effusion that can cause a pH <7.30. An abnormally high (alkaline) pH may rarely occur in the setting of *Proteus* pleural infection.

Pleural fluid triglyceride and cholesterol

Measure in turbid or milky effusions or where chylothorax is suspected.

Chylothorax

Chylothorax occurs following disruption of the thoracic duct, and pleural fluid may appear turbid, milky, serous, or blood stained. The presence of pleural fluid chylomicrons or a pleural fluid triglyceride level >110 mg/dL confirm the diagnosis. Causes of chylothorax incude the following:
- Malignancy (particularly lymphoma)
- Trauma
- Following thoracotomy
- Pulmonary lymphangioleiomyomatosis (LAM)

Cholesterol effusion

Cholesterol effusion occurs from cholesterol crystal deposition in chronic effusions, most commonly due to rheumatoid pleurisy or tuberculosis, and may cause a milky effusion. Raised pleural fluid (PF) cholesterol (>200 mg/dL), PF cholesterol/triglyceride ratio >1.0, and cholesterol crystals at microscopy distinguish it from chylothorax.

Pleural fluid amylase

This measure is abnormal if pleural fluid amylase is greater than the upper normal limit for serum amylase, or if the amylase pleural fluid/serum ratio is >1.0. Causes include the following:

- Pleural malignancy and esophageal rupture (both associated with raised *salivary* amylase)
- Pancreatic disease (acute and chronic pancreatitis with pancreatic pseudocyst; associated with raised *pancreatic* amylase).

It may be normal early in the course of acute pancreatitis or esophageal rupture.

Diffuse parenchymal lung disease

Causes

Diffuse parenchymal lung disease is relatively uncommon and its diagnosis is frequently challenging. This chapter describes a diagnostic approach based on clinical features, imaging, and other investigations; more detailed descriptions of the diseases themselves are presented later in the book.

The term *diffuse parenchymal lung disease* (DPLD) is used here to describe any widespread pulmonary disease process. Patients typically present with breathlessness and bilateral CXR infiltrates. The rate of onset and severity of breathlessness are extremely variable, and presentations range from an asymptomatic patient with longstanding radiographic changes to an acute onset of breathlessness over days leading rapidly to respiratory failure and death.

Anatomy of diffuse lung disease

An understanding of lung anatomy is helpful when considering the causes of DPLD and their radiographic appearance on HRCT.

Many diffuse lung diseases affect primarily the interstitium (interstitial lung disease [ILD]), a poorly defined term that refers to the connective tissue fibrous framework of the lung. Centrally, connective tissue surrounds bronchovascular bundles (each consisting of a bronchus and its accompanying pulmonary artery) that originate at the hila.

Peripherally, these connective tissue sheaths are in continuity with fibrous interlobular septa that organize the lung into units called "secondary pulmonary lobules," polyhedral structures with approximately 2-cm sides. Interlobular septa, which define and separate secondary pulmonary lobules, contain lymphatics and venules. A secondary pulmonary lobule contains around 5–12 acini and is supplied at its center by a bronchiole and pulmonary arteriole.

The term *interstitial lung disease* is confusing because many primarily interstitial processes also involve the airways, vasculature, and alveolar airspaces. Disease processes that primarily affect the airways (e.g., bronchiectasis), vessels (e.g., vasculitis), or airspaces (e.g., pneumonia) may also present with diffuse CXR shadowing and so are included in this chapter.

Causes

There are several hundred causes of diffuse lung disease, and it is useful to divide these into groups based on their rate of onset and etiology and disease mechanism (see Table 7.1).

Further information

American Thoracic Society/European Respiratory Society International Multidisciplinary Consensus Classification of the Idiopathic Interstitial Pneumonias. *Am J Respir Crit Care Med* 2002, **165**:277–304.

Table 7.1 Causes of diffuse lung disease

Disease onset	Cause or mechanism	Examples (common conditions in bold)
Acute (days–weeks)	Infection	**Bacterial** (pneumococcal, staphylococcal, Gram-negative, anaerobic, TB), viral (influenza, parainfluenza, adenovirus, RSV, measles, varicella, hanta), atypical, fungal (aspergillosis, histoplasmosis, *Pneumocystis jirovecii* pneumonia [PCP])
	Miscellaneous	**Adult respiratory distress syndrome**, acute interstitial pneumonia (AIP), acute hypersensitivity pneumonitis
Acute or chronic	Drugs	Immunosuppressants (methotrexate); treatment of connective tissue disease (gold, penicillamine, sulfasalazine); cytotoxics (chlorambucil, melphalan, busulfan, lomustine, carmustine, bleomycin, mitomycin); antibiotics (nitrofurantoin, cephalosporins); antiarrhythmics (amiodarone); illicit (cocaine inhalation, heroin, methadone, IV talc)
	Toxins	Radiotherapy, high-concentration oxygen, paraquat
	Vasculitis/ alveolar hemorrhage	Wegener's granulomatosis, Churg–Strauss syndrome, Goodpasture's syndrome, SLE, microscopic polyangiitis, idiopathic hemosiderosis
	Pulmonary venous hypertension	**Cardiogenic pulmonary edema**, pulmonary veno-occlusive disease
	Miscellaneous	**Sarcoidosis**, cryptogenic organizing pneumonia (COP), eosinophilic pneumonia, lipoid pneumonia
Chronic (months–years)	Idiopathic interstitial pneumonias	**Idiopathic pulmonary fibrosis (IPF)** nonspecific interstitial pneumonia (NSIP), desquamative interstitial pneumonia (DIP), lymphocytic interstitial pneumonia (LIP), respiratory bronchiolitis-associated interstitial lung disease (RB-ILD)
	Inhalational Inorganic	**Asbestosis**, coal workers' pneumoconiosis, silicosis, metals, e.g., cobalt, aluminum
	Organic	Hypersensitivity pneumonitis, e.g., bird fanciers' lung, farmers' lung
	Connective tissue disease	**Rheumatoid arthritis**, SLE, scleroderma, poly- and dermatomyositis, ankylosing spondylitis, Sjögren's syndrome, Behçet's disease
	Malignancy	Lymphangitic carcinoma, bronchoalveolar cell carcinoma, pulmonary lymphoma
	Miscellaneous	**Bronchiectasis**, Langerhans cell histiocytosis, amyloidosis, lymphangioleiomyomatosis (LAM), pulmonary alveolar proteinosis (PAP), microlithiasis

Clinical assessment and imaging

History

Clinical features may provide useful clues to the underlying diagnosis. Key points in the history are described below.

Presenting symptoms

- Breathlessness is the most common symptom, and its rate of onset may be useful diagnostically (see Table 7.1)
- Causes of truly *episodic* breathlessness and diffuse chest radiographic shadowing include eosinophilic pneumonia, vasculitis, Churg–Strauss syndrome, hypersensitivity pneumonitis, allergic bronchopulmonary aspergillosis, and pulmonary edema.
- Cough may occur, although its diagnostic value is uncertain; it may be a prominent symptom in lymphangitic carcinoma, hypersensitivity pneumonitis, cryptogenic organizing pneumonia, and sarcoid and eosinophilic pneumonia. Chronic production of purulent sputum suggests bronchiectasis. Bronchorrhea (production of large volumes of sputum) may occur with bronchoalveolar cell carcinoma. Hemoptysis suggests alveolar hemorrhage, malignancy, or pulmonary venous hypertension.
- Wheeze may occur in asthma associated with eosinophilic pneumonia or Churg–Strauss syndrome.
- Weight loss and fever are nonspecific symptoms associated with many diffuse lung diseases.

Other medical conditions

These include other accompanying conditions such as malignancy, connective tissue disease, HIV infection, or other immunosuppression, among others. Ask about old CXRs, which may be helpful in assessing disease duration.

Drugs and medications

- See Table 7.1 for common drug causes of diffuse lung disease.
- Delays of months or even years may occur between starting the drug and developing lung involvement.
- Illicit drug use (crack cocaine or heroin—pulmonary edema, eosinophilic pneumonia, diffuse alveolar hemorrhage, interstitial pneumonia; intravenous drug use—IV talcosis, septic emboli)
- Oily nose drops (lipoid pneumonia)

Occupation, lifestyle, hobbies, and pets

- May involve inhalation of inorganic or organic dusts. Document lifelong employment history, including probable exposure levels, use of protective equipment, and names of employers.
- Inorganic dusts associated with development of diffuse lung disease include asbestos, silica, cobalt, beryllium, aluminum, isocyanates, copper sulfate, iron, tin, barium, and antimony.
- Hypersensitivity pneumonitis may result from inhalation of organic dusts such as *Thermoactinomycetes* in moldy hay (farmers' lung), avian proteins or feathers (bird fanciers' lung), mushroom compost, moldy cheese, cork or sugar cane, and isocyanates.

- Risk factors for immunocompromise (opportunistic infection, LIP, lymphoma)
- Smoking history (pulmonary Langerhans cell histiocytosis, respiratory bronchiolitis-associated interstitial lung disease, desquamative interstitial pneumonia, and Goodpasture's syndrome are more common in smokers.)

Evidence of extrapulmonary disease
This includes manifestations of connective tissue disease, vasculitis, and sarcoidosis, e.g., arthralgia, skin rash, ocular symptoms, muscular pain and weakness, Raynaud's, nasal/sinus disease, hematuria.

Travel
- Tuberculosis, pulmonary eosinophilia from parasites (tropics), histoplasmosis (north and central United States, parts of South America and Africa), hydatid disease (Middle East, Australasia, Mediterranean).
- Family history
- α_1-antitrypsin deficiency, rare familial forms of pulmonary fibrosis and sarcoidosis

Examination
- Cyanosis and signs of cor pulmonale in severe disease
- Clubbing (usual interstitial pneumonitis, asbestosis, bronchiectasis)
- Basal crackles (usual interstitial pneumonitis, asbestosis, connective tissue disease, pulmonary edema, lymphangitis, drugs); crackles in bronchiectasis are characteristically coarse
- Absence of crackles despite a significant CXR abnormality may be suggestive of sarcoidosis, pneumoconiosis, hypersensitivity pneumonitis, or pulmonary Langerhans cell histiocytosis.
- Squeaks suggest the presence of bronchiolitis.
- Skin, joint, and eye disease (connective tissue disease, sarcoidosis, vasculitis)

Imaging
CXR
A CXR may occasionally be diagnostic. However, patients with a normal CXR can have biopsy-proven diffuse lung disease. Previous CXRs are helpful in assessing disease duration and progression.

High-resolution CT (HRCT) chest
HRCT is more sensitive and specific than CXR for diagnosing diffuse lung disease (see HRCT diagnosis and Appendix 4). HRCT is often in itself diagnostic, and should always precede biopsy in the investigation of diffuse lung disease.

HRCT also enables assessment of disease extent, and optimal biopsy site if required. HRCT appearance correlates with prognosis. Extensive reticulation and honeycombing are often associated with fibrosis, poor response to treatment, and a worse prognosis.

HRCT diagnosis

HRCT (and to a limited extent CXR) appearances can be classified according to the pattern of disease, and the presence of additional features (see also Appendix 4).

1. Imaging findings

Reticular (or linear) pattern

Causes include the following:

- Interstitial pulmonary edema
- Usual interstitial pneumonia (UIP; reticular shadowing is typically patchy, subpleural, and basal; other features include loss of architecture of secondary pulmonary lobules, honeycombing, and traction bronchiectasis)
- Asbestosis (similar features to UIP, often with pleural plaques)
- Connective tissue disease–associated fibrosis (similar features to UIP)
- Chronic hypersensitivity pneumonitis (often associated with regions of ground-glass change, air-trapping on expiration, and centrilobular micronodules)
- Drug-induced fibrosis
- Sarcoidosis

Nodular pattern

This consists of numerous discrete, round opacities 0.1–1 cm in diameter.

- Interstitial processes result in nodularity within interlobular septa, around bronchovascular bundles, and subpleurally (e.g., sarcoidosis, which may demonstrate associated perihilar reticular shadowing and lymphadenopathy).
- Airspace diseases may lead to affected acini becoming visible as nodules (e.g., hypersensitivity pneumonitis, miliary TB, COP, malignancy).

Ground-glass change

This is an increase in lung density through which pulmonary vasculature is still visible (compare the lung density with that of air within the bronchi). It may occur as a result of airspace or interstitial disease, and may be patchy or diffuse. Causes include the following:

- Pulmonary edema or hemorrhage, acute respiratory distress syndrome (ARDS)
- Hypersensitivity pneumonitis
- Drugs
- Certain idiopathic interstitial pneumonias (NSIP, RB-ILD, DIP, AIP)
- PCP
- Sarcoidosis
- Bronchoalveolar cell carcinoma
- Alveolar proteinosis

Ground-glass appearance may be artifactual, the increased density resulting from breath-holding during expiration. It may also be confused with mosaic perfusion, where densities vary in different regions of the lung as a result of variable perfusion, e.g., in chronic thromboembolic disease, small airways disease.

Consolidation

Consolidation (or airspace shadowing) is an increase in attenuation characterized by air bronchograms (air-filled bronchi superimposed against opacified alveoli) and the loss of visibility of adjacent vessels. It occurs as disease processes infiltrate and fill alveolar airspaces, for example, with water, blood, pus, malignant cells, or fibrous tissue. Causes include

• Pneumonia
• Pulmonary edema or hemorrhage, ARDS
• Drugs
• Cryptogenic organizing pneumonia (COP)
• Bronchoalveolar cell carcinoma, lymphoma
• Other rare conditions (eosinophilic pneumonia, alveolar proteinosis)

Cystic change refers to well-defined airspaces with a thin wall. Causes include the following:

• Pulmonary Langerhans cell histiocytosis (bizarrely shaped cysts and nodules, apical predominance)
• Usual interstitial pneumonitis (subpleural honeycomb cysts)
• PCP
• Lymphocytic interstitial pneumonia
• Septic emboli
• Lymphangioleiomyomatosis (thin-walled cysts, otherwise normal lung)
• Centrilobular emphysema may simulate cystic disease, but there is absence of a well-defined wall.

Interlobular septal thickening occurs as a result of processes affecting the lymphatics or venules within interlobular septa, such as

• Pulmonary edema (smooth thickening)
• Lymphangitic carcinomatosis (irregular, nodular thickening of interlobular septa and bronchovascular bundles, no architectural distortion)
• Sarcoidosis
• Usual interstitial pneumonitis

2. Imaging distribution

• *Upper zone*: Silicosis, pneumoconiosis, chronic sarcoidosis, hypersensitivity pneumonitis, ankylosing spondylitis, tuberculosis, pulmonary Langerhans cell histiocytosis
• *Lower zone*: UIP, connective tissue diseases, asbestosis
• *Mid-zone*: Sarcoidosis, pulmonary edema, PCP
• *Peripheral*: UIP, eosinophilic pneumonia, drugs (amiodarone), COP
• *Sharp borders*: Radiation pneumonitis

3. Additional imaging features

• *Lymphadenopathy*: Sarcoidosis, lymphoma, malignancy, infection, silicosis, berylliosis, LIP
• *Pleural effusion/involvement*: Pulmonary edema, connective tissue diseases, infection, malignancy, asbestosis, drugs, LAM

Further information

Ryu JH, Olson EJ, Midthun DE, Swensen SJ. (2002). Diagnostic approach to the patient with diffuse lung disease. *Mayo Clin Proc* **77**:1221–1227.

Further investigations

Urine and blood tests

Consider the following investigations:
- Urine dipstick and microscopy for detection of renal disease associated with vasculitis or connective tissue disease
- Erythrocyte sedimentation rate (ESR), C-reactive protein (CRP), full blood count (look specifically at the eosinophil count), renal and liver function, calcium (increased in >10% of patients with sarcoidosis)
- Autoantibodies (including anti-Jo-1, occurs with myositis-associated interstitial pneumonia; positive rheumatoid factor or ANA may occur in infection, malignancy, and UIP as well as in connective tissue disease)
- ANCA (vasculitis), anti-GBM (Goodpasture's syndrome)
- Serum precipitins (to antigens in hypersensitivity pneumonitis; poor specificity)
- Serum ACE levels may be increased in sarcoidosis, but this is a nonspecific and relatively insensitive test and is generally unhelpful diagnostically.

Sputum
- Cytology may be diagnostic in some lung cancers.
- Induced sputum may be useful in the diagnosis of PCP and TB.

Pulmonary function tests
- Useful in assessing physiologic pattern, severity of disease, and response to treatment
- Typically show restrictive pattern with reduced vital capacity and transfer factor. Normal values do not exclude disease.
- Obstructive pattern is rare, but may be seen in sarcoidosis, pulmonary Langerhans cell histiocytosis, and lymphangioleiomyomatosis among others; may see mixed picture if coexisting COPD
- Diffusing capacity may be increased transiently (days) in alveolar hemorrhage. Reduced diffusing capacity with preserved lung volumes in scleroderma is suggestive of pulmonary vascular disease (such as pulmonary arterial hypertension).
- Disease progression and response to treatment are best assessed by serial measurements of vital capacity and diffusing capacity.
- Check oxygen saturation and consider ABGs. A fall in oxygen saturation on simple exercise may be performed in the clinic setting, and is a useful clue to underlying lung disease in patients with normal saturation and lung function at rest and an unremarkable CXR.

Cardiac investigations
- *ECG:* Conduction abnormality in sarcoidosis. Cardiogenic pulmonary edema is unusual in the presence of a completely normal ECG.
- *Echocardiography:* Assess left ventricular and valvular function if cardiac pulmonary edema is suspected, and estimate pulmonary arterial pressure when pulmonary hypertension is suspected.

Bronchoalveolar lavage (BAL)

- Most useful in diagnosis of opportunistic infection (bacterial or fungal pneumonia, tuberculosis, PCP), malignancy, alveolar proteinosis, eosinophilic pneumonia, and alveolar hemorrhage
- BAL differential cell counts may be helpful diagnostically when combined with the entirety of the clinical data.

Lung biopsy

Which patients need a lung biopsy?

In cases of uncertain etiology, despite clinical assessment and HRCT, lung biopsies often provide a definitive diagnosis. Ideally they should be taken before treatment is started.

The decision to biopsy varies among clinicians, and should take into account the individual patient's clinical condition and wishes, and the likely benefit of a definitive diagnosis in terms of predicting treatment response and prognosis. Some take a pragmatic approach when a diagnosis (or group of diagnoses with the same treatment) is likely but not biopsy-proven, and treat empirically.

In some cases, the patient may be too unwell for biopsy and require empirical treatment. Biopsy of end-stage fibrosis is unhelpful in eliciting an underlying etiology.

Biopsy techniques

Transbronchial biopsy (TBB)

This technique provides small samples, but a relatively high diagnostic yield in diseases with a "centrilobular" distribution, e.g., sarcoidosis, hypersensitivity pneumonitis, malignancy, and infection (fungi, tuberculosis). Additional blind endobronchial biopsies may be diagnostic in sarcoidosis.

Open lung biopsy

Open lung biopsy via thoracotomy or video-assisted thoracoscopic (VATS) biopsy provide larger samples than those with TBB, and have diagnostic yields of at least 90%. Both require general anesthesia. VATS probably has a lower morbidity, and is generally preferred in stable patients; open biopsy is required in ventilator-dependent patients.

Percutaneous image-guided biopsy

This technique may be useful in the diagnosis of well-localized and dense peripheral infiltrates. A cutting needle biopsy technique is best and, if the lesion(s) abuts the pleural surface, pneumothorax is uncommon.

Chapter 8

Diffuse alveolar hemorrhage

Bleeding from the lungs can originate from the bronchial circulation, such as when a lung cancer erodes a bronchial vessel, or from the pulmonary microcirculation.

Injury to the microcirculation often resulting from a small-vessel vasculitis known as pulmonary capillaritis allows blood to enter the alveolar spaces, producing the clinical syndrome of diffuse alveolar hemorrhage (DAH).

Patients with diffuse alveolar hemorrhage may have a background history of vasculitis or it may be the presenting picture of a systemic vasculitis or connective tissue disease (see Table 8.1). It can present with slowly progressive dyspnea with possible hemoptysis, or represent an acute process with hypoxia, and acute respiratory failure.

Presentation

Abrupt-onset hemoptysis is the most common symptom, although this is not present in one-third of cases. There is also cough, dyspnea, low-grade fever, weight loss, arthralgia, and myalgia.

Examination

Findings may be nonspecific, or patients may have signs of underlying vasculitis with dermatologic leukocytoclastic vasculitis, nail fold infarcts, or digital gangrene. Episcleritis, corneal ulceration, epistaxis, nasal crusting, or deafness may occur. Patients may be breathless. Hematuria and proteinuria may be present as well as red blood cell casts in urine sediment examination.

Investigations

- May be hypoxic—check SaO_2 ± arterial blood gas (ABG)
- May have falling hemoglobin
- CXR showing bilateral alveolar infiltrates—difficult to distinguish from pulmonary edema or infection
- Consider chest HRCT
- Raised DLCO as increased intra-alveolar hemoglobin available to combine with carbon monoxide. Abnormal if raised by >30%. If the patient is breathless at rest, they will not be able to perform this test, as it requires breath-holding of an air, carbon monoxide, and helium mixture for 10 seconds. This test can be used to monitor disease progress.
- BAL shows a bloody bronchoalveolar lavage (BAL), which becomes sequentially more so with each aliquot of BAL fluid. Hemosiderin-laden macrophages are also seen on microscopic examination of the fluid.
- Renal involvement: blood and/or protein in the urine, raised urea and creatinine; and red blood cell casts
- Send blood for urgent ANA, ANCA, anti-GBM, dsDNA, and rheumatoid factor
- Consider biopsy of lung, kidney, or other affected sites if the patient is well enough for making a tissue diagnosis.

Management

- Admit patient to the hospital
- Provide support with intravenous (IV) fluids, blood transfusion, and oxygen if necessary
- Monitor, paying particular attention to oxygen saturation levels and keeping them above 92% with supplemental oxygen therapy. The patient may need respiratory support with intubation and ventilation or CPAP. Monitor hemoglobin with further transfusion if necessary. Monitor urine output and renal function.
- Treatment with plasma exchange, high-dose steroids and cyclophosphoamide, and dialysis if required.

Key questions

- Is the patient in respiratory failure?
- Is this isolated lung disease?
- Is there accompanying renal disease?
- Are there other features of a systemic disease?—ENT, joints, etc.

Table 8.1 Causes of alveolar hemorrhage

Cause	See page
Goodpasture's disease*	568
Wegener's granulomatosis*	562
SLE*	548
Rheumatoid arthritis	546
Microscopic polyangiitis	566
Progressive systemic sclerosis	554
Mixed connective tissue disease	
Polyarteritis nodosa	
Behçet's disease	
Essential mixed cryoglobulinemia	
Tumor-related vasculitis	
Endocarditis-related vasculitis	
Idiopathic rapidly progressive glomerulonephritis	
D-penicillamine induced	
Cocaine	
Idiopathic pulmonary hemosiderosis	
Chemicals: trimellitic anhydride, lymphangiography	
Leptospirosis	
Isolated pauci-immune pulmonary capillaritis	
Coagulopathy, such as disseminated intravascular coagulation	
Mitral stenosis	

* Most common causes of alveolar hemorrhage.

Pulmonary infiltrates in the immunocompromised host (non-HIV)

Clinical assessment

Respiratory disease is encountered most commonly in the setting of hematological malignancy, after chemotherapy or monoclonal antibodies, congenital or acquired immunodeficiencies, autoimmune diseases, post-transplant (particularly renal and bone marrow), prolonged corticosteroid use, and AIDS (see p. 84).

The finding of pulmonary infiltrates in the immunocompromised patient should be aggressively worked up, as it has significant morbidity and mortality. For example, 90% of those with hematological malignancies who die have pulmonary infections.

Immunocompromised patients may not display the typical symptoms of pulmonary infections and may only present with fever (pulmonary infections account for 30% of the causes of fever in immunocompromised patients). This, combined with the large number of possible causes, makes reaching a precise diagnosis difficult; the diagnosis remains unclear in up to 10% of cases even at autopsy.

Clinical evaluation

History

A history includes timing of symptoms (acute versus chronic), travel and work history, hobbies, sick contacts, recent hospitalization, and recent antibiotic exposure.

Physical exam

Assess fluid status. Mucositis is involved with an increased risk of infection. Indwelling lines are another important risk factor for infections. Chest **examination** may suggest the extent of pulmonary involvement, although this can be misleading and there are often no abnormal signs (e.g., PCP).

Extrapulmonary involvement may be helpful in suggesting a pathogen, e.g., cutaneous lesions (herpes simplex and varicella-zoster; necrotic lesions from *Pseudomonas* and other gram-negative bacteria, mycobacteria, and fungi; subcutaneous abscesses in *Staphylococcus aureus and Nocardia*), and central nervous system involvement (*Pseudomonas, Aspergillus, Cryptococcus, Nocardia, mycobacteria, S. pneumoniae, H. influenzae,* varicella zoster virus [VZV]).

Initial investigations

- *CBC with differential* to evaluate for neutropenia, which is the most common risk factor for bacterial and fungal infections
- *CXR:* Appearance is very variable; it may be normal or show consolidation (focal infiltrate, multiple nodules, cavitary lesion or diffuse shadowing). CXR is of limited diagnostic value, as appearances are nonspecific and atypical presentations are common; the first-choice diagnosis based on CXR is correct in only a third of cases. CXR may be helpful, however, in monitoring disease progression and response to treatment.
- *Blood and pleural fluid* (if available) staining and culture
- *Sputum examination* is often of little diagnostic value in immunocompromised patients, with the possible exceptions of invasive aspergillosis and tuberculosis. Send sputum for Gram stain and culture, AFB stain and culture, nocardial culture, fungal stain and culture, and cytology. Induced sputum has a low yield for PCP in non-HIV patients.
- The degree of *hypoxia* is often not appreciated; measure oxygen saturations and consider ABGs. Severe hypoxia tends to be more commonly associated with infection due to bacteria, viruses, or *Pneumocystis* than with mycobacteria or fungi.

Further investigations

More invasive diagnostic techniques are usually required for a definitive diagnosis.

CT chest
- Should be considered early, as it more sensitive than CXR in identifying the location and extent of pulmonary disease and aiding invasive sampling procedures.
- May be helpful in diagnosis, e.g., pulmonary embolism (CTPA); lymphangitis carcinomatosis; invasive aspergillosis ("halo" and "air crescent" signs)

Bronchoscopy with bronchoalveolar lavage (BAL)
- First-line investigation, consider early in management. Flexible bronchoscopy is diagnostic in about 56% of patients, with the yield increasing up to 81% in those with infection. BAL is diagnostic in 34% of bacterial infections, 22% of cytomegalovirus (CMV) infections, 15% of PCP infections, 6% in other viruses and mycobacterial infections, and 2% in invasive *Aspergillus* infections.
- BAL results in change to treatment in around 50% of cases overall. Complications are rare.
- Useful in the diagnosis of bacterial pneumonia, PCP (sensitivity 80%–90%), CMV (sensitivity 85–90%), aspergillosis (sensitivity 50%), tuberculosis, malignant disease, diffuse alveolar hemorrhage, and alveolar proteinosis
- BAL fluid analysis: routine microscopy and culture for bacteria; GMS and AFB stains and culture for fungi and mycobacteria, *Nocardia* culture; methenamine silver stain/immunofluorescence or polymerase chain reaction (PCR) for *Pneumocystis* and hemosiderin-laden macrophages if alveolar hemorrhage suspected
- BAL cytology (34% sensitivity for evaluating infectious etiology, which increases to 43% when CMV infection is excluded). It can also increase the sensitivity for diagnosing *Aspergillus* and PCP. Use flow cytometry to evaluate for malignant cells.
- Consider additional tests on BAL fluid, such as *Cryptococcus* antigen detection or CMV and other viral PCR. *Aspergillus* antigen detection or PCR and *Toxoplasma gondii* PCR are less well validated.
- Transbronchial biopsy (TBB) has similar sensitivity to BAL for the diagnosis of infection, but carries a risk of bleeding and pneumothorax, which can be serious complications in this patient group. TBB is not usually performed at initial bronchoscopy, although it may be considered, e.g., if lymphangitis is suspected. TBB in combination with BAL has a higher diagnostic yield of up to 70%.
- Protected specimen brush has no role in this patient population.

Other tests

- *Serum tests*: CMV antigenemia or PCR, HHV-6 PCR, *Aspergillus* galactomannan antigen or PCR, cryptococcal antigen (also on cerebrospinal fluid). Other viral PCR
- *Urine tests*: *Histoplasma* antigen, *Legionella* antigen
- Nasal washes or swabs for viral antigen or PCR
- Serologies are often not useful, given the difficulty of obtaining timely results.

Lung biopsy

Consider as a second-line investigation if BAL is nondiagnostic. Options include the following:

- **Repeat bronchoscopy with transbronchial lung biopsy** is useful in the diagnosis of malignancy, mycobacteria, fungi, organizing pneumonia, and drug-induced lung disease.

VATS or open lung biopsy has a greater diagnostic yield than that of TBB, although it is unclear if this can be directly translated into an improved survival. Either technique results in change to treatment in <50% of patients, and complications may be serious.

- **Percutaneous image-guided fine-needle aspiration or biopsy** for evaluation of peripheral nodules

Causes

Infectious causes

Infection accounts for >50%–75% of cases. The nature of immunological defect may provide clues to the likely infectious agent (see Table 9.1). For example, neutropenia is the most common risk factor, and these patients are more susceptible to enteric or pyogenic bacteria as well as fungi. However, considerable overlap exists, and this should serve only as a guide. The pattern of infection will be further modified by prophylactic treatment, e.g., CMV and PCP prophylaxis post-transplantation.

- Bacteria (incidence 37%)
  - Gram positives: *Staphylococcus aureus* and *epidermidis*, *Streptococcus pyognes* and *pneumoniae*, *Enterococcus faecalis*
  - Gram negatives: *Pseudomonas aerugenosa*, *Klebsiella pneumoniae*, *Escherichia coli*, and *Legionella*

Patients with T-cell defects (e.g., Hodgkin lymphoma) are more susceptible to intracellular organisms such as *Listeria* and *Salmonella*. Splenectomy patients are susceptible to encapsulated organisms such as *S. pneumoniae*, *H. influenzae*, and *N. meningitides*.

- Fungi (14%): *Aspergillus* (most common fungal infection, which occurs in 1% to >10% of transplant patients; can be angioinvasive in neutropenic patients), *Mucormycosis*, *Candida*
- Viruses (15%): CMV, VZV, herpes simplex virus (HSV) 1 and 2, Epstein–Barr virus (EBV), HHV 6, RSV, parainfluenza, influenza
- *P jirovecii* (8%)increased risk in patients on steroids dose as low as 15–20 mg/day for >3 weeks.
- *Nocardia* (7%)
- Mycobacteria (*Mycobacterium tuberculosis* and nontuberculous mycobacteria) (1%)
- Mixed infections (20%), especially in bone marrow transplant (BMT) and neutropenic patients

Hospital-acquired infections are most commonly *Staphylococcus aureus* (including MRSA), *Pseudomonas aeruginosa*, and other gram-negative bacteria. Fungi such as *Aspergillus and Candida* are particularly associated with hospital-acquired infection.

Noninfectious causes

Noninfection accounts for <25% of cases. Patients often present with clinical and radiological features similar to those of infection, and signs such as fever do not reliably differentiate between them. Causes include:

- **Pulmonary edema or pleural effusions**, particularly following renal or bone marrow transplant
- **ARDS**, e.g., secondary to sepsis or drugs (e.g., cytarabine, gemcitabine) or "engraftment syndrome" following bone marrow transplantation
- **Drug-induced disease** (allergy or toxicity) causes include all-*trans* retinoic acid (ATRA), antithymocyte globulin, azathioprine, bleomycin, busulfan, carmustine, chlorambucil, cyclophosphamide, cytosine arabinoside, dactinomycin, doxorubicin, fludarabine, gemcitibine, hydroxyurea,

interleukin-2, liposomal amphotericin B, lomustine, melphalan, mitomycin, methotrexate, procarbazine, sirolimus, taxanes, vinca alkaloids.

- *Respiratory involvement from the underlying disease*, e.g., lymphoma, leukemic infiltration or leukostasis, lymphangitis carcinomatosis, connective tissue disease
- *Diffuse alveolar hemorrhage (DAH)* is a relatively common complication of leukemia, bone marrow transplantation (rare in solid organ transplant), and thrombocytopenia. Hemoptysis is often absent, and there are diverse CXR appearances. Underlying infection is common.
- *Pulmonary embolism* is often complicated by secondary infection or with pulmonary infarct. Clinical and radiological features may be confused with invasive aspergillosis.
- *Radiation-induced pulmonary disease* includes pneumonitis, pneumothorax, effusion, airway obstruction, and COP.
- *Idiopathic pneumonia syndrome'*following bone marrow transplantation (breathlessness with hypoxia and diffuse CXR infiltrate, diagnosis of exclusion; high mortality)
- *Chronic graft-versus-host disease (GVHD)* following allogeneic bone marrow transplantation (dry cough, obstructive lung disease, rarely necrotizing bronchiolitis obliterans)
- *Post-transplant lymphoproliferative disease*
- *Secondary pulmonary alveolar proteinosis* (p. 606)
- *Transfusion-related acute lung injury (TRALI)*
- *Interstitial pneumonia (COP, diffuse alveolar damage [DAD], UIP)*
- *Hypersensitivity pneumonitis*
- *Pneumothorax/hemothorax* typically due to central-line complications
- *Mucositis* leading to upper airways obstruction.

Multiple disease processes

About a third of patients are thought to have two or more disease processes accounting for their respiratory involvement. Coinfection with multiple pathogens is common, and secondary infection with a different infectious agent (commonly *Aspergillus* or gram-negative bacteria such as *Pseudomonas*) may complicate either a primary respiratory infection or a noninfectious process such as pulmonary embolism.

Secondary infection is associated with a poor prognosis. It should be considered particularly in patients who deteriorate after an initial response to treatment and in patients who are neutropenic.

Onset of disease

The onset of disease may also suggest possible causes:
- *Acute onset* (<24 hours): Bacterial pneumonia, viral pneumonitis (e.g., CMV), pulmonary edema or hemorrhage, pulmonary emboli, ARDS
- *Subacute onset* (days): Fungi (e.g., *Aspergillus*), PCP, bacteria (e.g., *Nocardia*, *Legionella*), viral (e.g., CMV), drug-induced pneumonitis, TRALI and hemorrhage secondary to thrombocytopenia or DAH.
- *Chronic onset* (weeks): Malignancy, mycobacteria, fungi, PCP, CMV pneumonitis, *Nocardia*, drug toxicity, idiopathic pneumonia syndrome, GVHD, rejection, broncheolitis obliterans organizing pneumonia (BOOP)

Table 9.1 Infectious causes of pulmonary infiltrates based on underlying immunological defect and clinical condition

Clinical conditions	Immunological defect	Infectious agent
Leukemia Cytotoxic treatment Aplastic anemiaRare genetic conditions	Neutropenia or impaired neutrophil function	Bacteria (*Pseudomonas aeruginosa, Staphylococcus aureus, Escherichia coli, Klebsiella, Haemophilus influenzae, Nocardia*) Fungi (*Aspergillus*, p. 286; *Candida*, mucormycosis)
Post-transplantation Cytotoxic treatment High-dose steroids Lymphoma AIDS (p. 84) Renal impairment Rare genetic conditions	Impaired T-lymphocyte function	Fungi (PCP, *Cryptococcus neoformans, Candida, Histoplasma, Coccidioides, Blastomyces*)—pp. 285–310 Viruses (cytomegalovirus, herpes simplex, varicella zoster)—pp. 256–60 Bacteria (mycobacteria, *Listeria, Legionella, Nocardia*) Parasites (*Toxoplasma gondii*)
Myeloma Acute and chronic lymphocytic leukemia Lymphoma Common variable immunodeficiency Rare genetic conditions	Hypogammaglobulinaemia or impaired B-lymphocyte function	Encapsulated bacteria (*Streptococcus pneumoniae, Haemophilus influenzae*)
Genetic conditions (e.g., complement component deficiency, mannose-binding lectin deficiency)	Impaired complement activation	*Streptococcus pneumoniae*

Treatment

Antimicrobials

In general, neutropenic patients with fever or pulmonary infiltrates are at significant risk of developing overwhelming sepsis, and should receive prompt antibiotic cover, irrespective of the CXR appearance. In non-neutropenic patients, depending on the clinical circumstances, it is often possible to withhold treatment until definitive investigations have taken place.

Empirical treatment with broad-spectrum antibiotics should be chosen based on clinical presentation, the nature of immunological defect, prior infections, recent antibiotic use, epidemiological prevalence, and hospital antibiotic resistance patterns.

- In general, most neutropenic patients are treated with broad-spectrum antibiotics providing both gram-positive and gram-negative cover and MRSA, e.g., vancomycin/linezolid + β-lactam (antipseudomonal penicillin, cefepime, ceftazidime, or carbepenem) ± an aminoglycoside.
- Antifungal therapy can be considered when there is no significant improvement or if the patient deteriorates. Voriconazole and caspo-fungin are effective antifungal agents. Amphotericin B 1–1.5 mg/kg/day or liposomal amphotericin B 3–5 mg/kg/day should be initiated if *Aspergillus* is suspected.
- Treatment for CMV and PCP is associated with significant side effects, and ideally should be based on a definitive diagnosis or a high index of suspicion. BAL *Pneumocystis jirovecii* stains remain positive for up to 2 weeks of therapy.
- Antituberculous treatment should only rarely be administered in the absence of a microbiological diagnosis.
- Antiviral agents are initiated once a diagnosis has been established.

Diuretics

Fluid overload and pulmonary edema are common following renal and bone marrow transplantation, and typical clinical and radiological signs may be disguised; consider a trial of diuretics.

Steroids

Despite a lack of randomized, controlled trials, prednisone (1–2 mg/kg/day po, or up to 2 g methylprednisolone IV) is often considered in the treatment of drug- or radiation-induced lung disease, diffuse alveolar hemorrhage, and idiopathic pneumonia syndrome following bone marrow transplantation. Ideally, exclude underlying infection prior to starting steroids. Prednisone (40–80 mg daily po) is recommended for the treatment of PCP in patients with respiratory failure.

Supportive treatment

Administer oxygen to maintain saturations >87%. Respiratory failure in immunocompromised patients is associated with a poor outcome: mortality following intubation ranges from 60% to 100%. Early use of noninvasive ventilation (NIV) in immunocompromised patients with pulmonary infiltrates and hypoxia (defined as respiratory rate >30/min and PaO_2/FiO_2 ratio <200) has been shown to reduce the need for intubation and improve mortality. Before NIV is commenced, a decision regarding suitability for intubation and mechanical ventilation should be made.

Surgery

Surgical wedge resection or lobectomy may be considered in the treatment of invasive aspergillosis, either acutely for lesions adjacent to pulmonary vessels that are judged to have a significant risk of massive hemoptysis, or at a later date for residual lesions at risk of reactivation with further chemotherapy.

Prophylaxis

- Pneumococcal polysaccharide vaccine and annual influenza vaccine, especially in patients prior to splenectomy.
- CMV prophylaxis is indicated in allogeneic HSCT or in patients with solid organ transplant who are recipient negative and donor positive.
- Colony-stimulating factors when used empirically have not been show to reduce the morbidity and mortality of neutropenia-associated infections.

Further information

Hilbert G, Gruson D, Vargas F, et al. (2001). Non-invasive ventilation in immunosuppressed patients with pulmonary infiltrates, fever, and acute respiratory failure. *N Engl J Med* **344**:481–487.

Hughes WT, Armstrong D, Bodey GP, et al. (2002). 2002 guidelines for the use of antimicrobial agents in neutropenic patients with cancer. *Clinical infections diseases* **34**:730–751.

Jain P, Sandur S, Meil Y, et al. (2004). Role of flexible bronchoscopy in immunocompromised patients with lung infiltrates.*Chest.* **125**(2):712–722.

Raño A, Agustí C, Jimenez P, et al. (2001). Pulmonary infiltrates in non-HIV immunocompromised patients: a diagnostic approach using non-invasive and bronchoscopic procedures. *Thorax* **56**(5):379–387.

Shorr AF, Sulsa GM, O'Grady NP (2004). Pulmonary infiltrates in the non-HIV-infected immuno-compromised patient. *Chest* **125**:260–271.

Pulmonary infiltrates in the immunocompromised host (HIV)

Introduction

Widespread use of highly active antiretroviral therapy (HAART) and antimicrobial prophylaxis in HIV has resulted in a longer survival as well as a change in the epidemiology of infectious complications. Despite this, respiratory complaints remain a common manifestation of HIV.

Their etiology can be elucidated by considering the presentation of the patient, knowing the epidemiology of the various pulmonary diseases, interpreting common tests, and ordering further investigations when appropriate. It is important to remember that patients can have multiple etiologies of their respiratory complaints.

Causes of respiratory disease in the HIV-infected patient are listed on p. 84. Specific conditions are described separately. Steps in management are outlined below.

History
- As with other causes of immunocompromise, clinical features of respiratory disease in HIV-infected patients are nonspecific: breathlessness, cough, fever, weight loss, and fatigue are common, although chest symptoms are not always present.
- Ask about treatment and compliance with HAART and PCP prophylaxis as well as most recent CD4 count and viral load.
- The source of HIV infection may be relevant: Kaposi sarcoma occurs particularly in homosexual men and in African men and women; tuberculosis and bacterial pneumonia are more common in IV drug users.
- Detailed TB exposure history (if not in a country with high prevalence): incarceration, homelessness, IV drug abuse, health-care facilities, travel
- Travel history may be useful—infection with "endemic mycoses" (e.g., histoplasmosis, blastomycosis, coccidioidomycosis) is well recognized in parts of the United States.
- Subacute dyspnea and dry cough are more typical of *Pneumocystis* pneumonia while acute onset of productive cough and dyspnea are more typical of bacterial pneumonia.
- Subacute to chronic cough, fevers, night sweats, and weight loss are more typical of TB, a disseminated infection, or lymphoma.
- Headaches and meningismus would suggest cryptococcosis.
- Focal neurologic deficits may suggest toxoplasmosis.
- Chest X-ray findings without symptoms should be investigated thoroughly.

Physical examination
- Kaposi sarcoma is possible but unusual without skin manifestations.
- Palatal Kaposi sarcoma is particularly predictive of lung involvement.
- Decreased visual acuity may suggest cytomegalovirus.
- Lymphadenopathy may be from TB or lymphoma.
- Focal lung findings are suggestive of a bacterial pneumonia.
- Hepatomegaly or splenomegaly may be present in mycobacterial disease, fungal disease, or lymphoma..
- Patients with PCP will often have a normal examination.

Investigations

Labs

- CBC: WBC is often elevated in bacterial pneumonia; pancytopenia is seen in lymphoma or TB.
- LDH is nonspecific, but prognostic in PCP. It is also elevated in CMV.
- ABG helps to guide treatment (corticosteroids) in PCP based on PaO_2.
- Blood cultures may provide an etiology in bacterial pneumonia. They are also sensitive for disseminated *Mycobacterium avium* complex (MAC).
- CD4 count indicates risk of opportunistic infection (see By CD4 count, pp. 84–5)
- Sputum (may need induction, especially in PCP)
  - Always send for a bacterial Gram stain and culture
  - Sensitivity for PCP is around 80%, increased with direct fluorescent-antibody (DFA)
  - To look for TB, obtain 3 samples on 3 different days (induce only if otherwise unable to obtain)
    — Sensitivity of acid-fast staining is about 50%
    — Gold standard is culture
  - The finding of CMV or MAC in sputum is nonspecific
- DLCO is a sensitive test for PCP. If >75%, PCP is very unlikely.

CXR (findings in common infections)

- *Bacterial pneumonia* most commonly has segmental, lobar, or multi-lobar consolidation; diffuse reticulonodular pattern is less common. Cavitary lesions are rare and may suggest *Pseudomonas*.
- *TB:* With higher CD4 counts, upper-lobe cavitary lesions without lymphadenopathy; with lower CD4 counts, lower-lobe non-cavitary lesions with lymphadenopathy. CXR may be normal later in disease.
- *PCP:* bilateral symmetric perihilar reticular or granular opacities are the classical finding; may see pneumatoceles; may see pneumothorax. Many other findings are possible, but lymphadenopathy and pleural effusions suggest an alternative diagnosis.

Chest CT

- CXR may be normal in up to 17% of patients.
- If the patient is not critically ill, CXR is normal, and laboratory testing has not led to a diagnosis, a chest CT may suggest a diagnosis.
- A normal chest CT, CXR and laboratory testing make an infection unlikely.

Bronchoscopy and BAL

- Bronchoscopy and BAL are safe and frequently diagnostic in this patient group, and should be considered early in management, particularly in the presence of a diffuse CXR abnormality or following nondiagnostic induced sputum analysis. BAL should also be considered in patients with a localized CXR abnormality that has not responded to a trial of broad-spectrum antibiotics.
- BAL has higher sensitivity (98%) for PCP (with DFA) than induced sputum.
- BAL fluid analysis: routine microscopy and culture for bacteria; additional stains and culture for fungi, mycobacteria, *Nocardia*; silver or immunofluorescence stain for *Pneumocystis*; cytology, including flow cytometry for malignant cells; viral serology. Consider additional tests such as *Cryptococcus* antigen detection or CMV PCR.
- Both *Nocardia* and *Rhodococcus equi* stain weakly acid-fast, and may be confused with mycobacteria.
- Kaposi sarcoma appears as "raised bruises" in the trachea or bronchi on bronchoscopy. Routine biopsy is not recommended, as the diagnostic yield is low and significant hemorrhage may occur.

Lung biopsy

If bronchoscopy and BAL are nondiagnostic, consider repeat bronchoscopy with TBB or surgical lung biopsy. Additionally, if a prompt diagnosis of TB is necessary, TBB can be considered. Rarely, open lung biopsy may be required.

Treatment

- Treatment for bacterial pneumonia should be guided by local guidelines and antibiotic susceptibilities.
- Empiric coverage for *Pseudomonas* if CD4 <100, there is a history of bronchiectasis, or prior *Pseudomonas* infection.
- Four-drug therapy with isoniazid, rifampin, pyrazinamide, and ethambutol in patients with suspected tuberculosis.
- A macrolide can be added to the four-drug therapy used to treat tuberculosis if MAC is suspected.
- BAL *Pneumocystis* stains remain positive for up to 2 weeks despite treatment. Empirical treatment for PCP should not be delayed if the patient is unwell and this diagnosis is suspected.
- Treatment for CMV with gancyclovir can be considered if no other infectious etiologies are found, there are clear pulmonary symptoms, and CMV is clearly demonstrated in the lung. This may improve outcomes.
- Further antimicrobial treatment can be directed at specific pathogens isolated from BAL or biopsy.
- Provide supportive therapy with oxygen and noninvasive or mechanical ventilation if necessary.
- Steroids may be effective in the treatment of nonspecific interstitial pneumonitis and lymphocytic interstitial pneumonitis.

Causes of respiratory disease in HIV infection

Infectious

Bacteria
- *Streptococcus pneumoniae*
- *Haemophilus influenzae*
- *Staphylococcus aureus*
- Gram-negative bacteria
- *Nocardia*
- *Rhodococcus equi*

Mycobacteria
- *Mycobacterium tuberculosis*
- *Mycobacterium avium-intracellulare*
- *Mycobacterium kansasii*

Viruses
- Influenza
- Parainfluenza
- Respiratory syncitial virus (RSV)
- Herpes simplex
- Adenovirus
- Varicella

Fungi
- *Pneumocystis jiroveci*
- *Aspergillus*
- *Cryptococcus*
- Endemic mycoses

Parasites
- *Strongyloides stercoralis*
- *Toxoplasma gondii*

Noninfectious
- Kaposi sarcoma
- Lymphoma
- Drug-induced lung disease
- Nonspecific interstitial pneumonitis
- Lymphocytic interstitial pneumonitis
- Pulmonary edema
- Increased risk of lung cancer
- BOOP

By CD4 count

Any CD4 count
- Bacterial pneumonia: risk increases with lower CD4
- *Mycobacterium* tuberculosis

CD4 <200

- *Pneumocystis jiroveci*
- *Nocardia*
- *Cryptococcus neoformans*
- Endemic mycoses (often CD4 <50)
- Kaposi sarcoma
- Hodgkin or non-Hodgkin lymphoma

CD4 <50

- *Pseudomonas* more common
- *Mycobacterium avium-intracellulare*
- *Mycobacterium kansasii*
- CMV
- *Aspergillus*—usually with neutropenia or corticosteroids

The respiratory sleep patient

History

The problem

Sleep disorders are now a common reason for pulmonary consultation. This may be due in part to enhanced screening and recognition of these disorders. It may also reflect an increased incidence of these disorders related to the aging and increasing prevalence of obesity among the general population.

Although many pulmonologists care for patients with a variety of sleep disorders, such as restless legs syndromes, narcolepsy, and insomnia, evaluation for snoring and sleep-disordered breathing, particular obstructive sleep apnea (OSA), is more common. We will therefore concentrate on sleep-related breathing in this section.

History

A detailed clinical history is required. The clinician should review previous polysomnogram reports, if available, and inquire about previous diagnoses of sleep disorders, as well as their treatments and outcomes. Other medical problems that may be related to or are affected by OSA, such as systemic hypertension, acromegaly, hypothyroidism, cardiovascular disease, stroke, diabetes mellitus, epilepsy, COPD (i.e., "overlap syndrome") or nocturnal asthma, should be included in this assessment, since their presence may often guide treatment decisions.

Patients should be asked about daytime and nighttime symptoms (see below), sleep–wake patterns, and medication use. Nighttime symptoms may be reported by a bed partner.

A thorough review of family and social histories, particularly related to substance and alcohol use, should be included.

Inquire about the following presenting complaints of OSA:
- Daytime sleepiness—its duration, severity, and complications, especially related to work performance and its effect on driving. A subjective assessment using a standardized screening instrument, such as the Epworth Sleepiness Scale, is frequently useful (see Fig. 11.1). A score of ≥10 is suggestive of significant sleepiness. It is important to differentiate sleepiness from tiredness or fatigue
- Snoring—frequency and intensity, as well as change with weight loss or gain, alcohol intake, or sleep position
- Witnessed apneas, choking, or gasping occurring during sleep
- Other symptoms of OSA: morning headaches, nocturia, disrupted or restless sleep, sweating during sleep

The partial differential diagnosis of excessive sleepiness is listed in Box 11.1.

Box 11.1 Differential diagnosis of excessive sleepiness

- Sleep deprivation
- Inadequate sleep hygiene
- Obstructive sleep apnea
- Narcolepsy
- Idiopathic hypersomnia
- Recurrent hypersomnia
- Mood disorders
- Circadian rhythm sleep disorders
- Restless legs syndrome
- Periodic limb movement disorder
- Parasomnias
- Neurological disorders
- Substance abuse
- Medication and adverse effects of medications

Examination and investigations

Physical examination is not always predictive but should include an assessment of body habitus, facial anatomy (e.g., retrognathia), nasal and oropharyngeal airway, palatal length, dental occlusion and wear, neck circumference, and blood pressure. Other components related to cardiovascular and neurologic status should be included.

Related clinic tests are listed in Box 11.2.

> ### Box 11.2 Clinic tests to perform
>
> - Polysomnography is required for the diagnosis of OSA. Respiratory events associated with sleep apnea consist of obstructive apneas or hypopneas. This study may also demonstrate episodic oxygen desaturation, snoring, alterations in sleep architecture and sleep stages, cardiac rhythm abnormalities, and recurrent arousals.
> - An assessment of respiratory function including pulmonary function testing and arterial blood gas estimation may be necessary for those with other intrinsic lung disease.
> - Serum laboratory testing is usually not routinely indicated unless endocrinopathies, such as hypothyroidism, are suspected.

Treatment

Indications for specific treatments for OSA should be based on severity of the disorder, symptomatology, and comorbidities. Therapeutic options for OSA typically consist of continuous positive airway pressure (CPAP), mandibular advancement devices, and upper airway surgery. Although CPAP is generally regarded as the gold standard, its acceptance by patients is not universal. Education and the use of heated humidification may improve compliance. Mandibular advancement devices may be considered for patients with mild to moderate OSA who are unable to tolerate CPAP therapy.

Upper airway surgery may be indicated for patients with specific surgically correctable anatomic abnormalities. Patients whose OSA occurs exclusively or predominantly in the supine position may be advised to restrict sleep to a lateral or prone position.

Optimal weight management is important in those who are overweight, and may be particularly important in severely obese individuals.

Finally, patients should be counseled regarding the increased risk of vehicular accidents as well as cardiovascular and neurocognitive consequences of untreated OSA.

EPWORTH SLEEPINESS SCALE

Name:.................................Hospital number .... Date:.................

Your age (Yrs)...............Your sex (Male = M / Female = F)...............

- How likely are you to doze off or fall asleep in the situations described in the box below, in contrast to feeling just tired?
- This refers to your usual way of life in recent times.
- Even if you haven't done some of these things recently try to work out how they would have affected you.
- Use the following scale to choose the <u>most appropriate number</u> for each situation:-

0 = would <u>never</u> doze   2 = <u>Moderate</u> chance of dozing
1 = <u>Slight</u> chance of dozing   3 = <u>High</u> chance of dozing

Situation	Chance of dozing
Sitting and reading	☐
Watching TV	☐
Sitting, inactive in a public place (e.g. a theatre or a meeting)	☐
As a passenger in a car for an hour without a break	☐
Lying down to rest in the afternoon when circumstances permit	☐
Sitting and talking to someone	☐
Sitting quietly after a lunch without alcohol	☐
In a car, while stopped for a few minutes in the traffic	☐
Thank you for your cooperation Total score =	☐

Figure 11.1 Epworth Sleepiness Scale. Used with permission of American Academy of Sleep Medicine, from Johns MW. (1991). A new method for measuring daytime sleepiness: the Epworth Sleepiness Scale. *Sleep* **14**(6):540–545; permission conveyed through Copyright Clearance Center, Inc.

The breathless, pregnant patient

Causes

Normal physiological changes of pregnancy

Respiratory changes

Elevated serum progesterone stimulates respiratory drive. Tidal volume and resting minute ventilation increase, while respiratory rate is not changed. The subsequent fall in maternal PCO_2 (partial pressure of carbon dioxide) facilitates fetal CO_2 transfer across the placenta; any cause of maternal hypercapnia leads quickly to fetal respiratory acidosis.

The enlarging uterus pushes the diaphragm upward, reducing functional residual capacity by 20% by midterm. Bibasilar crackles are occasionally heard, due to compression of lower lung tissue. Diaphragm function, vital capacity, peak expiratory flow rate (PEFR), and FEV_1 (forced expiratory volume in 1 second) are not affected by pregnancy.

Cardiovascular changes

Blood volume increases 30%–50% by midterm. Cardiac output increases due to an increase in heart rate (by ~15 beats/minute) and stroke volume. Systemic vascular resistance falls. Blood pressure is reduced in the first and second trimesters by 10–20 mmHg, but is normal at term.

Peripheral pulses tend to be increased in volume. Dependent edema, a third heart sound, persistent splitting of the second heart sound, and systolic ejection murmurs are common. Continuous murmurs of cervical venous hum or mammary souffle may be heard.

Upper airway changes

Edema, hyperemia, and hypersecretion of the nasopharyngeal mucosa (with rhinitis), especially by the third trimester, may predispose to snoring, but frank obstructive sleep apnea is rare.

Hematological changes

Plasma volume increases more than red blood cell mass, resulting in a mild, dilutional anemia. Pregnancy is a hypercoagulable state.

Elevation of clotting factors and impaired fibrinolysis, combined with venous stasis, result in a 5-fold increased risk of venous thromboembolism. The risk is even higher in women with hereditary thrombophilias.

Causes of breathlessness in pregnancy

Causes are listed in Box 12.1. In general, breathlessness may be due to the following factors.

Normal physiological changes of pregnancy

Up to 75% of normal women experience some degree of breathlessness during pregnancy, perhaps from progesterone-induced hyperventilation. Normally, breathlessness occurs only with exertion and does not significantly impede daily activities. Tachypnea is a useful sign, as it is not normal in pregnancy and suggests an underlying disease process.

New disease process

Acute, severe, or progressive breathlessness should signal a new disease process. Pulmonary embolism is a major cause of maternal death. Other rare, but serious, causes are amniotic fluid embolism and ARDS.

Exacerbation of chronic respiratory or cardiac disease
Asthma is the most common. Unsuspected underlying cardiac or pulmonary disease may present for the first time in pregnancy, e.g., congenital heart disease, lymphangioleiomyomatosis.

Box 12.1 Causes of breathlessness in pregnancy

Pulmonary
- Exacerbation of preexisting lung disease, e.g., asthma (p. 134), cystic fibrosis, lymphangioleiomyomatosis
- Pneumonia
  - Bacterial: usual organisms (p. 208), including tuberculosis (p. 270) and aspiration (p. 230)
  - Viral: particularly varicella, influenza (pp. 250, 260)
  - Fungal: consider coccidioidomycosis (p. 308)
- Aspiration pneumonitis
- Pulmonary metastases from choriocarcinoma (very rare)

Pleural
- Pneumothorax (p. 316), particularly during labor
- Pleural effusion, e.g., parapneumonic, chylothorax in lymphangioleiomyomatosis, esophageal rupture
- Ovarian hyperstimulation syndrome (very rare)

Vascular
- Pulmonary embolism (p. 460)
- Amniotic fluid embolism (p. 462)
- Venous air embolism (p. 462)
- Pulmonary hypertension (p. 421)

Cardiogenic pulmonary edema
- Exacerbation of preexisting cardiac disease, e.g., mitral stenosis, atrial septal defect
- Cardiomyopathy, including peripartum cardiomyopathy
- Significant cardiac arrhythmia
- Ischemic heart disease (rare)
- Endocarditis
- Myocarditis

Non-cardiogenic pulmonary edema
- Iatrogenic fluid overload
- Tocolytic therapy (β-agonists used to inhibit preterm labor)
- ARDS due to preeclampsia, sepsis, multiple transfusions, amniotic fluid embolism, air embolism, gastric aspiration
- Renal failure

Other
- Anemia
- Hemidiaphragm rupture
- Pneumomediastinum
- Neuromuscular disease
- Sepsis

Investigations

Consult with OB-GYN, as well as pediatrics and anesthesia if delivery is approaching. If imaging involving ionizing radiation is needed, discuss with radiology how to best reduce radiation exposure. Management of specific conditions is discussed in the individual disease chapters in Part 2.

ABGs
Normal maternal PO_2 is >100 mmHg and PCO_2 is 25–32 mmHg.

A compensatory fall in serum bicarbonate (to 18–22 mmol/L) occurs, resulting in an average pH of 7.44. During the third trimester, perform ABGs in an upright position, as PO_2 may be 13 mmHg lower when supine. At term, mean A–a gradient increases to 14.3 mmHg while sitting and 20 mmHg while supine.

Blood tests
The "physiologic anemia of pregnancy" is reflected by a hematocrit of 33%–38%, with hemoglobin 11–12 g/100 mL. By the second or third trimester, total white blood cell count (WBC) is 9000–15,000 cells/μL, owing to an increase in blood neutrophils.

D-dimer is elevated in normal pregnancy and in the postpartum period, reaching a maximum of 685 ng/mL in one study. As in nonpregnant patients, an elevated D-dimer should be followed by further testing if pulmonary embolism is suspected.

CXR
CXR may show increased pulmonary vasculature because of the normal increase in blood volume. Small, asymptomatic pleural effusions are sometimes seen shortly after normal delivery. With proper abdominal shielding, radiation doses to mother and fetus are very small, and CXR should be performed when clinically necessary.

Spirometry and pulmonary function testing
This testing can be safely performed during pregnancy. Methacholine challenge is contraindicated in pregnancy.

ECG
Sinus tachycardia is common in the second half of pregnancy. Small T- and Q-wave inversions in lead III are common during the third trimester.

Echocardiogram
Small pericardial effusions, increased left atrial size, increased diastolic ventricular size, and tricuspid regurgitation are common late in pregnancy.

Venous ultrasound of the legs
When pulmonary embolism is suspected and the D-dimer is positive, detection of asymptomatic lower-extremity deep venous thrombosis by ultrasound may obviate the need for studies involving ionizing radiation. A negative venous ultrasound does not exclude pulmonary embolism, however, and further imaging is required.

Ventilation/perfusion (V/Q) scans

These scans are considered relatively safe in pregnancy and are considered by most experts to be the test of choice if pulmonary embolism is suspected. Radiation exposure may be decreased by reducing the dose of perfusion agent, or by eliminating ventilation images if perfusion images are normal.

CT pulmonary angiography

Angiography may be necessary in the evaluation for pulmonary embolism when the CXR is abnormal and/or the V/Q scan is nondiagnostic. Because of breast tissue changes during pregnancy, chest CT scanning increases the mother's risk of breast cancer. Although the estimated radiation dose to the fetus may be less than that with a V/Q scan, both mother and fetus are exposed to intravenous iodinated contrast.

Preoperative assessment of the pulmonary patient

Pulmonary physicians are often asked to assess patients prior to elective or emergency surgery, many of whom have known or occult preexisting respiratory disease. The preoperative pulmonary assessment should answer the following key questions:
- What is the patient's functional and pulmonary status?
- What is the patient's risk of postoperative complications?
- How may the patient's respiratory function be optimized, and the risk of pulmonary complications minimized?

Very often this assessment is characterized as "clearing" the patient for surgery. Don't be alarmed! The role of the pulmonary consultant is to *assess the risk of, and minimize the potential for, postoperative complications* such as pneumonia, prolonged mechanical ventilation, and COPD exacerbation.

Few pulmonary patients will have absolute contraindications to surgery. The decision of whether to perform surgery depends on the risk–benefit analysis, weighing the benefits of surgery against the risks of surgery. The decision to proceed to surgery is a collective one among the operating surgeon, anesthesiologist, other care providers, and the patient.

Assessing the preoperative patient

Patient-related risk factors
- General health and functional status (see Table 13.1 and Table 13.2)
  - Greater than ASA Class 2 = 2- to 3-fold ↑ risk of postoperative complication
- COPD doubles the risk of postoperative complications.
- Age: Older age may be associated with ↑ risk, but this is controversial.
- Obesity alone is not a risk factor, but may be associated with OSA.
- Asthma, unlike COPD, if well-controlled should not ↑ risk.
- Other: Cigarette smoking, impaired sensorium, recent weight loss, and history of stroke modestly ↑ risk.

Procedure-related risk factors
- The type of surgical procedure has more impact on risk assessment than patient-related factors, but generally cannot be modified.
- Higher risk for respiratory failure or pneumonia is seen with abdominal aortic aneurysm (AAA) repair, thoracic or upper abdominal surgery, emergent procedures, and prolonged procedures (>3 hours).

Preoperative testing
- Spirometry is indicated in patients undergoing lung resection to predict candidacy for surgery and postoperative FEV_1.
- CXR is indicated if patient age is ≥65, or if acute chest symptoms are present.
- Oxygen assessment should be performed at rest *and* with exertion.
- ABG, if history or risk factors for CO_2 retention
- ECG ± echocardiogram if cardiac disease known or suspected

Preoperative management of the pulmonary patient

- COPD/asthma
  - Inhaled β-agonist bronchodilators prn
  - Symptomatic COPD should receive inhaled anticholinergics
  - Inhaled steroids or oral steroids if not optimized
  - Do not initiate, but permissible to continue theophylline; check levels
  - Defer elective surgery if active exacerbation
- If evidence of infection, preoperative course of antibiotics
- Optimize volume status
- Optimize nutritional status
- CPAP for OSA
- Quitting tobacco use 8 weeks prior to surgery is optimal. If the patient quit or reduced use <8 weeks earlier, this may increase the risk for complications.
- Postoperative planning
  - Chest physiotherapy, breathing exercises, incentive spirometry
  - Pulmonary rehabilitation

Table 13.1 ASA classification for surgical candidates

Class 1	Normal healthy patient
Class 2	Mild systemic disease
Class 3	Severe systemic disease
Class 4	Severe systemic disease that is a constant threat to life
Class 5	Moribund, not expected to survive without operation

ASA = American Society of Anesthesiologists

Table 13.2 Risk index for postoperative respiratory failure

Preoperative variables	Points
Abdominal aortic aneurysm (AAA)	27
Thoracic surgery	21
Neurosurgical, upper abdomen, or vascular surgery	14
Neck surgery	11
Emergency surgery	11
Albumin <3 g/dL	9
Blood urea nitrogen >30 mg/dL	8
Functional dependency	7
History of COPD	6
Age ≥70	6
Age 60–69	4
Risk class	**Risk for respiratory failure**
Class 1 (≤10 points)	0.5%
Class 2 (11–19 points)	2.1%
Class 3 (20–27 points)	5.3%
Class 4 (28–40 points)	11.9%
Class 5 (>40 points)	30.9%

Adapted from Arozullah AM, Daley J, Henderson WG, Khuri SF (2000). Multifactorial risk index for predicting postoperative respiratory failure in men after major noncardiac surgery. *Ann Surg* **232**:242–253.

Further reading

Arozullah AM, Daley J, Henderson WG, et al. (2000). Multifactorial risk index for predicting postoperative respiratory failure in men after major noncardiac surgery. *Ann Surg* **232**:242–253.

Arozullah AM, Conde MV, Lawrence VA (2003). Preoperative evaluation for postoperative pulmonary complications. *Med Clin North Am* **87**:153–173.

Smetana GW (2006). Preoperative pulmonary evaluation: Identifying and reducing risks for pulmonary complications. *Cleve Clin J Med* **73**(1):s36–s41.

Postoperative breathlessness

The pulmonary physician is often asked to see patients postoperatively who have become dyspneic following an operative procedure. The incidence of postoperative pulmonary complications can range from 5% to 80% depending on the type of procedure performed. The risk of pulmonary complications is greatest with thoracic or upper abdominal surgery (see p. 102). Common causes of postoperative breathlessness are listed in Box 14.1.

> **Box 14.1 Causes of postoperative breathlessness**
>
> - Infection: bronchitis and pneumonia
> - Atelectasis
> - Pulmonary emboli
> - Left ventricular failure (fluid overload)
> - Aspiration
> - Exacerbation of underlying lung disease, such as COPD or IPF
> - Acute lung injury (ALI) or ARDS
>
> *Remember to always rule out upper airway obstruction.*

Points to consider when assessing these patients

- Is the patient acutely ill, needing immediate resuscitation and/or ventilatory support?
- Comorbid diseases, especially pulmonary, cardiac, or thromboembolic disease (or risk factors thereof)
- Type of surgery
- Amount of fluid and blood products the patient received
- Time since surgery
  - *Early complications (hours)* Differential diagnosis includes residual anesthetic effect not adequately reversed, laryngospasm, post-extubation pulmonary edema, infection, aspiration, pulmonary embolism (PE), fat embolism, air embolism, atelectasis, hypovolemic shock due to blood loss, drug-induced lung disease, transfusion-related acute lung injury (TRALI), left ventricular failure and fluid overload, and myocardial ischemia (MI)
  - *Later complications (hours–days)* Differential diagnosis includes PE, adult respiratory distress syndrome (ARDS), infection, atelectasis, and MI.

Initial tests to consider (see Table 14.1)

- Review the chart for preoperative vital signs, oximetry, and spirometry.
- Review the intraoperative record, which will include medications, fluids, and blood products given, vital signs, and oxygen saturations
- Oxygen saturations on room air and on oxygen
- ABG on room air
- ECG
- CXR—compare to preoperative CXR (if available)
- Complete blood count and clotting screen
- A D-dimer level is usually unhelpful, as it will be raised by many different intra- and postoperative mechanisms.

Table 14.1 Causes and management of dyspnea

Possible cause of dyspnea	Management options
Atelectasis (more common in smokers and following abdominal or transthoracic procedures)	Encourage expectoration (requires adequate analgesia), chest physiotherapy, deep breathing, and early mobilization
Pneumonia—also consider aspiration pneumonitis/pneumonia	If fever and infiltrate, cover with antibiotics for hospital-acquired pneumonia (see p. 226)
Thromboembolic disease	Oxygen as required. Start treatment dose of unfractionated heparin (if not contraindicated), check D-dimer (only helpful if negative), image pulmonary vasculature with VQ scan or CTPA, and/or image lower extremities with ultrasound. Consider IVC filter if heparin contraindicated (see p. 457)
Hypoventilation	Opiate overdose or anesthetic agents causing neuromuscular block not reversed
Metabolic acidosis	Check chemistries to look for underlying problem such as renal failure or sepsis
Myocardial ischemia	Oxygen, troponins, ECG, place on telemetry monitor. Start aspirin and beta-blocker. Give nitrates and morphine for pain. Consider heparin if not contraindicated
Myocardial infarction	Aspirin, beta-blocker, and referral for primary angioplasty
Cardiac failure/fluid overload	Oxygen, diuresis, and assessment of left ventricle (echocardiogram)
ARDS	Supportive care and lung-protective strategy with mechanical ventilation (see p. 588)
TRALI—history of transfusion of any blood product	CXR, oxygen, diuresis, supportive care, and mechanical ventilation if necessary
Phrenic nerve damage causing diaphragmatic paralysis. May occur with thoracic operations such as CABG	Diagnosed on fluoroscopy. Elevate head of bed for mechanical advantage when sleeping. Phrenic nerves may recover but can take 2+ years.
Fat embolism following long bone fracture, especially with manipulation	Oxygen, IV fluids, supportive care
Laryngeal spasm	Oxygen, heliox. May require reintubation
Negative pressure pulmonary edema (NPPE). Breathing against a closed glottis causes negative intrathoracic pressure.	Treat with diuretics, oxygen, noninvasive or mechanical ventilation
Myasthenia gravis crisis precipitated by anesthetic agents	May need intubation and ventilation. Stop all anticholinesterases. Consider plasma exchange and IV immunoglobulin. Urgent neurology input

Part II

Clinical conditions

Asthma

Definition, epidemiology, pathophysiology, etiology

Asthma is a chronic inflammatory disorder of the airways that is clinically characterized by recurrent episodes of respiratory symptoms including wheezing, cough, dyspnea, and chest tightness. These episodes are associated with and the result of variable airflow obstruction that is reversible either spontaneously or with therapy.

Causes of airflow obstruction

- *Bronchoconstriction*, in which bronchial smooth muscle rapidly contracts and narrows the airways. This can result from varied stimuli, including inhaled allergens and irritants.
- *Airway hyperresponsiveness*, in which the airways show an exaggerated narrowing response to irritating stimuli
- *Airway edema*, with inflammatory cell infiltration, extracellular fluid accumulation, and mucus hypersecretion
- *Airway remodeling*, with smooth muscle hypertrophy and hyperplasia, basement membrane thickening, collagen deposition, and epithelial desquamation. This occurs in chronic disease and may be irreversible.

Epidemiology

Asthma is the most common chronic lung disease worldwide, with an estimated 300 million affected individuals. The World Health Organization (WHO) has estimated that 15 million disability-adjusted life years are lost annually because of asthma, representing 1% of the total global disease burden.

There is a wide variation in disease prevalence, with highest levels seen in English-speaking countries (where there is also a high prevalence of sensitization to common aeroallergens). Best estimates suggest that the global prevalence of asthma ranges from 1% to 18% of the population in different countries, and has increased over the last few decades. The reason for the increasing worldwide prevalence remains unclear.

Pathophysiology

The clinical symptoms and physiological changes seen in asthma are a result of *airway narrowing*, with the pathological changes that lead to airway narrowing best described as either primary or secondary effects of *inflammation*.

A variety of cells play a role in this inflammatory response, including epithelial cells, eosinophils, mast cells, neutrophils, lymphocytes (both natural killer T cells and T helper 2 [Th2] lymphocytes), and macrophages. Multiple inflammatory cellular mediators are involved and mediate the complex inflammatory response in the airways; these include chemokines, leukotrienes, cytokines, histamines, nitric oxide (NO), and prostaglandin D2. Eosinophils appear to play a prominent role and are often present in increased numbers and release mediators that damage airway epithelial cells.

The inflammatory changes affect all airways, but are most pronounced in medium-sized bronchi. The airway inflammation is persistent even though symptoms are episodic. The relationship between the severity of asthma and the intensity of inflammation is not clearly established.

Etiology

The precise etiology of asthma remains unclear, but it is thought to be due to a combination of host factors and environmental exposures.

Genetic factors

The hereditary basis of asthma and atopy is well established. A number of chromosomes, genome-wide association studies, and linkage analyses have implicated in particular chromosomes 5, 13, and 14. However, given the multiple mechanisms and secondary messengers involved in asthma, the contribution of effects of specific genes is difficult to determine.

There is evidence that a functional single nucleotide polymorphism in the gene encoding CD14 may modify an individual's predisposition to developing allergic responses, depending on the level of environmental endotoxin exposure, and thus possibly alter susceptibility to asthma.

Environmental factors

Two major factors are considered most important in the development, persistence, and, potentially, the severity of asthma: inhaled allergens and viral respiratory infections. Additional environmental factors being studied include tobacco smoke, air pollution, and diet. The increasing prevalence of asthma appears to be associated with a rising standard of living worldwide, and not just in westernized societies.

Immunological mechanisms

Both the innate and adaptive immune systems have been implicated. A subgroup of asthmatics is atopic and therefore reacts to antigen challenge by producing specific IgE from B lymphocytes. This results in the formation of IgE–antigen complexes that bind to mast cells, basophils, and macrophages, leading to the release of preformed mediators such as histamine, and eosinophil chemotactic factor. These factors cause bronchoconstriction and airway edema.

Prostaglandins, leukotrienes, kinins, and platelet activating factor (PAF) are all important secondary messengers involved in the inflammatory response. The *hygiene hypothesis* suggests that early life exposure to allergens switches off the allergic response (by reducing Th2-mediated responses), leading to reduced allergen sensitivity later in life, therefore reducing allergen-driven diseases such as asthma. Large epidemiological studies support this hypothesis.

Obesity

Obesity has been shown to be a risk factor for asthma. Certain mediators, such as leptin, may affect airway function and increase the likelihood of asthma development.

Further information

Eder W, Ege MG, von Multius E (2006). The asthma epidemic. *N Engl J Med* **355**(21):2226–2235.

Global Initiative for Asthma: http://www.ginasthma.com.

National Asthma Education and Prevention Program Expert Panel Report 3. Guidelines for the Diagnosis and Management of Asthma. National Institutes of Health, 2007.

Diagnosis

This is usually a clinical diagnosis. Symptoms of recurrent episodes of airflow obstruction or airway hyperresponsiveness are present; airflow obstruction is at least partially reversible; and alternative diagnoses are excluded. Specific symptoms, their pattern, and precipitating and aggravating factors should be determined.

Symptoms and history (see Box 15.1, Box 15.2)
- Wheezing, particularly recurrent wheezing
- Cough
- Shortness of breath
- Chest tightness

Classically these are episodic, variable, worse at night, associated with both specific (e.g., tree and grass pollen, cat and dog dander) and non-specific triggers (e.g., cold air exposure, perfumes, bleaches, and other irritants), as well as exercise, viral infection, emotional responses, changes in weather, stress, and menstrual cycles.

Medical history
- Specific precipitating and aggravating factors (including aspirin sensitivity, see Box 15.3; psychosocial stressors; and exposures)
- Details of disease development and evolution, including history of exacerbations (prodromal signs and symptoms, rapidity of onset, duration, frequency, severity (urgent or emergent medical care, hospitalization, ICU admission, intubation), and previous beneficial treatment
- Family and social history and any occupational exposures (e.g., flour, soybean dust, latex, wood dust, diisocyanates)
- Impact on patient and their perception of disease

Don't forget to look for
- Concurrent sinusitis, rhinitis, nasal polyps
- Atopic dermatitis, eczema, hay fever
- Allergies (including food allergy)
- Gastroesophageal reflux disease (GERD)

Examination
- May be entirely normal
- Classically, expiratory wheeze is heard
- Chest deformity or hyperinflation (longstanding or poorly controlled disease)
- Severe, life-threatening acute asthma may have no wheeze and a silent chest on auscultation.

For the differential diagnosis for asthma see Box 15.4.

Box 15.1 Consider the diagnosis of asthma with the following:

- Episodic wheeze cough, and breathlessness
- Chest tightness
- Isolated or nocturnal cough
- Exercised-induced cough or breathlessness
- Hyperventilation syndrome (p. 600)

Box 15.2 Diagnostic questions to ask for asthma

- Has the patient had recurrent attacks of wheezing?
- Does the patient cough at night?
- Does the patient wheeze or cough after exercise?
- Does the patient experience wheezing, chest tightness, or cough after exposure to airborne allergens or pollutants?
- Do the patient's colds "go to the chest" or take more than 10 days to clear up?
- Are symptoms improved by appropriate asthma treatment (e.g., inhaled bronchodilators)?

Box 15.3 Aspirin-induced asthma (AIA)

- Defined as chronic rhinoconjunctivitis, nasal polyps, and asthma
- Asthma is precipitated by ingestion of aspirin or other nonsteroidal anti-inflammatory drugs (NSAIDs), with the onset of symptoms 0.5–3 hours after drug ingestion
- Occurs in up to 20% of asthmatics, and is more common in women
- The mechanism is thought to be via aspirin inhibition of the cyclooxygenase pathway, with excess leukotriene production via the lipooxygenase pathway
- BAL and urine in AIA patients show excess leukotrienes after aspirin exposure
- Loss of anti-inflammatory prostaglandin E2 may also be important

Box 15.4 Differential diagnosis for asthma in adults

- Chronic obstructive lung disease (COPD)
- Mechanical obstruction of the airway (e.g., neoplasm, foreign body)
- Congestive heart failure
- Pulmonary embolism (PE)
- Cough secondary to medications
- Vocal cord dysfunction (can be seen with asthma)
- Recurrent aspiration
- Bronchiectasis
- Bronchiolitis

Investigations

A correct diagnosis of asthma is essential if appropriate drug therapy is to be given. The number of investigations required depends on the certainty of the diagnosis from the history and spirometry. Further measurement of lung function, including testing for reversibility of airflow obstruction, may be necessary to enhance diagnostic certainty.

Spirometry is preferred to peak flow measurements because of the wide variability in peak flow meters and reference values. Peak flow meters are designed for monitoring, not as diagnostic tools.

Spirometry

Simple spirometry is used to look for airflow obstruction and reversibility in response to treatment. Airway obstruction decreases peak expiratory flow rate (PEFR) and forced expiratory volume in 1 second (FEV_1), but these may be normal between episodes of bronchospasm. Evidence of a fall in FEV_1 after exercise, or improvement in FEV_1 after the use of an inhaled bronchodilator (>12% and 200 mL) supports the diagnosis. If spirometry is consistently normal, the diagnosis should be questioned.

Additional investigations

- *CXR* if atypical symptoms; may show hyperinflation and airway wall thickening. Rarely, CXR can show evidence of a localized abnormality simulating wheezing (e.g., adenoma).

Blood tests

- *CBC with differential:* If eosinophilia is present (>1500 cells/μL), consider Churg–Strauss syndrome and/or another eosinophilic syndrome.
- *IgE:* Measurement of specific IgE in serum suggests associated allergic disease; however, measurement of total IgE has no value as a diagnostic test for atopy.
- *Aspergillus precipitins* (*Aspergillus* sensitivity, allergic bronchopulmonary aspergillosis [ABPA], see Chapter 22)
- *Skin tests* to define atopy and/or identify potential triggers
- *Metacholine/histamine challenge:* Measurements of airway responsiveness reflect the "sensitivity" of the airways; measures bronchial hyperresponsiveness (BHR) as a PC_{20} (the dose of agent provoking a 20% fall in FEV_1). Asthma is indicated by a PC_{20} below 8 mg/mL; normal subjects have a PC_{20} >16 mg/mL. The absence of BHR argues against the diagnosis of asthma (it is sensitive, but has limited specificity).
- *Specific bronchial provocation tests* aim to demonstrate bronchospasm to an inhaled agent, usually related to an occupation (e.g., flour in a baker). The response to an aerosolized sample of a suspected agent may be useful if the diagnosis of occupational asthma is suspected, but PEFR recordings at home, work, and on vacation may be more useful. This should only be carried out in a tertiary referral center, under expert supervision.

Noninvasive markers of airway inflammation

- *Sputum analysis:* Sputum eosinophilia may help confirm the diagnosis.
- *Exhaled nitric oxide (FeNO):* Levels of FeNO are elevated in people with asthma (who are not taking inhaled glucocorticosteroids) compared to those in people without asthma. These findings are not specific for asthma; they may be more useful in longitudinal measurements in response to treatment.
- *Laryngoscopy and ear, nose, throat (ENT) examination* are useful if there are concerns about nasal symptoms or obstruction (e.g., from polyps), or to exclude upper airway obstruction or a vocal cord abnormality.
- *Bronchoscopy* is occasionally needed; its main use is to exclude an obstructing airway tumor (e.g., carcinoid).
- *Lung biopsy* may be needed in those without an adequate explanation for persistent and minimally reversible airflow obstruction to exclude another cause (e.g., bronchiolitis obliterans).

Asthma exacerbations

Asthma exacerbations are acute or subacute episodes of progressively worsening symptoms of wheezing, cough, dyspnea, and chest tightness. These may occur individually or in combination. Exacerbations are the result of progressive airflow obstruction; objective measures of lung function (spirometry or PEFR) are more reliable indicators of the severity of the exacerbation than are symptoms.

While asthmatics that are well controlled with inhaled corticosteroids (ICS) have a decreased risk of exacerbations, they are still vulnerable. Effective management of exacerbations requires assessment of severity, close monitoring, medications, environmental control, and patient education.

Assessment of severity

Never underestimate the severity of an exacerbation. Severe exacerbations can be life threatening and occur in patients with any level of baseline asthma severity—i.e., intermittent, or mild, moderate, or severe persistent asthma. The exacerbation should be classified as mild, moderate, severe, or life threatening (see Table 15.1).

Table 15.1 Severity classification of asthma exacerbation

	Symptoms	Initial FEV$_1$ or PEF	Clinical course
Mild	Dyspnea with activity	PEFR ≥70% of predicted or personal best	Usually cared for at home Prompt relief with SABA Possible short course of oral systemic steroids
Moderate	Dyspnea limits usual activilty	PEFR 40%–69% of predicted or personal best	Usually requires office or ER visit Symptom relief with frequent SABA use Oral systemic steroids, symptoms may last for 1–2 days after therapy begun
Severe	Dyspnea at rest and with conversation	PEFR <40% of predicted or personal best	Usually requires ER visit and hospitalization Partial symptom relief with frequent SABA Oral systemic steroids, symptoms last for >3 days after therapy begun Adjunctive therapies
Life threatening	Too dyspneic to speak	PEFR <25% of predicted or personal best	Requires ER visit and hospitalization, possible ICU Minimal relief from frequent SABA Intravenous steroids Adjunctive therapies

ER, emergency room; SABA, short-acting β$_2$-agonist

Adapted from National Asthma Education and Prevention Program Expert Panel Report 3. Guidelines for the Diagnosis and Management of Asthma 2007.

Acute severe or life-threatening asthma

Asthma still accounts for over 4000 deaths in the United States annually. In 2002, the age-adjusted death rate associated with asthma was 1.5 per 100,000. Risk factors for fatal or near-fatal asthma are listed in Box 15.5.

Most asthma deaths occur outside hospital and are
- In patients with chronic severe disease
- In those receiving inadequate medical treatment
- In those who have been symptomatically deteriorating and may have already sought medical help
- Associated with adverse behavioral and psychosocial factors

The defining element of a near-fatal asthma attack is evidence of *hypercapnic respiratory failure* (see also Box 15.6).

Box 15.5 Risk factors for fatal or near-fatal asthma
- Previous severe exacerbation (e.g., ICU admission, intubation)
- Two or more hospitalizations or >3 ER visits in the past year
- Use of >2 canisters of SABA per month
- Limited perception of airway obstruction or severity of worsening
- Low socioeconomic status or inner-city residence
- Illicit drug use
- Major psychological or psychiatric disease
- Comorbidities (e.g., cardiovascular disease or other chronic lung disease)

Box 15.6 Recognition of near-fatal asthma

Potentially life-threatening features
- Too dyspneic to speak
- Full upright posture
- Diaphoresis
- Sternocleidomastoid retraction
- Respiratory rate >25 breaths/min
- Heart rate persistently >110 beats/min
- PEF <25% of predicted or personal best
- Pulsus paradoxus >10 mmHg

Imminently life-threatening features
- Silent chest on auscultation
- Cyanosis
- Bradycardia
- Exhaustion or severe diaphoresis
- Confusion or loss of consciousness

Patient groups at high risk for life-threatening asthma

- *Underperceivers:* This group of asthmatics does not sense worsening airflow limitation. These patients require ongoing monitoring with peak expiratory flow (PEF).
- *Brittle asthmatic* is characterized by tremendous variability in PEF
  - *Type 1:* Wide PEF variability (>40% diurnal variability that occurs >50% of the time over a period exceeding 150 days despite appropriate therapy)
  - *Type 2:* Sudden severe attacks on background of apparently good control (stable baseline peak flows); associated with a high incidence of food allergies and aspirin sensitivity. The patient should perform PEF monitoring twice daily.
- *Morning dippers:* There appears to be a group of asthmatics who are prone to life-threatening bronchospasm early in the morning. Episodes correlate with excessive diurnal variation in PEF (>50%). These individuals may benefit from transfer to a higher level of care to prevent a fatal event.
- *Aspirin sensitive:* Asthmatics with aspirin sensitivity are at increased risk for severe, acute, and potentially fatal episodes. These patients are also cross-sensitive to NSAIDs.

Further information

American Thoracic Society (2000). Proceedings of the ATS Workshop on Refractory Asthma: current understanding, recommendations, and unanswered questions. *Am J Respir Crit Care Med* **162**:2341–2351.

Treatment of acute asthma

For a summary of treatment of acute asthma, see Figure 15.1. Initial treatment consists of the following:

- **A**irway—ensure no upper airway obstruction
- **B**reathing—low-flow oxygen
- **C**irculation—gain IV access

Referral to an asthma specialist should be considered for all hospitalized patients.

- Administer supplemental oxygen to correct hypoxemia.
- Administer repetitive or continuous administration of short-acting β_2-agonist (SABA) to reverse airflow obstruction.
- Administer oral systemic corticosteroids to treat inflammation.
- Monitor response to therapy with regular serial assessments.

Monitoring

- Record PEF on arrival in the emergency department (ED), at 15–30 minutes after starting treatment, at 60 minutes, and at least hourly.
- Record O_2 saturation and maintain >92% with supplemental oxygen
- ABG for pH and $PaCO_2$ if saturation <93% or if other severe features are present
- Measure and document heart rate, respiratory rate, and electrolytes.
- CXR if concerns about infection/pneumothorax

$PaCO_2$ is often low (due to hyperventilation) in a mild asthma attack. A normal CO_2 may indicate a tiring patient. *A high CO_2 indicates a life-threatening attack and should precipitate urgent assessment for ventilatory support.*

Retention of CO_2 is not aggravated by treatment with oxygen in patients with severe acute asthma, and controlled oxygen therapy should be provided.

Treatment

Oxygen

Low-flow oxygen should be delivered via nasal cannula to provide a target saturation >92%.

Bronchodilators

Inhaled SABA bronchodilators remain the primary therapy to reverse bronchospasm rapidly, and can be delivered via a metered-dose inhaler (MDI) or a nebulizer (e.g., nebulized albuterol 2.5–5 mg driven by oxygen or 8 puffs of albuterol given by MDI with a spacer every 30–60 minutes). Nebulized anticholinergics (ipratropium bromide) added to SABA therapy may improve bronchodilation in the initial therapy of acute severe asthma. Systemic β_2-agonists should be reserved only for use in patients who fail to show an initial response to albuterol.

Glucocorticosteroids

Systemic corticosteroids remain the major definitive therapy for reducing inflammation—the earlier given in an attack, the better the outcome (they require at least 4 hours to produce clinical improvement). Oral therapy has been shown to be as effective as intravenous (typically 40–80 mg of prednisone daily). However, intravenous corticosteroids are recommended for at least 24 hours in patients who are hospitalized for an asthma exacerbation (e.g., 60 mg of methylprednisolone IV every 6 hours).

Therapy should be continued for at 5–10 days but duration is dependent on clinical response. Consider continuing oral steroids until peak flow is >70% of predicted or personal best.

The dose can be stopped abruptly (assuming the patient continues on inhaled steroid) depending on the duration of therapy. This does not apply to patients on repeated doses or long-term steroids, in whom a longer (tapered) course may be appropriate.

Magnesium sulfate

This is not recommended for routine use. If there is a poor response to glucocorticosteroids and bronchodilators, you can give a 2 g IV infusion over 20 minutes.

Helium oxygen therapy

There is no routine role for the use of combination helium–oxygen mixtures (HELIOX). Theoretically it reduces airflow resistance in areas of turbulence and may also increase bronchodilator availability by improving particle deposition. Consider its use for severe or life-threatening exacerbations unresponsive to initial treatments.

Not routinely recommended in severe exacerbations

Epinephrine

This is not routinely indicated during an asthma exacerbation, as there is no proven advantage over inhaled therapy. A subcutaneous or intramuscular injection of epinephrine (adrenaline) may be indicated for acute treatment of anaphylaxis and angioedema.

Theophylline

This is not recommended in the ED or hospital setting. Some patients may respond; consider it if there is a poor response to initial therapy. The use of theophylline requires therapeutic drug monitoring. Side effects include nausea, arrhythmias, and palpitations.

Antibiotics

Antibiotics are not recommended for routine use. Only if a concomitant bacterial infection is known or suspected should they be used.

IV fluids

Patients are often volume depleted, however aggressive hydration is not recommended.

Sedation, mucolytics, and chest physiotherapy are not recommended.

Decision of discharge from the ED versus hospitalization

No single measure is the best for assessing severity of predicting requirement for hospital admission.

Repeated lung function measures (PEF or FEV_1) at 1 hour after initial therapy and beyond are the strongest single predictor of hospitalization. Patients with a pretreatment FEV_1 or PEF <25% predicted (or personal best), or those with a post-treatment FEV_1 or PEF <40% predicted (or personal best) usually require hospitalization.

Patients with post-treatment lung function >70% can be discharged. Patients with post-treatment lung function of 40%–70% predicted generally may be discharged, provided that adequate follow-up is available and compliance is assured.

Pulse oximetry is useful in assessing initial severity. Repeated measures of <92%–94% after initial treatment predict the need for hospitalization.

Signs and symptom scores at 1 hour after initial therapy improve the ability to predict need for hospitalization. Drowsiness predicts impending respiratory failure.

If possible, at the time of discharge from the ER:
• Provide an asthma action plan
• Provide medications (SABA, oral corticosteroids, ICS)
• Refer to follow-up care
• Review inhaler technique

Decision to admit to the ICU

Early identification and treatment of patients at risk for a fatal or near-fatal event is the key factor in preventing further morbidity. It is better to discuss early a patient who does not subsequently need ICU input than to find you and your patient in difficulty, with no ICU bed. ICU admission should be considered for patients with one or more of the following:
• Lack of response to initial therapy
• Rapidly worsening disease or signs of impeding respiratory arrest
• Confusion, drowsiness, or loss of consciousness
• Hypoxemia (PO_2 <60 mmHg) despite supplemental oxygen (see Box 15.7)
• Hypercarbia with PCO_2 >45 mmHg

Box 15.7 Indications for mechanical ventilation

• Poor response to bronchodilator therapy
• Worsening airflows
• Worsening mental status
• $PaCO_2$ >55–77 mmHg
• Increasing $PaCO_2$ (>5 mmHg/hr) in association with PaO_2 <60 mmHg or metabolic acidosis
• Signs of muscle fatigue despite aggressive therapy

Decision to discharge from the hospital

Consider discharge when
- Reducing frequency of SABA
- Off nebulized drugs and on metered dose inhalers ≥24 hours
- PEF ≥70% predicted or personal best
- Minimal PEF diurnal variation

Prior to discharge consider
- Reason for the exacerbation—could it have been avoided?
- Checking patient's self-management plan and asthma action plan
- Checking inhaler technique (pp. 693–5)
- Scheduling an appointment with a primary care provider
- Referral to an asthma specialist

At the time of discharge
- Provide an asthma action plan
- Medications (SABA, oral corticosteroids, ICS)

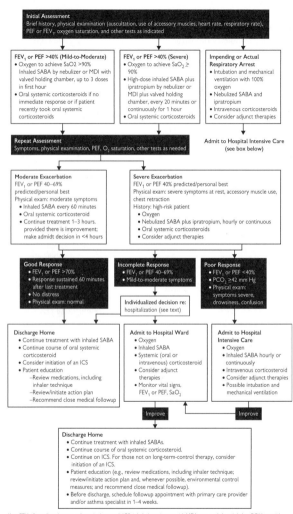

Initial Assessment
Brief history, physical examination (auscultation, use of accessory muscles, heart rate, respiratory rate), PEF or FEV$_1$, oxygen saturation, and other tests as indicated

FEV$_1$ or PEF >40% (Mild-to-Moderate)
- Oxygen to achieve SaO2 >90%
- Inhaled SABA by nebulizer or MDI with valved holding chamber, up to 3 doses in first hour
- Oral systemic corticosteroids if no immediate response or if patient recently took oral systemic corticosteroids

FEV$_1$ or PEF >40% (Severe)
- Oxygen to achieve SaO$_2$ ≥ 90%
- High-dose inhaled SABA plus ipratropium by nebulizer or MDI plus valved holding chamber, every 20 minutes or continuously for 1 hour
- Oral systemic corticosteroids

Impending or Actual Respiratory Arrest
- Intubation and mechanical ventilation with 100% oxygen
- Nebulized SABA and ipratropium
- Intravenous corticosteroids
- Consider adjunct therapies

Admit to Hospital Intensive Care
(see box below)

Repeat Assessment
Symptoms, physical examination, PEF, O$_2$ saturation, other tests as needed

Moderate Exacerbation
FEV$_1$ or PEF 40–69% predicted/personal best
Physical exam: moderate symptoms
- Inhaled SABA every 60 minutes
- Oral systemic corticosteroid
- Continue treatment 1–3 hours. provided there is improvement; make admidt decision in <4 hours

Severe Exacerbation
FEV$_1$ or PEF 40% predicted/personal best
Physical exam: severe symptoms at rest, accessory muscle use, chest retraction
History: high-risk patient
- Oxygen
- Nebulized SABA plus ipratropium, hourly or continuous
- Oral systemic corticosteroids
- Consider adjunct therapies

Good Response
- FEV$_1$ or PEF >70%
- Response sustained 60 minutes after last treatment
- No distress
- Physical exam: normal

Incomplete Response
- FEV$_1$ or PEF 40–69%
- Mild-to-moderate symptoms

Individualized decision re: hospitalization (see text)

Poor Response
- FEV$_1$ or PEF <40%
- PCO$_2$ ≥42 mm Hg
- Physical exam: symptoms severe, drowsiness, confusion

Discharge Home
- Continue treatment with inhaled SABA
- Continue course of oral systemic corticosteroid
- Consider initiation of an ICS
- Patient education
  - Review medications, including inhaler technique
  - Review/initiate action plan
  - Recommend close medical followup

Admit to Hospital Ward
- Oxygen
- Inhaled SABA
- Systemic (oral or intravenous) corticosteroid
- Consider adjunct therapies
- Monitor vital signs, FEV$_1$ or PEF, SaO$_2$

Admit to Hospital Intensive Care
- Oxygen
- Inhaled SABA hourly or continuously
- Intravenous corticosteroid
- Consider adjunct therapies
- Possible intubation and mechanical ventilation

Improve   Improve

Discharge Home
- Continue treatment with inhaled SABAs.
- Continue course of oral systemic corticosteroid.
- Continue on ICS. For those not on long-term-control therapy, consider initiation of an ICS.
- Patient education (e.g., review medications, including inhaler technique; review/initiate action plan and, whenever possible, environmental control measures; and recommend close medical followup).
- Before discharge, schedule followup appointment with primary care provider and/or asthma specialist in 1–4 weeks.

Key: FEV$_1$, forced expiratory volume in 1 second; ICS, inhaled corticosteroid; MDI, metered-dose inhaler; PC02, partial pressure carbon dioxide; PEF, peak expiratory flow; SABA, short-acting beta$_2$-agonist; SaO$_2$, oxyen saturation

Figure 15.1 Management of asthma exacerbations: emergency department and hospital-based care. Reprinted with permission from National Asthma Education and Prevention Program Expert Panel Report 3. Guidelines for the Diagnosis and Management of Asthma 2007.

Further information

British Thoracic Society. Scottish Intercollegiate Guidelines Network (2005). British guideline on the management of asthma. A national clinical guide. Revised edition.

Global Strategy for Asthma Management and Prevention. Revised 2006. Global Initiative for Asthma: http://www.ginasthma.com.

Rodrigo GJ, Rodrigo C, Hall JB (2004). Acute asthma in adults: a review. *Chest* **125**:1081–1102.

Chronic asthma: management

Goal of therapy

The goal of therapy in asthma is disease control as defined by minimizing the current impact of the disease on the patient (impairment) and future risk of problems due to asthma and its therapy. This means prevention of chronic and troublesome symptoms, maintenance of normal activity levels, infrequent requirement for the use of a short-acting bronchodilator for symptom control, and maintenance of near-normal pulmonary function, while preventing or minimizing: recurrent exacerbations, hospital and ER visits, loss of lung function, and adverse effects of medications.

Achieving and maintaining control includes the following four steps:
1. Assessment and monitoring of asthma severity and control
2. Education of the patient and family
3. Control of environmental factors and comorbid conditions
4. Medications

Assessment and monitoring

Assessment

- Determine and classify the severity of the asthma (see Fig. 15.2).
- Identify precipitating and aggravating factors.
- Identify comorbid conditions.
- Assess the patient's ability to self-manage the disease.

Use assessment of the severity of asthma to determine initial treatment, and use assessment of asthma control to monitor and adjust therapy.

Monitoring

- Symptom or peak-flow monitoring (benefits are similar). For patients with moderate or severe persistent asthma, a history of severe exacerbations, or poor perception of the severity of airflow limitation or worsening symptoms, peak-flow monitoring may be preferable.
- Assess asthma control, medication technique, adherence to the treatment plan, and specific concerns at each visit.
- See patients at 2- to 6-week intervals for those initiating therapy or require an increase in therapy.
- Once control is achieved, see the patient every 1–6 months to review maintenance of control.
- Consider seeing the patient at 3-month intervals with a decrease in therapy.

Education

The emphasis should be on the provision of self-management education and should occur at all points of care. Self-monitoring is used to assess the level of asthma control as measured by symptoms and/or peak flows.

Use a written asthma action plan. Confirm that the patient is taking their medication correctly and are avoiding environmental factors known to worsen asthma.

Control of environmental factors and comorbid conditions

Recommend measures to control exposures to allergens and pollutants or irritants known from previous and ongoing evaluation to make asthma worse. Avoidance of tobacco smoke is important. Consider allergen immunotherapy for patients who have persistent disease when there is confident evidence of a relationship between the exposure and asthma symptoms.

Identify and treat comorbid conditions, especially rhinosinusitis, gastroesophageal reflux disease, obesity, obstructive sleep apnea, allergic bronchopulmonary mycosis, and psychological or psychiatric disease.

Medications

Medications to treat asthma are classified as long-term *control medications* and faster-acting *relievers* (see Box 15.8). Controllers are taken daily on a long-term basis to keep asthma under clinical control through their anti-inflammatory effects. Relievers are used on an as-needed basis and act rapidly to reverse symptomatic bronchospasm.

Box 15.8 Long-term control and reliever medications

Controllers
- Inhaled glucocorticosteroids (e.g., fluticasone, budesonide)
- Leukotriene modifiers (e.g., montelukast, zileuton)
- Long-acting inhaled β_2-agonists (e.g., formoterol, salmeterol)
- Cromolyn sodium and nedocromil
- Methylxanthines (e.g., theophylline)
- Long-acting oral β_2-agonists (rarely used)
- Anti-IgE (omalizumab—limited to patients with elevated IgE)
- Systemic glucocorticosteroids (limited by adverse effects)

Relievers
- Rapid-acting inhaled β_2-agonists (e.g., albuterol, terbutaline)
- Inhaled anticholinergics (e.g., ipratropium bromide)
- Systemic glucocorticosteroids
- Short-acting oral β_2-agonists (limited by adverse effects)

Treatment is based on disease severity, using a step up/step down approach (see Fig. 15.3). Treatment is started at the level appropriate to disease severity based on the history, spirometry, and medication usage.

Components of Severity		Classification of Asthma Severity ≥12 years of age			
			Persistent		
		Intermittent	Mild	Moderate	Severe
Impairment Normal FEV₁/FVC: 8–9 yr 85% 20–39 yr 80% 40–59 yr 75% 60–80 yr 70%	Symptoms	≤2 days/week	>2 days/week but not daily	Daily	Throughout the day
	Nighttime awakenings	≤2x/month	3–4x/month	>1x/week but not nightly	Often 7x/week
	Short-acting beta₂-agonist for symptom control (not prevention of EIB)	2 days/week	>2 days/week but not daily, and not more than 1x on any day	Daily	Several times per day
	Interference with normal activity	None	Minor limitation	Some limitation	Extremely limited
	Lung function	• Normal FEV₁ between exacerbations • FEV₁ >80% predicted • FEV₁/FVC normal	• FEV₁ >80% predicted • FEV₁/FVC normal	• FEV₁ >60% but <80% predicted • FEV₁/FVC reduced 5%	• FEV₁ <60% predicted • FEV₁/FVC reduced >5%
Risk	Exacerbations requiring oral systemic corticosteroids	0–1/year (see note)	>2/year (see note) → ← Consider severity and interval since last exacerbation. → Frequency and severity may fluctuate over time for patients in any severity category. Relative annual risk of exacerbations may be related to FEV1.		
Recommended Step for Initiating Treatment (See "Stepwise Approach for Managing Asthma" for treatment steps.)		Step 1	Step 2	Step 3 and consider s of oral systemi	Step 4 or 5 hort course c corticosterioids
		In 2–6 weeks, evaluate level of asthma control that is achieved and adjust therapy accordingly.			

Figure 15.2 Classification of asthma severity. Reprinted with permission from National Asthma Education and Prevention Program Expert Panel Report 3. Guidelines for the Diagnosis and Management of Asthma 2007.

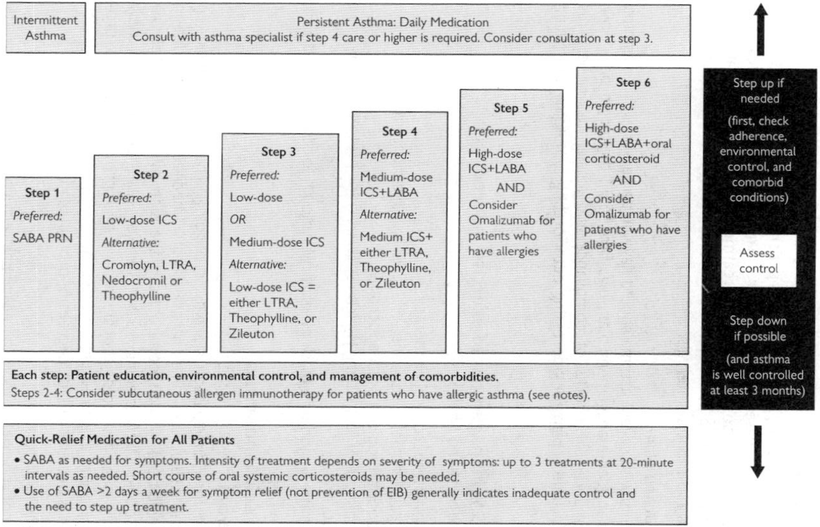
Intermittent Asthma
Persistent Asthma: Daily Medication
Consult with asthma specialist if step 4 care or higher is required. Consider consultation at step 3.
Step 1
Preferred:
SABA PRN
Step 2
Preferred:
Low-dose ICS
Alternative:
Cromolyn, LTRA, Nedocromil or Theophylline
Step 3
Preferred:
Low-dose
OR
Medium-dose ICS
Alternative:
Low-dose ICS = either LTRA, Theophylline, or Zileuton
Step 4
Preferred:
Medium-dose ICS+LABA
Alternative:
Medium ICS+ either LTRA, Theophylline, or Zileuton
Step 5
Preferred:
High-dose ICS+LABA
AND
Consider Omalizumab for patients who have allergies
Step 6
Preferred:
High-dose ICS+LABA+oral corticosteroid
AND
Consider Omalizumab for patients who have allergies
Step up if needed
(first, check adherence, environmental control, and comorbid conditions)
Assess control
Step down if possible
(and asthma is well controlled at least 3 months)
Each step: Patient education, environmental control, and management of comorbidities.
Steps 2-4: Consider subcutaneous allergen immunotherapy for patients who have allergic asthma (see notes).
Quick-Relief Medication for All Patients
• SABA as needed for symptoms. Intensity of treatment depends on severity of symptoms: up to 3 treatments at 20-minute intervals as needed. Short course of oral systemic corticosteroids may be needed.
• Use of SABA >2 days a week for symptom relief (not prevention of EIB) generally indicates inadequate control and the need to step up treatment.

Figure 15.3 Stepwise approach for managing asthma. Reprinted with permission from National Asthma Education and Prevention Program Expert Panel Report 3. Guidelines for the Diagnosis and Management of Asthma 2007.

Additional points

Regular review

Regular review is required to ensure patients are on appropriate treatment for their disease severity, and are maintained on the lowest possible inhaled steroid dose. Step down treatment if the patient is stable for 3 months or more. Step down inhaled steroid by reducing the dose by 25%–50% at 3-monthly intervals.

Asthma action plan

All patients with severe asthma should have an agreed-on written asthma action plan (self-management plan, e.g., Box 15.9), their own peak flow meter, and regular checks of compliance and inhaler technique. This should include a plan for addressing deteriorating symptoms and falling peak flows.

> **Box 15.9 Management of exercise-induced bronchospasm (EIB)**
>
> • Use long-term controller therapy
> • Pretreatment before exercise with SABA, leukotrience receptor antagonist, cromolyn, or nedocromil
> • Chronic use of long-acting β_2 agonist (LABA) for pretreatment is discouraged
> • Warm-up period or a mask or scarf over mouth for cold-induced EIB

Future developments

New steroids

Research for "dissociated" steroids is ongoing. These are steroids in which the useful, anti-inflammatory effects (mediated by transcription factor inhibition) are dissociated from the side effects (mediated via glucocorticoid DNA binding). Safer steroids (e.g., ciclesonide, a new once-daily inhaled steroid) appear to have an improved side-effect profile. Ciclesonide is a prodrug, activated by airway esterases, with fewer side effects because of high degrees of protein binding.

Eosinophil inhibitors

A variety of approaches to inhibit eosinophil recruitment are under investigation, including adhesion molecule inhibition and eosinophil chemotactic receptor inhibition.

Phosphodiesterase-4 (PDE4) inhibitors

New-generation PDE4 inhibitors (e.g., roflumilast) are being investigated in clinical trials. These drugs have a broad anti-inflammatory action, with neutrophil inhibitory effects.

Nonpharmacological therapies

Allergen and pollutant avoidance

This may reduce severity of disease in sensitized individuals. House dust-mite control measures need to be comprehensive; there is no current evidence to support it, although trials are ongoing. Pet removal may be useful if the history is suggestive and sensitivity has been demonstrated by skin-prick testing or elevated specific IgE levels. Multifaceted approaches are beneficial, while single steps are generally ineffective.

Smoking cessation may reduce asthma severity.

Complementary therapies have no current evidence for their use.

Dietary manipulation

There is no consistent evidence, and none supported by interventional trials. Low magnesium intake is associated with increased asthma prevalence. Fish oils may be beneficial.

Weight reduction in obese asthmatics leads to improved control.

Immunotherapy

Desensitization using allergen-specific immunotherapy may be beneficial in a small subgroup of patients with allergen-specific sensitivities.

Buteyko breathing technique

This technique is a series of breathing exercises that mimic yoga breathing techniques. A number of studies have shown a reduction in use of inhaled bronchodilator and in steroid use in asthmatics doing these exercises, with no change in lung function or bronchial hyperresponsiveness.

Further information

British Thoracic Society/Scottish Intercollegiate Guideline Network (2003). British guideline on the management of asthma. *Thorax* **58**:1–94.

Moore WC, Peters SP (2007). Update in asthma 2006. *Am J Respir Crit Care Med* **175**:649–654.

NAEPP Expert Panel Report: guidelines for the diagnosis and management of asthma- update on selected topics. National Asthma Education and Prevention Program. National Institutes of Health, 2007.

"Difficult/refractory" asthma

Patients with "refractory" asthma are a small subgroup of asthma patients (<5%). They have difficult-to-treat disease, reflected by high maintenance medication requirements or persistent symptoms and air flow obstruction, with multiple exacerbations, despite high medication use. This group encompasses asthma subgroups described as "severe," "steroid-dependent and/or steroid-resistant," "difficult-to-control," "poorly controlled," "brittle," or "irreversible."

Clinically, these patients present with separate and/or overlapping conditions, including widely varying peak flows ("brittle asthma"), severe and chronic airflow limitation, rapidly progressive loss of lung function, absent to copious mucus production, and varying response to corticosteroids.

The disease is usually defined on the basis of

- Medication requirements
- Asthma symptoms
- Frequency of exacerbations
- Severity of airflow limitation

These patients typically fail to completely reverse their airflow obstruction following a 2-week course of oral prednisone and demonstrate a poor bronchodilator response to inhaled β_2-agonists. The pathological mechanism is likely to be ongoing airway inflammation, with increasing airway fibrosis, but this is not proven. Other possibilities include steroid resistance, β_2-receptor down-regulation, or a different disease process altogether.

Before labeling a patient as "refractory," the diagnosis and medication compliance must be confirmed. This can be done by checking pharmacy prescription records, using inhaler devices that can monitor medication usage, or by measurement of plasma prednisolone levels.

Treatment

Treatment is that of nonrefractory asthma, using step 5 or 6 with inhaled long-acting β_2-agonists and high-dose inhaled corticosteroids and oral corticosteroids as necessary (see Fig. 15.3). In patients unable to tolerate a prednisone dose <20 mg/day, corticosteroid pharmacokinetic studies may be useful. However, <25% of patients with severe asthma show clinically significantly increased prednisone clearance (usually a specific reason can be identified, such as concomitant use of enzyme-inducing medication).

Diagnosis of refractory asthma

- Confirm that the diagnosis is correct: this means reviewing the previous medical record and retaking a thorough history.
- Confirm reversible airflow limitation (as for nonrefractory asthma; see p. 114)
- Consider alternative diagnoses and investigate for potential exacerbating comorbid conditions
  - COPD
  - Bronchiectasis or cystic fibrosis
  - Sinus disease
  - Churg–Strauss syndrome or eosinophilic syndromes: consider measuring serum IgE and ANCA
  - Allergic bronchopulmonary aspergillosis: consider *Aspergillus* precipitants, skin tests, IgE
  - Vocal cord dysfunction
  - Hyperventilation syndrome
  - Gastroesophageal reflux disease: consider further evaluation with tailored barium swallow, esophagram, 24-hour pH probe
  - Upper airway obstruction: consider CT or bronchoscopy
  - Obstructive sleep apnea: consider sleep study
  - Cardiac dysfunction: consider echocardiogram and/or referral to a cardiologist
  - Psychiatric or emotional issues, secondary gain: consider psychiatry or psychology review

Anti-inflammatory and immunomodulating drugs may be of benefit (through a specialized center only). These include methotrexate, cyclosporin, oral gold, intravenous gammaglobulin, and macrolide antibiotics. None of these have been studied in a randomized controlled trial in this group of patients, and none have demonstrated improvement in airway hyperresponsiveness.

"Steroid-resistant" asthma

This subgroup of patients represents a very small proportion of refractory asthmatics. Middle-aged, obese women, often with other additional diagnoses, are overrepresented in this group. Diagnoses other than asthma are likely and investigation should be directed toward these.

Further information

Robinson DS, Campbell DA, Durham SR, et al. (2003). Systematic assessment of difficult-to-treat asthma. *Eur Respir J* **22**:478–483.

Thomas PS, Geddes DM, Barnes SJ (1999). Pseudo-steroid resistant asthma. *Thorax* **54**:352–356.

Asthma in pregnancy

- Pregnancy can affect asthma.
- Asthma can adversely affect the outcome of pregnancy.
- During pregnancy, 1/3 of patients worsen, 1/3 of them improve, and 1/3 see no change.
- Asthma course is likely to be similar in successive pregnancies.
- Severe asthma is more likely to deteriorate than mild asthma.
- Albuterol is the preferred short-acting bronchodilator.
- Inhaled corticosteroids are the preferred long-term control medication (budesonide is preferred).

Pre-pregnancy counseling

- Asthmatics should continue normal asthma medication (it is safer for pregnant women to be treated with asthma medications than for asthma symptoms and exacerbations).
- Smoking cessation advice
- Monitor the pregnant asthmatic closely. Asthma control should be monitored at each prenatal visit. Monthly evaluations allow the opportunity to step up or step down therapy, based on the level of control.

Acute asthma in pregnancy

- Risk to the fetus of uncontrolled asthma outweighs any risk of drugs.
- Asthma medications are generally safe in pregnancy.
- If necessary for asthma control, steroids should be continued.

- Maintain oxygen saturation >95%
- Continuous fetal monitoring for acute severe asthma
- Liaise with the obstetrician

Leukotriene receptor antagonists
Limited safety data are available for pregnancy. It is recommended that patients not start taking these during pregnancy. Continue use in women who have previously demonstrated significant improvement in disease control prior to pregnancy.

Management during labor
- Acute asthma is rare in labor (due to high sympathetic drive).
- Regional anesthetic blockade is preferable to general anesthesia.
- Prostaglandin E_2 may be safely used for induction of labor.
- Prostaglandin $F_2\alpha$ (for postpartum bleeding) may cause bronchospasm.
- Give parenteral hydrocortisone 100 mg every 6–8 hours during labor if on oral prednisolone at >7.5 mg daily for >2 weeks prior to delivery.

Breast-feeding
- An asthmatic mother reduces the chance of atopy in her child by breast-feeding.
- Prednisolone is secreted in breast milk, but the infant is exposed to minimal, clinically irrelevant doses.

Further information

Managing asthma during pregnancy: recommendations for pharmacologic treatment- 2004 update. NAEPP expert panel report. *J Allergy Clin Immunol* 2005; **115**: 34-46

Occupational asthma

- This is asthma due to specific workplace sensitizers (see Table 15.2)
- It may account for up to 10% of adult-onset asthma.
- The diagnosis is often difficult.
- Early diagnosis is important, as earlier removal from the exposure in affected individuals leads to a better outcome.
- It is separate from preexisting asthma exacerbated by irritants in the workplace.

- Agents induce asthma through IgE and non-IgE mechanisms.
- The latency between first exposure and symptom onset can be long, and depends on the sensitizing agent. An accurate history is extensive and includes current and past exposures.
- Once sensitized, re-exposure to very low concentrations can provoke symptoms.
- May be associated with rhinitis and urticaria
- Improves away from work, but can take several days

Risk factors
- Atopy
- HLA type (e.g., HLA-DQB1*0503 is associated with isocyanate allergy)
- Smoking (especially for high-molecular-weight agents)

Diagnosis
- Requires a diagnosis of asthma
- Confirm a relationship between asthma and workplace exposures
- Find the specific cause (see Table 15.2)

Document lung function deterioration in the workplace, usually by serial peak-flow recording at work, at home, and on vacation.

Bronchial provocation/challenge testing using the suspected agent should only be conducted in specialized centers.

Skin-prick testing and specific IgE for certain sensitizers can also be performed.

Document
- Range of chemical exposures
- Specific job duties
- Use of personal protective equipment

Serial PEF recording in occupational asthma
- Record every 2 hours from waking to sleep
- For 4 weeks, while no changes in treatment
- Document home and work periods and any holidays.
- Analysis is best made by experts, usually with a criterion-based analysis system (e.g., OASYS, a computer program that plots and interprets serial peak-flow recordings; see www.occupationalasthma.com).
- Patients may be sensitized to more than one agent.

Table 15.2 Causes of occupational asthma

Sensitizing agent	Occupational exposure
Low-molecular-weight agents (act as haptens)	
Isocyanates	Paint sprayers, adhesives, polyurethane foams
Acid anhydrides	Epoxy paint, varnish, resins
Metals	Welders, plating, metal refiners
Glutaraldehyde and other disinfectants	Health-care workers
Drugs	Pharmaceutical industry
High-molecular-weight agents	
Amine dyes	Cosmetics, hair dyes, rubber works
Wood dusts, bark	Textile workers, joiners, carpenters
Animal-derived antigens	Veterinarians, laboratory workers (20% affected)
Biological enzymes	Detergent industry, pharmaceuticals
Plant products	Bakers, hairdressers
Fluxes	Solderers, electronics industry

Further information

Chan-Yeung M, Malo JL (1995). Occupational asthma. *N Engl J Med* **333**:107–112.

Management of occupational asthma

- Identify the cause.
- Remove the worker from exposure.
- Early diagnosis and removal from exposure are important factors for a good outcome.
- The decision to remove the patient from the workplace should not be taken lightly. Specifics concerning compensation and eligibility for disability vary from state to state. Early consultation with an occupational lung disease specialist should be considered.

Latex allergy is seen in up to 18% of health-care workers and is the leading cause of occupational asthma in this group, due to the widespread use of latex gloves. It is potentially serious, with avocado, bananas, kiwi, and chestnuts cross-reacting to give a similar clinical picture. Treatment is absolute avoidance; those affected should wear a medic-alert bracelet and always use non-latex gloves.

Vocal cord dysfunction

A small portion of patients labeled as having severe asthma will have vocal cord dysfunction (so-called upper airway hyperresponsiveness).

Patients typically present with asthma symptoms, with associated triggers (e.g., odors, cold air). They typically have little or no benefit from asthma medications (though it is possible). They typically will present with recurrent severe exacerbations resistant to standard treatments and often have been hospitalized several times.

A careful history will reveal that the shortness of breath is often abrupt in onset, worse on inspiration, and associated with symptom-free periods. Audible wheezing is generally prominent.

Pathogenesis
- Recent upper respiratory infection (URI)
- Postnasal drip or chronic sinusitis
- Gastroesophageal reflux disease with subclinical microaspiration
- Chronic laryngitis
- Hyperventilation in association with anxiety, panic
- It is postulated that the vocal cord closure may represent a reflex airway protective mechanism.

Diagnosis

Diagnosis is based on excluding other causes of wheeze, cough, and breathlessness. The gold standard is visualization of abnormal vocal cord movement (closure with inspiration) at laryngoscopy. Spirometry will often shows truncation of the inspiratory limb of the flow-volume loop.

Treatment (no randomized controlled trials)
- Panting (auto-PEEP)
- Coughing and cough suppression techniques
- Inspiratory resistance devices
- HELIOX, nebulized saline, lidocaine spray (for severe, acute episodes)
- Speech therapy

Further information

Newman KB, Mason UG 3rd, Schmaling KB (1995). Clinical features of vocal cord dysfunction. *Am J Respir Crit Care Med* **152:**1382–1386.

Allergic rhinitis (hay fever)

Asthma and allergic rhinitis or sinusitis are clinical manifestations of the same underlying syndrome of chronic inflammation of the upper and lower airways. There is clearly a pathological correlation between the two conditions.

Rhinitis and sinusitis are characterized by

- Rhinorrhea
- Itching
- Sneezing
- Nasal obstruction

Allergic rhinitis is defined as *perennial* if the symptoms occur year-round, *seasonal* if occurring at a particular time of year. The lifetime prevalence of allergic rhinitis is approximately the same as that of asthma. However, up to 50% of asthma patients will have allergic rhinitis. Nineteen percent of subjects with, but only 2% without, allergic rhinitis will have asthma.

Etiology

The lining of the nose is in continuum with the lower respiratory tract, and inflammation of the upper and lower airways often coexists. Common aeroallergens provoking seasonal allergic rhinitis are tree pollen (spring) and grass pollen (summer). Perennial rhinitis usually reflects allergy to indoor allergens such as house dust mite, cat salivary protein, cockroaches, or animal dander.

Pathophysiology

Symptoms occur following the inhalation of allergen to which the subject is sensitized, and against which they have IgE antibodies. These antibodies bind to mast cell IgE receptors, with the release of mediators, including tryptase and histamine, causing symptoms immediately after exposure.

Diagnosis

Diagnosis is usually made from the history, which should identify the triggers to the disease. The main differential diagnoses are sinusitis due to bacterial or viral infection and upper airway involvement due to vasculitis. Successful treatment of rhinosinusitis in association with asthma leads to improved asthma control.

Treatment

- Allergen avoidance. This may be easier said than done. It can take up to 20 weeks to remove cat allergen from a house. Pollen counts are highest in the afternoon and early evening
- Nonsedating antihistamines (e.g., terfenadine) improve sneezing and itching, but have no effect on nasal blockage.
- Topical intranasal steroid (e.g., budesonide, triamcinolone)
- Topical intranasal anticholinergics (e.g., ipratropium) may be useful for rhinorrhea, if uncontrolled with topical nasal steroids.
- Topical sodium cromoglycate may be beneficial, particularly for allergic conjunctivitis.
- Decongestant (e.g., oxymetazoline) may help, but rebound nasal blockage and tachyphylaxis are potential problems if used regularly.

Further information

Peters S (2007). The impact of comorbid atopic disease on asthma: clinical expression and treatment. *J Asthma* **44**:149–161.

Chronic obstructive pulmonary disease (COPD)

Definition, etiology, pathology, and clinical features

COPD is a common disease and is mostly due to smoking. Patients with COPD represent a large proportion of inpatient and outpatient work for the general pulmonary physician.

Definition
- Chronic airflow limitation
- Airflow limitation not fully reversible with bronchodilators
- Minimal variability in day-to-day symptoms
- Slowly progressive and irreversible deterioration in lung function, leading to progressively worsening symptoms
- Associated with systemic consequences

Etiology
About 85% of cases are related to cigarette smoking, typically >20 pack-years. Clinically significant COPD occurs in a minority of smokers (possibly 20%–25%); the exact reasons for the development of COPD in only some smokers are not understood.

COPD is increasing in frequency worldwide, particularly in developing countries where the disease is commonly related to heating and cooking with biofuels, in addition to the high levels of cigarette smoking. It can also be caused by environmental and occupational factors such as dust and chemicals. The only known genetic cause is α_1-antitrypsin deficiency.

Pathology
COPD is characterized by varying degrees of chronic inflammation of the small airways and destruction of the alveolar walls. There is often vascular involvement that may be associated with pulmonary hypertension.

- *Mucous gland hyperplasia* particularly in the large airways, with mucous hypersecretion leading to a chronic productive cough. Other mucosal damage from smoke includes
  - *Squamous metaplasia:* Replacement of the normal ciliated columnar epithelium by squamous epithelium
  - *Loss of ciliary function* leads to impairment of the normal functioning of the mucociliary escalator.
- *Chronic inflammation and fibrosis* of small airways, characterized by CD8 lymphocyte, macrophage, and neutrophil infiltration, with release of proinflammatory cytokines. Recurrent infections may perpetuate airway inflammation.
- *Emphysema* due to alveolar wall destruction causing irreversible enlargement of airspaces distal to the terminal bronchiole (the acinus), with subsequent loss of elastic recoil and hyperinflated lungs
  - Panacinar emphysema can occur with dilated airspaces evenly distributed across acini.
  - Centriacinar or proximal emphysema can occur with dilated airspaces found in association with the respiratory bronchioles.

- Periacinar or paraseptal emphysema can occur with dilated airspaces at the edge of the acinar unit and abutting a fixed structure, such as the pleura or a vessel.
- *Thickened pulmonary arteriolar wall and remodeling* occur with chronic hypoxia. Hypoxia leads to increased pulmonary vascular resistance, and pulmonary hypertension in some COPD patients.
- *Increase in airflow resistance* is multifactorial. Small-airway inflammation reduces the airway lumen. Secretions may be present in the airways. Emphysema destroys the radial attachments to the small airways, which normally hold airways open and resist dynamic compression.

Clinical features

COPD is a disease characterized by progressive airflow limitation and with a slow decline in function. Significant physiologic airflow obstruction may be present before the patient develops any symptoms, and when symptoms do develop their intensity generally correlates with the severity of the airflow limitation.
- Progressive dyspnea, generally first noticed with activity
- Decreased exercise tolerance
- Cough
- Wheeze
- Sputum production

Signs also depend on the severity of the underlying disease.
- Increased respiratory rate
- Hyperexpanded or barrel chest
- Prolonged expiratory time >5 seconds
- Pursed-lip breathing
- Use of accessory muscles of respiration
- Diminished breath sounds
- Wheeze
- Distant, quiet heart sounds (due to overlying hyperinflated lung)
- Possible basal crepitations (crackles/rales)
- Signs of cor pulmonale, which include ankle edema, raised jugular venous pressure, warm peripheries, plethoric conjunctivae, bounding pulse
- Flapping tremor (asterixis), uncommonly and only if $PaCO_2$ is acutely raised

α_1-Antitrypsin (α1-AT) deficiency

α1-AT deficiency is an autosomal recessive, inherited condition that is associated with the early development of emphysema. α1-AT is a glycoprotein protease inhibitor produced by the liver. It is secreted via the bloodstream into the lungs and inactivates neutrophil elastase. Neutrophil elastase destroys alveolar wall connective tissue.

Elastase is produced in increased amounts by pulmonary neutrophils and macrophages in response to smoking and lung infections. If α1-AT is deficient, the elastase cannot be opposed, and subsequently emphysema develops. This emphysema occurs primarily in the bases of the lung, in contrast to non-α1-AT deficiency emphysema, which occurs in the upper lung zones.

Disease presents earlier and more severely in cigarette smokers and can cause COPD at a young age. Nonsmokers are usually asymptomatic. There may also be associated liver dysfunction and cirrhosis, as abnormal protein secretion accumulates in the liver.

So far, about 75 different α1-AT alleles have been identified for this gene on the long arm of chromosome 4. The most common alleles are the M allele (the normal allele), the partially defective S allele, and the almost fully defective Z allele, common in Scandinavia.

In patients with the defective Z allele, lysine is substituted for glutamic acid at position 342, leading to abnormal folding of the α1-AT protein, preventing posttranslational processing, and resulting in intracellular protein accumulation.

- MM is the normal phenotype.
- MS and MZ have 50%–70% of normal α_1-protease inhibitor (Pi) levels and rarely develop COPD.
- SZ and SS have 35%–50% of normal levels and are at risk for developing COPD.
- Homozygous ZZ has only 10%–20% of normal levels and is the genotype most strongly associated with developing emphysema.

It has been recommended that screening for the defect should be carried out in all patients with COPD, especially in patients <40 years of age with COPD. Siblings of known α1-AT patients should be screened, and the importance of not smoking and avoiding passive smoking should be emphasized.

Treatment with enzyme augmentation to slow decline in lung function in patients with homozygous deficiency is currently used across the United States, but this is not the practice worldwide.

Further information

α_1-Antitrypsin deficiency support group, Alpha-1 Association: http://www.alpha1.org

Investigations

Pulmonary function tests

The following are required for the diagnosis:
- Obstructive spirometry and flow–volume loops
- FEV_1/FVC <0.7 post-bronchodilator defines the presence of chronic airflow limitation; COPD should be suspected in these subjects (see Table 16.1).
- Reduced post-bronchodilator FEV_1 to <80% predicted (FEV_1 is used to stage the severity of COPD; see Table 16.1)

Common features, but not required for the diagnosis:
- Usually minimal bronchodilator reversibility (<12%, or <200 cc), though some patients with COPD may have a significant response to bronchodilators
- Raised total lung volume, functional residual capacity, and residual volume because of emphysema, air trapping, and loss of elastic recoil
- Decreased diffusing capacity, because emphysema decreases surface area available for gas diffusion.

A CXR, though not required for diagnosis, is useful initially to exclude other disorders (see Box 16.1). Repeat CXR is unnecessary unless other new diagnoses are being considered (most importantly, lung cancer or bronchiectasis). Early in the disease, the CXR is normal.
- Hyperinflated lung fields with attenuation of peripheral vasculature— "black lung sign"
- Flattened diaphragms (best CXR correlate of postmortem degree of emphysema)
- More horizontal ribs; more than 7 posterior ribs seen
- May see bullae, especially in the lung apices, which, if large, can be mistaken for a pneumothorax due to the loss of lung markings (chest CT scan can differentiate bullae from pneumothorax)

Diagnosis is based on the history of smoking and progressive dyspnea, with evidence of airflow limitation on spirometry.

Table 16.1 COPD severity according to GOLD guidelines*

Mild	FEV_1/FVC <70%
	FEV_1 ≥80% predicted
Moderate	FEV_1/FVC <70%
	50% ≤ FEV_1 <80% predicted
Severe	FEV_1/FVC <70%
	30% ≤ FEV_1 <50% predicted
Very severe	FEV_1/FVC <70%
	FEV_1 <30% predicted or FEV_1 <50% predicted
	plus chronic respiratory failure

* All values are post-bronchodilator. GOLD, Global initiative for chronic Obstructive Lung Disease.

Box 16.1 Differential diagnosis of COPD

- Asthma
- Bronchiectasis
- Bronchiolitis
- Left ventricular failure

Nonpharmacological management of stable COPD

Aims of COPD management include the following:
- Assuring the correct diagnosis
- Smoking cessation to prevent disease progression
- Symptom reduction by optimizing treatment
- Improvement in quality of life

Comprehensive management is most effective when delivered by a multi-disciplinary team.

Smoking cessation is the only intervention proven to decrease the smoking-related decline in lung function. All patients with COPD who smoke should be encouraged to stop at every opportunity.

Figure 16.1 shows the accelerated decline in FEV_1 in susceptible smokers and the slowing of this rate of decline with smoking cessation. Susceptible smokers, however, never regain normal lung function.

Medications, including nicotine replacement therapy, buproprion, and varenecline, combined with ongoing counseling and psychological support should be used to aid smoking cessation.

Education can improve the ability to stop smoking and otherwise manage the illness.

Pulmonary rehabilitation is a multidisciplinary program, with evidence from randomized controlled trials that it improves dyspnea, exercise tolerance, quality of life, and reduces hospital admissions. The mainstay of rehabilitation is graded exercise, but it also incorporates education, breathing techniques, and psychosocial counseling.

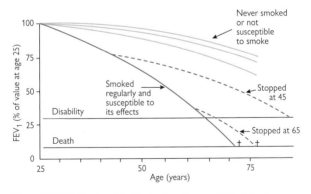

Figure 16.1 Modification of the Fletcher Peto diagram of FEV_1 decline in susceptible smokers.

Programs vary, but are usually run on an outpatient basis over 6–12 weeks, with multidisciplinary involvement. Pulmonary rehabilitation should be made available to all appropriate patients with COPD.

Diet

Weight loss is recommended if the patient is obese, to improve exercise performance and reduce dyspnea. If the patient is very breathless, calorific intake may be low and a catabolic state may exist. Nutritional supplementation may be necessary. Low body weight and decreased muscle mass are associated with reduced survival.

Psychosocial support, depression and anxiety are common in COPD and all patients should be assessed for these. Automotive disability signs may allow patients to be more active and functional in the community.

Pharmacological management of stable COPD

Pharmacological management aims to relieve symptoms and reduce exacerbations, but may not modify disease progression. Treatment should be increased in a stepwise fashion. Exacerbations require additional therapeutic support.

Bronchodilators

Simple pulmonary function testing may not show significant bronchodilator reversibility of FEV_1, but bronchodilators may provide therapeutic benefit in the long term, by reducing dyspnea, increasing exercise performance, and improving health-related quality of life.

- Initially prescribe short-acting β_2-agonists as required for symptom relief.
- If patients are still symptomatic, institute a therapeutic trial of regularly inhaled long-acting bronchodilator, either with a selective β_2 agonist or an anticholinergic. Also prescribe this if patients have a history of exacerbations.
- **Inhaler therapy** provides adequate bronchodilator doses for most patients, especially when used with a spacer device. It is important to have the patient trained in the use of the inhaler and to subsequently check the patient's inhaler technique.
- **Nebulizer therapy** is indicated if the patient is unable to use inhalers, or if they remain disabled or distressed by breathlessness despite maximal inhaler therapy. Only those with a clear and measurable response to nebulized therapy, a reduction in symptoms, or improvement in activities of daily living should continue with long-term nebulized treatment.
- **Bronchodilators are more effective when used in combination,** i.e., a long-acting β-agonist plus a long-acting anticholinergic.

Inhaled steroids

These should be considered for patients with an $FEV_1 \leq 50\%$ predicted, and who have had two or more exacerbations per year requiring treatment with antibiotics or oral steroids. Clinical trials of inhaled steroids have shown a reduction in exacerbation frequency in severe COPD.

In patients with breathlessness and exercise limitation, inhaled steroids can be added to long-acting β-agonists for a 4-week trial, to see if their symptoms improve.

Warn patients about possible steroid side effects. Screen for osteoporosis and prescribe treatment if present. Encourage regular ophthalmologic examinations.

Combined inhaled long-acting bronchodilator/steroids

In COPD patients with 1–2 exacerbations per year, combination inhaled therapy reduces the rate of exacerbations, improves quality of life, symptoms, and lung function, and appears to reduce mortality. These benefits are accompanied by an increase in the risk of pneumonia. Because of these findings, combination therapy should be considered in all patients with clinically significant COPD.

Oral steroids

These are not recommended as maintenance therapy in COPD because of their side effects. They may, however, be used to treat exacerbations.

Oxygen

Oxygen can be administered as long-term oxygen therapy (LTOT) via an oxygen concentrator, compressed gas tank, or liquid oxygen. The criteria for therapy are a PaO_2 ≤55 mmHg or PaO_2 of 56–59 mmHg with either secondary polycythemia (Hct >56%), peripheral edema, or pulmonary hypertension.

Patients who use oxygen continuously have improved survival. Additional ambulatory delivery devices can be provided for periods of activity away from a stationary source. Low-flow oxygen, such as 2–4 L/min via nasal prongs, is usually adequate to increase oxygen saturation to 90% or greater.

Vaccination

Influenza vaccine annually and pneumococcal vaccine once every 5 years are recommended.

Mucolytics

Mucolytics may benefit a few patients with chronic productive cough. Prescribe them for a trial period and only continue use if there is evidence of symptomatic improvement.

Palliative care and respiratory sedation

Use of low-dose sedatives, such as alprazolam or lorazepam twice daily, can be used as a palliative care measure. The aim is to relieve the sensation of dyspnea and associated anxiety, when the patient has very severe COPD and is on maximal treatment.

Further information

Buist AS, Anzueto A, Calverley P, deGuia TS, Fukuchi Y, Jenkins C, et al. (2006). Global strategy for the diagnosis, management and prevention of chronic obstructive pulmonary disease. Available at: www.goldcopd.com.

Sutherland ER, Cherniack RM (2004). Management of chronic obstructive pulmonary disease. N Engl J Med **350**:2689–2697.

Management of exacerbations

An *exacerbation* is a clinical diagnosis and defined as an increase in respiratory symptoms beyond the normal daily variation that lead to a change in therapy. Increases in at least two symptoms such sputum volume, sputum purulence, and dyspnea are present for a day or more.

Exacerbations may cause mild symptoms in those with relatively preserved lung function, but may cause considerable morbidity in those with limited respiratory reserve. It has been increasingly recognized that significant numbers of patients do not regain their premorbid lung function or quality of life following an exacerbation.

Causes may be infective organisms, either viral or bacterial, or noninfective causes, such as pollution or temperature changes. Common bacterial pathogens are *Haemophilus influenzae, Streptococcus pneumoniae,* and *Moraxella catarrhalis.* The most common viral pathogens are rhinovirus, influenza, coronavirus, and adenovirus.

Symptoms may include increased sputum volume and/or purulence, increasing dyspnea or wheeze, and chest tightness.

Management
Assessment
Assess the severity of the exacerbation: increase in dyspnea, tachypnea, use of accessory muscles, new cyanosis, pedal edema, or confusion. Can the patient provide self-care and self-medicate? In the presence of severe symptoms, with possible comorbid disease and decreased functional activities, the patient is likely to need inpatient hospital management.

Investigations
These are with CXR, arterial blood gases, oxygen saturation, electrocardiogram, complete blood count, and basic chemistry blood tests.

Admission arterial pH is the best predictor of survival. A pH <7.25 is associated with a rapidly rising mortality. A *raised* pH may imply an alternative diagnosis, not associated with worsening airways limitation, such as pulmonary edema. Consider sputum for culture if purulent.

Antibiotics
Give antibiotics if sputum is purulent, the patient is febrile, or new changes on CXR are present.

Systemic steroids
These are for all patients with exacerbations of COPD who are admitted to the hospital or are significantly more breathless than usual. Give prednisone 40 mg/day for 3 days followed by a quick taper over 10 days. Use intravenous methylprednisolone for patients admitted to the ICU.

Long-term steroid treatment should be avoided due to side effects.

Inhaled or nebulized bronchodilators
Breathless patients may benefit from nebulizer therapy with a combination of albuterol and ipratropium in the acute period every 2–4 hours until improvement is noted. The interval between treatments may then be spaced out more liberally.

Oxygen therapy
Monitor with pulse oximetry and/or arterial blood gases, and titrate to maintain arterial saturation >90%. Falling consciousness level is a clinical marker of significant CO_2 retention and acidosis.

Noninvasive ventilation (NIV)
Bilevel positive airway pressure is effective in supporting patients during an exacerbation, helps reduce the work of breathing, and may help prevent intubation. Use of NIV should be considered early in patients with an exacerbation who are admitted to the hospital. It is appropriate for conscious patients who can tolerate a tight-fitting facemask.

Nausea and vomiting are contraindications to its use. Once titrated correctly, arterial blood gas should show a decrease in hypercapnia and correction of pH.

Intubation and intensive care
If the patient is not responding to medical therapy (systemic steroids, bronchodilator, oxygen, NIV), a decision regarding invasive mechanical ventilation needs to be made. This may be considered appropriate if the patient has a good premorbid functional status with few comorbidities. The decision to intubate should be discussed with the patient and/or their family. Resuscitation decisions should also be made.

Further information
Stoller JK (2002). Clinical practice. Acute exacerbation of chronic obstructive pulmonary disease. N Engl J Med **346**:988–994.

Summary of approaches to medical treatment

> **Box 16.2 An approach to a patient with exacerbation of COPD in the hospital setting**
>
> - Assess severity of the exacerbation by measuring respiratory rate, degree of air entry, tachycardia, peripheral perfusion, blood pressure, and oxygen saturation.
> - If the patient is hypoxic, give oxygen. Titrate to achieve SaO_2 >90%.
> - Albuterol and ipratopium by nebulizer
> - Establish venous access.
> - Check arterial blood gas, CXR, blood count, and blood chemistries.
> - Perform an electrocardiogram.
> - Exclude other treatable causes of deterioration, e.g., tension pneumothorax, myocardial infarction, pulmonary embolus,
> - Optimize volume status.
> - Take a *history* if possible. It is important to know the patient's normal functional status, such as exercise tolerance and the need for help with activities of daily living. Old hospital notes are helpful regarding severity of disease and whether previous decisions have been made about assisted ventilation or resuscitation.
> - Nebulized bronchodilators: albuterol 2.5–7.5 mg and ipratropium 500 µg on arrival and 2–4 hourly
> - Start NIV early to help with work of breathing. Repeat blood gases after 60 minutes to ensure improvement if the patient is hypoxic or acidotic. Repeat if clinical deterioration is noted.
> - Start antibiotics.
> - Oral or intravenous steroids
> - Consider intensive care—ideally a consultant-led decision is made with the patient and their family about invasive mechanical ventilation. Document this in the medical notes. Consider resuscitation status.
> - Deep venous thrombosis prophylaxis

Box 16.3 An approach to COPD in the outpatient clinic

- Establish diagnosis and severity—pulmonary function tests, CXR
- Evaluate for other causes for symptoms, e.g., anemia, pulmonary emboli, heart failure, interstitial lung disease, thyroid dysfunction, pneumothorax, large bulla, depression.
- Focus on smoking cessation.
- Review current treatment and inhaler technique—optimize bronchodilators and inhaled steroids.
- Assess whether there is any need for a nebulizer.
- Check oxygen saturation and consider arterial blood gas.
- Consider long-term oxygen therapy, if appropriate.
- Consider pulmonary rehabilitation.
- Make sure vaccinations are up to date.
- Consider lung volume reduction surgery and lung transplantation evaluation, if appropriate (high-resolution CT scan of chest, maximal exercise test).
- Follow up patient in clinic for ongoing medical issues
- Inform the primary care physician of all of the above decisions.

Surgical treatment

Lung transplant

In patients (generally below 60–65 years of age) with severe disease, including α_1-antitrypsin deficiency, lung transplantation may be an option. Local transplant teams will advise regarding local criteria.

Bullectomy

Bullectomy is suitable for selected patients with isolated bullae. It improves chest hyperinflation and gas trapping.

Lung volume reduction surgery (LVRS)

LVRS involves resection of areas of emphysema to reduce chest hyperinflation, improve elastic recoil, and improve physiology of the lungs and functional status. Patients considered for LVRS are those with FEV_1 20%–45% predicted, hyperinflation on pulmonary function testing, symptomatic dyspnea despite maximal medical therapy, and heterogeneous areas of emphysema on CT (predominantly upper lobe disease) giving target areas to resect.

Preoperative assessment includes pulmonary function tests, chest CT scan, and maximal cardiopulmonary exercise test. Surgery is performed in specialized centers via median sternotomy or by thoracoscopy. The most emphysematous areas are removed.

In responders, improvements are seen in exercise capacity, dyspnea, and quality-of-life scores. Symptomatic improvement is sustained for 2–4 years.

Postoperative complications include persistent air leak >7 days in 30%–40%, pneumonia in up to 22%, and respiratory failure in up to 13%. Postoperative mortality of 2.4%–17% has been reported.

The group most likely to benefit are those with a poor preoperative exercise capacity (<40 watts in men and <25 watts in women), and upper lobe–predominant emphysema.

Patients with FEV_1 and/or DLCO <20% predicted, or with homogeneous emphysema and a good preoperative exercise capacity are significantly less likely to benefit from surgery and have an associated increased surgical mortality. Surgery is thus not recommended for this group.

Bronchoscopic lung volume reduction

This treatment is being investigated, such as with valve implants placed within the segmental bronchi that supply the hyperinflated lobes. It is a minimally invasive variation on lung volume reduction surgery, with the aim of improving lung function and quality of life.

Further information

Benditt JO (2004). Surgical therapies for chronic obstructive pulmonary disease. *Respir Care* **49**:53–63.

MacNee W, Calverley PMA (2003). Chronic obstructive pulmonary disease. 7: Management of COPD. *Thorax* **58**:261–265.

National Collaborating Centre for Chronic Conditions (2004). Chronic obstructive pulmonary disease. National clinical guideline on management of COPD in adults in primary and secondary care. *Thorax* **59**(Suppl. 1):1–232.

Naunheim KS, Wood DE, Mohsenifar Z, Sternberg AL, Criner GJ, et al. (2006). Long-term follow-up of patients receiving lung-volume-reduction surgery versus medical therapy for severe emphysema by the National Emphysema Treatment Trial Research Group. *Ann Thorac Surg* **82**:431–443.

Toma TP, Hopkinson NS, Hillier J, et al. (2003). Bronchoscopic volume reduction with valve implants in patients with severe emphysema. *Lancet* **361**:931–933.

Patient information Web site: www.copd-international.com

For families of patients with COPD: www.copd-support.com

Lung cancer

Epidemiology and types

Epidemiology

- Lung cancer is the most common cause of cancer deaths in men and women in the United States.
- Nearly 215,000 new cases are diagnosed per year in the United States, and an estimated 160,000 deaths from lung cancer.
- The male–female ratio is 2:1, but numbers are decreasing for men and increasing for women because of changing smoking patterns—the rate of smoking is increasing among women.
- 90% of cases are smoking related (clear dose–response relationship). Passive smoking causes up to 25% of lung cancer in nonsmokers.
- Smoking cessation decreases risk, but risk remains higher in smokers than in nonsmokers.
- Risk of lung cancer may be increased by asbestos exposure, arsenic and heavy metal exposure, and coexistent usual interstitial pneumonitis (UIP) pattern interstitial lung disease (ILD).

Types of lung cancer

In practical terms, lung cancer is divided into two groups, non-small cell and small cell, which influence management and treatment decisions (see also Box 17.1).

Non-small cell lung cancer (NSCLC)

- Accounts for at least 75%–80% of all lung cancers
- *Adenocarcinoma* is the most common histological type. Although this tumor is mostly smoking related, there are patients in whom this is not smoking related. It can occur in scar tissue or sites of fibrosis. It can be a lung primary, or a secondary from adenocarcinomas at other sites, especially if causing pleural infiltration and subsequent pleural effusion.
- *Squamous cell carcinoma* usually presents as a central mass on CXR, but may cavitate and look radiologically like a lung abscess. Rarely there may be multiple cavitating lesions. Patients with hypercalcemia are most likely to have squamous cell carcinoma.
- *Bronchoalveolar carcinoma (BAC)* can rarely cause copious sputum production (bronchorrhea). It may present as a unifocal or multifocal ground-glass density(ies) on CXR or chest CT.

Small cell lung cancer (SCLC)

- Accounts for approximately 18% of all lung cancers
- Usually disseminated by the time of diagnosis (hematogenous spread)
- Frequently *metastasizes* to liver, bones, bone marrow, brain, adrenals, or elsewhere
- Syndrome of inappropriate secretion of antidiuretic hormone (SIADH) is common in small cell lung cancer
- Surgery usually not appropriate
- Chemo- and radiosensitive
- Untreated extensive small cell lung cancer is rapidly progressive and has a median survival of 6 weeks.

Box 17.1 WHO classification of lung tumors (1999)

- Squamous cell carcinoma
- Small cell carcinoma
- Adenocarcinoma
- Large cell carcinoma
- Adenosquamous carcinoma
- Pleomorphic/sarcomatoid

Clinical features

Smokers with chest symptoms, especially those aged over 50, need investigation.

Symptoms and signs

These may be due to local tumor effects, metastatic tumor effects, or paraneoplastic manifestations. Many patients have no specific signs. In some patients, lung cancer is found as an incidental finding on CXR performed for another reason. Only 5%–10% is asymptomatic, and 15% of patients have extrapulmonary symptoms.

Local tumor effects
- Persistent cough, or change in usual cough
- Hemoptysis
- Chest pain (suggests chest wall or pleural involvement)
- Unresolving pneumonia or lobar collapse
- Unexplained dyspnea (due to bronchial narrowing or obstruction)
- Wheeze or stridor
- Shoulder pain (due to diaphragm involvement)
- Pleural effusion (due to direct tumor extension or pleural metastases)
- Hoarse voice (tumor invasion of left recurrent laryngeal nerve)
- Dysphagia
- Raised hemidiaphragm (phrenic nerve paralysis)
- Superior vena cava obstruction (SVCO)
- Horner syndrome (miosis, ptosis, enopthalmos, anhidrosis) due to apical or Pancoast tumor
- Pancoast tumors can directly invade sympathetic chain and brachial plexus and rib. They cause weakness of small muscles of the hand—C5/6, T1 motor loss, and shoulder pain.

Metastatic tumor effects
- Cervical or supraclavicular lymphadenopathy (common, present in 30%, and may be an easy site for diagnostic biopsy)
- Palpable liver edge
- Bone pain or pathological fracture due to bone metastases
- Neurological sequelae secondary to cerebral metastases (median survival of NSCLC with brain metastases is 2 months)
- Hypercalcemic effects (due to bony metastases or direct tumor production of parathyroid hormone [PTH]-related peptide)
- Dysphagia (compression from large mediastinal nodes)

Paraneoplastic syndromes
- Cachexia and wasting
- Clubbing (any cell type, more common in squamous and adenocarcinoma)
- Syndrome of inappropriate ADH (SIADH; mainly SCLC)
- Ectopic adrenocorticotropic hormone (ACTH; Cushing syndrome, but due to rapid development, biochemical changes predominate; mainly SCLC)

- Hypertrophic pulmonary osteoarthropathy (HPOA, often in association with clubbing, any cell type; more common in squamous and adenocarcinoma), Eaton–Lambert myasthenic syndrome—both with SCLC. Affects proximal limbs and trunk, with autonomic involvement and hyporeflexia and only a slight response to edrophonium. Repeated muscle contraction may lead to increasing strength and reflexes. Symptoms may predate lung cancer by up to 4 years.
- Cerebellar syndrome (usually SCLC)
- Limbic encephalitis (usually SCLC)

Lymphangitic carcinomatosa

This is characterized by infiltration of pulmonary lymphatics by tumor. It may be due to lung cancer or breast, prostate, stomach, or pancreatic malignancies. It causes shortness of breath and cough, and is often associated with systemic signs of advanced malignancy.

Lymphangitic carcinomatosa may be visible on CXR as fine linear shadowing throughout both lung fields. Septal lines are present. It may look like pulmonary edema, and is easily diagnosed on CT.

Oral steroid treatment and diuretics can give symptomatic relief, but it is usually a short-lived response. Often this condition is part of a rapid decline.

Investigations

Patients should be referred under the "2-week cancer wait" scheme and be seen within 14 days of referral. The aim of the investigations is to reach a histological diagnosis and tumor stage, in order to determine the most appropriate treatment.

Outpatients

- **History and examination**, including smoking and occupational histories
- **Pulmonary function test/spirometry** before biopsy or surgery
- **CXR** (posteroanterior [PA] and lateral) for location of lesion, pleural involvement, pleural effusion, rib destruction, intrathoracic metastases, mediastinal lymphadenopathy. The CXR can be normal.
- **Blood tests**, including sodium, calcium, and liver function tests. Check coagulation profile if biopsy is planned.
- **Sputum cytology** is indicated only in patients who are unfit for bronchoscopy or biopsy.
- **Diagnostic pleural tap** if effusion present
- **Fine needle aspiration (FNA)** of enlarged supraclavicular or cervical lymph nodes

Radiology

CT chest, liver, adrenals (contrast-enhanced)

These are done to assess tumor site and size. Lung cancers frequently metastasize to the mediastinal lymph nodes, liver, and adrenals. CT can show lesions amenable to biopsy (either primary tumor or a metastasis).

CT can be used to assess the size of local and regional lymph nodes; it is poor at assessing whether enlarged nodes are reactive (inflammatory) or represent metastatic spread (79% sensitive, 78% specific). It can be used to assess tumor invasion to the mediastinum and chest wall.

Ultrasound scan

Ultrasound of the neck or liver may provide information about enlarged lymph nodes or metastases suitable for biopsy.

MRI

MRI is used to answer specific questions relating to tumor invasion and borders. It is good for assessing brachial plexus involvement, but has no role in nodule assessment.

Bone scan

A bone scan is indicated with any suggestion of metastatic disease, such as bony pain, pathological fracture, hypercalcemia, or raised alkaline phosphatase. It is highly suggestive of bony metastases if there are multiple areas of increased uptake. Solitary lesions may require further evaluation.

CT head

This is indicated only if there is neurological evidence of metastatic disease, such as persistent vomiting, focal neurological signs, headache, unexplained confusion, or personality change.

Positron emission tomography (PET scanning)

PET is an imaging technique in which metabolically active tissues such as tumors take up more of a radiolabeled 18-fluorodeoxyglucose (FDG) molecule. They then show as a "hot spot."

Use of PET improves the rate of detection of local and distant metastases in patients with NSCLC. It is useful for assessing regional and mediastinal lymph nodes (88% sensitive, 93% specific). PET is becoming more widely used and should be interpreted with the CT.

PET-positive nodes that would exclude a patient from surgery should be confirmed as malignant with a biopsy, unless the pre-test probability of malignancy is high. False negatives occur in tumors with low metabolic activity (such as carcinoids and bronchoalveolar carcinoma), small nodules, and hyperglycemic patients. False positives occur in patients with benign pulmonary nodules with a high metabolic rate, such as infective granulomata.

Multidisciplinary team (MDT)

The MDT should include a chest physician, radiologist, thoracic surgeon, oncologist, radiation oncologist, pathologist, lung cancer nurse, and palliative care specialist, who meet regularly to discuss patients' conditions and needs and plan the most appropriate course of management.

Most health-care institutions take advantage of the MDT in decision making for the treatment and investigation of all patients with lung cancer.

Diagnostic procedures

Aspects of further investigation may be inappropriate if the patient has advanced disease, is frail with comorbid conditions, or does not want to pursue diagnosis.

Bronchoscopy

This method of obtaining histological and cytological specimens is suitable for central tumors. Tumors can be washed, brushed, and biopsied. Transbronchial needle aspiration of lymph nodes is performed to aid staging. Bronchoscopic samples are more likely to be histologically positive if there is

- An ill-defined lesion on CXR
- An endobronchial component to the tumor
- Tumor <4 cm from the origin of the nearest lobar bronchus
- A segmental or larger airway leading to the mass

Bronchoscopy has greater diagnostic yield if it is performed after the CT scan, as radiologically abnormal areas can be targeted.

Tumor position bronchoscopically may contribute to operative decisions: tumor confined to a lobar bronchus may be resectable with lobectomy, tumor <1 cm from the main carina requires pneumonectomy, left vocal cord paralysis indicates inoperability due to tumor infiltration of the left recurrent laryngeal nerve, and a splayed carina occurs secondary to enlarged mediastinal nodes.

Image-guided biopsy

Image guidance is used to perform biopsy of tumor or an enlarged lymph node, especially in the neck, or of a metastasis. This technique has 85%–90% sensitivity in lesions >2 cm. Modalities include CT scanning and ultrasound via transthoracic, esophageal (EUS), and endobronchial (EBUS) routes.

Mediastinoscopy

This biopsy of enlarged mediastinal lymph nodes is used to determine whether they are inflammatory or have malignant invasion. The method entails suprasternal notch incision under general anesthetic, blunt dissection, palpation, and endoscopic visualization and biopsy of nodes: paratracheal, prevascular, tracheobronchial, and anterior subcarinal.

Mediastinoscopy has 93% sensitivity and 96% specificity. It is technically more difficult with SVCO. Bleeding occurs in <0.3%, left recurrent laryngeal nerve injury in 1%. Pneumothorax, mediastinal emphysema, infection, and esophageal perforation can also occur (all rare). Repeat mediastinoscopies have a lower positive yield and higher complication rate.

Mediastinotomy

Mediastinotomy is used for biopsy of aortopulmonary, subaortic, phrenic, or hilar nodes. Metastatic involvement of these nodes does not necessarily preclude curative surgical resection with a pneumonectomy. It is also used to assess direct tumor invasion of the central pulmonary artery or thoracic aorta, which would preclude curative surgery. The method entails right or left parasternal incision, blunt dissection, palpation, and endoscopic visualization and biopsy of nodes.

Thoracoscopy

Thoracoscopy may be required to determine whether a pleural effusion contains malignant cells or is inflammatory, for example, due to pneumonia caused by an obstructing lesion. Malignant effusions are evidence of T4 disease and are hence a contraindication to surgery.

Operative

It is sometimes difficult to obtain definitive cytology or histology preoperatively. If there is high suspicion of malignancy, surgery can be performed regardless. Patients undergoing surgery are given a pathological stage, which is sometimes different from the clinical stage, because resection margins, lymph nodes, and the pleura can be sampled histologically.

Box 17.2 Radiologically guided lung biopsy

Indications
- New or enlarging mass, not amenable to bronchoscopy
- Multiple chest nodules in patient not known to have malignancy
- Persistent undiagnosed single or multiple focal infiltrates
- Hilar mass

Pre-biopsy preparation
- Discuss with MDT
- Recent spirometry, with FEV_1>35% predicted
- Check APTT and PT <1.4 and platelets >100,000/mL. If not, discuss with hematologist to determine whether it is safe to proceed.
- Recent imaging available
- High-risk patients should have overnight admission following biopsy.
- Written information for patient, with informed signed consent

Biopsy preparation
- Perform without sedation if possible
- Use ultrasound scanning if possible
- Local anesthetic to skin and subcutaneous tissue
- Perform at least two passes, may use FNA or cutting needle. FNA has a high diagnostic yield for malignant lesions (95%), but less for benign ones (10%–50%). Cutting needles are good for malignancy and better for benign diagnoses. Use of either is the operator's decision.

Post-biopsy
- Observation by staff for 1 hour in case of complications
- Upright CXR 1 hour after biopsy
- Small pneumothoraces often resolve spontaneously, but may need inpatient admission if there are concerns. Chest tube drainage may be necessary for larger pneumothoraces.

Complications
- 20% chance of pneumothorax, 3% of patients require a chest drain
- Hemoptysis 5%, death 0.15%

Manhire A, Charig M, Clelland C, et al. (2003). Guidelines for radiologically guided lung biopsy. *Thorax* **58**: 920–934.

Staging

The current staging systems employ a two-stage (limited, extensive) system for SCLC, and the TMN approach for NSCLC, using clinical and radiological tools to categorize tumor size, location, and regional and distant spread (see Table 17.1 and Table 17.2). The currently used system is due to be revised in January 2009, with recommendations from the International Association for the Study of Lung Cancer.

Small cell lung cancer is staged as

• *Limited* is confined to ipsilateral hemi-thorax, including ipsilateral hilar, mediastinal, and supraclavicular lymph nodes. The area is encompassed by one radiation port.

• *Extensive* is everything else.

Non-small cell lung cancer is commonly classified using the TNM staging system. Frequency of patient stage at diagnosis:

• I and II—20%
• III—35%
• IV—45%

Table 17.1 TNM staging of lung cancer

Extent of primary tumor (T)

Tx	Primary tumor cannot be assessed, or tumor proven by malignant cells in sputum or bronchial washings but not visualized by imaging or bronchoscopy
T0	No evidence of primary tumor
T1	Tumor <3 cm surrounded by lung or visceral pleura, without bronchoscopic evidence of invasion more proximal than the lobar bronchus
T2	Tumor >3 cm, or in main bronchus, >2 cm distal to carina or invading visceral pleura or associated with atelectasis or obstructive pneumonitis that extends to the hilar region, but does not involve whole lung
T3	Tumor of any size that invades chest wall, diaphragm, parietal pericardium, or mediastinal pleura, or tumor in main bronchus <2 cm distal to carina, or associated atelectasis or obstructive pneumonitis of the entire lung
T4	Tumor of any size invading mediastinum, heart, great vessels, trachea, esophagus, carina, or vertebral body, or separate nodules in the ipsilateral lobe as primary tumor, or malignant pleural or pericardial effusion

Regional lymph nodes (N)

Nx	Cannot be assessed
N0	No regional lymph node metastasis
N1	Ipsilateral peribronchial and/or ipsilateral hilar nodes and intrapulmonary nodes involved by direct extension of tumor
N2	Ipsilateral mediastinal and/or subcarinal nodes
N3	Contralateral mediastinal, hilar nodes, or any scalene or supraclavicular nodes

Distant metastasis (M)

Mx	Cannot be assessed
M0	No distant metastasis
M1	Distant metastasis present, including separate nodules in different lobes

Table 17.2 Lung cancer clinical staging and survival

Stage	TNM subset	After treatment survival (%)	
		1 year	5 years
IA	T1 N0 M0	72	61
IB	T2 N0 M0		38
IIA	T1 N1 M0	79	34
IIB	T2 N1 M0	61	24
	T3 N0 M0	55	22
IIIA	T1 N2 M0	50	13
	T2 N2 M0	50	13
	T3 N1–2 M0	56	9
IIIB	T4 N0–2 M0	37	7
	T1–4 N3 M0	32	3
IV	Any T, Any N, M1	20	1

Although not recognized by the American Joint Committee on Cancer (AJCC), stage IIIA (N2) disease can be divided into the following:
• IIIA1 = (+) nodes found on final resection specimen
• IIIA2 = (+) nodes (single station) found intraoperatively
• IIIA3 = (+) nodes (single/multiple stations) on preoperative staging
• IIIA4 = (+) bulky or fixed multistation nodes

The role of neoadjuvant chemotherapy and radiotherapy given prior to surgery in stage IIIA3 (N2) disease in NSCLC is currently being studied. The concept is that such therapy may result in tumor shrinkage and eradication of micrometastases, thus allowing for possible complete resection.

Lymph node stations

Superior mediastinal nodes
1. Highest mediastinal
2. Upper paratracheal
3. Pre-vascular and retrotracheal
4. Lower paratracheal (including azygos nodes)

Aortic nodes
1. Subaortic (aortopulmonary [AP] window)
2. Para-aortic (ascending aorta or phrenic)

Inferior mediastinal nodes
1. Subcarinal
2. Paraesophageal (below carina)
3. Pulmonary ligament

N1 nodes
1. Hilar
2. Interlobar
3. Lobar
4. Segmental
5. Subsegmental

Further information

Hensing TA (2005). Clinical evaluation and staging of patients who have lung cancer. *Hematol Oncol Clin North Am* **19**:219–235.

Mountain CF (2000). The international system for staging lung cancer. *Semin Surg Oncol* **18**:106–115.

Robinson LA, Wagner H Jr, Ruckdeschel JC, et al. (2003). Treatment of stage IIIA non-small cell lung cancer. *Chest.* **123**:202S–220S.

Non-small cell lung cancer (NSCLC): surgery

Much of the investigation of lung cancer is to determine whether a patient has potentially curable disease by surgery. Other treatment options consist of chemotherapy, radiotherapy, and best supportive care, i.e. symptom-based conservative management. The MDT decides on the most appropriate choice of treatment to be discussed with the patient.

Surgery

The aims of surgery for lung cancer are to completely excise the tumor and local lymphatics, with minimal removal of functioning lung parenchyma.

- Stages I and II non-small cell lung cancers are usually amenable to surgery if the patient is fit enough. This has a high chance of cure in stage I (70% in IA), and a reasonable chance in stage II. Following surgical resection, postoperative chemotherapy is administered for stage II patients.
- In Stage IIIA tumors, options include neoadjuvant chemotherapy and radiation therapy followed by surgery, or chemotherapy and radiation therapy only.
- Stages IIIB: Except for some with T4N0M0 disease, treatment is chemotherapy and radiation. For patients with poor performance status, treatment is radiation only.
- Stage IV disease is almost always inoperable, and chemotherapy improves survival time. For good performance status, chemotherapy provides 4-month survival and quality-of-life benefits. For poor performance status, provide best supportive care.

Resectability of a tumor implies the likelihood of complete removal by surgery; this is different from patient *operability*, which is determined by the patient's fitness for surgery.

Fitness for surgery

Age

Age is not a contraindication, although increasing age is associated with an increased preoperative morbidity. There is a higher mortality risk if the patient is over 80 and if pneumonectomy rather than lobectomy is performed (14% mortality vs. 7%, respectively). Right pneumonectomy has a higher mortality than left pneumonectomy (more lung is removed). Two-year postoperative survival is similar to that of other age groups.

Lung function

Patients need FEV_1 >1.5 L post-bronchodilators for lobectomy, and >2 L post-bronchodilator for pneumonectomy or >60% of predicted. Borderline cases may require further lung function assessment (arterial saturation, full pulmonary function tests [PFTs] including DLCO, isotope perfusion scan, exercise testing), to calculate whether the predicted postoperative FEV_1 >40% is in association with DLCO >40%.

If both are below <40% predicted, exercise testing can be used to identify surgical candidates for those with VO_2max >15 mL/kg/min. Those with VO_2max <15 mL/kg/min are at high risk of perioperative complications and mortality and are best managed by nonsurgical modalities.

Cardiovascular

Postpone surgery if the patient has had a myocardial infarction (MI) within 6 weeks. Get a cardiology opinion if the patient has had an MI within 6 months. Order an echocardiogram (Echo) if they have heart murmur. Order a preoperative ECG for all surgical patients.

CNS

If there is any history of transient ischemic attacks (TIAs), strokes, or carotid bruits the patient will need carotid Doppler studies, and a vascular surgeon's opinion if necessary.

Nutritional

Nutritional requirements should be optimized, with advice from a dietitian if necessary.

Types of surgery

Lobectomy or bilobectomy

These techniques are used for localized tumor, or pneumonectomy for tumor involving more than one or two lobes. If hilar nodes are infiltrated by tumor a more radical lobectomy or a pneumonectomy is required. The local lymph nodes are removed in each procedure for pathological staging.

Wedge excision

Wedge excision is used to remove only the tumor with minimal surrounding lung parenchyma, and may be performed for a localized peripheral lesion with clear regional lymph nodes, especially if the postoperative respiratory function is predicted to be borderline. There is a higher local recurrence rate, however (up to 23%).

Sleeve resections

Sleeve resections involve a lobectomy and the removal of a section of bronchus affected by tumor, forming an anastomosis between the airway proximal and distal to it. This may avoid a pneumonectomy. Resection margins should be macroscopically free from tumor.

If there is limited local tumor invasion to the chest wall, this can be resected with a 5 cm margin. Reconstruction with prosthetic material may be necessary if two or more ribs are resected, aiming to preserve chest wall function.

Postoperative complications

These include bronchopleural fistula, respiratory failure, infection, phrenic nerve damage causing diaphragmatic paralysis, recurrent laryngeal nerve damage causing hoarse voice, and prolonged chest wall pain.

Mortality is 1%–3.5% for wedge excision, 2%–4% for lobectomy, and 6%–8% for pneumonectomy. Risk increases with increasing age, associated ischemic heart disease, impaired respiratory function, and poor performance status.

Following surgery
Patients are often followed up by the chest clinic every 6 months for CXR or chest CT review. This is to ensure that they are radiologically clear of tumor recurrence, and that there is not a second primary tumor. They should also be advised to seek earlier review if they have symptoms of persistent hemoptysis or new cough, weight loss, or new chest pain.

Further information

Beckles MA, Spiro SG, Colice GL, Rudd RM (2003). The physiologic evaluation of patients with lung cancer being considered for resectional surgery. *Chest* **123** :105S–114S.

British Thoracic Society, Society of Cardiothoracic Surgeons of Great Britain, and Ireland Working Party (2001). Guidelines on the selection of patients with lung cancer for surgery. *Thorax* **56**:89–108.

Detterbeck FC, DeCamp MM Jr, Kohman LJ, Silvestri GA (2003). Invasive staging: the guidelines. *Chest* **123**: 167S–175S.

NSCLC: chemotherapy

- Consider chemotherapy in patients with stage II, III, or IV disease, Eastern Cooperative Oncology Group (ECOG) performance status 0 to 2 (see also Box 17.3), even if they are asymptomatic from their cancer (greater toxicity in those with poorer performance status).
- 40% respond temporarily
- Small improvement in symptom control and quality of life compared to that with best supportive care
- Limited survival gains, 6–7 weeks compared to best supportive care
- Combination chemotherapy (the use of more than one drug) is superior to single-agent chemotherapy.
- Commonly used **first-line regimens** include gemcitabine or vinorelbine plus a platinum-based drug (carboplatin or cisplatin), usually given for 4 cycles.
  - *Side effects*: Nausea, myelosuppression, ototoxicity, peripheral neuropathy, nephropathy if dehydrated. No alopecia
- Treatment is given for 4–6 cycles, which takes about 4–5 months to complete.
- Patients are monitored during chemotherapy with repeat CT, usually after 2 cycles, to establish whether they have partial response, stable disease, or progressive disease (see Box 17.4), despite chemotherapy. This CT finding influences decisions regarding further chemotherapy.

Second-line treatments can be given in patients who relapse and are of good performance status. Taxanes (paclitaxel, docetaxel) are the most commonly used agents. These cause alopecia. Erlotinib, an epidermal growth factor receptor (EGFR)-tyrosine kinase inhibitor, has recently been used, showing 2-month survival benefit. There is no role for combination therapy in second-line treatments.

- Neoadjuvant chemotherapy is used with surgery in stage IIIa disease, in some centers, usually as part of a clinical trial.

Box 17.3 ECOG performance status

0 = Fully active, able to carry on all pre-disease performance without restriction

1 = Restricted in physically strenuous activity but ambulatory and able to carry out work of a light or sedentary nature, e.g., light house-work, office work

2 = Ambulatory and capable of all self-care but unable to carry out any work activities. Up and about more than 50% of waking hours

3 = Capable of only limited self-care, confined to bed or chair more than 50% of waking hours

4 = Completely disabled. Cannot carry out any self-care. Totally confined to bed or chair.

Oken MM, Creech RH, Tormey DC, et al. (1982). Toxicity and response criteria of the Eastern Cooperative Oncology Group. *Am J Clin Oncol* **5**:649–655.

Box 17.4 Response evaluation criteria in solid tumors

Evaluation of target lesions

- **Complete response (CR)**—disappearance of all target lesions
- **Partial response (PR)**—at least a 30% decrease in the sum of the longest diameter of target lesions
- **Progressive disease (PD)**—at least a 20% increase in the sum of the longest diameter of target lesions
- **Stable disease (SD)**—neither sufficient shrinkage to qualify for PR, nor sufficient increase to qualify for PD

Evaluation of non-target lesions

- **Complete response**—disappearance of all non-target lesions and normalization of tumor marker level
- **Incomplete response/stable disease**—persistence of one or more non-target lesion(s) or/and maintenance of tumor marker level above the normal limits
- **Progressive disease**—appearance of one or more new lesions and/or unequivocal progression of existing non-target lesions

Further information

Chemotherapy and non-small-cell lung cancer. *Drug Ther Bull* 2002; **40**(2):9–11.
Molina JR, Adjei AA, Jett JR (2006). Advances in chemotherapy of non-small cell lung cancer. *Chest* **130**:1211–1219.

NSCLC: radiotherapy

Radiotherapy may be given for
• Curative intent (high dose)
• Palliative control (high dose)
• Symptom relief (low dose)

Radiotherapy has a role in the treatment of early but medically inoperable but potentially curable stage I disease, tumors with positive margins, or incompletely resected tumors. Neoadjuvant radiotherapy is used in Pancoast tumors, locally advanced unresectable disease (such as stage IIIA3–4, IIIB, often with concurrent or sequential chemotherapy), and in the palliation of advanced lung cancer of all types for control of pain, hemoptysis, SVC syndrome, and atelectasis.

CHART (continuous hyperfractionated accelerated radiotherapy) is high-dose radiotherapy given with curative intent.
• Recommended for patients with localized chest disease >5 cm, stage I to II with performance status 0 to 1, who are resectable but unfit for surgery or do not want surgery
• Small radiation doses three times a day for 12 days (54 Gy in 36 fractions over 12 days)
• Patients are often inpatients for the duration of their therapy, to facilitate their frequent radiotherapy sessions.
• Less morbidity than that with conventional radical radiotherapy
• A large, randomized control trial has shown an improvement in 2-year survival from 20% with conventional radical radiotherapy to 29% with CHART. The largest benefits were in patients with squamous cell carcinoma.
• Severe dysphagia is more likely with CHART in the first 3 months than with conventional radiotherapy.

High-dose palliative radiotherapy is given to patients with symptomatic disease, good performance status, and no evidence of metastases, and who will be able to tolerate a high-dose regimen. An example of such a regimen is 36–39 Gy in 12–13 fractions over 6 weeks.

Low-dose radiotherapy is given for symptom relief in patients who would be unable to tolerate high-dose palliative radiotherapy or those with evidence of metastases. Symptoms may include pain, hemoptysis, breathlessness, or cough.

Urgent radiotherapy is used in combination with oral steroids for relief of superior vena cava obstruction by tumor, although stenting performed via CT angiography is the treatment of choice. Radiotherapy has no benefit following complete primary tumor surgical resection.

Chemoradiotherapy is used to improve tumor radiosensitization for localized disease. There may be some additional advantages with treatment of potential distant micrometastases. Some early survival benefits have been shown, and further studies are underway.

Further information

Saunders M, Dische S, Barrett A, et al. (1997). Continuous hyperfractionated accelerated radiotherapy (CHART) vs. conventional radiotherapy in non-small-cell lung cancer: a randomised
multicentre trial. CHART Steering Committee. *Lancet* **350**: 161–165.
Senan S, lagerwaard FW (2005). Role of radiotherapy in non-small cell lung cancer. *Ann Oncol*
16(Suppl 2): 223–228.

Small cell lung cancer: treatment

Chemotherapy

Combination chemotherapy is used for limited and extensive SCLC.

- Etoposide with either cisplatin or carboplatin is the standard regimen.
- Given 3-weekly, commonly initially for 2 cycles for induction and up to 6 cycles for consolidation
- Different regimens are selected according to performance status.
- Patients with performance status 3 may benefit from less intensive outpatient chemotherapy on a 3-weekly basis.
- Patients are carefully assessed and, if there is no sign of a response to treatment based on CXR or CT scan, they are switched to second-line agents.
- Complete response in 20%–30% in extensive disease; 45%–75% in limited disease with radiotherapy
- Chemotherapy may increase survival to 14 months in limited disease.

Radiotherapy

- Patients with limited stage disease who are reasonably well and obtain a partial response or better from chemotherapy should go on to have consolidation radiotherapy to the chest disease.
- Prophylactic cranial radiotherapy is advised at completion of chemotherapy. This improves survival by 5.4% as well as quality of life. It may decrease metastases by 50%.
- In patients with extensive disease, including cerebral metastases, or poorer performance status, chemotherapy is given first. If there is a good response, palliative radiotherapy may be given on an individual patient basis.

Lung cancer: emerging areas

Target therapy

This therapy is aimed at specific molecular targets. Examples include EGFR-tyrosine kinase inhibitors such as gefitinib and erlotinib, and anti-angiogenesis antibodies such as bevacizumab (humanized anti-VEGF monoclonal antibody that neutralizes vascular endothelial growth factor [VEGF]).

Further information

- www.cancer.org
- www.cancerguide.org
- www.lungcanceronline.org
- www.lungusa.org
- www.thoracic.org

Superior vena caval obstruction (SVCO): etiology and clinical assessment

Obstruction of the flow of blood in the superior vena cava results in the symptoms and signs of SVCO. It is caused by two different mechanisms (which may coexist): 1) *external compression* or *invasion* of the superior vena cava by tumor extending from the right lung (four times more common than the left lung), lymph nodes, or other mediastinal structure, or 2) thrombosis within the vein.

Etiology

The most common cause is malignancy. Lung cancer and lymphoma together cause 94% of SVCO.

Malignant causes

Lung cancer

Up to 4% of lung cancer patients will develop SVCO at some point during their disease. Up to 10% of small cell lung cancers present with SVCO.

Lymphoma

Up to 4% of lymphoma patients will develop SVCO, most commonly in non-Hodgkin lymphoma. This usually occurs from extrinsic compression of the SVC by enlarged lymph nodes.

Other malignant causes

These include thymoma, mediastinal germ cell tumors, and tumors with mediastinal metastases (most common is breast cancer).

Benign causes

Benign causes include granulomatous disease, intrathoracic goiter, and central venous lines, portacaths, and pacemaker wires (causing thrombosis). SVCO was commonly due to untreated infection, such as syphilitic thoracic aortic aneurysm or fibrosing mediastinitis (due to actinomycosis, tuberculosis, blastomycosis, or aspergillus); these are all now rare.

Clinical features

- Facial and upper body edema with facial plethora, often with increased neck circumference, and a cyanotic appearance
- Venous distension of the face and upper body. SVCO due to malignancy usually develops over days to weeks, so an adequate collateral circulation does not have time to develop. Pemberton's sign, facial plethora, distress, and sometimes stridor after lifting the arms above the head for a few minutes may clarify the diagnosis.
- Breathlessness
- Headache—worse on bending forward or lying down
- Cough/hemoptysis or other signs of an underlying lung malignancy
- Hoarse voice
- Dysphagia
- Syncope/dizziness (reduced venous return)
- Confusion

Diagnosis is usually made clinically from the signs of facial and upper body swelling, with distension of superficial veins across the chest wall, neck, and upper arms.

Investigations

Previously considered a medical emergency, SVCO is now not thought to be immediately life threatening, making treatment less urgent and allowing a definitive diagnosis to be made prior to treatment. The exception to this rule is the patient who presents with stridor or laryngeal edema, which is a medical emergency.

CXR

Up to 85% of patients have an abnormal CXR (as lung malignancy is the most common underlying disorder). Mediastinal widening is common.

CT chest with contrast

This can be used to stage the underlying malignancy and image the venous circulation and collateral blood supply.

Tissue diagnosis

Usual practice is to obtain a tissue diagnosis of the underlying disease before starting treatment, as the underlying diagnosis can alter treatment markedly. Symptomatic obstruction will have been developing for some weeks prior to presentation. In the clinically stable patient, a delay of 24–48 hours is warranted to obtain the correct underlying diagnosis.

Radiotherapy prior to biopsy can lead to problems in making a subsequent histological diagnosis. Similarly, high-dose steroids can make the diagnosis of lymphoma difficult.

Cytological diagnosis

This may be obtained from the following:

- Pleural fluid
- Biopsy of an extrathoracic lymph node (e.g., supraclavicular nodes)
- Bronchoscopy, or mediastinoscopy if there is no endobronchial disease, may be needed, depending on CT features. There may be an increased risk of bleeding post-biopsy because of venous congestion, and anesthesia is theoretically more risky because of possible associated tracheal obstruction or pericardial effusion (potentially leading to hemodynamic compromise due to cardiac tamponade). These complications can be anticipated from the CT scan.
- Sputum

SVCO: management

This is usually in two phases:
- *Initial general treatment*: Oxygen, analgesia, sitting the patient upright (to reduce venous pressure), and steroids (in some)
- Followed by *treatment of the underlying disease* causing the SVCO, which depends on the tissue diagnosis. The major differential in terms of treatment is small cell carcinoma (initial chemotherapy), non-small cell carcinoma (initial radiotherapy), and lymphoma (chemotherapy). The presence of SVCO usually means that surgical resection of a NSCLC is not possible.

Steroids

There are limited trial data supporting the use of steroids in SVCO, prior to definitive treatment, but most clinicians would start them fairly promptly. Steroids may be useful in reducing edema and improving symptoms.

Ideally, a tissue diagnosis should be obtained before commencing steroids, but this may not always be possible. The problem arises when the underlying diagnosis is lymphoma; steroids may alter the histology, making a definitive diagnosis more difficult.

In an older smoker with an obvious CXR mass (in whom the diagnosis is likely to be lung cancer), steroids can probably be started without risk to the underlying histology.

Radiotherapy

Most (90%) patients are edema-free by 3–4 weeks. In those with a poor response to radiotherapy, only 25% survive 1 year.

Intraluminal stents

Stents are used for malignant SVCO, and will often be a first-line treatment while radiotherapy is planned. These are successful in 90% of cases, with relief of symptoms in most patients within 48 hours. They do not preclude subsequent radiotherapy or chemotherapy. It is not clear whether post-procedure anticoagulation is required.

Some centers advocate the use of low-dose warfarin anticoagulation (i.e., 1 mg/day), aiming for an international normalized ratio (INR) of <1.6. Thrombosis in the superior vena cava is not a contraindication to the procedure, as clot can be dispersed mechanically or with thrombolysis at the time or the procedure.

Stent complications

Stent migration is the major complication, but most patients do not live long enough for this to be a major problem.

Anticoagulation

Some recommend prophylactic anticoagulation in the presence of SVCO. There is a small increased risk of intracerebral bleeding, but the benefits of SVCO treatment may be limited by subsequent SVC thrombus if anticoagulation is not started. This treatment is controversial.

SVCO due to thrombosis

This is usually in association with central venous lines or pacemaker wires. If the clot is <5 days old (as judged by symptoms) thrombolysis is warranted. Subsequent oral anticoagulation may reduce recurrence.

Prognosis

Prognosis depends on the underlying disease and is unrelated to the duration of SVCO at presentation. The majority of SVCO cases are due to mediastinal spread of lung carcinoma, so the overall prognosis is generally poor. It depends on the patient's performance status, stage and extent of disease, and the cell type.

Further information

Rowell NP, Gleeson FV (2002). Steroids, radiotherapy, chemotherapy and stents for SVCO in carcinoma of the bronchus: a systematic review. *Clin Oncol (R Coll Radiol)* **14**:338–351.

Wilson LD, Detterbeck FC, Yahalom J (2007). Clinical practice. Superior vena cava syndrome with malignant causes. *N Engl J Med* **356**:1862–1869.

Hypercalcemia

Definition and etiology

A serum calcium level over 10.5 mg/dL is considered abnormal; border-line values need repeating. In malignancy a raised calcium level is due to increased osteoclast activity, either from bony metastases or the ectopic production of a PTH-like hormone. A serum level over 13 mg/dL is rare outside malignancy, although it can occur in sarcoidosis.

Clinical features

Values over 12 mg/dL are usually symptomatic. Common symptoms are confusion, weakness, nausea, reduced fluid intake, and constipation. There may be a short QT interval on ECG, and renal failure. These features are most commonly seen in squamous cell carcinomas.

Investigations

Exclude other causes of hypercalcemia and identify the tumor, although in most patients with malignant hypercalcemia the diagnosis of malignancy will already be known. The PTH will be suppressed in malignant hypercalcemia, but raised in hyperparathyroidism.

Phosphate will tend to be low in hyperparathyroidism and hypercalcemia due to ectopic PTH, and low or normal in sarcoidosis, metastatic bone disease, and with excess vitamin D. Check for renal failure.

Management

- Isotonic saline infusion (250 mL/hr initially, to reverse dehydration, but avoid fluid overload, reducing to 150 mL/hr) with furosemide to increase calcium excretion
- Steroids help, but less so than in sarcoid-associated hypercalcemia, partly through reduced intestinal absorption

In addition to this initial management:
- Reduce bone reabsorption with bisphosphonates (they take a few days to work maximally)
  - *Intravenous preparations*: Disodium pamidronate, sodium clodronate, zoledronic acid
  - *Oral preparations*: Clodronate. The bisphosphonates can also reduce the pain of secondary bony deposits and may reduce pathological fracture rate.

Syndrome of inappropriate ADH secretion (SIADH)

Definition and etiology

SIADH is excessive retention of water relative to electrolytes due to inappropriate production of ADH. Hence there is hyponatremia (<135 mEq/L), hypo-osmolality, urine osmolality >100 mOsmol/kg, urine sodium concentration usually above 40 mEq/L, normal acid–base (and potassium), and usually a low plasma urea concentration. Diuretic-induced hyponatremia will be accompanied by evidence of dehydration, e.g., raised urea.

Causes of SIADH include the following:

- Drugs, e.g., carbamezepine, fluoxetine, high-dose cyclophosphamide
- After major surgery
- Pneumonia
- HIV infection
- CNS disorders, e.g., stroke, infection, psychosis
- Small cell lung cancer, either ectopic ADH production or, rarely, stimulation of normal ADH production

Clinical features

Lethargy and confusion occur, often when sodium levels fall below 130 mEq/L and nearly always when below 120 mEq/L.

Investigations

A low sodium level in the presence of low urea and an appropriate clinical setting may be adequate to make a diagnosis. If sodium depletion and water overload are possible alternative causes of hyponatremia, they should be accompanied by a urine osmolarity <100 mOsmol/kg (or a specific gravity <1.003, or a urine sodium <40 mEq/L). Therefore, values increasingly above this are suggestive of SIADH (unless the patient is on loop diuretics, when urinary sodium concentration will be higher).

Management

- Fluid restriction (0.5–1.0 L/day) will help, but is often unpleasant for the patient.
- Demeclocycline blocks ADH action at the distal renal tubules and can be used long term.
- Salt tablets or extradietary salt
- May resolve over a few weeks following chemotherapy
- Hypertonic saline is rarely indicated and can provoke brainstem damage (demyelination) through rapid changes in osmolality.

Spinal cord compression

Prompt treatment is needed for spinal cord compression to prevent irreversible paraplegia and loss of bowel and bladder function.

Definition and etiology

Spinal cord compression occurs commonly in patients with metastatic cancer (in about 5% of all cancer patients, particularly breast, lung, and prostate cancer). It may be the first presentation of cancer, but often occurs with a known primary tumor.

Cord compression is commonly caused by direct spread from a vertebral metastasis into the extradural space. It is less commonly caused by pressure on the cord from a primary tumor in the posterior mediastinum or retroperitoneum, or pressure from a mass of retroperitoneal nodes.

It is unusual to have a metastasis within the cord itself, although meningeal spread can occur. Spinal cord compression causes interruption of the arterial supply to the cord and subsequent infarction.

Clinical features

Patients frequently experience back pain initially, due to associated vertebral collapse. This precedes any neurological signs. Pain is not, however, universal.

Neurological signs may be nonspecific: weak legs, constipation, and urinary incontinence. Leg weakness develops over hours to days, with associated sensory loss. Loss of bladder and bowel sensation is a late sign and usually herald irreversible paraplegia within hours or a few days.

Examination reveals bilateral upper motor neuron signs in the legs, with increased tone, weakness, brisk reflexes, and extensor plantars. There may be sensory loss in the legs, particularly with a loss of proprioception and a sensory level on the trunk. Sensory loss in the saddle area, with decreased rectal tone suggests a cauda equina lesion. The bladder may be palpable.

Investigations

Have a low threshold for investigating a patient with known cancer with back pain

- **MRI** of the spine is the investigation of choice to demonstrate the level of the cord compression
- **CT** is less reliable, but can also be helpful, if MRI is not available
- **Plain spine XR** may show vertebral metastases, but this is usually unhelpful, as there is no imaging of the spinal cord. Time should not be wasted in getting a plain XR
- **Bone scan** shows vertebral metastases, but again does not image the spinal cord. Earlier scans showing bony metastases may alert the physician to the possibility of future cord compression
- If patient is not known to have an underlying malignant disease, a search for a primary tumor should be performed, but must not delay treatment of the spinal cord compression. Take full history (weight loss, anorexia, specific symptoms) and perform full examination, CXR, blood tests, PSA, and myeloma screen.

Management

Management depends on tumor type and overall prognosis. Discuss with the oncologist and/or neurosurgeon to determine which definitive treatment(s) is the most appropriate for the patient.

- High-dose steroids (dexamethasone IV 4 mg/6 hours). These should be started while waiting for the MRI scan, if the clinical picture suggests cord compression.
- Radiotherapy to the metastasis or tumor causing cord compression, particularly if there are multiple sites of cord compression or if surgery is not advised
- Surgical decompression of the cord, reconstruction, and stabilization of the spinal column
- Catheter for urinary retention
- Care for pressure areas
- Deep vein thrombosis (DVT) prevention
- Consider chemotherapy if appropriate, for underlying cancer causing the spinal cord compression, once the initial treatment has taken place
- Rehabilitation, ideally in facilities with spinal cord expertise

A recent Dutch study showed 66% of patients with metastatic cord compression (from all cancers) admitted to rehabilitation centers were discharged. Average survival post-discharge was 808 days, and 52% were alive at 1 year.

Prognosis

Patients who are mobile at presentation have the best prognosis and are likely to have preserved neurological function following treatment. If there is some preserved motor function, 25% will be able to walk post-treatment. If paraplegia is present pretreatment, less than 10% of patients will be able to walk afterward. Loss of bladder function for more than 24–48 hours cannot be reversed.

Further information

Abdi S, Adams CI, Foweraker FL, O'Connor A (2005). Metastatic spinal cord syndromes: imaging appearances and treatment planning. *Clin Radiol* **60**:637–647.

Pulmonary carcinoid tumors

These are uncommon primary lung tumors, accounting for 1%–2% of all lung tumors. It has equal male–female incidence, with typical age at presentation being 40–50 years. They are a form of neuroendocrine tumor and can have a similar histological appearance to that of small cell lung cancer.

Pathophysiology

Although these tumors are typically slow growing and benign, more aggressive subtypes do exist, with metastatic potential. Commonly they are located endobronchially, but can also be located peripherally in the lung parenchyma.

Clinical features

- Endobronchial carcinoids can cause isolated wheeze, dyspnea, infection, hemoptysis, or persistent lobar collapse.
- Parenchymal carcinoids are often asymptomatic, being detected on routine CXR.
- Carcinoid syndrome, with flushing, tachycardia, sweats, diarrhea, wheeze, and hypotension, occurs in 1% of pulmonary carcinoid tumors.
- Carcinoid tumors can also be associated with Cushing's syndrome, due to ectopic tumor ACTH production.

Investigations

CXR

CXR may reveal a well-defined tumor, which should be further characterized on CT. *Tumorlets* is the description given to multiple endobronchial or parenchymal carcinoid tumors.

Bronchoscopy

Bronchoscopy is performed for accessible endobronchial carcinoid tumors. They typically appear to be intraluminal, cherry red, and covered with intact epithelium. Bronchial brushings may be adequate for a histological diagnosis.

Bronchial biopsy can be associated with brisk or torrential bleeding, so care should be taken. Some clinicians avoid biopsy altogether and proceed to surgical resection based on a clinical diagnosis. CT-guided biopsy may be preferred for peripheral tumors.

Histological diagnosis

Such diagnosis can be difficult, as the appearances can be similar to those of small cell lung cancer. Special stains and immunohistochemistry are used to help differentiate between the two conditions. Clinically, however, these tend to be quite different conditions and clinical details can aid pathological diagnosis.

Carcinoid tumors are characterized as being *typical* or *atypical*. They each have a characteristic pattern:

- *Typical carcinoids* have no necrosis, occasional nuclear pleomorphism, and absent or late mitoses. Distant metastases are rare and metastasis to lymph nodes occurs in 5%–15% of cases. The 5-year survival is 100% and 10-year survival is 87%.

- *Atypical carcinoids* may show focal necrosis and often have nuclear pleomorphism. There is increased mitotic activity. They have distant metastases in 20% and metastasize to the lymph nodes in up to 48% of cases. The 5-year survival is 69%, and 10-year survival is 52%.

Management

Patients with isolated pulmonary carcinoid tumors should be considered for surgical resection. Resection is ideally limited, removing minimal amounts of normal lung parenchyma. Tumor resection is associated with resolution of any features of the carcinoid syndrome

If the tumor is atypical or close to the resection margin, patients should be followed up with repeat CXR or chest CT annually. Radiotherapy is not performed.

Tumor size does not relate to the presence of lymph node metastases, thus local lymph nodes should be sampled perioperatively.

In the 1% with carcinoid syndrome, serotonin antagonists, such as octreotide, can be used for treatment. Isolated liver metastases can be treated with arterial embolization. Metastatic aggressive carcinoid tumors can be treated with chemotherapy, such as etoposide, cisplatin, 5-fluorouracil, and streptozotocin.

Further information

Hage R, de la Rivière AB, Seldenrijk SA, van den Bosch JM (2003). Update in pulmonary carcinoid tumors: a review article. *Ann Surg Oncol.* **10**:697–704.

Pulmonary nodules

Pulmonary nodules are focal, round, or oval areas of increased opacity in the lung, measuring <3 cm in diameter. They are detected on CXR or CT.

Greater use of CT and thinner slice spiral CT scanning has led to increased detection rates. CT allows the precise localization of a nodule and reliable determination of its features. It has a high sensitivity of detecting nodules of <5 mm in diameter.

Volumetric analysis using CT-aided software means that a 3D nodule can be simulated, to aid nodule characterization and assess whether its volume has increased over time. It is important to search for old imagings for comparison.

• Most pulmonary nodules are benign, although exact numbers depend on the characteristics of the population screened (see Table 17.3).
• 20%–30% of patients with lung cancer may present with a solitary pulmonary nodule.
• Of the nodules detected on CT in smokers with a normal CXR, between 1% and 2.5% will be malignant.
• The Early Lung Cancer Action Project screening program of CT scans in 60+ year-olds with at least a 10-pack year history of smoking in the United States found noncalcified nodules in 23%, which were seen on CXR in 7%; 11% of these nodules were malignant on biopsy.
• Early detection of these malignant nodules might alter patient management, with surgical resection of a stage 1 cancer.

Table 17.3 Causes of solitary pulmonary nodules

Benign	Malignant
Infectious granulomata	Lung cancer
Noninfectious granulomata	Solitary metastasis
Bronchial adenoma	
Benign hamartoma*	

* A developmental abnormality, benign hamartomas contain cartilage, epithelium, and fat. They can contain smooth muscle, and are slow growing. They can be seen at any age, especially 40+ years. They often calcify.

Management options for patients with pulmonary nodules
Observation/serial CT scans
Two-year nodule stability generally rules out neoplasms except for slow-growing indolent tumors such as bronchoalveolar carcinoma (BAC).

Incidentally found nodules can be followed serially with CT scanning based on Fleischner Society guidelines (see Table 17.4). Low-risk patients have no history or minimal history of smoking and other risk factors.

Note: The guidelines in Table 17.4 are not applicable for patients <35 years old, or patients with unexplained fevers or with extrathoracic malignancy.

If the nodule has increased in size or is showing features of malignancy, consider biopsy or proceed straight to surgical resection. A PET scan may be helpful in combination with CT if the nodule is increasing in size but cannot be biopsied.

Biopsy Difficult on small nodules <7 mm

Resection If nodule has features of malignancy and biopsy is not possible

Chemotherapy or radiotherapy If nodule is proven to be malignant, but surgical treatment is not indicated due to performance status

Combined-modality treatment

Table 17.4 Recommendation for follow-up and management of nodules *incidentally* detected at nonscreening CT

Nodule size (mm)	Low-risk patients	High-risk patients
≤4	No follow-up needed	Follow-up CT at 12 months; if unchanged, no further follow-up needed
>4–6	Follow-up CT at 12 month	Follow-up CT at 6–12 months, then 18–24 months
>6–8	Follow-up CT at 6–12 months, then 18–24 months	Follow-up CT at 3–6 months, then 9–12 months, and 24 months
>8	Follow-up CT at 3, 9, and 24 months (can consider other modalities such as PET, contrast-enhanced CT, and/or biopsy	Same as low-risk patient

Factors that suggest a pulmonary nodule is malignant

- Size >1 cm
- Smokers, older age
- Increasing volumetrically determined growth rates over time
- Increased enhancement with contrast, suggesting increased vascularity (>15 Hounsfield units)
- Irregular or spiculated margin, with distortion of adjacent vessels
- Associated ground-glass shadowing
- Cavitation with thick, irregular walls
- Pseudocavitation within nodule—bronchoalveolar cell carcinoma

Factors that suggest a pulmonary nodule is benign

- Stable or decreasing size for 2 years
- Nodule resolves during follow-up
- Nonsmoker
- Lack of enhancement with contrast
- Smooth, well-defined margins (although 21% of smooth nodules may be malignant)
- Benign pattern of calcification: central, diffuse solid, laminated, or popcorn like—related to prior infections or calcification in a hamartoma
- Intranodular fat—likely hamartoma
- Cavitation with thin smooth walls
- Younger age
- Resident in histoplasmosis endemic areas

Pulmonary nodule with extrathoracic malignancy

In a patient with preexisting malignancy, a pulmonary nodule could be a metastasis, new lung cancer, or benign disease. The histology of the extra-pulmonary neoplasm and the patient's smoking history influence this. These cases need discussion with the cancer MDT to determine whether nodule biopsy or treatment of the underlying primary cancer would be the most appropriate management.

One study determined the likelihood of a pulmonary nodule being a new primary or metastasis on the basis of site of the original cancer:

- **New lung primary more likely** if primary tumor is head and neck, bladder, breast, bile ducts, esophagus, ovary, prostate, or stomach
- **Metastasis more likely** if primary tumor is melanoma, sarcoma, or testes
- **Either new primary or metastasis possible** if primary tumor is salivary gland, adrenal, colon, parotid, kidney, thyroid, thymus, or uterus

Further information

Henschke CI, McCauley DI, Yankelevitz DF, et al. (1999). Early Lung Cancer Action Project: overall design and findings from baseline screening. *Lancet* **354**: 99–105.

Libby DM, Smith JP, Altorki NK, et al. (2004). Managing the small pulmonary nodule discovered by CT. *Chest* **125**:1522–1529.

MacMahon H, Austin J, et al. (2005). Guidelines for management of small pulmonary nodules detected on CT scans: a statement from the Fleischner Society. *Radiology* **237**:395–400.

Ost D, Fein A (2004). Management strategies for the solitary pulmonary nodule. *Curr Opin Pulm Med* **10**:272–278.

Quint LE, Park CH, Iannettoni MD (2000). Solitary pulmonary nodule with extra pulmonary neoplasms. *Radiology* **217**:257–261.

Lung cancer screening

This is an area that is actively being studied. Screening programs are based on the theory that early detection of lung cancer and any subsequent intervention will improve the patient's outcome.

There is no evidence yet of reduction in lung cancer mortality from screening studies. To be detectable on CXR, a lung cancer needs to be 1 cm in diameter, and 3–4 mm in diameter to be detectable on CT.

Screening studies

Four previous CXR screening studies in the 1970s were negative, of which the **Mayo Lung Project** has been the most studied. This compared 4-monthly CXR and sputum cytology for 6 years in 45+ year-old smokers of 20+ cigarettes per day, with infrequent or no screening in a control group. A total of 206 cancers were found in the study group and 160 in the control group, but all-cause mortality was not affected by screening, even at 20 years.

More recent studies have used low-dose spiral CT scanning. The **Early Lung Cancer Action Project (ELCAP)** in New York recruited 1000 symptom-free volunteers aged 60+ with a 10 pack-year history of smoking who would be fit for a thoracotomy. There was no control group. Baseline CXR and CT were performed. Noncalcified nodules were present in 23% of patients at baseline on CT. Repeat CT was performed for nodules <5 mm; nodules >6 mm were biopsied and nodules >11 mm received standard care. Of all the patients entered, 2.7% had malignant nodules, with stage 1 disease in 2.3%. All but one patient had their cancer surgically resected.

The National Institutes of Health (NIH) is currently conducting a multicenter randomized trial to assess the potential efficacy of lung cancer screening with chest CT in high-risk individuals with a significant smoking history. As yet, it is not clear whether chest CT screening improves mortality rates.

Further information

Kawahara M (2004). Screening for lung cancer. *Curr Opin Oncol* **16**:141–145.
McWilliams A, Lam S (2005). Lung cancer screening. *Curr Opin Pulm Med* **11**:272–277.

Mediastinal abnormalities

The *mediastinum* is the central area of the chest between the pleural cavities. It contains the heart, great vessels, nerves, lymph nodes, trachea, esophagus, and thymus.

Clinical presentations of mediastinal disease include masses (see Box 18.1), mediastinitis, and pneumomediastinum. Mediastinal disease may be asymptomatic or may present with cough or chest pain, as well as symptoms relating to any structure being compressed or invaded, such as dysphagia, stridor, or SVC obstruction. Nerve involvement may cause hoarseness, Horner's syndrome, or dyspnea due to diaphragmatic paralysis. Often asymptomatic masses are incidentally noted on CXR or other imaging study.

Diagnosis of most mediastinal abnormalities requires a tissue diagnosis (see also Box 18.2). This may be obtained via needle aspiration (transesophageal, transcutaneous, or transbronchial biopsy). More commonly, a surgical procedure is required; mediastinoscopy, video-assisted thoracoscopic surgery (VATS), or open thoracotomy is frequently employed.

Anatomy

Anterior mediastinum The area behind the body of the sternum, below the thoracic inlet and in front of the pericardium and great vessels. Contains the thymus and lymphatic tissue, and may contain portions of the thyroid and parathyroid glands. Some clinicians define a superior mediastinum that is the superior portion of this anterior compartment.

Middle mediastinum The area containing the heart and pericardium, the aortic arch, great vessels, the pulmonary arteries and veins, the trachea, phrenic nerves, and lymph nodes.

Posterior mediastinum The area posterior to the heart and trachea; it reaches to the posterior ribs and paravertebral gutters from the first rib to the diaphragm. It contains the esophagus, descending aorta, azygous and hemiazygous veins, paravertebral lymph nodes, thoracic duct, spinal nerve roots, the vagus nerve, and the sympathetic chain.

These areas are easily seen on a lateral CXR (see Fig. 18.1).

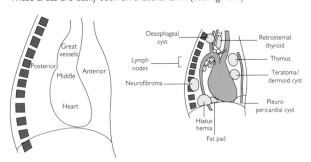

Figure 18.1 Anatomy of the mediastinum.

Box 18.1 Likely nature of mediastinal mass according to anatomic site

Anterior mediastinal mass
- Thymoma and other thymic neoplasms
- Germ cell tumors: teratoma, seminoma, nonseminomatous tumors
- Lymphoma
- Thyroid neoplasm
- Parathyroid neoplasm
- Mesenchymal tumor
- Ascending aortic aneurysm
- Pericardial fat pad
- Morgagni anterior diaphragmatic hernia

Middle mediastinal mass
- Lymphoma
- Lymphadenopathy
- Developmental cysts: foregut duplication cysts
- Vascular enlargement
- Hiatal hernia

Posterior mediastinal mass
- Neurogenic tumor
- Esophageal lesions
- Meningocele
- Descending aortic aneurysm
- Bochdalek posterior diaphragmatic hernia (p. 660)

Box 18.2 Approach to patients with a mediastinal mass

- Full history
- Examination, including skin and lymphadenopathy (neck, axillae, groin)
- Examine testes
- Look for fatigability: ptosis, ophthalmoplegia, unable to maintain upward gaze
- Look for signs of SVC obstruction or stridor
- Blood tests, including CBC, chemistry, and tests bases on clinical suspicion: thyroid studies (goiter), anti-acetylcholine receptor antibodies (thymic disease), AFP, β-hCG (germ cell tumor), catecholamine levels (neurogenic tumor)
- Chest CT scan
- Consider additional imaging: PET scan, MRI, or nuclear study
- Obtain a tissue biopsy

Mediastinal abnormalities

Primary mediastinal masses

These masses occur with an overall annual incidence of approximately 1 per 100,000. Neurogenic tumors, thymoma, duplication cysts, lymphoma, and germ cell tumors account for the most common causes in roughly descending order.

The epidemiology of mediastinal masses varies with age: children and young adults are more likely to have neurogenic tumors, while older adults are more likely to have thymoma or thyroid disease. Children are more likely to have malignant tumors (40%) than adults (25%). Persons with HIV have an increased incidence of reactive lymphadenopathy, granulomatous disease, and lymphoma.

Neurogenic tumors

These tumors occur mostly in the posterior mediastinum. They are named according to tissue of origin, and 75% are benign in adults.

- *Schwannomas and neurofibromas* are benign peripheral nerve sheath tumors. They may be multiple. Usually asymptomatic, they can cause segmental pain. They are treated with surgical excision.
- *Malignant peripheral nerve sheath tumors, or neurogenic fibrosarcomas,* may cause systemic features of malignancy and can invade locally or metastasize. Treatment is wide excision and adjuvant radiotherapy. Half of these tumors occur in a setting of neurofibromatosis.
- *Autonomic nervous system tumors,* including ganglioneuromas and neuroblastomas, range from benign to malignant. Resection is indicated, as is radiation and chemotherapy if the tumor is malignant.

Thymoma

Thymoma is the most common anterior mediastinal mass. Peak incidence is 40–60 years of age, with no gender predilection.

Myasthenia gravis is present in 30%–50% of patients with a thymoma; conversely 10%–12% of patients with myasthenia gravis have a thymoma, while 60%–70% have thymic hyperplasia.

The mechanism of myasthenia gravis is not completely known, but involves antibodies directed against acetylcholine receptors at the postsynaptic motor endplate, decreasing available acetylcholine binding sites and causing nerve fatigability.

Patients with thymomas are usually asymptomatic, but 1/3 may present with cough, chest pain, dyspnea, or myasthenia gravis symptoms. They are also associated with red cell aplasia, hypogammaglobulinemia, and other paraneoplastic syndromes.

CT scans are suggestive of thymoma, usually showing round or oval masses with smooth or lobulated margins. Diagnosis depends on tissue biopsy. Thymic neoplasms are defined as invasive if they cross tissue planes.

Surgical excision is the mainstay of treatment. Consider postoperative radiotherapy for invasive tumors, especially those not completely excised. Thymectomy is indicated in patients with myasthenia gravis even without thymoma, as it may lead to symptomatic improvement.

Thymic carcinoid

This is not associated with myasthenia gravis. It behaves aggressively, with local recurrence and metastasis. It may be associated with Cushing's syndrome, and is associated with MEN1 syndrome in 25% of cases.

Thymic carcinoid has a much worse prognosis than that of pulmonary carcinoid. Treatment with surgery or chemotherapy is not very effective.

Thymic carcinoma, thymic cyst, thymic lipoma, and thymic hyperplasia also occur.

Germ cell tumors

Germ cell tumors arise from immature germ cells during development. They tend to be in an anterior and mid-line location. They account for 10% of primary mediastinal masses.

Mature cystic teratomas

These teratomas represent 52%–75% of germ cell tumors. They are benign and occur primarily in young adults, with no gender predilection. They are defined as tissue foreign to an area where they are located.

Cystic teratomas are often asymptomatic, but can erode surrounding structures and cause symptoms. CXR shows a well-defined mass, which may contain flecks of calcification.

Treatment is by surgical excision. Teratocarcinoma is the malignant counterpart.

Seminoma

Seminoma occurs in men age 20–40 years. Mediastinal seminomas are malignant and almost always arise within the thymus and are histologically indistinguishable from those occurring in the testes. They can be a primary mediastinal tumor or metastasis from testicular tumor; therefore, always examine the testes.

Patients frequently present with chest pain. CXR shows a noncalcified, lobulated anterior mediastinal mass, confirmed with CT. Characteristically, human chorionic gonadotrophin, β subunit (β-hCG) is elevated, along with a normal serum α-fetoprotein (AFP). Diagnose with surgical biopsy.

Treatment is with chemotherapy and radiation. Even widely disseminated disease may be cured with aggressive cisplatin-based regimens. Long-term survival is expected in 80% of patients. Seminoma has a better prognosis than that of nonseminomatous germ cell tumors.

Nonseminomatous germ cell tumors

These include choriocarcinoma, embryonal cell carcinoma, and yolk sac tumors. They are malignant and occur in men in their 30s. Klinefelter syndrome is associated with increased risk of nonseminomatous germ cell tumors.

They are symptomatic due to local invasion and often disseminated at initial presentation. CXR shows mediastinal mass. Diagnosis is with surgical biopsy. β-hCG and AFP are elevated.

Treatment is with cisplatin-based chemotherapy. β-hCG and AFP are markers of disease and their levels will fall with tumor response. Long-term survival is 50%.

Thyroid

Retrosternal goiter occurs as an extension of a cervical goiter or arises from ectopic thyroid tissue. It is usually asymptomatic unless large and compressing the trachea or SVC.

It may be seen on plain CXR. Radioactive iodine isotope scans will demonstrate thyroid tissue. Flow-volume loops are abnormal if there is tracheal compression. Surgery is recommended if there is airway compromise; this can often be done via a transcervical approach.

Parathyroid

Mediastinal parathyroid adenomas and carcinomas are often functional. Mediastinal adenomas account for 10% of cases of hyperparathyroidism and are a primary cause of surgically resistant hyperparathyroidism.

Occasionally cysts are large enough to appear on plain films of the chest. Usually localization is improved by using a technetium-99m sestamibi nuclear imaging study, which localizes parathyroid activity. Treatment is resection.

Lymphoma

Primary mediastinal lymphoma is rare and accounts for <10% of cases. The mediastinum is involved in combination with extrathoracic sites in 60% of patients with Hodgkin disease and 10%–25% of non-Hodgkin disease. Lymphoma typically occurs in the anterior compartment followed by the middle mediastinum.

A CT scan is necessary to stage the extent of disease and assess response to treatment. To establish the histological diagnosis of lymphoma, an adequate tissue sample is required. This should be from a biopsy, rather than from a fine needle aspirate, and may be best achieved surgically, via mediastinoscopy.

Examine the patient for peripheral lymph nodes, as these may be easier to biopsy. Treatment is with radiation and/or chemotherapy initially.

Enlarged lymph nodes

Metastases from lung, breast, esophageal, and other primary cancers occur.

Granulomatous disease may include tuberculosis, sarcoidosis, or silicosis. Patients with HIV will present with increased mediastinal lymphadenopathy.

Castleman disease
Also known as angiofollicular lymph node hyperplasia, this disease is a lymphoproliferative disorder. There are two forms of the disease.

Unicentric or localized, asymptomatic disease occurs in the mediastinum or lungs. Focal disease presents as a smooth, lobulated mass.

The multicentric disease has significant systemic symptoms including fever, night sweats, weight loss, and neuropathy. Multicentric Castleman disease is associated with HIV infection and has been associated with HHV-8 infection. Diagnosis is based on surgical biopsy. It often requires an excisional biopsy to obtain enough tissue to clearly define the disease.

Treatment of focal disease is primarily resection and results in excellent long-term results. Multicentric disease does not respond well to treatment. Immune reconstitution with antiviral treatment for AIDS patients is beneficial in some cases.

Developmental cysts

These include pericardial, bronchogenic, and enteric cysts. They are named according to the type of tissue lining the cyst

Foregut duplication cysts

These cysts comprise bronchogenic and enteric cysts. They are derived from the ventral and dorsal embryologic foregut, and are often located posterior to the trachea. Usually asymptomatic, they may occasionally become infected or cause complications due to mass effects.

They can be identified on CT scan and diagnosed by needle aspiration for cytology. They are often diagnosed in childhood, as they cause dyspnea, stridor, or cough due to limited space to expand. Cysts are seen on CXR and CT, and are treated with surgical excision.

Pericardial cysts

Pericardial cysts occur mostly at the cardiophrenic angles and can measure up to 25 cm diameter. There is no gender predilection. They are usually asymptomatic, but may cause chest pain. CXR shows a smooth, round shadow abutting the heart. Excision can be carried out at thoracoscopy, but conservative management is often favored.

Mesenchymal tumors

These tumors comprise lipomas, fibromas, mesotheliomas, and lymphangiomas. Unless they are very large, symptoms suggest malignancy.

Inflammation

Mediastinitis

Mediastinitis describes infection or inflammation of the mediastinum. Most commonly it occurs after instrumentation leads to esophageal perforation. Classically, Boerhaave syndrome describes esophageal rupture due to forceful vomiting. Infections can also extend into the mediastinum from the neck (e.g., odontogenic infections) or from other intrathoracic infections.

Penetrating trauma, cardiac surgery, foreign-body ingestion, or erosion due to cancer or necrotizing infection may cause mediastinitis. Pancreatitis has been reported as a cause of mediastinitis, and pancreatic pseudocysts can develop in the mediastinum.

Patients with mediastinitis are severely ill, with pain and fever. CXR may show widened mediastinum or air in the mediastinum. Pneumothorax with or without pleural effusion may also be seen.

Treatment includes early surgical exploration, parenteral feeding, and antibiotics. Mediastinitis has high morbidity and mortality.

Mediastinal fibrosis

This rare, idiopathic condition occurs in middle age. Symptoms depend on which aspects of the mediastinum are involved, but may include dyspnea, wheeze, hemoptysis, hoarse voice, dysphagia, pulmonary hypertension, or SVC obstruction. CXR shows a widened mediastinum. Diagnosis is made on biopsy, particularly to exclude malignancy.

Treatment is supportive; steroids and surgical debulking are ineffective. Prognosis is variable, depending on the sites involved.

Mediastinal fibrosis is most commonly attributed to prior histoplasma infection in the United States. It is also associated with past tuberculosis infection, retroperitoneal fibrosis, autoimmune disease, prior radiotherapy, silicosis, or certain drug exposures (methysergide is best described).

Pneumomediastinum

Pneumomediastinum or mediastinal emphysema results from air escaping into the mediastinum. Air may originate from alveolar rupture related to barotraumas or may be spontaneous. It may result from sneezing, straining, Valsalva maneuvers, vomiting, substance abuse, parturition, positive pressure ventilation, instrumentation, or transbronchial biopsy.

Usually this condition is asymptomatic, but occasionally there is chest pain. Hamman's sign is positive (click or crunch with each heart beat on auscultation over precordium).

Treat with high-flow oxygen. Pneumomediastinum resolves spontaneously as the underlying insult resolves. Be prepared to emergently manage pneumothorax if a patient develops pneumomediastinum while receiving positive pressure ventilation.

Vascular

Aortic aneurysms are usually asymptomatic, but symptoms can arise from compression of adjacent structures. CXR may show a widened mediastinum. This is best imaged via CT or MRI. Surgery should be considered to prevent death from rupture.

Coarctation of the aorta, aneurysms of pulmonary vessels, and other vascular abnormalities may also give the appearance of a mediastinal mass on initial imaging.

Bacterial respiratory infection

Community-acquired pneumonia (CAP)

Community-acquired pneumonia is a common disease, associated with significant morbidity and mortality.

Definition CAP is a syndrome of infection with symptoms and signs of consolidation of part(s) of the lung parenchyma.

Epidemiology
- CAP is the most common infectious cause of death and the eighth leading cause of death in the United States.
- Overall incidence increases with age.
- Up to 20% of U.S. adults with CAP require hospital admission. Hospital mortality varies, between 5% and 12%.
- Mortality is up to 50% in those admitted to the ICU.
- CAP managed in the community has a mortality of 1%.

Pathophysiology
The lung and tracheobronchial tree are usually sterile below the level of the larynx, so an infecting agent must reach this site via a breach in host defenses. This may be by microaspiration (which occurs in around 45% of healthy individuals overnight), hematogenous spread, direct spread from an adjacent structure, inhalation, or activation of previously dormant infection. The development of CAP is suggestive of an overwhelming inoculum, a particularly virulent organism, or a defect in host defenses.

Etiology
Streptococcus pneumoniae is the most common cause; however, a broad range of microorganisms (bacterial, mycobacterial, viral, fungal, and parasitic) capable of causing disease (see Box 19.1). Bacteria have traditionally been divided into "typical" (*S. pneumoniae, H. influenza, S. aureus, M. catarrhalis*, group A streptococci, anaerobes, and aerobic gram-negative bacteria) and "atypical" (*Legionella* species, *M. pneumoniae, C. pneumoniae, C. psittaci*) organisms.

Risk factors for CAP
- *Aspiration* may be related to a multitude of predisposing conditions. Infection is typically caused by gram-negative organisms; oral anaerobes and mixed infections are more common.
- *Alcoholism and diabetes* are typically associated with bacteremic pneumococcal pneumonia. Anaerobes, gram-negative organisms, and mixed infections are more common in alcoholics because of their predisposition for aspiration with decreased levels of consciousness.
- *Oral steroids/immunosuppression* A variety of organisms are more common.
- *COPD Haemophilus influenzae* and *Moraxella catarrhalis, Pseudomonas aeruginosa*, and *Legionella* species are more common. Underlying COPD is more common in those with bacterial pneumonia.
- *Nursing home residents* have an increased frequency of pneumonia with aspiration, gram-negative organisms and anaerobes being more common than in age-matched elderly people. Drug-resistant organisms are a major concern in this population.

Box 19.1 Organisms causing community-acquired pneumonia

- *Streptococcus pneumoniae* (pneumococcus) is the most frequently identified organism, being most common in winter. Data suggest it is the cause of many culture-negative infections.
- *Legionella pneumophilia* is most common in autumn. Frequency is significantly higher in patients with severe CAP than in ambulatory patients, who have a rate of <1%. Epidemics occur in relation to exposure to aerosol-producing devices, including air conditioners, showers, whirlpool spas, and grocery store mist machines
- *Staphylococcus aureus* is most common in winter months. Community-acquired cases usually occur in the elderly or in younger patients as post-influenza infections. Increasing incidence of community-acquired methicillin-resistant *S. aureus* (MRSA) is an increasing concern and may be associated with influenza infection, often causing a severe, necrotizing pneumonia.
- Gram-negative bacilli, as a group, are the most commonly isolated organisms after pneumococcus. It includes *Klebsiella pneumoniae, Escherichia coli, Enterobacter* species, *Serratia* species, *Proteus* species, *Acinetobacter* species, and *Pseudomonas aeruginosa.*
- *Haemophillus Influenza* is an important cause of pneumonia in the elderly and in patients with underlying lung disease such as COPD.
- *Mycoplasma pneumoniae* is the most common organism seen in ambulatory cases (up to 15%). Infection rates are highest in military recruits, college students, and school-aged children and their contacts.
- *Pseudomonas aeruginosa.* Community-acquired cases most commonly occur in immunocompromised patients or in those with structural lung disease such as COPD and bronchiectasis.
- *Chlamydophila* (formerly *Chlamydia*) *pneumoniae* is most common in those aged 65–79 years, with very little seasonal variability.
- *Acinetobacter* species is an increasing cause of community-acquired infections and long seen as causative in resistant health-care-associated infections. Very high mortality rates are seen with this species and infections are much more common in tropical climates.

CAP: clinical features

- Fever
- Cough
- Mucopurulent sputum production
- Shortness of breath
- Pleuritic chest pain
- Nonspecific features in the elderly. May present with confusion and absence of fever

Examination

- Fever
- Tachypnea (may be the only sign in the elderly)
- Tachycardia
- Localizing signs on chest examination. Reduced chest expansion on the affected side, with signs consistent with consolidation (reduced air entry, with bronchial breathing, dullness to percussion, increased vocal resonance) and crackles. A normal chest examination makes the diagnosis less likely.

Diagnosis

Diagnosis of CAP is made on the basis of the following:
- Symptoms and signs of an acute lower respiratory tract infection
- New focal chest signs
- New radiographic shadowing, for which there is no other explanation
- At least one systemic feature (e.g., sweating, fevers, aches, and pains)
- No other explanation for the illness

Most helpful in diagnosis
- Fever, pleuritic pain, dyspnea, and tachypnea
- Signs on chest examination

Specific clinical features of pathogens

The etiological agent cannot be accurately predicted from the clinical features alone, although some features are more statistically likely with one pathogen than with another. The exception to this is the presence of chest pain or fever (>39°C) in those admitted to ICU, which predicts a higher likelihood of streptococcal pneumonia.

- *Streptococcus pneumoniae:* Increasing age, comorbidity (especially cardiovascular), acute onset, high fever, and pleuritic chest pain
- *Bacteremic Streptococcus pneumoniae:* Alcohol, diabetes, COPD, dry or no cough, female
- *Legionella:* Younger patients, smokers, absence of comorbidity, more severe infection, neurological symptoms, evidence of multisystem disease (e.g., abnormal liver enzymes and raised creatine kinase)
- *Mycoplasma pneumoniae:* Younger patients, prior antibiotics, less multisystem involvement, but extrapulmonary involvement, including hemolysis and skin and joint problems
- *Staphylococcus aureus:* Recent influenza-like illness

- *Chlamydia psittaci:* Longer duration of symptoms prior to admission, headache
- *Coxiella burnetti* (Q fever): Dry cough, high fever, male
- *Klebsiella pneumoniae:* Low platelet count and leukopenia, male

Rare causes
- *Acinetobacter:* Older patients, history of alcoholism, high mortality
- *Streptococcus milleri:* Dental or abdominal source of infection
- *Streptococcus viridans:* Aspiration is a risk factor

CAP: severity assessment

CAP has a wide range of severity. An assessment of severity enables the most appropriate care to be delivered in the most appropriate clinical setting.

Early identification of patients at high risk of death aids in decision making about hospital admission and the possible need for assisted ventilation.

Assessment of disease severity depends on the experience of the clinician. A number of predictive assessment models have been developed and evaluated, and should be regarded as adjuncts to clinical assessment. Regular reassessment of the disease is required.

Prognostic tools

The 2007 consensus guidelines from the Infectious Diseases Society of America (IDSA) and the American Thoracic Society (ATS) recommend using either the CURB-65 or pneumonia severity index (PSI) (see Table 19.1) as an aid in guiding decisions regarding the initial site of treatment for adults with CAP. These criteria are meant to be used within the clinical setting as a tool for assisting in the clinician's decision-making.

The CURB-65 scoring system is by far simpler, with a higher score predicting a higher risk of dying, but fails to take into account comorbid illness. Thus it may be of limited utility in older populations. The PSI has been best validated as a way to identify patients with low mortality.

CURB score core factors

- **C**onfusion—new mental confusion
- **U**rea—$\geq$7 mmol/L
- **R**espiratory rate $\geq$30/min
- **B**lood pressure—systolic BP $\leq$90 and/or diastolic BP $\leq$60
- **65** age $\geq$ 65

One point is given for each factor present. A score of 2 or more suggests need for inpatient treatment. Presence of the four "core" CURB factors correlates with mortality:

- 4 factors present gives a mortality of 83%; 3 factors, 33%; 2 factors, 23%, 1 factor, 8%, and no core factors, 2.4%
- Low risk of death: age <50, no coexisting disease, CURB score of zero

The CURB-65 score provides a complimentary guide to the PSI for the identification of the more severely ill.

Severe CAP

The ATS and IDSA have modified the criteria used to define severe CAP requiring admission to the ICU. *Severe CAP* is defined as a total of three of the following criteria: (major) need for mechanical ventilation or septic shock; (minor) respiratory rate >30, confusion, blood urea nitrogen (BUN) >20 mmol/L, leukopenia resulting from the infection, acidemia, hypothermia, multilobar disease, PaO_2/FiO_2 ratio below 250, or hypotension requiring aggressive volume resuscitation.

Table 19.1 Pneumonia severity index (PSI): criteria

Age	
Male	Age (years) − 0
Female	Age (years) − 10
Nursing home resident	10
Comorbidity illness	
Neoplastic disease	30
Hepatic disease	20
Congestive heart failure	10
Cerebrovascular disease	10
Renal disease	10
Physical findings	
Mental confusion	20
Respiratory rate > 30/min	20
Systolic blood pressure <90 mmHg	20
Temperature <35 or >40°C	15
Tachycardia >125 b.p.m.	10
Laboratory abnormalities	
Arterial pH<7.35	30
PaO_2 <60 mmHg	10
SaO_2 <90%	10
Blood urea nitrogen >11 mmol/l	20
Sodium <130 mmol/l	20
Glucose >250 mg/dl	10
Hematocrit <30%	10
Radiographic abnormalities	
Pleural effusion	10

Risk class I: age <50 years without cormorbidity or vital signs abnormality
Risk class II: <70 points
Risk class III: 71–90 points
Risk class IV: 91–130 points
Risk class V: >130 points

Classes I and II should not require hospital admission if without evidence of arterial oxygen desaturation (oxygen saturation <90% or PaO_2 <60 mm Hg), class III may be suitable for outpatient care, and classes IV and V require admission. Classes IV and V are considered to have a high mortality and to be at greater risk of requiring admission to the intensive care unit (ICU). The presence of arterial oxygen desaturation (oxygen saturation <90% or PaO2 <60 mm Hg) may warrant hospitalization regardless of PSI risk class.

Adapted from Fine MJ, Auble TE, Yealy DM, et al: A prediction rule to identify low-risk patients with community-acquired pneumonia. *N Engl J Med* **336**:243–250, 1997.
Copyright © 1997 Massachusetts Medical Society. All rights reserved.

CAP: investigations

General investigations

Investigations are aimed at confirming the diagnosis, assessing disease severity, guiding appropriate treatment, assessing presence of underlying disease, enabling identification of complications, and monitoring progress.

Oxygenation assessment

Those with an oxygen saturation of <92% on admission or with features of severe pneumonia should have arterial blood gases (ABGs) measured. The inspired oxygen concentration must be documented.

CXR

- Consolidation—most commonly in the lower lobes. Also interstitial infiltrates and cavitation
- Multilobe involvement—more common in bacteremic pneumococcal infection
- Pleural effusion—more common in bacteremic pneumococcal infection
- Lymphadenopathy—uncommon, most likely with mycoplasma infection
- Multilobe involvement, cavitation, or spontaneous pneumothorax suggest *Staphylococcus aureus* infection
- Upper lobe preponderance—*Klebsiella*

CT chest

This is unlikely to add additional information. It may be useful if the diagnosis is in doubt or the patient is severely ill and failing to respond to treatment, in order to exclude abscess formation, empyema, underlying malignancy, or other interstitial processes.

Blood tests

- CBC—a white cell count >15 x 10^9 suggests bacterial (particularly pneumococcal) infection. Counts >20 or <4 indicate severe infection.
- Deranged renal and liver function tests (LFTs) can be indicative of severe infection or point to the presence of underlying disease. LFTs may be abnormal, particularly with right lower lobe pneumonia. A raised urea level is a marker of more severe pneumonia.
- Metabolic acidosis is associated with severe illness.
- C-reactive protein (CRP) may be useful in management, with high levels being a more sensitive marker of infection than the white cell count or temperature. Serial measures may be useful in assessing response to treatment.
- Procalcitonin (PCT), when assessed serially, seems to correlate with outcome and may be a reliable indicator of when it is safe to discontinue antibiotics or change to an oral regimen.

Microbiological investigations

The microbiological cause for CAP is not found in 25%–60% of patients, and thus often does not contribute to patient management. Microbiological investigations can help to aid selection of optimal antibiotics, hence limiting antibiotic resistance as well as the possible problems of *antibiotic*-associated diarrhea.

They also inform public health or infection control teams, aiding in the monitoring of pathogen trends causing CAP over time. Routine diagnostic tests, looking for an etiology for CAP, are optional in the outpatient setting.

Blood cultures
These are recommended for all patients with severe CAP. If they are to be obtained, samples should be drawn prior to initiating antibiotic therapy and before the patient leaves the emergency department.

Sputum culture and sensitivity
These are useful for patients who have failed to improve with empirical antibiotic treatment, and in those admitted to hospital with non-severe pneumonia who are expectorating purulent samples and have not received prior antibiotics. These tests are also useful for investigating severe pneumonia.

They are not routinely recommended for those treated in the community. Sputum examination is recommended for possible tuberculosis (TB) in those with weight loss, a persistent cough, night sweats, and risk factors for TB, e.g., ethnic origin, social factors.

Pleural fluid (if present) for microscopy, culture, and sensitivity (M, C, & S) and pH to exclude empyema (see p. 334)

Viral and atypical pathogens in severe CAP

Serological testing
Paired samples (from within 7 days of the onset of illness, repeated 7–10 days later) should be tested together, in those with severe CAP, and in those unresponsive to β-lactam antibiotics.

Specific serological tests

Legionnaires' disease
A number of immunological tests exist to aid in the prompt and accurate diagnosis of Legionella pneumophilia:
- Urinary antigen detection is sensitive and specific, and rapid results can be obtained early.
- Direct immunofluorescence tests (DIF)—Legionella pneumophilia can be detected on bronchial aspirates.
- Culture is 100% specific (sputum, endotracheal aspirate, BAL, pleural fluid, lung)
- Serology—antibody levels and PCR are also available.

Mycoplasma pneumonia
The complement fixation test (CFT) is the most common serological assay and is regarded as the gold standard. Culture of Mycoplasma pneumoniae is not generally available.

Chlamydia
Chlamydial antigen can be detected by DIF in respiratory samples or by CFT.

Others
- Influenza A and B, adenovirus, and respiratory syncytial virus (RSV)

CAP: management

General management

Oxygen

Hypoxia is due to V/Q mismatching, as blood flows through unventilated lung. Aim for oxygen saturation >92%. If there is severe concomitant COPD, controlled oxygen therapy and close monitoring of blood gases are mandatory.

A rising CO_2 in a patient without prior respiratory disease may indicate that the patient is tiring and needs respiratory support. Consider mechanical ventilation early to avoid an emergent procedure.

Fluids

Assessment of volume status, by jugular venous pressure (JVP; with or without central venous access), urine output, and blood pressure is paramount. Encourage oral fluids. Intravenous fluids may be needed if the patient is volume depleted and severely ill. Consider use of central venous oxygen saturation as an indicator of perfusion (goal >70%).

Analgesia

Give acetaminophen or NSAIDs initially if required.

Nutrition

Nutritional status is important to the patient's outcome, and nutritional supplements may be of benefit in treating prolonged illness. Poor nutritional status may increase the risk of acquiring pneumonia.

Physiotherapy

This is of no proven benefit in treating acute pneumonia.

Additional treatments

Bronchoscopy

Bronchoscopy may be helpful, especially after intubation to suction retained secretions. If these are causing lobar collapse, obtain further samples for culture and to exclude an endobronchial abnormality.

Steroids

There is early but increasing evidence that low-dose corticosteroid therapy in the setting of severe CAP may be beneficial.

Drotrecogin-α

Patients should be considered for this therapy if they have pneumococcal infection, a PSI class of IV or V, a CURB-65 score ≥3, or an acute physiology and chronic health evaluation (APACHE) II score of >25.

Monitoring

Temperature, respiratory rate, heart rate, blood pressure, mental status, oxygen saturation, and inspired oxygen concentration should be monitored at least twice daily, and more often in the severely ill.

ICU admission

Those fulfilling criteria for severe CAP on admission or who fail to respond rapidly to treatment should be considered for transfer to a higher level of care for close monitoring. Persisting hypoxia, acidosis, hypercapnia, hypotension, or depressed conscious level, despite maximal therapy, are indications for assisted ventilation.

When to discuss mechanical ventilation

- Always sooner rather than later
- Respiratory failure (PaO_2 <8 kPa), despite high-flow oxygen
- Tiring, with a rising CO_2
- Worsening metabolic acidosis, despite antibiotics and optimum fluid management
- Hypotension despite adequate fluid resuscitation

CAP: antibiotics

Most antibiotics are used empirically at the diagnosis of CAP, in the absence of microbiological information. The clinical scenario also guides antibiotic choice, such as the addition of anaerobic cover in an alcoholic who has a high chance of aspiration.

Severity assessment guides antibiotic therapy and the method of antibiotic administration.

Local protocols and antibiotic resistance patterns may also guide choice of antibiotic.

General points

- Early administration of antibiotics is associated with an improved outcome (see Table 19.2).
- Antibiotics given before admission can influence the results of subsequent microbiological investigations, but this should not delay antibiotic administration in the community if the patient is ill.
- It is vital that there be no delay in administration of the first antibiotic dose in patients admitted to the hospital.

IV antibiotics

Consider IV antibiotics if the following occur:

- Severe pneumonia
- Loss of swallow reflex
- Impaired absorption
- Impaired conscious level

Oral antibiotics should be used in those with community-managed pneumonia, or those with non-severe hospital-managed pneumonia, with no other contraindications.

Add anaerobic antibiotic cover, e.g., clindamycin, for possible aspiration pneumonia in an unconscious patient or one with poor dentition. This should also be given if there is suspicion of a lung abscess on CXR/CT.

Switch from IV to oral antibiotics as soon as possible, usually when a patient has shown a clear response to treatment, with a normal temperature for 48–72 hours. Data suggest that observation in the hospital overnight after switching from an IV to an oral agent is unnecessary and does not improve outcomes.

Length of treatment

There is no evidence to guide treatment length, but consensus suggests

- 5–7 days: non-severe, uncomplicated pneumonia
- 10 days: severe microbiologically undefined pneumonia
- 14–21 days: *Legionella*, staphylococcal, or if gram-negative pneumonia suspected

The decision of when to stop treatment should be based on clinical criteria such as resolution of fever, leukocytosis, inflammatory marker (CRP) elevation, etc.

Table 19.2 Suggested initial antibiotics for CAP treatment

	Preferred treatment	**Alternative (if intolerant of, or allergic to, preferred treatment)**
Community treatment (no antibiotic therapy in last 3months)	Macrolide	Doxycycline
Outpatient treatment: comorbid condition(s) present or recent antibiotic therapy	Fluoroquinolone **OR** β-lactam with macrolide	
Hospital treatment: non-ICU	β-lactam (cefotaxime, ceftriaxone, or ampicillin-sulbactam) **plus** azithromycin **OR** fluoroquinolone	
Hospital treatment: ICU	β-lactam (cefotaxime, ceftriaxone, or ampicillin-sulbactam) **plus** azithromycin OR fluoroquinolone	If penicillin allergic: fluoroquinolone **plus** aztreonam
Hospital treatment: ICU **with risk** for *Pseudomonas* infection	β-lactam (pipercillin-tazobactam, cefepime, imipenem or meropenem) **plus** ciprofloxacin or levofloxacin OR β-lactam plus an aminoglycoside plus azithromycin **OR** β-lactam **plus** aminoglycoside **plus** antipneumococcal fluoroquinolone	

CAP: treatment failure

A CRP level that does not fall by >50% at 4 days suggests either treatment failure or development of a complication such as a lung abscess or empyema.

Causes of failure to improve

- Slow clinical response, particularly in the elderly patient
- Incorrect initial diagnosis
  - Pulmonary thromboembolic disease
  - Pulmonary edema
  - Bronchial carcinoma
  - Bronchiectasis
  - Also consider eosinophilic pneumonia, foreign-body aspiration, alveolar hemorrhage, cryptogenic organizing pneumonia, vasculitis or connective tissue disease, drug-induced lung disease
  - Review the history, examination, and radiology
  - Consider repeat imaging, e.g., CT chest
- Secondary complication
  - Pulmonary, e.g., parapneumonic effusion (occurs in 36%–57%; most cases resolve spontaneously; thoracentesis is recommended), empyema, abscess formation, ARDS
  - Extrapulmonary, e.g., septicemia, metastatic infection (e.g., meningitis, endocarditis, septic arthritis), sequelae of initial insult, e.g. renal failure, myocardial infarction
- Inappropriate antibiotics or unexpected pathogen (see Table 19.3)
  - Review dose, compliance, and route of administration. Send further microbiological specimens
  - Review microbiological data, exclude less common pathogens, e.g., *Legionella, Mycoplasma*, staphylococcal disease
  - Pathogen may be resistant to common antibiotics; 10% of CAP will have a mixed infection
  - Consider tuberculosis, fungal infection
- Impaired immunity
  - Systemic, e.g., hypogammaglobulinemia, HIV infection, myeloma
  - Local, e.g., bronchiectasis, aspiration, underlying bronchial carcinoma
  - Overwhelming infection

Table 19.3 Recommended antibiotic treatment of specific causative organisms

Pathogen	Preferred antibiotic	Alternative antibiotic
Streptococcus pneumoniae	Amoxicillin or benzylpenicillin	Erythromycin or clarithromycin or cefuroxime or cefotaxime or ceftriaxone
Mycoplasma pneumoniae and *Chlamydia pneumoniae*	Erythromycin or clarithromycin	Tetracycline or fluoroquinolone
Chlamydia psittaci and *Chlamydia burnetti*	Tetracycline	Erythromycin or clarithromycin
Legionella species	Clarithromycin and rifampin	Fluoroquinolone
Haemophilus influenzae	Non-β-lactamase-producing amoxicillin or ampicillin	Cefuroxime or cefotaxime
	β-lactamase-producing amoxicillin-clavulanate	Ceftriaxone or fluoroquinolone
Gram-negative enteric bacilli	Cefuroxime or cefotaxime IV or ceftriaxone	Fluoroquinolone or imipenem or meropenem
Pseudomonas aeruginosa	Ciprofloxacin or ceftazidime *plus* gentamicin or tobramycin (NB therapeutic drug monitoring)	Ciprofloxacin or piperacillin *plus* gentamicin or tobramycin
Staphylococcus aureus	Non-MRSA nafcillin	
	MRSA vancomycin	Teicoplanin and rifampin or linezolid
	(NB therapeutic drug monitoring)	

CAP: follow-up

CXR resolution

Radiographic improvement lags behind clinical improvement. There is no need to repeat a CXR before hospital discharge in those who have made a satisfactory clinical recovery.

- In one study of CAP, complete radiographic resolution occurred after 6 weeks in 74% of patients, but only in 51% at 2 weeks.
- Radiographic resolution is slower in the elderly, those with multilobe involvement at presentation, smokers, and hospital inpatients.
- *Legionella* and pneumococcal pneumonia are slower to resolve (may take 12 weeks or more).

CXR follow-up

Around 6 weeks after clinical improvement, CXR should be considered

- In all patients with persisting symptoms or clinical signs
- In all patients at higher risk of underlying lung malignancy, i.e., smokers and those over the age of 50.

This is to exclude an underlying condition that may have led to CAP, such as lung cancer. Further investigations such as bronchoscopy should be considered at this time in patients with persisting symptoms and/or a persistently abnormal CXR.

- One study showed that lung cancer is diagnosed on follow-up in 17% of smokers aged over 60 treated for CAP in the community.
- Other studies have shown an incidence of lung cancer of 11% in current and ex-smokers aged over 50, who are inpatients with CAP, and who undergo bronchoscopy prior to discharge.

Vaccination

Influenza vaccination

This reduces hospital deaths from pneumonia and influenza by about 65% and respiratory deaths by 45%. It also leads to fewer hospital admissions.

Recommended for "high-risk" individuals

- Chronic lung disease
- Cardiac, renal, and liver disease
- Diabetes
- Immunosuppression due to disease or treatment
- Age over 65
- Long-term residential care
- Health-care workers
- Contraindicated in people with egg hypersensitivity (the virus is cultured in chick embryos)

The vaccination contains both A and B subtype viruses and provides partial protection against influenza illnesses. It is modified annually, based on recent viral strains. The protection rate from influenza by vaccination is over 75% for influenza A and 51%–97% for influenza B. It gives protection of around 66%, though antibody levels appear to reduce about 6 years after vaccination.

Pneumococcal vaccination

Recommended for

- Asplenic individuals (including celiac disease and sickle cell disease)
- Chronic renal, cardiac, and liver disease
- Diabetes
- Immunodeficiency or immunosuppression (due to disease, including HIV infection, or drugs)

It should not be given during acute infection or during pregnancy.

Further information

British Thoracic Society Standards of Care Committee, et al. (2001). BTS guidelines for the management of community acquired pneumonia in adults. *Thorax* **56** (Suppl. 4): v1–v64.
An updated version of the 2001 guidelines is on the BTS Web site:
www.brit-thoracic.org.uk/docs/MACAPrevisedApr04.pdf
Thomas MF (2003). Community-acquired pneumonia. *Lancet* **362**:1991–2001.

Hospital-acquired pneumonia: clinical features

Definition

Hospital-acquired pneumonia is defined as new radiographic infiltrate in the presence of infection (fever, purulent sputum, leucocytosis) with onset at least 72 hours after hospital admission. It represents around 15% of hospital-acquired infections. Most cases occur outside the ICU, but those at highest risk are mechanically ventilated patients.

Hospital-acquired pneumonia is expensive to treat and prolongs hospital stay. It requires different antibiotic treatment from that for community-acquired pneumonia, and is the leading cause of death from hospital-acquired infection. It is also known as nosocomial pneumonia.

Pathophysiology

Hospital-acquired pneumonia occurs from hematogenous spread of organisms, aspiration of infected upper airway secretions, or the inhalation of bacteria from contaminated equipment.

Aspiration is thought to be the most important cause. Around 45% of normal people aspirate during sleep, and this rate is increased in hospital inpatients (who may be more frail) and those with chronic disease. These patients' upper airways become colonized with gram-negative bacteria (in up to 75% within 48 hours of admission). This proportion is even higher among those who have received broad-spectrum antibiotics. In addition, the severely ill may have impaired host defenses, making them more susceptible to hospital-acquired pneumonia.

Alteration in the gastric pH with illness and various drugs means that the gastrointestinal tract is no longer sterile, thereby providing a potential source of bacterial infection. A cerebrovascular event and reduced level of consciousness are the major risk factors for aspiration (see also Box 19.2).

Box 19.2 Risk factors for nosocomial pneumonia

- Age >70
- Chronic lung disease and/or other comorbidity (especially diabetes)
- Reduced level of consciousness or cerebrovascular accident
- Chest or abdominal surgery
- Mechanical ventilation
- Nasogastric feeding
- Previous antibiotic exposure
- Poor dental hygiene
- Steroids and cytotoxic drugs

Risk factors for specific organisms

- *Streptococcus pneumoniae* and *Haemophilus influenza*—increased risk in trauma
- Staphylococcus aureus—increased risk in ventilated neurosurgical patients (especially closed head injury), blunt trauma, and coma
- *Pseudomonas aeruginosa*—increased risk with intubation >8 days, COPD, prolonged antibiotics
- *Acinetobacter* species—increased risk with prolonged ventilation and previous broad-spectrum antibiotics
- Anaerobic bacteria—increased risk with recent abdominal surgery, aspiration

Clinical features

It presents typically with the following:
- Fever
- Productive cough
- Raised serologic markers of inflammation
- New CXR infiltrate
- Deterioration in gas exchange

Diagnosis

Diagnosis is often a clinical one, and identification of the infecting agent can be difficult, especially if the patient has already received broad-spectrum antibiotics.

Investigations

- CXR usually shows a nonspecific infiltrate
- Blood, sputum, and pleural fluid should be cultured
- Arterial blood gas to determine severity
- Renal and liver function tests to assess other organ dysfunction
- Serological tests are of little use in nosocomial pneumonia.
- Bronchoalveolar lavage should be considered in all intubated patients with quantitative culture.

Hospital-acquired pneumonia: management

Severity assessment

The CURB or CURB-65 pneumonia severity score (see p. 212) for community-acquired pneumonia has not been validated in hospital-acquired pneumonia, but may be useful in guiding the treatment needed.

Microbiology

- About 50% of cases are mixed infections.
- 30% are due to aerobic bacteria alone (most commonly gram-negative bacilli and *Pseudomonas*)
- Anaerobes alone are found in about 25%
- *Pseudomonas aeruginosa* and *Staphylococcus aureus* are common causes.
- *Peptostreptococcus, Fusobacteroides,* and *Bacteroides* species are commonly isolated, as well as *Enterobacter* species, *Escherichia coli, Serratia marcescens, Klebsiella,* and *Proteus* species.
- *Acinetobacter* is a new emerging pathogen.
- MRSA is increasing in prevalence.
- Viruses are recognized as causes.

Management

- Patients developing pneumonia within 48 hours of arrival in the hospital can be treated with standard community-acquired pneumonia antibiotics (see p. 218), as the pneumonia is likely to be due to bacteria acquired in the community.
- Patients developing pneumonia more than 48 hours after hospital admission need antibiotics to cover different organisms.
- Intravenous, prolonged treatment is usually needed, with coverage for gram-negative, anaerobic bacteria. This is best done using a second-generation cephalosporin, e.g., cefuroxime, with an aminoglycoside (unless there is renal impairment).
- Supportive treatment is also required, with oxygen, fluids, and ventilation if necessary.
- In penicillin-allergic patients, clindamycin or ciprofloxacin can be used (as long as *Streptococcus pneumoniae* is not thought to be the infecting agent). Levofloxacin has better pneumococcal coverage.
- Complications of nosocomial pneumonia are the same as for community-acquired pneumonia, including lung abscess and empyema. Drug fever, sepsis with multiorgan failure, and pulmonary embolus with secondary infection are all more common in nosocomial pneumonia.
- In this situation, chest ultrasound (to look for empyema) or CT may demonstrate abscess, underlying tumor, or infection at extrathoracic sites.

Prognosis

It has a high mortality, ranging between 20% and 50%.

Prevention

Meticulous hygiene and hand washing by medical staff, in addition to careful infection control measures, have been shown to reduce incidence of hospital-acquired pneumonia.

Postoperatively, early mobilization and careful cleaning and maintenance of respiratory equipment, and preoperative smoking cessation reduce infection rates. Some intensive care units use antibiotics to selectively decontaminate the gastrointestinal tract of gram-negative bacilli. This has been shown to reduce infection rates, but there is no proven effect on mortality or length of ICU admission.

Ventilator-acquired pneumonia (VAP)

Definition

VAP is pneumonia in a mechanically ventilated patient that develops 48 hours after intubation. It has a prevalence of up to 65% in some units. It is an independent predictor of mortality, with mortality up to 50% in some series.

The major cause is bacterial contamination of the lower respiratory tract from aspiration of oropharyngeal secretions, which is not prevented by cuffed endotracheal tube or tracheostomy.

Diagnosis

Diagnosis is
- Suggested by new or progressive CXR infiltrate
- Associated with fever, high WBC, and purulent secretions

There are many noninfectious causes of fever and CXR infiltrate in ICU patients, so the diagnosis is not always straightforward (see Box 19.3).

Investigations

CXR often shows a nonspecific infiltrate, with air bronchograms being the best predictor of the disease.

Airway sampling for microbiology

Bronchoscopic sampling

Protected specimen brush (PSB) samples or BAL samples (from a sub-segmental bronchus, ideally >150 mL saline wash) are the best methods to obtain lower airway samples with minimal contamination. VAP is diagnosed when an arbitrary threshold of organisms is grown on a BAL or PSB sample.

The usual cutoffs are 1000 colony-forming units/mL (CFU/mL) for PSB samples and >10,000 CFU/mL for BAL samples. The thresholds will vary from unit to unit, and the threshold for starting treatment will also vary. Airway neutrophil counts may also aid in making the diagnosis.

Box 19.3 Differential diagnosis of fever and CXR infiltrate in the ICU

- Chemical aspiration without infection
- Atelectasis
- ARDS
- Left ventricular failure
- PE with lung infarction
- Pulmonary hemorrhage
- Cryptogenic organizing pneumonia (COP)
- Drug reaction
- Tumor
- Lung contusion

Nonbronchoscopic airway sampling
This type of sampling, e.g., blind bronchial sampling of lower respiratory tract secretions, is less sensitive and specific than bronchoscopic sampling. It does not need an expert operator and is cheaper.

Serial sampling
Serial sampling is favored in some units. Regular noninvasive serial airway sampling may aid early diagnosis of VAP. It needs careful interpretation, as the microbiology of the respiratory tract changes over time in critically ill mechanically ventilated patients.

Tracheal aspiration samples
These samples are easy to obtain, but nonspecific in diagnosing VAP, as upper airway colonization is very common.

Additional sources of fever are common in ventilated patients, including infected lines, sinusitis, urinary tract infection, and pseudomembranous colitis, and may warrant further investigation.

Antibiotic treatment

The emergence of resistant bacteria (see Box 19.4) means that empirical treatment with antibiotics is used less commonly. Local policies are often in place, and advice should always be sought from microbiology and infection control.

Antibiotics should be chosen on the basis of
- Recent antibiotic treatment
- Local policy and known local flora
- Culture data

Antibiotics should cover anaerobes and MRSA, *Legionella* (if there is a long hospital stay), *Pseudomonas aeruginosa*, and *Acinetobacter*.

Failure to respond should lead to a change of antibiotics and a search for additional infection or another cause of the radiographic infiltrate. Further cultures should be sent.

Box 19.4 Risk factors for resistant organisms

- Ventilation >7 days
- Prior broad-spectrum antibiotic use (e.g., third-generation cephalosporin)

Aspiration pneumonia

Definition
This is pneumonia that follows the aspiration of exogenous material or endogenous secretions into the lower respiratory tract.

Epidemiology
Aspiration pneumonia is the most common cause of death in patients with dysphagia due to neurological disorders, and is the cause of up to 20% of pneumonias in nursing home residents. It occurs in about 10% of patients admitted to the hospital with a drug overdose.

Pathophysiology
Microaspiration is common in healthy individuals. For an aspiration pneumonia to occur, there must be compromise of the normal defenses protecting the lower airways (i.e., glottic closure, cough reflex), with inoculation of the lower respiratory tract of a significant amount of material. Most pneumonias are a result of aspiration of microorganisms from the oral cavity or nasopharynx.

Situations predisposing to aspiration pneumonia
Reduced level of consciousness (impaired cough reflex and glottic closure)
- Alcohol
- Drug overdose
- Post-seizure
- Post-anesthesia
- Massive CVA

Dysphagia
- Motor neuron disease
- Following a neurological event—those with impaired swallow reflex post-CVA are seven times more likely to develop pneumonia than those in whom the gag reflex is unimpaired.

Upper gastrointestinal tract disease
- Surgery to the stomach or esophagus
- Mechanical impairment of sphincter closure, e.g., tracheostomy, nasogastric feeding, bronchoscopy
- Pharyngeal anesthesia

Increased reflux
- Large-volume vomiting
- Large-volume nasogastric feeding
- Feeding gastrostomy
- Recumbent position

Nursing home residents

- The risk of aspiration is lower in those without teeth, who receive aggressive oral hygiene.
- There is a higher incidence of silent aspiration in the otherwise healthy elderly than in younger adults
- There is a high correlation between volume of aspirate and risk of developing pneumonia

Aspiration pneumonia: clinical features

Three pulmonary syndromes result from aspiration. The amount and nature of the aspirated material, the site and frequency of aspiration, and the host's response to it will determine the type of pulmonary syndrome that occurs.

1. Chemical pneumonitis

This is aspiration of substances toxic to the lower airways, in the absence of bacterial infection.

This aspiration causes a chemical burn of the tracheobronchial tree, resulting in an intense parenchymal inflammatory reaction, with release of inflammatory mediators that may lead to ARDS. Animal studies show that an inoculum with a pH <2.5 is needed to initiate an inflammatory reaction; if of a relatively large volume, about 25 mL is required in adults.

Animal models show rapid pathological changes within 3 minutes, with atelectasis, pulmonary hemorrhage, and pulmonary edema. (This was first described by Mendelson, referring to the aspiration of sterile gastric contents and its toxic effects. The original case series was in obstetric anesthesia.)

Clinical features
- Rapid onset of symptoms, with breathlessness (within 1–2 hours)
- Low-grade fever
- Severe hypoxemia and diffuse lung infiltrates involving dependent segments
- CXR changes within 2 hours.

Treatment
- If aspiration is observed, suction and/or bronchoscopy to clear aspirated secretions or food. This may not prevent chemical injury from acid, which is similar to a flash burn.
- Support of cardiac and respiratory function with intravenous fluids, oxygen ± ventilation.
- Steroids are controversial; no benefit has been shown in human studies
- Antibiotics are usually given, even in the absence of evidence of infection, because secondary bacterial infection is common and may be a contributing or primary factor in the aspiration. Acid-damaged lung is more susceptible to the effects of secondary bacterial infection; up to 25% will develop secondary bacterial infection. Activity against gram-negative and anaerobic organisms is needed, e.g., cefuroxime plus metronidazole, penicillin plus clindamycin.

2. Bacterial infection

This results from the aspiration of bacteria normally resident in the upper airway or stomach. While less virulent than the bacteria that cause CAP, in a susceptible host they can cause infection.

Clinical features
Features depend on the infecting organism:
- Cough, fever, purulent sputum, breathlessness
- The process may evolve over weeks and months rather than hours.
- May be more chronic, with weight loss and anemia
- Absence of fever or rigors
- Foul-smelling sputum
- Periodontal disease
- Involvement of dependent pulmonary lobes
- Anaerobic bacteria are more difficult to culture, so they may be present but not identified in microbiological culture.
- May present with later manifestations, e.g., empyema, lung abscess

Major pathogens are *Peptostreptococcus, Fusobacterium nucleatum*, and *Prevotella* and *Bacteroides* species. Mixed infection is common.

Treatment
- Antibiotics, to include anaerobic cover, e.g. amoxicillin-clavulanate or metronidazole plus penicillin
- Swallow assessment and neurological review if no obvious underlying cause is found

3. Mechanical obstruction

Aspiration of matter not directly toxic to the lung may lead to damage by causing airway obstruction or reflex airway closure. Causative agents include the following:
- Saline
- Barium
- Most ingested fluids, including water
- Gastric contents with a pH >2.5
- Mechanical obstruction, as can occur in drowning, or in those unable to clear a potential inoculum, e.g., neurological deficit, impaired cough reflex, reduced level of consciousness
- Inhalation of an object, with the severity of the obstruction depending on the size and site of the aspirated particle. This is more common in children but does occur in adults, e.g., teeth, peanuts.

Treatment
- Tracheal suction
- No further treatment is needed if there are no CXR infiltrates.

Lung abscess: clinical features

Definition

A lung abscess is a localized area of lung suppuration leading to necrosis of the pulmonary parenchyma, with or without cavity formation.

Lung abscesses may be single or multiple, acute or chronic (>1 month), primary or secondary. They may occur spontaneously, but more commonly an underlying disease exists. Although lung abscess is now rare in the developed world, it has a high mortality of 20%–30%. They are most common in alcoholic men aged >50.

Pathophysiology

Most abscesses are the result of aspiration pneumonia. Predisposing factors for abscess are those for aspiration pneumonia (p. 230).

- Dental disease
- Impaired consciousness—alcohol, post-anesthesia, dysphagia
- Diabetes
- Bronchial carcinoma (with bronchial obstruction)
- Secondary to pneumonia (cavitation occurs in about 16% of *Staphylococcus aureus* pneumonia)
- Immunocompromise—abscesses due to *Pneumocystis jiroveci* (PCP), *Cryptococcus neoformans, Rhodococcus* species, and fungi in HIV-positive patients
- Septic embolization (right heart endocarditis due to *Staphylococcus aureus* in intravenous drug abusers)

The bacterial inoculum reaches the lung parenchyma, often in a dependent lung area. Cavitation occurs when parenchymal necrosis leads to communication with the bronchus, with the entry of air and expectoration of necrotic material, leading to formation of an air–fluid level. Bronchial obstruction leads to atelectasis with stasis and subsequent infection, which can predispose to abscess formation.

Presentation

- Often insidious onset
- Productive cough
- Emoptysis
- Breathlessness
- Fevers
- Night sweats
- Nonspecific feature of chronic infection—anemia, weight loss, malaise (especially in the elderly)
- Foul sputum, or purulent pleural fluid

Lemierre's syndrome (necrobacillosis)

Lemierre's syndrome is characterized by jugular vein suppurative thrombophlebitis. This is a rare pharyngeal infection in young adults, most commonly due to the anaerobe *Fusobacterium necrophorum*.

It presents with a classical history of painful pharyngitis, in the presence of bacteremia. Infection spreads to the neck and carotid sheath, often leading to thrombosis of the internal jugular vein. This may not be obvious clinically (neck vein ultrasound or Doppler imaging may be needed).

Septic embolization to the lung with subsequent cavitation, leads to abscess formation. Empyema and abscesses in the bone, joints, liver, and kidneys can complicate.

Lung abscess: diagnosis

The diagnosis is usually made from the history along with the appearance of a cavity with an associated air–fluid level on CXR. See Box 19.5 for the differential diagnosis.

Investigations

These include microbiological culture, ideally before commencing antibiotics. It is useful to exclude tuberculosis.

• Blood cultures
• Sputum or bronchoscopic specimen (BAL or brushings rarely needed)
• Transthoracic percutaneous needle aspiration (CT- or ultrasound-guided) may provide samples. There is a risk of bleeding, pneumothorax, and seeding of infection to pleural space if the abscess is not adjacent to the pleura.

In practice, blood cultures and sputum microbiology usually suffice. Samples are usually only obtained by more invasive means if appropriate antibiotics are not leading to an adequate clinical response.

Imaging

Exclude aspirated foreign body, underlying neoplasm, or bronchial stenosis and obstruction.

CXR

CXR may show consolidation, cavitation, and air–fluid level (if the patient is ill, the CXR is likely to be taken in a semi-recumbent position, so an air–fluid level may not be visible). Some 50% of abscesses are in the posterior segment of the right upper lobe, or the apical basal segments of either lower lobe.

CT

CT is useful if the diagnosis is in doubt and cannot be confirmed from the CXR appearance, or if the clinical response to treatment is inadequate. It can also help to define the exact position of the abscess (which may be useful for physiotherapy or if surgery is being considered—it is rarely needed).

CT is also useful to differentiate an abscess from a pleural collection—a *lung abscess* appears as a rounded intrapulmonary mass, with no compression of adjacent lung, with a thickened irregular wall, making an acute angle at its contact with the chest wall. An *empyema* typically has a "lenticular" shape, and compresses adjacent lung, which creates an obtuse angle as it follows the contour of the chest wall.

CT can determine the presence of obstructing endobronchial disease due to malignancy or foreign body, and may be useful in defining the extent of disease in a very sick patient who has had significant hemoptysis. Even with CT, differentiation of an abscess from a cavitating malignancy can be very difficult (no radiological features differentiate them).

Microbiology

Commonly there is mixed infection, usually anaerobes.

- The most common organisms are those colonizing the oral cavity and gingival crevices: *Peptostreptococcus, Prevotella, Bacteroides*, and *Fusobacterium* species.
- Aerobes: *Streptococcus milleri, Staphylococcus aureus, Klebsiella species, Streptococcus pyogenes, Haemophilus influenzae, Nocardia*
- Nonbacterial pathogens are also reported: fungi (*Aspergillus, Cryptococcus, Histoplasma, Blastomyces*) and mycobacteria
- Opportunistic infections in immunocompromised patients include *Nocardia, Mycobacteria,* and *Aspergillus*.

Box 19.5 Differential diagnosis of a cavitating mass, with or without an air–fluid level

- Cavitating carcinoma—primary or metastatic
- Cavitatory tuberculosis
- Wegener's granulomatosis
- Infected pulmonary cyst or bulla (can produce a fluid level, usually thinner walled)
- Aspergilloma
- Pulmonary infarct
- Rheumatoid nodule
- Sarcoidosis
- Bronchiectasis

Lung abscess: management

Antibiotics

Antibiotics for covering aerobic and anaerobic infection include β-lactamase inhibitors, e.g., amoxicillin-clavulanate and clindamycin. Long courses are needed. There is a risk of *Clostridium difficile* or antibiotic-associated diarrhea.

- Infections are usually mixed, therefore use antibiotics to cover these.
- Metronidazole to cover anaerobes
- No data exist to guide length of treatment. Common practice would be 1–2 weeks intravenous treatment, with a further 2–6 weeks of oral antibiotics, often until the outpatient clinic review.

Drainage

Spontaneous drainage is common, with the production of purulent sputum. This can be increased with postural drainage and physiotherapy.

- There are no data to support use of bronchoscopic drainage.
- Percutaneous drainage with radiologically placed small percutaneous drains for peripheral abscesses may be useful in those failing to respond to antibiotic and supportive treatment. These are usually placed under ultrasound guidance (although are rarely indicated).

Surgery

Surgery is rarely required if appropriate antibiotic treatment is given. It is usually reserved for complicated infections failing to respond to standard treatment after at least 6 weeks of treatment.

Surgery may be needed if the following occur:

- Very large abscess (>6 cm diameter)
- Resistant organisms
- Hemorrhage
- Recurrent disease

Lobectomy or pneumonectomy is occasionally needed if severe infection with an abscess leaves a large volume of damaged lung that is hard to sterilize.

Complications

Hemorrhage (erosion of blood vessels as the abscess extends into the lung parenchyma) can be massive and life threatening (see p. 678), and is an indication for urgent surgery.

If slow to respond, consider

- Underlying malignancy
- Unusual microbiology, e.g., *Mycobacterium*, fungi
- Immunosuppression
- Large cavity (>6 cm)—may require drainage
- Nonbacterial cause, e.g., cavitating malignancy, Wegener's granulomatosis
- Other cause of persistent fever, e.g., *Clostridium difficile* diarrhea, antibiotic-associated fever

Prognosis

There is an 85% cure rate in the absence of underlying disease. Mortality is reported to be as high as 75% in immunocompromised patients. The prognosis is much worse in the presence of underlying lung disease, and with increasing age and large abscesses (>6 cm) with *Staphylococcus aureus* infection.

Nocardiosis

Definition
Nocardia are gram-positive, partially acid-fast, aerobic bacilli that form branching filaments. They are found in soil, decaying organic plant matter, and water, and have been isolated from house dust, garden soil, and swimming pools. Infection typically follows inhalation, although percutaneous inoculation also occurs. The *Nocardia asteroides* species complex accounts for the majority of clinical infections.

> Consider *Nocardia* infection when soft-tissue abscesses and/or CNS manifestations occur in the setting of a pulmonary infection. The combination of respiratory, skin, and/or CNS involvement may lead to a misdiagnosis of vasculitis, and the respiratory manifestations may mimic cancer, tuberculosis, or fungal disease.

Epidemiology
Nocardia occurs worldwide. The frequency of subclinical exposure is unknown. Clinically apparent infection is rare, and usually occurs in patients with immunocompromise (hematological malignancy, steroid therapy, organ transplant, diabetes, alcoholism, and HIV infection, especially IV drug users) or preexisting lung disease (particularly pulmonary alveolar proteinosis, tuberculosis). Infection also occurs in apparently healthy people (10%–25% of cases). Nosocomial infection and disease outbreaks have been reported.

Clinical features
Pulmonary disease
- The lung is the most common site of involvement.
- Patients typically present with productive cough, fever, anorexia, weight loss, and malaise; dyspnea, pleuritic pain, and hemoptysis may occur but are less common.
- Empyema occurs in up to a quarter of cases, and direct intrathoracic spread causing pericarditis, mediastinitis, rib osteomyelitis, or SVCO is also reported.

Extrapulmonary disease
- Dissemination from the lungs occurs in 50% of patients.
- The central nervous system is the most common site of dissemination, occurring in 25% of pulmonary nocardiosis cases. Single or multiple abscesses occur and may be accompanied by meningitis.
- Other sites include the skin and subcutaneous tissues, kidneys, bone, joints and muscle, peritoneum, eyes, pericardium, and heart valves.

Investigations

- Identification by smear and culture is the principal method of diagnosis. *Nocardia* grow on routine media usually within 2–7 days, although more prolonged culture (2–3 weeks) may be required.
- Direct smear of appropriate specimens (e.g., aspirates of abscesses, biopsies) is highly sensitive and typically shows gram-positive, beaded branching filaments, which are usually acid-fast on modified Ziehl–Neelson stain. Examination of BAL fluid may also be diagnostic.
- Sensitivity testing of isolates and identification to species level is done by reference laboratories.
- Biopsies typically show a mixed cellular infiltrate; granulomata occur rarely, and may result in misdiagnosis as tuberculosis or histoplasmosis
- CXR and CT may demonstrate parenchymal infiltrates, single or multiple nodules (sometimes with cavitation), or features of pleural infection.
- Sputum smear is usually unhelpful. Sputum culture has a greater yield, but *Nocardia* growth may be obscured in mixed cultures. The significance of *Nocardia* growth on sputum culture in asymptomatic patients is unclear; it may represent contamination or colonization in the setting of underlying lung disease.
- Blood cultures are almost always negative, although *Nocardia* bacteremia may occur in the setting of profound immunocompromise.
- Consider MRI of the brain to exclude asymptomatic CNS involvement in patients with pulmonary nocardiosis.

Management

Discuss treatment with an infectious diseases specialist.

Drug treatment choices include sulfonamides/co-trimoxazole, minocycline, imipenem, cefotaxime, ceftriaxone, or amikacin. Sulfa drugs, in particular co-trimoxazole, have traditionally been the mainstay of therapy. Imipenem and amikacin combination therapy has been shown to be active in vitro and in animal models, and is recommended for pulmonary nocardiosis and for very ill patients. Extended-spectrum cephalosporins such as ceftriaxone and cefotaxime have the advantages of good CNS penetration and low toxicity.

Optimal treatment duration is unclear: typically it is given for 6 months in non-immunocompromised patients and for 12 months or longer for CNS involvement or immunocompromised patients.

Surgery may be required for abscess drainage.

Prognosis

Clinical outcome is dependent on the site and extent of disease and on underlying host factors. Disease remissions and exacerbations are common. Cure rates are approximately 90% for pleuropulmonary disease and 50% for brain abscess. Mortality of *Nocardia* infection is generally low, although it approaches 50% in cases of bacteremia.

Further information

Lerner PI (1996). Nocardiosis. *Clin Infect Dis* **22**;891–905.
Saubolle MA, Sussland D (2003). Nocardiosis: review of clinical and laboratory experience. *J Clin Microbiol* **41**:4497–4501.

Actinomycosis

Definition

Actinomycosis is caused by a group of anaerobic gram-positive bacilli, of which *Actinomyces israelii* is the most common. These organisms are present in the mouth, gastrointestinal tract, and vagina. Clinical infection may follow dental procedures or aspiration of infected secretions. Infection is slowly progressive and may disseminate via the bloodstream or invade tissue locally, sometimes resulting in sinus tract formation.

Consider this diagnosis particularly in patients with pulmonary disease accompanied by soft tissue infection of the head and neck. The diagnosis of actinomycosis is often unsuspected, and the clinical and radiological features may mimic cancer, tuberculosis, or fungal disease.

Epidemiology

Actinomycosis is rare. It can occur at any age, and is more common in men. Predisposing factors include corticosteroid use, chemotherapy, organ transplant, and HIV infection.

Clinical features

Thoracic disease

Thoracic disease occurs in about 15% of cases. Symptoms of pulmonary involvement are nonspecific and include cough, chest pain, hemoptysis, fever, anorexia, and weight loss. Chest wall involvement may occur, with sinus formation and rib infection, and empyema is common. Mediastinal involvement is documented.

Extrathoracic disease

Soft tissue infection of the head and neck, particularly the mandible, is the most common disease presentation (about 50% of cases). Discharging sinuses may form. Other extrathoracic disease sites include the abdomen (particularly the ileocecal region), pelvis, liver, bone, and CNS (manifest as single or multiple abscesses).

Investigations

CXR and CT appearances are variable, including masses (sometimes with cavitation), parenchymal infiltrates, consolidation, mediastinal disease, and/or pleural involvement.

Diagnosis is based on microscopy and anaerobic culture of infected material. Inform the microbiology laboratory when the diagnosis is suspected, as specific stains and culture conditions are required.

Examination of infected material may reveal yellow "sulfur granules" containing aggregated organisms. Sample sputum, pleural fluid, and pus from sinus tracts, inoculate into anaerobic transport media, and rapidly transport them to the laboratory. Endobronchial biopsies have a low sensitivity. Most infections are polymicrobial, with accompanying aerobic or anaerobic bacteria.

Management

- Discuss treatment with an infectious diseases specialist.
- Drug treatment choices include penicillin, amoxicillin, clindamycin, or erythromycin. Administration should initially be intravenous. Optimal treatment duration is unclear (typically given for 6–12 months).
- Surgery may be required for abscess drainage.
- Monitor response to treatment with serial CT or MRI scans.
- Treat any associated periodontal disease.

Prognosis

Disease relapse is common if prolonged treatment is not administered.

Further information

Mabeza GF, Mcfarlane J (2003). Pulmonary actinomycosis. *Eur Respir J* **21**: 545–551.

Anthrax

Definition and epidemiology

Bacillus anthracis is an aerobic, gram-positive, spore-forming bacterium that causes human disease, principally following either inhalation or cutaneous contact. Spores can survive in soil for many years. Person-to-person transmission does not occur.

Considerable recent interest has focused on the use of anthrax in bioterrorism.

Anthrax infection also occurs very rarely in association with occupational exposure to *Bacillus anthracis* in animal wool or hides. The majority of occupational cases result in cutaneous disease, and a diagnosis of inhalational anthrax strongly suggests a bioterrorist attack.

Clinical features

Inhalational anthrax

The incubation period is variable, typically ranging from 4 to 6 days following exposure.

Patients typically experience a prodrome of flu-like symptoms such as fever and cough. Gastrointestinal symptoms (vomiting, diarrhea, abdominal pain), drenching sweats, and altered mental status are often prominent symptoms. Breathlessness, fever, and septic shock develop several days later. Hemorrhagic meningitis is a common complication.

Large hemorrhagic pleural effusions are a characteristic feature.

Cutaneous anthrax

Initial symptoms include itch and development of a papule at the infection site. A necrotic ulcer with a black center and often surrounding edema subsequently develops. Systemic symptoms such as fever and sweats may be present.

Investigations

- *Bacillus anthracis* grows on conventional media and is readily cultured if sampling precedes antibiotic treatment; a definitive diagnosis requires specialized laboratory tests.
- Blood tests typically reveal leukocytosis.
- Blood cultures are positive in nearly all cases of inhalational anthrax when taken prior to antibiotic treatment. Staining and culture of pleural fluid may be diagnostic.
- CXR in inhalational anthrax classically shows a widened mediastinum; pleural effusions and pulmonary infiltrates may be present. CT may also demonstrate mediastinal and hilar lymphadenopathy.
- Gram stain and culture of the ulcer is usually diagnostic in cutaneous anthrax, although biopsy is sometimes required.

Management

Discuss with infectious diseases and public health specialists if the diagnosis is suspected.

Antibiotic treatment should be administered immediately after taking blood cultures. Recent recommendations are for initial treatment with either ciprofloxacin or doxycycline IV, in combination with 1–2 additional antibiotics (choices include clindamycin, vancomycin, meropenem, or penicillin). Subsequent treatment should be with either ciprofloxacin or doxycycline orally for 60–100 days. Oral treatment alone may be sufficient in cases of mild cutaneous disease.

Corticosteroid treatment should be considered in patients with meningitis or severe neck or mediastinal edema.

Supportive care, including ventilatory support, treatment of shock with intravenous fluids and/or inotropes, and chest tube drainage of large pleural effusions, may be needed.

Prognosis

Inhalational anthrax is associated with a high mortality: 5 of the recent 11 patients in the United States died. The mortality of previously documented cases has been even higher, perhaps reflecting a delay or lack of antibiotic treatment.

Prophylaxis

Recent U.S. recommendations advise prophylaxis with oral ciprofloxacin or doxycycline for individuals considered to have been exposed to anthrax spores in contaminated areas. A vaccine is available, although its value in post-exposure prophylaxis is unknown.

Viral respiratory infection

Viral pneumonia: overview

- Viral upper respiratory tract infections (URIs) are common but typically self-limiting, and only a subset of patients with URIs seeks the attention of medical providers. Care, when required, is generally supportive and symptom directed.
- Lower respiratory tract infections (LRIs) from viruses are less common but often more serious and may require hospitalization. Viral LRIs include tracheobronchitis, bronchiolitis, and pneumonia. Viral pneumonia is a subset of the pneumonitides, or atypical pneumonias.
- Viral pneumonia classically affects children and elderly, immunosuppressed, or immunocompromised patients, and those with chronic illness. It also occurs in pregnant women, and more commonly in smokers than in nonsmokers. There is increasing appreciation for a significant burden of disease in healthy adults, most commonly influenza. About 8% of patients hospitalized with community-acquired pneumonia have a viral pneumonia.
- Diagnosis of viral pneumonias is difficult and they commonly go undetected.
- The clinical and radiological features of viral pneumonia are non-specific and can be difficult to distinguish from bacterial pneumonia. Worsening cough and breathlessness following a URI suggest the development of pneumonia, while wheezing may accompany bronchitis or bronchiolitis. CXR typically shows a nonspecific, diffuse interstitial infiltrate. Secondary bacterial infection may complicate viral pneumonia.
- If viral pneumonia is suspected, a variety of diagnostic techniques are available, including PCR, viral culture, immunofluorecence staining (e.g., of BAL fluid), and serology.
- Viral pneumonias are spread by aerosols (influenza and adenovirus) or by person-to-person contact. Infection with certain viruses may require isolation.
- Treatment generally consists of supportive care and, in some cases, antivirals, particularly for severe disease. Secondary bacterial infections need to be treated with appropriate antibiotics.

Influenza

Influenza is caused by a single-stranded RNA virus from the *Orthomyxo viridae* family.

Epidemiology

Influenza is the most common cause of viral pneumonia in immunocompetent adults. It is the seventh leading cause of death in the United States, with 10,000 to 40,000 excess deaths during the flu season (typically occurring in the late winter and early spring in the United States and Europe). It is transmitted by aerosolized virus or direct contact with respiratory secretions, and is extremely contagious.

There are three pathogenic serotypes: A, B, and C. Type A, causing more severe disease, is associated with annual epidemics and intermittent pandemics. Type B causes less severe disease in closed populations such as boarding schools. Type C is uncommon and causes sporadic cases.

The influenza virus particle has two important envelope glycoproteins: hemagglutin, which binds to cellular siasilic acid residues and facilitates viral entry, and neuriminidase which cleaves siasilic acid to allow viral spread. Different mutations of each protein are denoted by numbering (e.g., A/H2N3), which is the influenza serotype.

Genetic mutations in preexisting serotypes result in antigenic drifts that cause annual seasonal epidemics, while genetic reassortment of serotypes results in novel combinations called antigenic shifts and is associated with infrequent but devastating pandemics. Antigenic shifts can occur in non-human animal reservoirs and subsequently be transferred to humans, as with the avian-derived strain A/H5N1, which has recently raised fears of a new pandemic. A/H5N1 has a reported case-mortality rate of about 60%.

Individuals with chronic lung disease or congestive heart failure (CHF), those who are immunocompromised, and elderly or institutionalized persons are at particular risk of contracting influenza. Mitral stenosis may also increase susceptibility. Most deaths and hospitalizations due to influenza are in patients older than age 65.

Influenza causes decreased mucociliary clearance and suppression of the local immune system, promoting bacterial superinfection.

Clinical features

Influenza has a 1- to 4-day incubation period after exposure. The symptoms of influenza infection are variable but can be severe and debilitating even in healthy individuals.

URI symptoms include myalgias, arthraligas, rhinorrhea, sore throat, diarrhea, fever, and cough.

LRI infections include tracheobronchitis, bronchiolitis, and pneumonia (either primary from influenza virus itself, or secondary from bacterial infection), which can progress to pulmonary hemorrhage, diffuse alveolar damage (DAD), and acute respiratory distress syndrome (ARDS). Symptoms can progress rapidly from minor to severe disease.

Avian influenza is associated with leukopenia and thrombocytopenia in addition to severe pneumonia.

In patients with poor baseline health status, the symptoms of influenza can be only fever and mental status change, without cough.

CXR can show a perihilar or bronchiolar infiltrate that progresses to a diffuse interstitial infiltrate in severe disease. However, the CXR can resemble and be mistaken for CHF.

Elderly patients who recover from influenza infection often have a permanent decline in functional status.

Diagnosis

Diagnostic tests for influenza include viral culture, immunofluorescence, or enzyme-linked immunosorbent assay (ELISA) of nasopharyngeal washes, throat swabs, sputum, or lung tissue. Rapid and effective PCR-based tests are available.

The clinical setting is important: if a local outbreak is ongoing and the symptoms are classic for influenza, the pretest probability is much higher.

Treatment

In addition to supportive care, antiviral treatment with amantadine or rimantadine (which are effective only against type A influenza) may shorten the duration of illness if started within 48 hours of symptom onset. Early treatment with inhaled zanamivir or oral oseltamivir may also shorten symptom duration.

Secondary bacterial infections need to be treated appropriately.

In severe influenza pneumonia, starting treatment with antivirals after 48 hours is likely warranted, but not supported by data.

Administration of amantadine or rimantadine to high-risk individuals (such as nursing home residents and health-care workers during a nursing home epidemic) after known exposure and throughout an ongoing period of exposure may also prevent infection.

Inhaled zanamivir can worsen respiratory function in patients with underlying COPD or asthma.

Avian influenza is intrinsically resistant to amantadine and rimantadine, and has been reported to develop resistance to oseltamivir. Patients with suspected avian influenza should be isolated, given the very high case-fatality rate, but it is unclear if this is effective in preventing transmission.

Vaccination

The inactivated influenza vaccine contains two A serotypes and one B serotype and is modified annually based on prediction of the important serotypes during the next flu season. Antibodies generated are directed against the H and N proteins. The vaccine provides partial protection against LRIs, with decreased rates of hospitalization and death.

Indications to vaccinate are age over 65, chronic comorbidity, nursing home residents, or health-care workers. Contraindication to vaccination is anaphylactic allergy to egg or other components of the vaccine.

Live inhaled attenuated influenza vaccines are available but should be used in younger, healthy adults who have no respiratory comorbidities.

Further information

Oliveira EC, Lee B, Colice GL (2003). Influenza in the intensive care unit. *J Intensive Care Med* **18**(2):80–91.

Smith NM, Bresee JS, Shay DK, et al. (2006). Prevention and control of influenza: recommendations of the Advisory Committee on Immunization Practices. *MMWR Recomm Rep* **55**(RR-10):1–42.

WHO Web site for updated information: www.who.int/csr/disease/avian_influenza/en/

Respiratory syncytial virus

Respiratory syncytial virus (RSV) is a single-stranded RNA member of the *Paramyxoviridae* family.

Epidemiology

RSV is a common cause of bronchiolitis and pneumonia in children. In infected day care centers the case rate approaches 100%. RSV is easily spread by large droplets (from coughing and sneezing) and person-to-person contact or through fomites.

The role of RSV in adult respiratory disease is more significant than previously appreciated, and infection often goes unrecognized.

Postinfectious immunity is incomplete and wanes, thus reinfection is common.

RSV is a seasonal illness, with increased incidence in the fall, peaking in the winter, and declining in the spring.

Adult infection occurs particularly in the setting of underlying cardiac disease, respiratory disease, malignancy, or after bone marrow or solid organ transplants. Outbreaks affecting adults in hospitals and nursing homes also occur.

Clinical features

Approximately 25%–40% of infections with RSV involve the lower respiratory tract.

Symptoms of an RSV URI are rhinorrhea, fever, and cough. Progression to LRI can include bronchitis, bronchiolitis (which is most classic for RSV), or pneumonia, with symptoms of wheezing, tachypnea, rales, and hypoxia.

RSV can cause severe respiratory distress and failure in immunosuppressed patients.

Bacterial superinfection may be a complication.

Diagnosis

RSV can be detected by antigen detection using ELISA. Bronchoscopy with BAL can help make the diagnosis: detection of RSV antigen in BAL fluid has a sensitivity of nearly 90%. PCR for viral RNA and viral culture can also be used.

If there is a known outbreak of RSV and the clinical symptoms are characteristic of RSV infection, confirmatory testing may not be necessary.

Treatment

Treatment of RSV infection is principally supportive.

In children, ribavirin and palivizumab are used in preventing and treating RSV infection. Ribivarin is a broad-spectrum antiviral. Palivizumab is a monoclonal humanized antibody against a fusion protein on the viral particle. Similarly, aerosolized ribavirin and palivizumab have been used for severe disease in adults, but the efficacy of these therapies in adults has not been formally tested.

Steroids and immunoglobulin have also been used as adjunctive therapy to treat severe disease.

Further information

Falsey AR (2007). Respiratory syncytial virus infection in adults. *Semin Respir Crit Care Med* **28**(2):171–81.
Greenberg SB (2002). Respiratory viral infections in adults. *Curr Opin Pulm Med* **8**(3):201–208.

Parainfluenza

Parainfluenza is caused by single-stranded RNA viruses belonging to the *Paramyxovirus* family.

Epidemiology

Parainfluenza is composed of four distinct serotypes: 1, 2, 3, and 4. Type 3 is most common. Type 4 causes a milder disease than the others, principally at the extremes of age.

Parainfluenza is the second most common viral infection in children after RSV, and is also very common in adults as immunity wanes.

Parainfluenza can cause severe disease in the immunosuppressed. The prevalence of parainfluenza is highest in the late fall and winter.

Clinical features

Parainfluenza URI symptoms are similar to influenza URI symptoms, with severe myalgias, arthralgias, fatigue, rhinorrhea, sore throat, fever, and cough.

Parainfluenza LRI includes bronchiolitis and pneumonia, with symptoms of fever, cough, wheezing, tachypnea, retractions, and cyanosis.

CXR can show a range from focal interstitial infiltrate to diffuse alveolar or interstitial infiltrates depending on the severity of disease.

Diagnosis

Viral culture, reverse transcriptase polymerase chain reaction (RT-PCR) for viral RNA, and ELISA for viral antigens can be used to detect the virus.

Treatment

Supportive care is the mainstay of treatment. Ribivarin can be used in severe illness, but without evidence to support its efficacy.

Further information

Barton TD, Blumberg EA (2005). Viral pneumonias other than cytomegalovirus in transplant recipients. *Clin Chest Med* **26**(4):707–720, viii.

Adenovirus

Adenovirus is a double-stranded DNA virus in the family *Adenoviridae*.

Epidemiology

Adenovirus is most commonly associated with URIs. It occasionally causes pneumonia particularly in closed settings such as military camps.

Adenovirus is spread by aerosolized viral particles, making infection common in close living quarters.

Adenovirus LRI is more common in immunosuppressed patients.

Adenovirus accounts for 15% of post-transplant pneumonias, with a mortality rate in that patient population of 50%. It accounts for only 1%–3% of pneumonias in healthy adults, and mortality is rare.

Clinical features

Adenovirus causes typical URI symptoms of fever, malaise, headache, sore throat, and cough. In immunosuppressed patients it causes higher fevers and more GI symptoms.

Adenovirus LRI includes pneumonia, which has signs and symptoms of high fever and cough, dense infiltrate on CXR, and leukopenia and thrombocytopenia.

Diagnosis

RT-PCR, ELISA, and viral culture can all be used to diagnose adenovirus infection.

The virus is shed in the stool, thus a stool viral culture can be diagnostic.

Treatment

Supportive care is the mainstay of therapy. Ribivarin has in vitro activity against adenovirus but has not been studied in human disease, so it may have a role in serious cases.

Further information

Pham TT, Burchette JL, Jr, Hale LP (2003). Fatal disseminated adenovirus infections in immunocompromised patients. *Am J Clin Pathol* **120**(4):575–583.

Cytomegalovirus

Cytomegalovirus (CMV) is a double-stranded DNA virus of the *Herpesviridae* family and is also known as human herpes virus 5 (HHV-5).

Epidemiology

CMV is the most common serious viral pathogen in the immunocompromised population, and is a particular problem following bone marrow and solid organ transplantation. Prophylaxis starting before transplant is now widely used to decrease the incidence of infection.

Individuals are seropositive for CMV if they have IgG antibodies indicating latent infection after prior exposure. The prevalence of seropositivity is 40%–100%, with higher rates in populations of lower socioeconomic status.

Infection in transplant recipients results from either transmission of the virus from a CMV-positive donor to a CMV-negative recipient or reactivation of latent CMV in a seropositive recipient as a result of immunosuppression.

CMV infection occurs most frequently during the first 4 months following organ or bone marrow transplantation, during the period of maximal T-cell suppression. Graft-versus-host disease increases the risk of CMV infection.

Clinical features

CMV causes flu-like URI symptoms in immunocompetent patients.

Symptoms of CMV pneumonia in the immunocompromised are non-specific: fever, dry cough, dyspnea, hypoxia, and malaise. Leukopenia, thrombocytopenia, and abnormal liver function tests are common.

Extrapulmonary manifestations of CMV infection include enterocolitis, retinitis, bone marrow suppression, encephalitis, and hepatitis. The presence of these conditions may provide clues to the overall diagnosis.

CXR typically shows a bilateral lower-lobe predominant interstitial infiltrate, although lobar consolidation or localized haziness can also be seen. Occasionally the CXR can be normal.

CT of CMV pneumonia can have two different appearances: a *multifocal or military pattern* of small spheres <4 mm in diameter (from alveolar hemorrhage and fibrin deposition), or a *diffuse interstitial pneumonia* with interstitial edema and fibrosis.

Diagnosis

Antibody serology tests are used to diagnose latent infection prior to transplantation.

Diagnosis of active disease requires evidence of either viremia (by antigen or PCR testing of blood) or tissue invasion (by biopsy).

Early antigen fluorescence test on BAL fluid has a high sensitivity but low specificity, i.e., a high false-positive rate.

Qualitative PCR on blood or BAL fluid is highly sensitive, but unable to differentiate between latent and replicating CMV: a negative result practically excludes the diagnosis, but a positive result is unhelpful.

Quantitative PCR on the blood or BAL fluid differentiates between latent and replicating virus. The presence of CMV antigen in the blood by ELISA indicates active infection.

Histology of lung tissue from transbronchial or surgical biopsy that demonstrates CMV inclusion bodies—the "owl's eye" appearance—within infected cells is considered the gold standard to diagnose infection. The tissue can also have a monocytic interstitial infiltrate with thickened alveoli, fibrinous exudates, and hemorrhage, which can make CMV inclusion bodies hard to find.

CMV can be grown on culture but this can take over 2 weeks.

Treatment

Ganciclovir is the first-line treatment for CMV infection. In severe disease anti-CMV hyperimmune globulin can be used. Oral valganciclovir can be used to suppress relapsing disease. Foscarnet is an alternative to ganciclovir for resistant cases, but toxicity can limit treatment.

Opportunistic infection can arise (e.g., PCP, aspergillosis) due to further suppression of T-cell function by the CMV infection itself.

CMV is associated with increased risk of organ rejection, as allografts are more susceptible to CMV infection than native organs.

The reported mortality from CMV pneumonia varies, although may be as high as 85%. Relapse occurs in up to one-third of patients.

Further information

de la Hoz RE, Stephens G, Sherlock C (2002). Diagnosis and treatment approaches of CMV infections in adult patients. *J Clin Virol* **25**(Suppl. 2):S1–S12.

Ison MG, Fishman JA (2005). Cytomegalovirus pneumonia in transplant recipients. *Clin Chest Med* **26**(4):691–705, viii.

Herpes simplex virus

Herpes simplex viruses 1 and 2 (HSV-1 and HSV-2) are two strains of the *Herpesviridae* family, and are also referred to as human herpes virus 1 and 2 (HHV-1 and HHV-2).

Epidemiology

HSV pulmonary infections occur through direct extension of oral mucocutaneous disease with focal or multifocal necrosis, or by hematogenous spread from oral, genital, or cutaneous sources.

Populations at risk for HSV pulmonary disease include patients receiving chemotherapy or with other forms of immunosuppression, such as those with HIV or congenital deficiency, and burn victims.

HSV accounts for 1%–10% of post-transplant pneumonias.

Clinical features

The presence of mucocutaneous or esophageal HSV disease increases the probability that HSV is causing pulmonary disease.

The symptoms of HSV LRI include dyspnea, cough, fever, tachypnea, wheezing, chest pain, and hemoptysis.

HSV involves other organs as well, and can cause meningitis, encephalitis, and keratoconjunctivitis.

CXR in HSV pneumonia can show focal or diffuse infiltrates and peripheral nodules that coalesce with progression to severe disease.

Diagnosis

HSV infection is best identified by viral culture. Serology using ELISA does not distinguish between past exposure and current infection. PCR can also be used to identify viral DNA and is particularly used in testing cerebrospinal fluid (CSF).

Airway inspection on bronchoscopy can reveal tracheitis, bronchitis, and punctate mucosal lesions.

On biopsy, the pathology of HSV pulmonary infection is a monocytic infiltrate with necrosis and hemorrhage. There may also be giant cells with intranuclear inclusions.

Treatment

Intravenous acyclovir is the primary treatment for HSV pulmonary infections and is preferred for severe disease. Famciclovir and valacyclovir can also be used.

Further information

Simoons-Smit AM, Kraan EM, Beishuizen A, Strack van Schijndel RJ, Vandenbroucke-Grauls CM (2006). Herpes simplex virus type 1 and respiratory disease in critically ill patients: real pathogen or innocent bystander? *Clin Microbiol Infect* **12**(11):1050–1059.

Varicella zoster virus

Varicella zoster virus (VZV) is a double-stranded DNA virus of the *Herpesviridae* family, and referred to as human herpes virus 3 (HHV-3).

Epidemiology

VZV is typically associated with chicken pox on primary infection or shingles with reactivation.

VZV pneumonia occurs in a small proportion of adults who have chicken pox or shingles. Risk factors for LRI complicating VZV infection include pregnancy, steroid treatment, and immunocompromised state.

VZV is spread by large respiratory droplets or by direct contact with cutaneous lesions.

Clinical features

VZV LRI symptoms occur 1–6 days after the onset of rash. The rash is characterized by erythematous macules progressing to papules and then vesicles. The rash and vesicles may be present simultaneously on different parts of the body. The rash classically begins on the trunk and spreads to the face and extremities.

VZV LRI symptoms include cough, fever, dyspnea, and tachypnea. Pleuritic pain and hemoptysis may also occur.

The pneumonia course is more severe in smokers, pregnant women, and the immunocompromised.

CXR typically shows a diffuse fluffy, reticular, or small nodular infiltrate. Hilar lymphadenopathy and pleural effusions may uncommonly occur. The nodules may subsequently calcify and persist.

Multiorgan involvement may occur with encephalitis and hepatitis. Reye syndrome can also occur with concurrent aspirin use.

Bacterial superinfection can complicate the underlying viral infection.

Diagnosis

The diagnosis of VZV pneumonia is usually based on a history of exposure, presence of the typical rash, and CXR features.

Cytological examination using Tzanck smears from skin lesions can identify viral infection but does not distinguish between HSV and VZV.

Serology, or viral culture or PCR on BAL fluid can be used to confirm the diagnosis.

Treatment

Acyclovir is used to treat varicella pneumonia. Vidarabine, interferon-α, and foscarnet have also been used for adjunctive therapy. Valacyclovir and famciclovir have been used to treat zoster, but have not been studied for use in VZV LRI.

Varicella is very infectious until all cutaneous lesions enter the "crusting" stage. Hospitalized patients should be placed in respiratory isolation.

VZV live virus vaccinations are now widely administered to children. Adults can also be vaccinated if they have no history of prior VZV infection and if they work in a high-exposure setting (e.g., health-care workers).

VZV vaccine can also be administered to healthy individuals as post-exposure prophylaxis. Varicella-zoster immune globulin can by used in immunocompromised or pregnant patients exposed to varicella who cannot receive the live virus vaccine.

Most cases of VZV infection resolve spontaneously, but a minority progress to respiratory failure and death. Mortality due to VZV LRI may be as high as 40% in pregnancy.

Further information

Harger JH, Ernest JM, Thurnau GR, et al. (2002). Risk factors and outcome of varicella-zoster virus pneumonia in pregnant women. *J Infect Dis* **185**(4):422–427.

Measles

The measles, or rubeola virus, is a single-stranded RNA member of the *Paramyxovirus* family.

Epidemiology

Measles is much less common since vaccination has become widespread, but outbreaks still occasionally occur in unimmunized populations. Measles infection is very rare in adults.

A small portion (5%) of measles cases involves pneumonia. The mortality rate of measles is 1 death per 1000 cases, most of which are due to severe pneumonia.

Clinical features

Typical measles infection is characterized by a fever and URI followed by a diffuse maculopapular rash.

Pathognomonic for measles is the presence of Koplik spots, which are gray spots on a red base on the buccal mucosa.

Measles pneumonia is characterized by rales, wheezing, and a barking cough, and leukopenia is common.

The severity of the pneumonia parallels the intensity of the rash.

CXR in measles pneumonia may show reticulonodular infiltrates, hilar lymphadenopathy, and pleural effusions.

Diagnosis

Measles can generally be diagnosed on the basis of rash and symptoms.

ELISA for IgM to the measles virus can confirm acute infection, but will not be positive for the first 2 days of infection.

PCR and immunofluorescence can be used to identify the virus in BAL or tissue specimens.

Pulmonary biopsy during measles pneumonia shows an interstitial infiltrate with monocytes and multinucleated giant cells.

Treatment

First-line treatment for measles pneumonia is supportive. Ribivarin can be used for severe pneumonia in adults, similar to its application for RSV pneumonia.

Secondary bacterial infection is common and should be treated appropriately.

Post-exposure prophylaxis for pregnant women and immunosuppressed patients can be provided with intravenous immunoglobulin (IVIG).

Further information

Yang E, Rubin BK (1995). "Childhood" viruses as a cause of pneumonia in adults. *Semin Respir Infect* **10**(4):232–243.

Epstein–Barr virus

Epstein–Barr virus (EBV) is a double-stranded DNA virus, a member of the *Herpesviridae* family, and is also known as human herpes virus 4 (HHV-4).

Epidemiology

EBV is spread by oral–oral contact with infected saliva, and typically causes infectious mononucleosis.

Less than 10% of primary EBV infections are complicated by pneumonia.

EBV targets lymphocytes and the epithelium of the nasopharynx, oropharynx, and salivary glands.

Clinical features

Infectious mononucleosis is characterized by fever, pharyngitis, laryngitis, and occasionally splenomegaly.

The symptoms of EBV pneumonia are nonproductive cough, tachypnea, malaise, and fever.

Diagnosis

The heterophile test is most commonly used to diagnose EBV infection.

EBV antibody tests can also be used to detect a new infection, based on IgM and IgG levels.

Treatment

There is no specific treatment for mild EBV infection other than supportive measures.

In severe infection, acyclovir can be used. Other antivirals have efficacy against EBV in vitro, but have not been tested in clinical trials. IVIG can be used as adjunctive therapy.

EBV pneumonia is associated with a high incidence of bacterial superinfection, thus there should be a low threshold to start broad-spectrum antibiotics if there is no clinical response to antivirals.

Further information

Gautschi O, Berger C, Gubler J, Laube I (2003). Acute respiratory failure and cerebral hemorrhage due to primary Epstein-Barr virus infection. *Respiration* **70**(4):419–422.

Hantavirus

Hantaviruses are single-stranded RNA viruses in the *Bunyaviridae* family. Several different hantaviruses (particularly the Sin Nombre virus) have been associated with this syndrome.

Epidemiology

Hantavirus pulmonary syndrome was first described following an outbreak in the southwestern United States in 1993.

Previously described hantavirus-associated diseases have occurred in Scandinavia and northeastern Asia, and tended to cause hemorrhagic fever and renal failure with relative sparing of the lung.

Hantavirus pulmonary syndrome is very rare, with approximately 200 reported cases. Affected individuals are almost exclusively from the United States, particularly the "Four Corners Region" where Arizona, Colorado, Utah, and New Mexico meet.

The animal reservoir is the deer mouse, which is chronically infected with the virus. The mouse excretes the virus in urine and feces, and human disease develops following inhalation of aerosolized viruses from rodent feces or urine. The disease can also be acquired through saliva from bites.

Hantavirus typically affects previously healthy young adults.

Clinical features

Hantavirus pulmonary syndrome goes through five stages:
1. *Prodrome*: The first stage lasts 3–6 days and consists of fever, chills, cough, myalgias, and gastrointestinal symptoms such as nausea, vomiting, and abdominal pain.
2. *Fulminant infection*: This stage is characterized by breathlessness, which is quickly followed by respiratory failure due to noncardiogenic pulmonary edema and pulmonary capillary leakage with the development of ARDS. There is a decrease in circulatory volume causing shock, resulting in diminished cardiac output and lactic acidosis.
3. *Oliguric stage*: If patients survive the fulminant infection stage, it is followed by a period of 3–7 days of low urinary output and renal failure.
4. *Diuresis*: After the oliguric phase, patients have a diuresis of 3–6 L/day, which can last from 2 days to weeks.
5. *Convalescence*: This is a period of slow recovery back to normal, lasting weeks to months.

CXR is initially clear during the prodrome phase, and changes to pulmonary edema and fullness of the pulmonary hila, alveolar infiltrates, and often effusions.

Laboratory testing classically reveals neutrophilia and thrombocytopenia, sometimes with renal impairment and mildly abnormal liver function tests.

Diagnosis

The diagnosis may be confirmed using serology or PCR for the virus, or by detection of viral antigen using immunochemistry.

Treatment

Treatment is supportive within an ICU. Mechanical ventilation is often required. Extracorporeal membrane oxygenation (ECMO) has been used to stabilize patients during the fulminant phase.

It is unclear if person-to-person transmission of hantavirus occurs, but given the severity of disease, patients should likely be in respiratory isolation.

Intravenous ribavirin is commonly administered, although it is unclear if this improves outcome.

Bacterial superinfection is common, and patients in the fulminant phase should be empirically treated with broad-spectrum antibiotics.

Mortality is approximately 50%, with death usually occurring within several days of presentation, during the fulminant stage.

Further information

Borges AA, Campos GM, Moreli ML, et al. (2006). Hantavirus cardiopulmonary syndrome: immune response and pathogenesis. *Microbes Infect* **8**(8):2324–2330.

Chang B, Crowley M, Campen M, Koster F (2007). Hantavirus cardiopulmonary syndrome. *Semin Respir Crit Care Med* **28**(2):193–200.

Severe acute respiratory syndrome

Severe acute respiratory syndrome (SARS) is caused by a single-stranded RNA virus belonging to the *Coronavirus* family.

Epidemiology

SARS was first recognized in November 2002 in the Guangdong Province of China, and had spread internationally by late February 2003. The disease began waning by May 2003, and by July 2003 the epidemic had ended.

Further cases have been reported in laboratory workers in Singapore and Beijing who were exposed to previously obtained samples.

The masked palm civet is a host for a similar coronavirus, and is thought to be the original source of SARS.

SARS is spread by large droplets and person-to-person contact, but is also shed in large quantities in the stool and has been transmitted through contaminated sewage.

The first outbreak affected primarily health-care workers and their contacts. Overall, one-fifth of those infected by SARS were health-care workers, and nosocomial infection was common. The use of aerosol-generating procedures (e.g., endotracheal intubation and bronchoscopy) may amplify transmission.

A total of 8422 cases were reported to the WHO, with 916 deaths, for a case fatality rate of 11%. The fatality rate for those older than 60 was 43%, but 0% in those younger than 12.

Twenty-nine countries in Asia, Europe, and North America were affected, with 83% of the worldwide cases occurring in China and Hong Kong. There were 251 cases and 41 deaths in Canada. No deaths occurred in the United States.

Clinical features

The incubation period of SARS is 2–10 days after exposure.

The first symptom is typically fever, and may be accompanied by malaise, headache, and myalgias.

The respiratory stage of SARS starts 3–7 days after the prodromal phase with a dry cough and breathlessness. This often rapidly progresses to respiratory failure requiring mechanical ventilation.

Up to 70% of patients develop large-volume watery diarrhea without blood or mucus.

Patients can have a normal or low white blood cell count, thrombocytopenia, elevated CK and LDH, and transaminitis.

CXR ranges from normal to focal consolidation or diffuse bilateral interstitial infiltrate.

CT may reveal areas of interstitial infiltrate in those with a normal CXR. Spontaneous pneumothorax, pneumomediastinum, subpleural fibrosis, and/or cystic changes can occur in later disease stages.

Diagnosis

The WHO-defined case definition criteria for SARS are as follows:

- Fever over 38°C *plus*
- One or more symptoms of LRI (cough, difficulty breathing, shortness of breath) *plus*
- Radiographic evidence of lung infiltrate consistent with pneumonia or ARDS, or autopsy findings consistent with the pathology of pneumonia or ARDS without identifiable cause *plus*
- No alternative diagnosis to explain the illness.

Laboratory testing should be used to diagnose SARS if it is locally available. Testing that has been developed includes PCR, ELISA for seroconversion, or viral culture.

Destruction of lung tissue is thought to result from an excessive immune response to the virus, rather than from the direct effects of the virus.

An initial positive result on PCR should be confirmed by another clinical sample to avoid false positives.

Treatment

There is no specific treatment for SARS other than general supportive care.

Some patients have been treated with oseltamivir and/or intravenous ribavirin, but a series from Toronto showed a trend toward worsening outcome in those treated with ribavirin due to elevated transaminases and hemolysis. There are no in vitro data to show any anti-SARS virus activity of ribavirin.

Steroids reduce fever and improve oxygenation and CXR appearance, but do not alter the need for mechanical ventilation, or mortality.

Experimental animal models show reduced viral replication with pegalated interferon-α, and human studies using interferon and corticosteroids have shown no adverse effects.

Known and suspected cases of SARS should be in respiratory and contact isolation.

The SARS epidemic ended largely due to public health measures, including avoidance of exposure, and effective infection control by closing public gatherings and the use of quarantine.

Further information

Peiris JS, Yuen KY, Osterhaus AD, Stohr K (2003). The severe acute respiratory syndrome. *N Engl J Med* **349**(25):2431–2441.
WHO Web site for continuously updated information: www.who.int/csr/sars/en

Mycobacterial respiratory infection

Tuberculosis (TB): epidemiology and pathophysiology

Despite being curable, tuberculosis is the second leading infectious cause of death worldwide (after AIDS), taking nearly 2 million lives per year. In the United States, TB rates have fallen substantially over the last 15 years, largely because of enhanced professional awareness and the widespread use of directly observed therapy (DOT).

Following an upsurge of multidrug-resistant TB (MDR-TB) in the early 1990s, the prevalence of such cases has also fallen. Although small in number, cases of extensive drug-resistant TB (XDR-TB) have caused concern.

Epidemiology

There were 13,299 cases of TB in the United States in 2007, a case rate of 4.4 per 100,000 population; 58% of these cases occurred among foreign-born individuals; the case rate in this population was 20.7 vs. 2.1 per 100,000 in the U.S. born.[1] Mexico, the Philippines, Vietnam, India, and China accounted for over half of the foreign-born cases.

Case rates among the U.S. born varies widely by race: 1.1 per 100,000 for whites vs. 8.5 for Hispanics, 9.4 for blacks, 23 for native Hawaiians or Pacific Islanders, and 26.3 among Asians. Among white Americans, TB is more prominent in the elderly. Among minorities and immigrants, TB is most prevalent among young adults and children.

Transmission and pathophysiology

TB is spread almost exclusively via the airborne route. Typically, patients with pulmonary disease generate small-particle aerosols while coughing. Desiccated particles, or "droplet nuclei," roughly 1 μm in size, are inhaled by indoor contacts. These particles can drift down the branching airways to be deposited in the alveoli, beyond the protective barrier of the ciliated epithelium.

The bacillus is taken up there by alveolar macrophages, which ultimately interact with pulmonary dendritic cells to initiate a cascade of host defenses that involves chemokines, cytokines, and lymphocytes. This process usually includes a pulmonary focus, "the primary lesion," and ipsilateral hilar lymph nodes. Before effective cellular immunity evolves, there is a widespread bacillemia.

In most cases, acquired cell-mediated immunity results in involution of these scattered foci. In most normal hosts the only vestige of this primary infection is the development of delayed-type hypersensitivity (DTH) to TB antigens. DTH evolves in 4–12 weeks, and may be detected by the traditional Mantoux skin test or the newer interferon-gamma release assays.

In persons with poor immune capacity (the very young, the very old, those with AIDS, or those immunosuppressed from organ transplantation or oncological therapy), there may be uninterrupted progression to clinically active TB.

---

1 Centers for Disease Control and Prevention (CDC) (2007). *Reported Tuberculosis in the United States, 2007.* Atlanta, GA: U.S. Department of Health and Human Services.

Most infected persons never develop disease. However, even among "normal hosts," there is an approximately 10% lifetime risk of "reactivation" TB. This most commonly involves the apices of the lungs or extrapulmonary sites that were seeded during the primary infection.

TB: clinical manifestations

Symptoms of pulmonary tuberculosis:
- Cough, increasingly productive
- Hemoptysis
- Malaise
- Night sweats
- Weight loss
- Chest pain

Extrapulmonary tuberculosis (XPTB)

Annually, 20% of U.S. patients *without* HIV infection present with tuberculosis disease outside the lungs.

Pleura
Pleural TB may occur with either primary or reactivation disease. Symptoms include chest pain, dyspnea and cough. An exudative, lymphocyte-rich fluid is typical. AFB smear and culture of the pleural fluid are often negative; biopsy has a high yield.

Lymphadenitis
Lymphadenitis is typically unilateral and painless. Inflamed anterior or posterior cervical and/or supraclavicular nodes are the most common presentation.

Genitourinary
GU TB may involve the kidneys, ureters, bladder, epididymis, prostate, or fallopian tubes. Flank pain, hematuria, pyuria and fever are common presenting manifestations. Urine culture is a standard diagnostic test.

Spinal
Spinal TB may infect the intervertebral disc space and/or the vertebra(e) proper. Among younger patients, the higher thoracic spine is typically involved, while among older subjects the lumbar spine is more common. Back pain and "cold abscesses" (minimal inflammation, non-tender) are the usual presentation.

Osseous
Weight-bearing joints such as the knees or hips are most frequently involved, although a variety of long or flat bones may be involved.

Meningeal
The most disabling and potentially lethal form of TB is meningitis. It may occur as part of disseminated TB or as isolated CNS involvement. Classically, there are three stages in clinical evolution: (1) behavioral changes, irritability, cognitive slippage; (2) focal neurological deficits; and (3) global neurological dysfunction including coma.

Early diagnosis is critical, for the prognosis worsens as the stages advance. Lumbar puncture is central to recognition: moderate leukocytosis, usually lymphocytic, with lowered glucose and elevated protein levels is found. An MRI indicating basilar meningeal enhancement, ventricular dilatation, and focal infarction is characteristic.

If TB meningitis is suspected, empirical therapy should be initiated. Corticosteroids are of proven efficacy in TB meningitis.

Miliary
Multiorgan TB tends to involve the very young, the elderly, and immunocompromised, including persons with AIDS. However, it can appear in otherwise healthy individuals. Among African Americans, a disproportionate share of TB morbidity involves disseminated disease.

Early, plain CXR may be normal; CT scan is more sensitive. Bone marrow biopsy is a highly sensitive test.

TB: diagnostics studies

Tuberculin skin test (TST)
The intradermal Mantoux test is neither sensitive nor specific for TB. Among those not HIV-infected, roughly 20% of active TB cases do not have significant (5 mm or more) reactions. Up to 85% of those with advanced AIDS and TB do not react to the TST.

Due to cross-reactivity from BCG vaccination or nontuberculous mycobacterial infection, a reactive TST does not clearly indicate infection with *M. tuberculosis*.

Interferon gamma release assays (IGRAs)
Whole-blood assays of the production of IFN-γ by peripheral blood monocytes stimulated by two antigens found in *M. tuberculosis* (but not BCG or most pathogenic nontuberculous mycobacteria) may well supplant the TST. However, to date, the IGRAs have proven more specific but only modestly more sensitive than the TST.

Chest X-ray
The overwhelming majority of those with pulmonary TB have abnormal CXRs. Two-thirds involve typical upper-lobe fibronodular findings; cavities are seen in half of these cases. Lower-lobe abnormalities are more common among Asian patients.

Among those with AIDS, the more advanced the immunosuppression the more atypical are the radiographic features, including large pleural effusions.

Drug susceptibility testing (DST)
DST should be done on all new isolates and repeated in cases with delayed conversion of sputum (positive cultures beyond 3 months of therapy). Particular attention must be given to cases among immigrants from regions with high rates of drug resistance (Mexico, Asia, Pacific Rim nationals, the Indian subcontinent, Russia, and former Soviet republics).

TB: treatment

Treatment of latent TB infection (TLTI)

There are two major components of TLTI: (1) performing contact investigations around new cases to identify those who are newly infected and, thus, at high risk of progressing to active disease, and (2) identifying other subjects who, due to various factors, are at risk for active disease. These factors include the following:

- HIV infection
- Immunosuppression, including cancer chemotherapy, organ transplantation
- TNF-α inhibition such as infliximab, etanercept, or adalimumab
- Upper-lobe fibronodular opacities consistent with prior, healed TB infection
- Being an immigrants from a high-risk region

For those at particularly great risk, TST reactions of 5 mm or greater are deemed positive or significant. For lower-risk subjects, TST reactions of 10 mm or more are deemed positive.

Many immigrants from areas with high rates of TB give a history of BCG vaccination in childhood. However, the tuberculin reactivity induced by BCG usually wanes within 5–10 years. Thus, an adult with a strongly reactive TST may reasonably be inferred to have had intercurrent TB infection and be a candidate for TLTI. IGRAs may be useful here.

Regimens for TLTI identified in the 2000 ATS/CDC guidelines[1] include (1) isoniazid (INH) daily for 9 months, (2) INH daily for 6 months, or (3) rifampin (RIF) daily for 4 months. Given the disproportionate risk for acquired resistance to the rifamycins, RIF monotherapy should not be used in persons with HIV infection.

The 2000 Guidelines originally identified 2–3 months of RIF and pyrazinamide (PZA) as an option for TLTI. However, because of unanticipated hepatotoxicity, including deaths, this recommendation was subsequently withdrawn.

Treatment of active TB

Multidrug therapy is employed to prevent acquired resistance and accelerate the time to cure (see Table 21.1). Rifampin is the keystone of modern therapy; cases involving RIF-resistance entail prolonged treatment and are less predictably responsive to therapy.

The 2003 American Thoracic Society/Centers for Disease Control (ATS/CDC) guidelines[2] advocate an initial four-drug regimen: RIF, INH, PZA, and ethambutol (EMB) (see Table 21.2). Most programs commence with daily therapy, although one of the ATS/CDC options employs a thrice-weekly schedule throughout.

---

1 American Thoracic Society (2000). Targeted tuberculin testing and treatment of latent tuberculosis infection. *Am J Respir Crit Care Med* **161**:S221-S247.
2 American Thoracic Society/Centers for Disease Control and Prevention/Infectious Diseases Society of America (2003). Treatment of tuberculosis. *Am J Respir Crit Care Med* **167**:603–662.

Directly observed therapy is used in the United States in the great majority of potentially communicable (respiratory tract) TB cases. A public-health worker delivers all doses to patients and observes them ingesting the meds. Such ensured therapy prevents nonadherence and reduces treatment failure, post-therapy relapses, and acquired drug resistance.

To be effective, DOT programs employ patient-centered strategies including incentives and enablers. The ATS/CDC guidelines clearly assign responsibility for ensuring therapy to the caregivers, not the patients.

Reporting

All proven or *suspected* cases must be reported to local public-health agencies. In possibly infectious cases, contact investigations are initiated in the home, workplace, or other situations where transmission seems likely.

Although not regarded as capable of transmitting TB to others, infants and children with suspected TB are reported so that investigations can be done to find the adult who presumably infected them.

Treatment of drug-resistant TB

M. tuberculosis has the capacity to spawn mutants resistant to all known drug families used in treatment. These mutants are rare and unlinked; on average, they occur in 1 in 10^6–10^8 replications.

The risk for acquired drug resistance is greatest in the early phase of therapy, especially in cavitary diseases, when there are immense numbers of bacilli rapidly multiplying. Hence three or more active agents are needed during the initial 2 months. If patients take some but not all of their medications, or if they have suboptimal drug levels due to malabsorption or substandard products, selection for drug resistance may occur.

Resistant to RIF and INH, MDR-TB requires extended therapy with expensive second-line drugs that are hard to tolerate and relatively toxic. MDR-TB substantially increases the risks for treatment failure (inability to achieve negative cultures during therapy) or relapses (reactivated disease following cessation of therapy).

Extensive drug-resistant TB (XDR-TB) was recognized by the CDC and WHO in 2007 to represent a unique threat to global health. XDR-TB entails resistance to not only RIF and INH but also the fluoroquinolones and one or more of the second-line injectable agents (amikacin, kanamycin, or capreomycin). XDR-TB cases in developing nations, especially in persons with AIDS, represent an immense management challenge.

Patients with drug-resistant forms of TB represent high risks for nosocomial transmission, further acquired drug resistance, and treatment failures. They must be reported promptly to public-health authorities and referred for specialized management.

Table 21.1 ATS/CDC 6-month regimens for TB (2003)*

Initial 2 months	Continuation phase, 4 months	
I. Daily	*IA. Daily*	
RIF 600 mg	RIF 600 mg	
INH 300 mg	INH 300 mg	
PZA 25 mg/kg	*IB. Twice weekly*	
EMB 15 mg/kg	RIF 600 mg	
	INH 900 mg	
II. Daily or twice-weekly		
Daily x 2 weeks	Twice-weekly x 6 weeks	Twice-weekly x 18 weeks
RIF 600 mg	RIF 600 mg	RIF 600 mg
INH 300 mg	INH 900 mg	INH 900 mg
PZA 25 mg/kg	PZA 40 mg/kg	
EMB 15 mg/kg	EMB 40 mg/kg	
III. Thrice-weekly		
Thrice-weekly x 8 weeks	Thrice-weekly x 18 weeks	
RIF 600 mg	RIF 600 mg	
INH 600 mg	INH 600 mg	
PZA 30 mg/kg		
EMB 30 mg/kg		

EMB, ethambutol; INH, isoniazid; PZA, pyrazinamide; RIF, rifampin.

*For details, including potential use of rifapentine or rifabutin, see ATS/CDC Guidelines.[1]

1 American Thoracic Society/Centers for Disease Control and Prevention/Infectious Diseases Society of America (2003). Treatment of tuberculosis. *Am J Respir Crit Care Med* **167**:603–662.

Table 21.2 Drug profiles for agents used in TB treatment

Agent	Toxicities*	Comments
Rifampin	Hepatitis Thrombopenia Drug interactions	RIF is a highly potent inducer of hepatic cytochrome P450 pathways; it may result in clinically significant reductions in the levels of many categories of drugs, including calcium channel blockers, beta-blockers, sulfanylurea hypoglycemics, coumadin, corticosteroids, oral contraceptives, opiates, azoles, anticonvulsants, protease inhibitors, and some NNRTIs (see ATS Guidelines 2003 for additional drugs and details).
Isoniazid	Hepatitis CNS effects Peripheral neuritis	Modest, asymptomatic elevations of transaminases are common early in therapy and do not require cessation. However, abnormal LFTs with symptoms should lead to prompt cessation. Mood alterations and problems with concentration may be problematic. Pyridoxine (B6) supplementation is advised in pregnancy and malnutrition (20–50 mg/day).
Pyrazinamide	Hepatitis Hyperuricemia with arthralgias or arthritis in gouty subjects Impaired glucose control	Hyperuricemia is less problematic in bi-weekly or thrice-weekly schedules. May cause sustained hepatocellular damage
Ethambutol	Optic neuritis Peripheral neuritis Hyperuricemia	Cleared renally; dosage must be adjusted with reduced GFR

*See ATS Guidelines[1] or PDR for comprehensive reviews of the side effects or toxicity

Monitoring for drug toxicity
Hepatitis
Monitor for symptoms, use baseline liver chemistries. Be alert for underlying chronic viral hepatitis B and/or C.

Optic neuritis
Alert patients to possible visual effects. Use baseline then monthly Snellen (acuity) and Ishihara (color) testing.

Other
Warn patients that their urine and tears will appear red-orange while on rifampin (can stain soft contact lenses). The effect will lessen over time; this is not a toxic reaction.

1 American Thoracic Society (2001). Update: Fatal and severe liver injuries associated with rifampin and pyrazinamide for latent tuberculosis infection, and revisions in American Thoracic Society/CDC recommendations—United States 2001. *Am J Respir Crit Care Med* **164**:1319–1320.

Isolation of TB suspects and patients

TB is spread by infectious aerosols, which are typically generated by patients with sputum that is smear-positive for pulmonary or laryngeal TB. However, transmission can and does occur with smear-negative cases.

Transmission also occurs in these settings:
- Sputum induction facilities
- Bronchoscopy suites
- Autopsy facilities
- Debridement of soft-tissue wounds associated with TB

Appropriate policies include the following:
- All hospital patients with suspected or proven potentially communicable forms of TB should be isolated in rooms with negative pressure, non-recirculated ventilation (6 or more air changes per hour are desirable).
- Upper room air ultraviolet germicidal irradiation may provide additional protection.
- All staff entering the room should wear fit-tested N95 personal respirators.

For release from isolation, most patients with drug-susceptible TB will have a rapid reduction in the number of viable bacilli and the frequency of cough during the first 2 weeks of therapy. Hence, this time has been historically regarded as the period to release from isolation.

However, patients with MDR-TB do not enjoy these effects and constitute a particular hazard for nosocomial transmission. For proven or suspected MDR cases, release should depend on clear-cut clinical and bacteriological (reduced number of AFB on smear) improvements. Modern laboratories can report drug susceptibility results in 18–21 days, while others take up to 2 months. Molecular techniques which identify the *rpo*B mutation associated with resistance to the rifamycins may allow identification of rifampin resistance and, thereby, MDR-TB in 24 to 48 hours.

Nontuberculous (environmental) mycobacterial (NTM) lung disease

In many regions of the United States, Canada, and Western Europe, the prevalence of NTM lung disease is equal to or greater than that of TB (see Table 21.3). Extrapolating from systematic data derived in Ontario, Canada, Iseman and Marras calculated that the annual incidence of TB modestly exceeded that of MAC and other NTM diseases.[1] However, since 80% or more of TB cases are cured in 6 months, whereas the normal MAC case requires 18 months of therapy and still poses up to 50% risk of relapse, the prevalence of NTM disease may be an order of magnitude greater than TB.

Surveys indicate that NTM are widely distributed in the water, particularly in potable water systems. Hence it is reasonable to infer that NTM infections are acquired from the environment and are not spread human to human.

Geographically, early experience indicated the preponderance of NTM disease was in the Southeast United States. However, cases are being seen in all contiguous 48 states, Alaska, and Hawaii. A high prevalence of NTM disease has also been noted in Canada, Western Europe and Japan.

Broadly, there are two forms of pulmonary NTM disease:
1. TB-like upper-lobe fibronodular opacities with prominent cavitation
2. Scattered bronchiectasis, particularly involving the right middle lobe (RML) and lingular segment of the left upper lobe

The TB-like disease is more common among males, largely with underlying COPD or silicosis. The bronchiectatic variety of disease is far more common among women. Disproportionately Caucasians in the aggregate, these women tend to be slender with a variety of phenotypic features: subtle scoliosis, straight back syndrome, pectus excavatum, narrow anteroposterior diameter, and/or mitral valve prolapse.[2]

Heritable risk factors include adult variants of cystic fibrosis (CF) and anomalous α_1-anti-trypsin phenotypes. As children with classic CF have survived longer, NTM infections have become more prevalent.

Symptoms patterns are divergent as well. Those with cavitary disease commonly present with productive cough ± hemoptysis, fever, chills and sweats, and weight loss. By contrast, variably productive cough, fatigue, and malaise are the more typical presentation with bronchiectasis.

1 Iseman MD, Marras TK (2008). The importance of nontuberculous mycobacterial lung disease. *Am J Respir Crit Care Med* **178**(10):999–1000.

2 Kim RD, Greenberg DE, Ehrmantraut ME, Ding L, Shea Y, Chernick M, et al. (2008). Pulmonary nontuberculous mycobacterial disease: prospective study of a distinct preexisting syndrome. *Am J Respir Crit Care Med* **178**(10):1066–1074.

Table 21.3 Common NTM pathogenic species

Species	Comments
M. avium, M. intracellulare (M. avium complex [MAC])	MAC is before the most frequent NTM pathogen.
M. kansasii (MK)	More often associated with TB-like disease, MK is seen more frequently in the U.S. Southeast.
M. chelonae, M. abscessus, M. fortuitum (rapidly growing mycobacteria [RGM])	M. abscessus is the most common RGM pathogen. The RGM are more commonly associated with the bronchiectasis pattern.
M. xenopi, M. malmoense, M. simiae	There are a large number of NTM species that occasionally are pathogenic.
M. gordonae*	This species is the most common contaminant among the NTM. In most cases, the contaminant occurs in the laboratory. In rare instances it may be pathogenic.

Diagnostic criteria for NTM lung disease

Because these organisms are environmental, isolated sputum culture is not regarded as diagnostic. Rather, the 2007 ATS guidelines identify the following criteria:

- Abnormal CXR and/or CT lung scan
- Two or more positive sputum cultures for one of the more common NTM pathogens
- Chronic symptoms
- Absence of other pathogens such as TB

Tuberculin skin tests are generally nonreactive in persons with NTM infection; however, there is considerable cross-reactivity with M. kansasii and, to a lesser extent, MAC.

Treatment of NTM lung disease

Drug regimens are described in detail in the 2007 ATS guidelines[1]; typical regimens are listed in Table 21.4.

Table 21.4 Drug regimens for treatment of NTM lung disease according to the 2007 ATS guidelines

MAC	Azithromycin or clarithromycin, rifamycin and ethambutol. Amikacin may be used in the initial therapy with cavitary disease. For non-cavitary disease, thrice-weekly regimens are efficacious. Duration: 18 months
M. kansasii	Isoniazid, rifampin, and ethambutol comprise the standard regimen. Usual duration is 15–18 months. An alternative would be to substitute a macrolide for isoniazid.
RGMs	There is very little systematic information regarding regimen selection for these species. Infection due to M. chelonae or M. abscessus is rarely curable. Regimens of imipenem or cefoxitin plus amikacin are generally effective in suppressing infection. Episodic therapy based on symptomatic, radiographic, and/or bacteriological deterioration is the usual practice.

Surgery in NTM lung disease

In some cases there is such severe damage to the lungs that resectional surgery may be considered. The right middle lobe and the lingular segment of the left upper lobe are particularly vulnerable to severe bronchiectasis, which predisposes to chronic refractory infections including the NTM or other opportunistic pathogens including Pseudomonas or other gram-negative rods. Resection has been made more acceptable by video-assisted thoracoscopic surgical (VATS) techniques.

1 American Thoracic Society (2007). An official ATS/IDSA statement. Diagnosis, treatment, and prevention of nontuberculous mycobacterial diseases. *Am J Respir Crit Care Med* **175**:367–416.

Fungal respiratory diseases

Aspergillus lung disease: classification

Introduction

The *Aspergillus* spp. are ubiquitous molds whose habitat includes soil and vegetable materials. Disease associated with *Aspergillus* is related to the inhalation of airborne conidia. Dust and water droplets have been implicated as vectors of transmission. All humans inhale several hundred conidia per day, according to environmental surveys, but few have related disease.

Aspergillus fumigatus is the most commonly implicated *Aspergillus* species in causing human disease, making up over 90% of documented infections.

Classification

Pulmonary disease related to *Aspergillus* can be broken down into three broad classifications:

1. Allergic diseases
   - Extrinsic asthma
   - Allergic bronchopulmonary aspergillosis (ABPA)
   - Hypersensitivity pneumonitis—rarely occurs; associated with massive exposure to *Aspergillus* spores; less common etiology for farmer's lung
   - Bronchocentric granulomatosis—characterized by necrotizing granulomas that obstruct and destroy bronchioles. Clinically shares many similarities with ABPA, including eosinophilia and increased IgE. Typically steroid responsive
   - Eosinophilic pneumonitis
2. Airway- and tissue-invasive disease
   - Invasive pulmonary aspergillosis
   - Chronic necrotizing aspergillosis
   - Invasive pleural disease
3. Infestation of airways, cavities, and necrotic tissue
   - Aspergilloma

1. Atopic allergy to fungal spores

Approximately 10% of asthmatics are skin-prick positive to *Aspergillus* species, compared to about 70% being positive to house dust mite. It is assumed that this allergy contributes to allergic inflammation in the airways but, in the few relevant studies, symptoms have not correlated with exposure.

2. Allergic bronchopulmonary aspergillosis

Clinical features and investigations

Associated features may include the following:

- Serum IgE >1000 ng/mL
- Blood eosinophilia >500/mm^3
- Skin sensitivity testing positive to *Aspergillus*
- IgG precipitins to *Aspergillus*

Definition

Allergic bronchopulmonary aspergillosis (ABPA) is a hypersensitivity reaction to *Aspergillus* antigens. It is most commonly seen in patients with long-standing asthma and cystic fibrosis. ABPA is usually suspected on clinical grounds with supporting laboratory and radiological findings. Patients can present with wheezing, cough often productive of brown sputum, and eosinophilia, with evidence of pulmonary infiltrates.

Some authors have chosen to subdivide ABPA into two groups based on the presence or absence of central bronchiectasis.

The prevalence of ABPA in asthmatic populations has varied considerably between studies. It probably occurs in about 1%–2% of asthmatics but is present in approximately 10% of corticosteroid-dependent patients. A related condition occurs in patients with cystic fibrosis, of whom up to 15% meet diagnostic criteria for ABPA.

Pathophysiology

The factors promoting the evolution from atopic asthmatic to ABPA are not known.

Aspergillus conidia persist in the airway and germinate, leading to presence of hyphae within mucus plugs, but there does not appear to be actual bronchial invasion. Exoproteases are released as well as other cellular products that affect clearance, damage the airway mucosa, and activate innate immune response to secrete a number of cytokines. This host defense response is believed to be responsible for most of the damage induced in ABPA.

A. fumigatus reactive CD4+ TH2 cells responding to chemokine signals are felt to be an important part of the pathogenesis of the disease. Genetic factors including major histocompatibility complex (MHC) restricted-phenotype expression are also related to the TH2 response. Cytoplasmic allergens *Asp f3* and *f4* are associated with ABPA.

The immune inflammatory activity induced by these mechanisms produces local and systemic eosinophilia, granular exoproducts, and an antigen-specific humoral response that histopathologically appears as mucoid impaction in the airways, eosinophilic pneumonitis, bronchocentric granuloma formation, and hyphae-filled microabscesses.

Main criteria for diagnosis

- History of asthma
- Immediate skin reactivity to *Aspergillus fumigatus*
- Serum precipitins to *A. fumigatus*
- Total serum IgE >1000 mg/mL
- Current or previous pulmonary infiltrates
- Increased serum IgG and IgG to *A. fumigatus*
- Peripheral eosinophilia (1000 cell/μL)
- Central bronchiectasis (absent in patients with seropositive ABPA)

Staging

Patients may not progress through all stages.

Stage 1 (acute stage)

- Asthma, elevated IgE, peripheral eosinophilia, pulmonary infiltrates, positive IgE and IgG to *A. fumigatus*

Stage 2 (remission stage)

- IgE falls but does not normalize, normal eosinophil count, normalization of CXR

Stage 3 (exacerbation stage)

- Similar to stage 1 in patients with known ABPA

Stage 4 (corticosteroid-dependant stage)

- Tapering of steroids leads to worsening symptoms and recurrent infiltrates. IgE may be normal in this phase. Bronchiectasis may be present.

Stage 5 (fibrotic stage)

Many patients are not diagnosed until they reach stage 4. Only a minority of patients progress to the fibrotic stage.

Clinical features

- History of asthma with recent deterioration
- Fever/malaise
- Expectoration of brown sputum occasionally with visible plugs
- Eosinophilia (sputum and blood)
- Pulmonary infiltrates

Investigations

Spirometry

- Airway obstruction

CXR

- Fleeting pulmonary infiltrates often of the upper lobe and central areas
- Gloved-finger appearance (band-like opacities radiating from the hilum)
- Tram lines, parallel lines, and ring shadows
- Central bronchiectasis and interstitial fibrosis

CT

- Central bronchiectasis with upper lobe predominance

Management

Corticosteroids are the mainstay of treatment. Typically, treatment is initiated at 0.5–1.0 mg/kg for 14 days with prolonged taper over 3–6 months. Inhaled corticosteroids do not prevent progression to bronchiectasis.

Itraconazole has been documented to reduce airway eosinophilia, decrease rates of exacerbation, and decrease serum IgE- and IgG-specific precipitants. It is currently recommended for use only in patients that are slow to respond to corticosteroids, suffer dose-limiting side effects from steroids, or are unable to be weaned from steroids.

Treatment with 200 mg/day has been documented to be efficacious. Initial studies used a dose of 5 mg/kg. Treatment course is typically 3–6 months. Liver function monitoring is necessary.

Olamizumab has been used in two cystic fibrosis patients with clinical improvement.

Differential diagnosis

• Churg–Strauss syndrome
• Pulmonary parasitic disease
• Drug-induced eosinophilic pneumonia
• Eosinophilic pneumonia
• Loeffler's pneumonia

3. Invasive aspergillosis

Definition

Invasive aspergillosis (IA) is characterized by the invasion of pulmonary tissue by aspergillus hyphae. IA is most commonly associated with significantly immunosuppressed hosts, most notably patients with prolonged neutropenia.

Aspergillus can involve any organ, but the lung is most commonly involved and is the port of entry for *Aspergillus* species. The species most commonly seen are *Aspergillus fumigatus* (56%), *A. flavus* (19%), *A. terreus* (16%), and *A. niger* (8%). These recent data indicate diversification of pathogenic organisms, as prior data indicated *A. fumigatus* as the etiology of 90% of IA.

Pathogenesis

Alveolar macrophages are the first line of defense against *Aspergillus conidia*. If macrophages are unable to prevent germination of spores, neutrophils are the primary host defense against the invasive phase. Inadequate neutrophil function allows invasion across tissue planes into blood vessels.

Angioinvasion can lead to vascular thrombosis, tissue infarction, and coagulative necrosis. This is most commonly seen in IA associated with profound neutropenia. Angioinvasion can also lead to distant spread of disease.

Virulence factors intrinsic to the hyphae appear to cause injury, in contrast to the inflammatory response of the host. Medications that affect neutrophil levels and mediators of inflammation such as TNF-α are associated with increased rates of invasive aspergillosis.

Clinical features

Typical setting
Fever, pleuritic chest pain, cough, hemoptysis, dyspnea, and pulmonary infiltrate in a neutopenic patient failing to respond to broad-spectrum antibiotics.

Risk factors
- Neutropenia (increased risk associated with increased severity and duration of neutropenia)
- Stem cell transplant patients (allogeneic > autologous)
- Solid organ transplant (lung transplant patients are at greatest risk; direct association with degree of immunosuppression)
- Immunosuppressive medications (including prednisone, calcineurin inhibitors, anti-TNF-α agents)
- AIDS (CD4 count <100)
- Phagocyte-associated immunodeficiencies

Sites of disease

Aspergillus can invade blood vessels, leading to distant spread. Frequent sites of disease outside the lung include the following:

- Sinus involvement with local spread to the brain
- Endocarditis
- Endopthalmitis and keratitis
- Cutaneous disease
- Kidney, liver, and spleen are all commonly involved in disseminated aspergillosis.

Investigations

CXR

- Nodules, patchy infiltrates, and cavitary lesions can all be seen, although CXR is often normal.

CT

- The most common finding is one or more pulmonary macronodules >1 cm in diameter (present in 90% of confirmed cases).
- "Halo sign": An area of ground-glass appearance surrounding a nodule is a classic finding and represents hemorrhage into tissue surrounding an invading focus (present in approximately 60% of confirmed cases).
- "Crescent sign": An area of air within a density which suggests cavitation and is associated with recovering neutrophil response in existing disease (present in only 10% and is of little diagnostic utility)
- Frequency of halo sign decreases, crescent sign frequency increases, and size of nodules increases routinely in the first week to 10 days after identification and treatment despite clinical response.

Others

- Sputum culture
- Bronchoalveolar lavage (50% sensitivity)

Laboratory studies

Galactomannan

An ELISA test is used for detecting this constituent of the fungal cell wall. Antigenemia can precede radiographic and clinical findings by 1 week. In a recent meta-analysis, the sensitivity was only 71% with a specificity of 89%. The negative predictive value was 92%–98%, but the positive predictive value was only 25%–62%. It is useful as an adjunctive test at this time. Efficacy is affected by concurrent anti-mold therapy and antibiotics, including pipericillin-tazobactam.

B-glucan

This is a fungal cell wall constituent that has been found to be elevated in early invasive fungal disease (not specific to *Aspergillus*). Efficacy has been proven in patients with acute myeloid leukemia (AML) and myelodysplastic syndrome.

Management

Azoles

- Voriconazole is the current standard of care after increased efficacy over amphotericin B was proven (71% to 58% survival at 12 weeks with less side effects in the voriconazole group)
- Posaconzale shares similarities with voriconazole, as it has shown benefit as salvage therapy.
- Itraconazole can be used as second-line therapy.

Amphotericin B formulations
Echinocandins

- Caspofungin has shown efficacy in salvage therapy and in patients intolerant of prior standard therapy. Retrospective analysis also suggests benefit in combination use with voriconazole.
- Micafungin
- Anidulafungin
- 5-flucytosine, used as adjunctive therapy

Surgical removal

- There have been no clinical trials to validate benefit of removal of infected tissue.

Immune modulation

- Colony-stimulating factors
- Recombinant interferon-γ
  - Augments innate and Th1-dependant immunity in vitro

~mocystis pneumonia (PCP)

~on

~ystis pneumonia (PCP) is the clinical syndrome of pneumonia
from infection with the fungus *Pneumocystis jiroveci* (previously
Pneumocystis carinii). *Pneumocystis jiroveci* is widespread in the
~ent, and 75% of people are infected by the age of 4 years.
~ansmission of PCP is not completely understood. It was widely
~t clinical infection was a result of reactivation. Animal studies
~ed into question this presumption, as immunosuppressed animals
~ared the trophozooite and were not chronic carriers.

~ors for PCP include: HIV infection (particularly with CD4 coun
10^6/L), treatment with chemotherapy (T-cell-depleting agent
~ludarabine), corticosteroids, or other immunosuppressive agents
~es are directly affected by the use of chemical prophylaxis t
infection.
~hreshold steroid dose for predisposition to PCP is unclear, an
~pend on the underlying condition. A retrospective analysi
a median dose of 30 mg in patients who were on corticosteroid
~oximately 8 weeks at the time of initial diagnosis of PCP. How
significant minority (25%) of patients who developed PCP wer
~dnisone doses of 16 mg daily.

~al features

~oms include subtle onset of progressive dyspnea, cough, and lo~
~ever. PCP in non-HIV patients may present more acutely and m~
~porally associated with the tapering of their immunosuppressi~
~tions. Tachycardia, tachypnea, and hypoxemia are also presen
~s may also present with pneumothorax.

~tigations

~ pattern is highly variable. The classic manifestation are diffuse,
~eral interstitial or alveolar infiltrates; 25% of patients will present
~ a normal CXR. Less common appearances include lobar infiltrates
~monary cystic lesions, and pulmonary nodules. There is an increased
~dence of pneumothorax and upper lobe disease in patients on
~led pentamidine. **Pleural effusions and lymphadenopathy are rare**
~rial blood gas should be drawn to determine PaO_2 and A–a
~dient (patients with PCP with PaO_2 <70 mmHg or A–a gradient
~ benefit from concurrent steroid treatment).
~ite blood count is usually normal.
~um lactate dehydrogenase is typically raised (sensitive but nonspecific)
~uced sputum has a diagnostic yield of about 60%–90%. There is
~reased specificity and sensitivity when immunoflorescent staining
~h antibodies is used. Diagnostic yield is impaired by prior use of
~ophylaxis.

4. Chronic necrotizing aspergillosis

Definition

This form of aspergillosis is a chronic low-grade locally invasive process
that occurs in patients with preexisting cavitary lung disease and mild
immunodeficiency. This process is poorly defined and carries a variety of
names including semi-invasive aspergillosis, complex aspergilloma, chronic
cavitary and fibrosing pulmonary aspergillosis, and pseudomembranous
tracheobronchitis.

Pathogenesis

As described in the introduction (p. 286), *Aspergillus* is a ubiquitous mold
that all humans are exposed to on a daily basis. Patients with existing
cavitary disease have decreased clearance of inhaled spores.

To progress to CPA, a factor that influences local macrophage or
neutrophil response to allow airway and alveolar invasion, such as tobacco
use, alcohol abuse, debilitation, diabetes, or low-dose use of inhaled or
oral corticosteroids, must be present. Histopathologically, there is no or
only minimal vascular invasion. A mild granulomatous reaction occurs
along with low rate of distant spread.

Clinical features (see Box 22.1)

> **Box 22.1 Suspect chronic necrotizing aspergillosis when**
>
> - Reason for mild immunosuppression
> - A preexisting chronic lung disease
> - Fever
> - Productive cough
> - Hemoptysis
> - Patchy, indolent, CXR changes.

Invasion into the pleural space can occur.

Investigations

- Sputum samples may show hyphae.
- CT will show an airway-centered type of picture with an initial
  "tree-in-bud" appearance. It may show infiltrate associated with
  cavitary lesion or mycetoma.
- The majority have IgG precipitins to *Aspergillus*.

Management

On the assumption that mild immune suppression is the dominant cause,
steroids are not usually recommended for fear of further immune
suppression.

Itraconazole has been used with clinical improvement in 50%–60% of
patients and radiographic improvement in approximately 20%. It has been
used as effective monotherapy and as perioperative treatment for patients
undergoing lung resection.

Voriconazole has also been used with clinical benefit in a retrospective
case series.

5. Aspergilloma/mycetoma

Definition
The term *aspergilloma* is used to describe a ball of fungal hyphae within a preexisting cavity in the lung.

Pathogenesis
Multiple disorders can lead to pulmonary cavitary lesions. Aspergilloma is a result of the noninvasive growth of hyphae within a preexisting cavity. Routinely, patients are immunocompetent, which prevents invasive disease. Hemoptysis frequently occurs. This is felt to be due to local invasion of bronchial blood vessels lining the cavity, endotoxin release, and mechanical friction.

Risk factors
Preexisting cavitary disease, including the following:
- Tuberculosis
  - Approximately 11% had aspergilloma in one series of 544 patients
- Sarcoidosis
- Bronchiectasis
- COPD
- Ankylosing spondylitis
- Neoplasm
- Pulmonary infarction
- Bronchial cysts or bullae

Clinical features
Aspergillomas are often asymptomatic. A significant percentage is found on CXR obtained for other purposes. A majority of patients will ultimately develop varying degrees of hemoptysis.

Chronic cough and dyspnea are more likely related to other underlying lung diseases. Fever is rarely associated and likely represents secondary bacterial infection.

Investigations
- *CXR:* Cavity with associated opacity. Opacity may change position if CXR is performed decubitus
- *CT:* Opacity within a preexisting cavity
- *Sputum culture*
- *Aspergillus* IgG precipitins: Often higher levels than seen in other *Aspergillus* diseases

Management
- Most patients do not require treatment.
- If symptoms such as cough and fever are thought to be related, a trial of itraconazole could be performed.
- Hemoptysis may require aggressive management by bronchial embolization or surgical resection depending on the severity. Stable patients can be treated with itraconazole.

- Itraconazole will not eradicate the fungus, but size and lessen the tendency to hemoptysis. It any fungus in the walls and inhibits growth in t
- No medicine has shown consistent benefit in r
- Bronchial arteriograms should reveal a blush of the cavity wall that can be embolized, even Due to large degrees of collateralization of blo offers only temporary control of symptoms.
- Surgery can be highly successful for control of many patients have compromised lung function management due to their underlying lung disease high surgical mortality of 5.7%.

Differential diagnosis
The most important consideration in the managel to not overlook alternate diagnoses that may share
- Lung malignancy
- Wegener's granulomatosis

Summary of *Aspergillus* lung disease
Aspergillus is associated with a broad spectrum o manifestations of the disease are related to the host to the spores. The host defense response is dir disease manifestations in the allergic disorders, and th tion of the immune system is associated with manifes diseases.

Pneu

Defini*
*Pneumo
resultin;
termed
environ

The
held th
have ca
have cl

Cause
Risk fa
<200 :
such as
PCP r
preven

The
may (
showe
for ap
ever,
on pre

Clini
Symp
grade
be te
medic
Patie

Inve
- *CX
  bil
  wi
  pu
  inc
  inl
- Ar
  gr
  >:
- W
- Se
- In
  in
  w
  p*

Further information
Aspergillus Trust (for patients): www.aspergillustrust.org

- *Bronchoscopy with BAL* is the diagnostic investigation of choice in non-HIV-infected patients and in patients with HIV in whom induced sputum analysis is nondiagnostic. BAL with silver or immunofluorescent staining has a specificity of nearly 100% and sensitivity of 80%–90%. This sensitivity is lower in non-HIV-infected immunocompromised patients, reflecting their lower pathogen loads.
- *Transbronchial lung biopsy* has a slightly higher sensitivity (around 95%) but is associated with an increased risk of complications, so is reserved for cases where BAL is nondiagnostic.

PCP: treatment

Antimicrobial

- High-dose trimethoprim-sulfamethoxazole (TMP-SMX) remains the drug of choice. Administer 15–20mg/kg of the trimethoprim portion of the medication. Use IV route initially and then po during clinical improvement; po administration may be used initially in mild cases. Side effects (e.g., rash, nausea, vomiting, blood disorders) are common, particularly in HIV-infected patients.
- Second-line choices if the patient is intolerant or unresponsive to TMP-SMX include intravenous pentamidine, clindamycin and primaquine, dapsone and trimethoprim, atovaquone, trimetrexate.
- All treatments should be for 3 weeks
- Empiric treatment can be started immediately without compromising subsequent BAL results. *Pneumocystis* stains remain positive for up to 2 weeks.
- In new cases of HIV presenting with PCP, subsequent early introduction of highly active antiretroviral therapy (HAART) may rarely be associated with acute respiratory failure related to immune reconstitution syndrome.

Steroids

High-dose steroids are recommended for patients who present with a PaO_2 of <70 mmHg or A–a gradient >35. This serves to temper the inflammatory response that occurs with the initiation of treatment of the infection.

Initial dose is prednisone 40 mg twice daily for 5 days, with a taper to once-daily therapy for 5 days, followed by 20 mg for 11 days. It should be administered 30 minutes prior to the TMP-SMX.

Supportive therapy

Hypoxia is common: administer supplementary high-flow oxygen, and consider use of continuous positive airway pressure (CPAP). Mechanical ventilation may be required.

Outcome

Mortality is <10% in the setting of HIV, but around 30% in patients with cancer in a series of patients from 1985 to 1995. Mortality from PCP requiring mechanical ventilation in HIV-infected patients is about 60%.

The relapse rate in AIDS is high (60% in 1 year), so secondary prophylaxis with TMP-SMX is recommended. Primary prophylaxis is offered to HIV-positive patients with CD4 count <200 × 10^6/L, although new data suggest that patients with control of their viral replication on HAART with a CD4 count of <200 × 10^6/L do not require prophylaxis.

The indications for prophylaxis in non-HIV patients are less well defined; consider prophylaxis for patients who are likely to receive prednisone doses of >20 mg for >1 month.

Future directions

B-glucan, a cell wall component, can be measured in blood and BAL and appears to be a reliable marker for PCP. It can be used for patients who are too ill to undergo bronchoscopy.

The use of PCR to detect *Pneumocystis* may further increase diagnostic sensitivity, although in a proportion of cases, detection with PCR is not accompanied by evidence of clinical infection.

There is emerging TMP-SMX resistance.

Endemic mycoses

Several types of dimorphic fungi are known to commonly cause pulmonary disease in endemic regions, particularly in North America: **histoplasmosis, blastomycosis, coccidioidomycosis**, and **paracoccidioidomycosis**. Endemic fungi can rarely present in nonendemic areas, and diagnosis is often delayed because of their nonspecific and varied clinical features, and the failure to obtain a detailed travel history.

Fungal infection may mimic other diseases such as tuberculosis and lung cancer, often leading to inappropriate investigations and treatment. Fungal infections can also cause granulomata on lung biopsy, which sometimes results in diagnostic confusion (e.g., with sarcoidosis).

Infection in immunocompetent individuals is usually either asymptomatic or mild and self-limiting, although severe infection may rarely occur in apparently immunocompetent individuals. Outbreaks of disease may occur as well as sporadic cases.

Unlike invasive candidiasis and aspergillosis, where neutrophils are the key host defense mechanism, T-cell-mediated immunity is essential for defense against the endemic mycoses. Patients with impaired T-cell-mediated immunity (e.g., AIDS, lymphoma, steroid use) are therefore at particular risk of developing severe or disseminated infection.

Histoplasmosis

Epidemiology

Histoplasma capsulatum is found in bird and bat dropping–contaminated soil in the Midwest and southeastern United States, particularly the Ohio and Mississippi valleys, as well as in Mexico and parts of South America. The mycelial form is inhaled and subsequently develops into the yeast form ("dimorphism") within the lung, before spread via the lymphatics and activation of T-cell-mediated immunity with granuloma development.

Clinical features

Manifestations of infection are highly variable:

- **Asymptomatic** infection occurs in the majority of cases. CXR may be normal or demonstrate single or multiple nodules, which may calcify in a characteristic "target-lesion" pattern. Lymphadenopathy may occur with eggshell calcification.
- **Acute** symptoms may follow heavy or recurrent exposure (e.g., pigeon fanciers, cavers). They range from a self-limiting flu-like illness with fever, cough, and malaise to fulminant disease and respiratory failure. CXR may be normal or show consolidation, bilateral alveolar shadowing, multiple small nodules, and sometimes lymphadenopathy.
- **Chronic**, progressive lung disease occurs particularly in patients with underlying COPD; lung cavitation is common, sometimes leading to an incorrect diagnosis of tuberculosis or cancer.
- **Disseminated** disease may affect the immunocompromised (particularly those with AIDS) and the elderly. Presentation may be acute or chronic, and manifestations include fever, weight loss, and diffuse lung involvement, although almost any organ system may be affected. Other features may include hepatosplenomegaly, gastrointestinal symptoms, headache and meningisms, cytopenias, endocarditis, and adrenal failure.
- Other, unusual manifestations include broncholithiasis, mediastinal fibrosis (with compression of large airways, esophagus, or superior vena cava), or isolated extrapulmonary disease (e.g., arthritis, pericarditis, erythema nodosum, erythema multiforme).

Diagnosis

Obtain smears or culture of infected material, e.g., sputum or BAL fluid (for chronic pulmonary disease, insensitive for acute disease), blood, urine, or bone marrow (for disseminated disease). Results may take several weeks.

Serology in acute disease is typically negative at presentation, and becomes positive after several weeks. A variety of serological tests are in use, including the following:

- *Complement fixation* is designed to detect antibodies to *Histoplasma* mycelial antigen or *Histoplasma* yeast antigen. A positive result (serum titer ≥1:16 for mycelial antigen, ≥1:32 for yeast antigen) for either antigen, in a compatible clinical setting, is considered diagnostic of active disease.

- *Immunodiffusion* may distinguish active disease from previous exposure, but is less sensitive than complement fixation, and a negative result does not exclude the diagnosis.
- *Serum or urine Histoplasma polysaccharide antigen test* is useful for diagnosis of disseminated disease and also pulmonary disease. It is positive in 85%–95% of AIDS patients. Antigenuria is seen in 90%, and antigenemia in <50% of non-AIDS patients.

Treatment

Infection in immunocompetent individuals is typically self-limiting, and symptoms usually resolve within 2–4 weeks without treatment.

Indications for antifungal treatment are
- Persistent symptoms (usually lasting >1 month)
- Progressive disseminated disease
- Heavy exposure leading to ARDS
- Infection in the setting of immunocompromise

Oral itraconazole is appropriate for persistent symptoms in mild to moderate disease and for disseminated disease, including in patients with AIDS who have mild disease. Treat for 6–12 weeks in the setting of acute histoplasmosis, and for 1–2 years in chronic disease.

In the setting of AIDS, treatment should be lifelong or until the CD4 count is >200 for at least 6 months after starting HAART. Check itraconazole drug interactions and monitor liver function (ideally monthly) if the patient is taking it for >1 month. Hypokalemia may be associated with long-term use.

Intravenous amphotericin B should be used to treat severe infection in the setting of ARDS or immunocompromise.

Blastomycosis

Epidemiology

Infection with *Blastomyces dermatitidis* follows the inhalation of spores from contaminated soil, and clinical infection may follow outdoor activities. Blastomycosis is endemic in a distribution similar to that of histoplasmosis in the United States, although extending further north: it is endemic in the southeastern United States, and the Mississippi, Ohio, and St. Lawrence river valleys. Blastomycosis also occurs in Africa, India, and the Middle East. It is significantly less common than histoplasmosis.

Clinical features

Clinical presentation is variable and may mimic other diseases such as bacterial pneumonia, tuberculosis, and lung cancer. Clinical manifestations include the following:

- **Asymptomatic** in at least 50% of those infected
- **Acute** presentation is typically with fever, cough productive of mucopurulent sputum, and sometimes pleuritic chest pain; misdiagnosis as bacterial pneumonia is common. Acute presentation with fulminant respiratory disease and ARDS may occur. Other acute presentations include a flu-like illness with fever, myalgia, arthralgia, and erythema nodosum.
- **Chronic** presentation with fever, productive cough, and weight loss
- **Disseminated** disease occurs in a minority of patients (especially in the immunocompromised), and most commonly involves the lungs, skin, bone, joints, and CNS.

CXR

Airspace infiltrates are the most common finding, but a wide range of appearances is seen, including nodular pattern, lobar consolidation, diffuse infiltrates, and large, peripheral masses (often with air bronchograms). Lymphadenopathy and pleural effusions may rarely occur.

Diagnosis

Diagnosis is by staining or culture of infected material. A pyogenic inflammatory response to the fungus is common (unlike in histoplasmosis) and facilitates diagnosis

Culture of sputum has a high yield and is diagnostic in most cases of acute pulmonary disease. Multiple specimens may be required, however. A drawback of sputum culture is that several weeks may elapse before the fungus is identified. Cytological examination of sputum may provide a rapid diagnosis if the examiner is trained appropriately and alerted to the possible diagnosis

Bronchoscopy has similar diagnostic yield to that of sputum culture (92% in one study), and is recommended for patients with negative sputum results. Note that lidocaine may inhibit the fungal growth, thus minimal amounts should be used.

More invasive procedures such as surgical lung biopsy or thoracoscopy are only rarely needed. Histological specimens require particular stains (e.g., silver stain) to facilitate identification of the fungus.

Currently available serological tests lack sensitivity and are rarely helpful.

Treatment

Treatment is usually with itraconazole for at least 6 months. Observation without treatment is not generally recommended, although this is controversial and symptoms are usually self-limiting in immunocompetent individuals. Amphotericin B should be used to treat very ill patients.

Coccidioidomycosis

Coccidioidomycosis is endemic in parts of southwestern United States (Arizona, California, Texas, New Mexico, Utah, Nevada), northern Mexico, and Central and South America. Infection follows inhalation of *Coccidioides immitis* spores from the soil. Manifestations of infection are variable:

- **Asymptomatic** infection appears to be common in endemic regions.
- **Acute** pulmonary disease presents in a similar manner to bacterial pneumonia, with fever, cough, pleuritic chest pain, and often skin rash (e.g., erythema nodosum or erythema multiforme). Eosinophilia may be present. CXR appearance is variable, and may show areas of consolidation, lymphadenopathy, or pleural effusion, or it may be normal. The disease is self-limiting in most cases; a minority progress to ARDS or chronic disease.
- **Chronic** pulmonary disease is uncommon and may be asymptomatic. CXR typically shows single or multiple nodules that may cavitate. Upper lobe infiltrates similar to those seen in tuberculosis may develop.
- **Disseminated** disease is rare, occurring particularly in the immuno-compromised. Presentation may be acute or chronic. Pulmonary disease occurs in association with involvement of the skin, bones, joints, genitourinary system, or CNS.

Diagnosis

Diagnosis is with stains or culture of infected tissues. Sputum cultures are often positive in cavitating disease. BAL fluid culture and lung biopsies may also be diagnostic. Serological tests are also available.

Treatment

Treatment is not required in most patients who have mild, self-limiting disease. Fluconazole is the antifungal of choice when required.

Paracoccidioidomycosis

- Paracoccidioidomycosis is endemic in parts of Central and South America and Mexico.
- It typically presents as a chronic pulmonary disease, although acute disseminated disease may occur in the immunocompromised.
- Diagnosis is made on culture of sputum or BAL fluid, or following staining of lung biopsy samples.
- Treatment is with itraconazole, and long courses of up to 6 months may be needed.

Cryptococcosis

Epidemiology

Cryptococcus neoformans is found worldwide in bird droppings. Following inhalation, yeasts propagate within the alveoli without usually causing symptoms. Migration to the central nervous system may then occur, and meningoencephalitis is the most common clinical manifestation of infection.

Patients with impaired cell-mediated immunity (e.g., AIDS, steroid use, lymphoma) are particularly vulnerable to cryptococcal infection.

Clinical features

Clinically evident cryptococcal lung disease is rare but well described, even in HIV-negative patients. Symptoms are nonspecific, including fever and cough, and presentations may be acute or chronic. CXR patterns extend from nodules to interstitial or pleural involvement

Pulmonary involvement is often associated with meningitis, and clinical signs of meningismus are characteristically absent. CT of the head (to exclude a space-occupying lesion) followed by lumbar puncture should therefore be considered in all patients with pulmonary cryptococcal disease.

Diagnosis

Diagnostic techniques include the following:
- India ink stain of CSF, or latex agglutination test for capsular antigen in BAL or pleural fluid, blood, or CSF
- Stains and culture of sputum, blood, urine, or BAL fluid. Positive culture from sputum may indicate colonization rather than active disease, and should be interpreted within the clinical context.
- Serum cryptococcal antigen test is extremely sensitive and specific for the diagnosis.

Treatment

Treatment of cryptococcal infection in the immunocompromised is with amphotericin B IV and flucytosine IV for 2–3 weeks, followed by fluconazole. The natural history of disease in immunocompetent patients is poorly understood, and observation alone is often recommended. Disseminated disease may occur, however, and some clinicians advise treatment with fluconazole.

Candida

- *Candida* occurs as part of the normal human flora and is found in the gastrointestinal tract and on the skin. Invasive disease may occur in the immunocompromised, particularly in neutropenic patients.
- *Candida* is often isolated from respiratory secretions, but very rarely causes respiratory disease. Definitive diagnosis of pulmonary disease requires identification of tissue invasion by *Candida* on TBB or surgical lung biopsy.
- In a case series of biopsy-confirmed candidal pneumonia, the sensitivity and specificity of bronchoalveolar lavage was 71% and 57%, respectively.
- The two most common causes of candidal lung infection are aspiration (rare) and hematogenous dissemination into the lung.
- Risk factors for candidemia include immunocompromise, central venous lines, parenteral nutrition, and gastrointestinal surgery. In lung transplant recipients a positive donor tracheal culture for *Candida* is a marker for post-transplant candidal infection.
- The clinical and radiological features of pulmonary involvement are nonspecific. In a series of patients with histologically confirmed diagnosis, a majority had multiple nodules and associated air-space consolidation. A small number had a halo sign.
- Definitive diagnosis of pulmonary disease requires identification of tissue invasion by *Candida* on TBB or surgical lung biopsy.
- Treat with amphotericin B 0.7 mg/kg/day IV or fluconazole 400 mg daily. Treatment of underlying candidemia along with central venous catheter removal is critical for a response to therapy.

Parasitic lung disease

A wide variety of parasitic organisms may infect the lung. In general, parasites may cause lung disease by two mechanisms:
- Hypersensitivity reactions, e.g., Löffler's syndrome and eosinophilic lung disease, most commonly from helminths such as ascariasis, toxocara, and liver flukes
- Direct infection and invasion, e.g., amoebic disease, pulmonary hydatid disease

Some of the more important examples are noted below.

Hyadatidosis

Hyadatidosis is the most common parasitic lung disease worldwide.

Human infection follows ingestion of parasite eggs, with the adult worm found in dogs, sheep, goats, horses, camels, and moose. Infection is common in sheep-raising regions, particularly Central Europe and the Mediterranean, as well as Alaska and Arctic Canada.

There are two main forms:
- *Echinococcus granulosus*, which causes cystic hydatid disease as the larvae grow in the lungs. It is common. Symptoms include cough (sometimes producing cyst contents, "hydatidoptysis"), hemoptysis, and chest pain. CXR shows rounded cysts, sometimes with calcified walls, most commonly in lower lobes. CT may show daughter cysts. Cyst rupture may occur, with wheeze, eosinophilia, and bronchial or pleural spread.
- *Echinococcus multilocularis*, which leads to alveolar hydatid disease following tissue invasion. This form is rare. Lung masses are less clearly delineated on CT than in cystic disease.

Hyadatidosis is diagnosed from serology or sputum analysis. Serology is insensitive for the diagnosis of pulmonary disease (around 50%). Demonstration of liver cysts supports the diagnosis. Avoid needle aspiration of cysts, which may result in a hypersensitivity reaction or dissemination.

Treatment is with surgical excision in most cases. Medical treatment is with albendazole if the patient is unfit for surgery or following cyst rupture and dissemination.

Amebiasis

- Intestinal and liver infection is common, with lung involvement in a minority of patients.
- Lung disease can develop either directly from the liver or via the bloodstream or lymphatics.
- Pulmonary manifestations are right lower lobe infiltrate, mass, empyema, lung abscess, or hepatobronchial fistulae (with large volumes of brown or "anchovy" sputum) and may be associated with pericardial disease.
- Diagnose using serology or following identification of trophozoites in stool, sputum, or pleural fluid
- Treatment is with metronidazole plus iodoquinol or diloxanide.

Ascariasis

- Distributed worldwide
- Lung involvement occurs during maturation of *Ascaris lumbricoides*, and is typically manifest as a hypersensitivity reaction with cough, wheeze, fever, CXR infiltrates, and peripheral eosinophilia.
- Examination of stool for eggs may confirm the diagnosis.
- Usually resolves spontaneously after 1–2 weeks. Consider treatment with mebendazole for gastrointestinal infection.

Strongyloidiasis

- Caused by *Strongyloides stercoralis*, found in Central and South America and Africa
- Uncomplicated infections in immunocompetent patients are minimally symptomatic. When present, pulmonary involvement may lead to a Löffler-type syndrome with wheeze, skin rash, eosinophilia, and CXR infiltrate. Altered cellular immunity such as with long-term steroid therapy, lymphoma, and in transplant recipients may be associated with disseminated infection leading to the "hyperinfection syndrome." ARDS may develop, and secondary bacterial sepsis is common.
- Diagnose using serology or following microbiological analysis of stool or duodenal fluid.
- Treatment is with thiabendazole.

Toxocara canis

- Caused by *Toxocara canis*, distributed worldwide. Dogs are the primary host.
- Ingestion of eggs from contaminated soil may result in visceral larva migrans. Migration of larvae through the lungs results in an immune response, with wheeze, cough, dyspnea, hypergammaglobulinemia, and eosinophilia.
- Diagnosis may be made from serology. Lung biopsy may show granulomas.
- Treatment is often not required; steroids may be useful in severe cases.

Dirofilariasis

- Found in the United States, Japan, South America
- Infection is caused by *Dirofilaria immitis* following mosquito transfer from animals, especially dogs. Worms lodge in the pulmonary arteries and elicit an inflammatory response, leading to a necrotic nodule.
- Presentation is classically asymptomatic with a single peripheral nodule on CXR, mimicking cancer. Patients may present with cough, chest pain, and hemoptysis, presumably due to pulmonary infarction.
- Definitive diagnosis requires lung biopsy. Serology lacks sensitivity and specificity.
- Treatment is not usually needed.

Schistosomiasis

- Found in the Middle East, South America, Southeast Asia, Africa, and the Caribbean
- *Schistosoma* species are carried by snails, and infection follows skin penetration, often during swimming.
- Pulmonary involvement may reflect acute tissue migration, causing cough, wheeze, and CXR infiltrates, or chronic infection, leading to interstitial infiltrates, pulmonary hypertension, or AV fistulae.
- Diagnosis is from observation of ova in sputum, BAL, urine, or stool, or from lung biopsy. Granulomas may be seen on lung biopsy.
- Treatment is with praziquantel.

Paragonimiasis

- Caused by *Paragonimus westermani*, distributed in West Africa, the Far East, India, and Central and South America
- Following ingestion, flukes migrate to the lung or pleura. Clinical features may be acute or chronic, and include chest pain, pneumothorax, pleural effusion, and Löffler's syndrome; 90% of patients have blood-stained, coffee-colored, or rusty sputum. Serum eosinophilia is common.
- Diagnose with serology or observation of eggs in sputum, TBB, BAL, or pleural fluid.
- Treatment is with praziquantel.

Tropical pulmonary eosinophilia

- Endemic areas include India, Pakistan, Sri Lanka, Burma, Thailand, and Malayasia.
- Follows infection with *Wuchereria bancrofti* or *Brugia malayi*
- Pulmonary involvement is common and represents a hypersensitivity reaction to the organism, with cough, wheeze, CXR infiltrates, and raised serum IgE (>1000 U/mL), and absolute blood eosinophilia of >3000.
- Treatment is with diethylcarbamazine.

Pneumothorax

Clinical features and investigations

Definition
A *pneumothorax* is defined as air in the pleural space. It may occur with apparently normal lungs (primary pneumothorax) or in the presence of underlying lung disease (secondary pneumothorax). It may occur spontaneously or following trauma.

Epidemiology
The annual incidence of primary pneumothorax is around 9 per 100,000.

Primary pneumothoraces occur most commonly in tall, thin men between 20 and 40 years of age. They are less common in women (male–female ratio is 5:1), but if they do occur, consider the possibility of underlying lung disease (e.g., lymphangioleiomyomatosis, catamenial pneumothorax).

Cigarette smoking is a major risk factor for pneumothorax, increasing the risk by a factor of 22 in men and 9 in women. The mechanism is unclear; a smoking-induced influx of inflammatory cells may break down elastic lung fibers (causing bulla formation) and cause small airways obstruction (increasing alveolar pressure and the likelihood of interstitial air leak).

Pneumothorax may rarely be familial.

Causes and pathophysiology
Primary
The pathogenesis is poorly understood; they are presumed to occur following an air leak from apical bullae, although small airway inflammation is often also present and may contribute by increasing airway resistance.

Secondary
Underlying diseases include COPD (60% of cases), asthma, interstitial lung disease, necrotizing pneumonia, tuberculosis, PCP, cystic fibrosis, Langerhans cell histiocytosis, lymphangioleiomyomatosis, Marfan syndrome, esophageal rupture, lung cancer, catamenial pneumothorax, and pulmonary infarction.

Pneumothorax may be the first presentation of the underlying disease.

Clinical features
Classically pneumothorax presents with acute onset of pleuritic chest pain and/or breathlessness. Breathlessness is often minimal in young patients and is more severe in secondary pneumothorax.

Signs of pneumothorax include tachycardia, reduced expansion, hyper-resonant percussion note, and quiet breath sounds on the pneumothorax side. These are frequently absent in small pneumothoraces. Hamman's sign refers to a "click" on auscultation in time with the heart sounds, due to movement of pleural surfaces with a left-sided pneumothorax.

The patient may be asymptomatic or present with breathlessness if there is subcutaneous emphysema.

Pneumothorax presents in ventilated patients with acute clinical deterioration and hypoxia or increasing inflation pressures.

Investigations

CXR

CXR is the diagnostic test in most cases, revealing a visible lung edge and absent lung markings peripherally. Blunting of the ipsilateral costophrenic angle due to bleeding into the pleural space is common. Pneumothoraces are difficult to visualize on supine films: look for a sharply delineated heart border, hemidiaphragm depression, and increased lucency on the affected side.

The width of the rim of air surrounding the lung on CXR may be used to classify pneumothoraces into small (rim of air <2 cm) and large (≥2 cm). A 2 cm rim of air approximately equates to a 50% pneumothorax in volume.

Tiny pneumothoraces not apparent on PA CXR may be visible on lateral chest or lateral decubitus radiographs.

The CXR appearance may also show features of underlying lung disease, although this can be difficult to assess in the presence of a large pneumothorax.

CT chest

This may be required to differentiate pneumothorax from bullous disease, and is useful in diagnosing unsuspected pneumothorax following trauma and in looking for evidence of underlying lung disease.

ABGs

ABGs frequently show hypoxia and sometimes hypercapnia in secondary pneumothorax.

Prognosis

On average, 30% (range 16%–54% in studies) of primary pneumothoraces recur, most within 2 years. Continued smoking increases the risk of recurrence. The risk of recurrence increases with each subsequent pneumothorax: 30% after a first pneumothorax, about 40% after a second one, and >50% after a third one.

Mortality of secondary pneumothorax is 10%.

Recurrence of secondary pneumothorax occurs in 39%–47% of patients, and is associated with age, pulmonary fibrosis, and emphysema. Recurrence rates may be as high as 80% in patients with Langerhans cell histiocytosis or lymphangioleiomyomatosis.

Further information

Sahn SA, Heffner JE (2000). Spontaneous pneumothorax. *N Engl J Med* **342**(12):868–874.

Initial management

There is considerable variation among clinicians regarding optimal pneumothorax management. The treatment algorithms presented on pp. 322–3 follow the British Thoracic Society (BTS) guidelines.

General management points

- Management is determined by the degree of breathlessness and hypoxia, evidence of hemodynamic compromise, presence and severity of any underlying lung disease, and, to some extent, size of the pneumothorax.
- Severe breathlessness out of proportion to pneumothorax size may be a feature of impending tension pneumothorax.
- Secondary pneumothorax has a significant mortality rate (10%), and should be managed more aggressively. Treat both the pneumothorax and the underlying disease.

Aspiration

- Procedure is described on p. 774
- Halt the procedure if painful, or if the patient coughs excessively; do not aspirate >2.5 L of air, as this suggests a large air-leak and aspiration is likely to fail.
- Ideal timing of repeat CXR following aspiration is unknown; it may be advisable to wait several hours before performing the CXR, to detect slow air leaks
- Aspiration is successful if the lung is fully or nearly reexpanded on CXR.
- If initial aspiration of a primary pneumothorax fails, repeat aspiration should be considered (unless ≥2.5 L has already been aspirated). At least one-third of patients will respond to second aspiration, although the optimal timing of repeat aspiration is unclear.

Chest drainage

- Procedure is described on pp. 782–3
- Associated with significant morbidity and even mortality, and not required in most patients with primary spontaneous pneumothorax
- Small (10–14F) drains are sufficient in most cases; consider a large-bore (24–28F) drain in secondary pneumothorax with large air leak, in severe subcutaneous emphysema, or in mechanically ventilated patients.
- Never clamp a bubbling chest drain (risk of tension pneumothorax).
- When air leak appears to have ceased, clamping of the drain for several hours followed by repeat CXR may detect very slow or intermittent air leaks, thereby avoiding inappropriate drain removal. This is controversial, however, and should only be considered on a specialist ward with experienced nursing staff.
- If the drain water level does not swing with respiration, the drain is kinked (check underneath the dressing, as the tube enters the skin), blocked, clamped, or incorrectly positioned (drainage holes are not in the pleural space; check CXR).

- Heimlich valves (or thoracic vents) are an alternative to underwater bottle drainage and are being used increasingly in some centers. They allow greater patient mobilization, and sometimes outpatient management of pneumothorax.

Oxygen

All hospitalized patients should receive high-flow (10 L/min) inspired oxygen (unless CO_2 retention is a problem). This reduces the partial pressure of nitrogen in blood, encouraging removal of air from the pleural space and speeding up resolution of the pneumothorax.

Persistent air leak

This is defined as continued bubbling of the chest drain 48 hours after insertion.

Consider drain suction (−10 to −20 cm H_2O), insertion of large-bore drain, and/or thoracic surgical referral.

Check that persistent bubbling is not the result of "outside" air being sucked down the drain, e.g., following drain displacement such that a hole lies outside the pleural cavity, or, if enlargement of the drain track occurs, allowing outside air to enter and then be released down the drain.

Discharge

Prior to patient discharge, discuss precautions for flying and diving (see p. 320), and advise patient to return to the hospital immediately if breathlessness worsens. Document this in the medical notes.

Further management

Outpatient follow-up

Repeat CXR to ensure resolution of pneumothorax and normal appearance of underlying lungs.

Discuss the risk of recurrence and emphasize smoking cessation, if appropriate.

Ascent in altitude with a pneumothorax is potentially hazardous. Guidelines recommend that patients not fly for at least 6 weeks from the resolution of pneumothorax on CXR or surgical treatment. This time interval is arbitrary, however, and patients should understand that there is a high initial risk of recurrence that falls with time, and they may wish to avoid flying for a longer period, e.g., 1 year.

Advise patients that they should never dive in the future, unless they have undergone a definitive surgical procedure.

Surgical management

Indications for cardiothoracic surgical referral

- Second ipsilateral pneumothorax
- First contralateral pneumothorax
- Bilateral spontaneous pneumothorax
- Persistent air leak (>5–7 days of drainage)
- Spontaneous hemothorax
- Professions at risk (e.g., pilots, divers) after first pneumothorax.

Note that these are guidelines only, and patient choice will also influence the decision for surgical intervention.

Surgical treatments are aimed at repairing the apical hole or bleb and closing the pleural space (pleurodesis). Options include the following:

- *Video-assisted thoracoscopic surgery* (*VATS*) Recurrence rates are higher than those for open thoracotomy (4% vs. 1.5%), although VATS is a less invasive procedure and probably requires a shorter hospital stay. Pleural abrasion (rather than talc poudrage) is usually favored for pleurodesis. Often it is the procedure of choice in young patients with primary pneumothorax.
- *Open thoracotomy* An apical bleb is resected, and pleural space closed by pleural abrasion or parietal pleurectomy. This is an effective procedure with a recurrence rate <1%, but probably prolonged recovery rates compared to those for VATS.
- *Transaxillary minithoracotomy* uses a relatively small axillary incision and may be a less invasive alternative to open thoracotomy.

Chemical pleurodesis

Talc or tetracycline is most commonly used; the procedure is described on p. 785. It can be performed via intercostal drain or at VATS.

Failure rates are around 10%–20%, and there is some concern about the long-term safety of intrapleural talc. Its use is therefore not recommended in younger patients. However, long-term follow-up after talc pleurodesis has not documented an increased risk of lung cancer, mesothelioma, or fibrothorax.

Consider pleurodesis via intercostal drain only as a last resort in older patients with recurrent pneumothorax in whom surgery would be high risk (e.g., patients with severe COPD).

The likelihood of successful pleurodesis in the setting of an incompletely re-expanded lung with a persistent air leak remains uncertain, although it may be attempted if surgery is not an option.

Treatment algorithm for primary pneumothorax

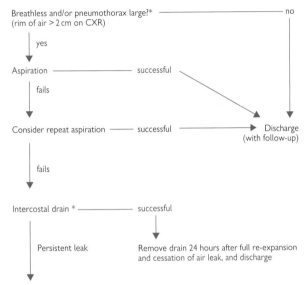

Figure 24.1 Treatment algorithm for primary pneumothorax. *Some disagreement exists regarding this point: in the setting of a relatively asymptomatic patient with a large pneumothorax, the risk of intervention may outweigh the risk of the pneumothorax, and conservative management may be considered.

Treatment algorithm for secondary pneumothorax

Consider inpatient observation without aspiration in relatively asymptomatic patients with small (<1 cm) pneumothoraces.

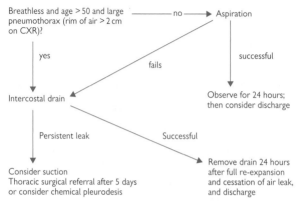

Breathless and age > 50 and large pneumothorax (rim of air > 2 cm on CXR)?

— no —→ Aspiration

yes

fails

successful

Intercostal drain

Observe for 24 hours; then consider discharge

Persistent leak

Successful

Consider suction
Thoracic surgical referral after 5 days
or consider chemical pleurodesis

Remove drain 24 hours after full re-expansion and cessation of air leak, and discharge

Figure 24.2 Treatment algorithm for secondary pneumothorax.

Further information

M Henry, T Arnold, et al. (2003). BTS guidelines for the management of spontaneous pneumothorax. *Thorax* **58** (Suppl. II):ii39–ii52.

Specific situations

Tension pneumothorax

Pneumothorax acts as a one-way valve, with air entering the pleural space on each inspiration and unable to escape on expiration. The progressive increase in pleural pressure compresses both lungs and mediastinum and inhibits venous return to the heart, leading to hypotension and potentially cardiac arrest.

Occurrence is not related to pneumothorax size, and tension can occur with very small pneumothoraces in the context of air trapping in the lung from obstructive lung disease.

Tension pneumothorax typically presents with acute respiratory distress, agitation, hypotension, raised jugular venous pressure, and tracheal deviation away from the pneumothorax side. There is reduced air entry on the affected side. It may present with cardiac arrest (pulseless electrical activity), or with acute deterioration in ventilated patients.

If suspected, give high-flow oxygen and insert a large-bore cannula into the second intercostal space in a midclavicular line on the side of the pneumothorax. Do not wait for a CXR if cardiac arrest has occurred or the diagnosis is clinically certain. The hiss of escaping air confirms the diagnosis. Aspirate air until the patient is less distressed and then, leaving cannula in place, insert a chest drain in a midaxillary line.

Iatrogenic pneumothorax

Causes include transbronchial biopsy, transthoracic needle lung biopsy, subclavian line insertion, mechanical ventilation, pleural aspiration, pleural biopsy, external cardiac massage, and percutaneous liver biopsy Presentation may be delayed, even several days after the procedure.

Most cases do not require intervention and improve with observation, although aspiration is sometimes required.

Drainage is seldom needed, although it is more commonly required in patients with COPD. The exception is mechanically ventilated patients, who will require an intercostal drain in most cases.

Traumatic pneumothorax

Up to half of cases may not be clinically apparent or visible on CXR; chest CT is required for diagnosis.

Most patients require an intercostal drain. Consider VATS early if there is a persistent air leak.

Subcutaneous (or "surgical") emphysema

This occurs as air tracks below the skin under pressure from the pleural space. It may result from large air-leaks, particularly in the presence of underlying lung disease such as COPD. It also may occur if a chest drain is blocked or displaced so that holes lie subcutaneously.

Subcutaneous emphysema is harmless in most cases, although rarely it may result in significant respiratory compromise from upper airway compression.

Treat with high-flow (10 L/min) inspired oxygen (unless CO_2 retention is a problem). Check that the drain is patent (swinging, bubbling).

Management if the patient is unwell is with oxygen, and a large-bore chest drain on suction. If the airway is compromised, consider anesthetizing and incising areas of affected skin and "milking" out subcutaneous air. Subcutaneous drains are sometimes used, and in rare cases tracheostomy is required.

Pneumothorax in HIV

This most commonly occurs as a result of PCP. Empirical treatment of PCP is advised (see p. 298).

Use of nebulized pentamidine may increase the risk of pneumothorax.

Consider early intercostal drainage and surgical referral.

Pneumothorax in cystic fibrosis

This pneumothorax is associated with severe underlying lung disease. Subsequent ipsilateral and contralateral pneumothorax is common.

Manage as for secondary pneumothorax, although intercostal drainage is frequently required. Give a course of intravenous antibiotics.

In cases of persistent air leak despite suction, discuss management with the cardiothoracic surgical team at the local transplant center. Partial pleurectomy is effective in preventing recurrence. Pleurodesis renders later transplant technically more difficult, but it is not an absolute contraindication to transplantation.

Catamenial pneumothorax

This is pneumothorax occurring at the same time as menstruation. It is usually recurrent but does not recur with each menstrual cycle.

The pathogenesis is unknown; possibilities include pleural endometriosis or transfer of air into pleural spaces through a diaphragmatic defect from the peritoneal cavity at menstruation.

Treatment options include VATS, pleurodesis, and ovulation-suppressing drugs (high recurrence rate).

Re-expansion pulmonary edema

This occurs in up to 14% of cases following treatment, and causes breathlessness and cough with evidence of edema in the re-expanded lung (and sometimes both lungs) on CXR.

Pulmonary edema is more common in young patients with large primary pneumothoraces, and may be associated with late presentations to the hospital.

It may be precipitated by early use of suction (<48 hours).

The edema is self-resolving in most cases, although it may rarely be fatal.

Pleural effusions

Clinical features and imaging

Pleural effusions are common and are associated with many different diseases—see Chapter 6 for a step-by-step approach to the diagnosis of a patient with a pleural effusion, differential diagnosis of transudates and exudates, and details of pleural fluid analysis.

Clinical features

The patient may be asymptomatic or present with breathlessness, dry cough, pleuritic chest pain (suggesting pleural inflammation), chest "heaviness," and sometimes pain referred to the shoulder or abdomen.

Signs on examination include reduced chest expansion, reduced tactile vocal fremitus, a dull percussion note, quiet breath sounds, and sometimes egophony or bronchial breathing above the fluid level. A friction rub may be heard with pleural inflammation.

Imaging

CXR

- Sequential blunting of posterior, lateral, and then anterior costophrenic angles are seen on radiographs as effusions increase in size.
- PA CXR will usually detect effusion volumes of 200 mL or more; lateral CXR is more sensitive and may detect as little as 50 mL pleural fluid.
- Classical CXR appearance is of basal opacity obscuring hemidiaphragm, with concave upper border. Massive effusion may result in a "whiteout" of the hemithorax, with mediastinal displacement away from the effusion. Lack of mediastinal shift in such cases raises the possibility of associated volume loss due to bronchial obstruction from a primary lung cancer.
- Other CXR appearances include rounded or lentiform shadowing in loculated interlobar effusions, and diffuse shadowing throughout the hemithorax on supine films.
- CXR appearance may suggest the underlying diagnosis, e.g., bilateral effusions with cardiomegaly in cardiac failure; massive effusions are most commonly due to malignancy.

Ultrasound is extremely sensitive for even very small fluid volumes and is useful for distinguishing pleural fluid from pleural masses or thickening and for demonstrating loculation.

CT chest with contrast is useful in distinguishing benign and malignant pleural disease: nodular, mediastinal, or circumferential pleural thickening all suggest malignant disease. CT may also reveal evidence of extrapleural disease, e.g., lymphadenopathy or parenchymal change, which may suggest a diagnosis such as cancer or tuberculosis.

The role of *MRI* is unclear. It may have an increasing role in distinguishing benign from malignant pleural disease.

Pleural thickening

Pleural fibrosis and thickening may follow previous episodes of pleural inflammation. Causes include previous empyema, tuberculous pleuritis, rheumatoid pleuritis, hemothorax, thoracotomy, and asbestos exposure (diffuse pleural thickening, p. 349)

Pleural thickening may be asymptomatic or cause breathlessness.

CXR features include blunting of the costophrenic angle or apices, sometimes with associated calcification. Ultrasound or CT may be required to distinguish this from a pleural effusion.

Treatment is problematic and usually unnecessary; decortication may be considered.

Malignant pleural effusion: causes and investigations

Epidemiology

Malignant effusion is the most common cause of exudative pleural effusion in patients older than 60 years.

Causes

Most malignant effusions are metastatic, with lung and breast being the most common primary sites (see Table 25.1).

Table 25.1 Most common primary sites for malignant pleural effusion

Primary site	Approximate frequency (%)
Lung	37
Breast	16
Lymphoma	10
Mesothelioma	10
Genitourinary tract	9
Gastrointestinal tract	7
Unknown primary	10

Other, rarer tumors include sarcoma, melanoma, leukemia, and myeloma; almost any malignant tumor may spread to the pleural cavity. *Mesothelioma* is an important cause of malignant effusions and is discussed on p. 352.

Clinical features

Breathlessness is the main symptom; chest pain, cough, weight loss, and anorexia may also be present. A small proportion of patients are asymptomatic. Effusions may be unilateral or bilateral, and are frequently large volume.

Differential diagnosis

Consider other potential (direct and indirect) causes of pleural effusion (paramalignant effusion) in patients known to have cancer, e.g., causes due to pneumonia, pulmonary embolism, radiotherapy, pericardial disease, or drugs.

Investigations

A strategy for investigating the patient with an undiagnosed pleural effusion is detailed on p. 44. Key investigations in patients suspected to have a malignant effusion are listed below. The sensitivity of all tests increases with the stage of the malignancy.

1. Pleural fluid cytology

Sensitivity for malignancy is about 60%; yield is increased by analysis of a second, but not a third, sample. Immunostaining of malignant cells may provide clues as to the likely primary site. Detection of a monoclonal cell population in fluid on flow cytometry may support a diagnosis of lymphoma.

2. CT chest with contrast

Nodular, mediastinal, or circumferential pleural thickening on CT is highly specific for malignant disease. It may also demonstrate extrapleural disease, e.g., lymphadenopathy.

3. Pleural biopsy histology

This is required in cytology-negative cases. Options are as follows:

- *CT-guided* cutting needle biopsy has been demonstrated to be a more effective diagnostic test for malignant pleural disease than Abrams pleural biopsy (sensitivity 87% in CT-guided biopsy group vs. 47% in the Abrams group).
- *Ultrasound-guided* needle biopsies are also effective and relatively straightforward to perform.
- *Thoracoscopy* is an extremely useful investigation allowing direct visualization of the pleural space with a high sensitivity (>90%) for biopsies. Therapeutic talc poudrage (talc is insufflated directly onto the pleural surfaces) may be performed at the same time, with a pleurodesis success rate >80%. It can be performed under general anesthesia, although it is well tolerated with sedation and local anesthesia. Complications (such as empyema) are rare.

Serum tumor markers

Serum tumor markers (CEA, CA19-9, CA15-3, CA125, PSA) may be helpful in the investigation of patients with malignant effusion of unknown primary, although their diagnostic and prognostic value is limited.

Prognosis

Median survival 3–12 months from diagnosis is shortest for lung cancer, and longest for mesothelioma and ovarian cancer. Pleural fluid pH <7.30 tends to be associated with shorter survival (median survival 2.1 months) and decreased success of pleurodesis.

Further information

Antunes G, Neville E, Duffy J, et al. (2003). BTS guidelines for the management of malignant pleural effusions. *Thorax* **58** (Suppl. II):ii 29–38.

Maskell NA, Gleeson FV, Davies RJ. (2003). Standard pleural biopsy versus CT-guided cutting-needle biopsy for diagnosis of malignant disease in pleural effusions: a randomised controlled trial. *Lancet* **361**:1326–1331.

Malignant pleural effusion: management

Key points influencing the management of malignant effusions are
- Symptoms, performance status, and wishes of the patient
- Sensitivity of the primary tumor to chemotherapy, e.g., small cell lung carcinoma, lymphoma, and ovarian and breast carcinoma, which may respond to chemotherapy, although in some cases pleural effusions remain problematic and require additional treatment
- Extent of lung re-expansion following effusion drainage

Treatment options

Observation and follow-up are sufficient if the patient is asymptomatic.

Therapeutic pleural aspiration

Pleural aspiration is used to improve breathlessness. It can be performed at the bedside as an outpatient procedure. It is useful in the palliation of breathlessness in patients with a poor prognosis, and in rare cases where effusion reaccumulates very slowly.

Most effusions recur within 1 month of aspiration, and these patients should be considered for pleurodesis. Repeated aspiration may be inconvenient and uncomfortable for the patient, and carries a risk of complications such as empyema, pneumothorax, and tumor seeding (in mesothelioma).

If breathlessness does not improve following fluid aspiration, there is little to be gained by repeated aspiration, and other causes of breathlessness should be considered, e.g., lymphangitis carcinomatosa, pulmonary embolism, and microscopic tumor emboli.

Intercostal chest drainage and pleurodesis

The aim of pleurodesis is to achieve pleural symphysis to prevent pleural fluid accumulation. The success of pleurodesis depends on the degree of apposition of the visceral and parietal pleura, which in turn depends on the degree of lung re-expansion following drainage of the effusion.

Malignant lung entrapment occurs when tumor encases the visceral pleura and prevents lung expansion. Lung expansion may also be inhibited by a proximal airway obstruction or by a persistent air leak (e.g., after tearing of a friable, tumor-infiltrated lung on re-expansion). Trapped lung may also be caused by remote inflammatory insults such as nonmalignant, fibrotic processes, e.g., rheumatoid pleuritis, hemothorax, and tuberculosis.

The patient should be admitted and the effusion drained with an intercostal tube. If the lung fully re-expands on CXR, pleurodesis may be considered (see p. 785).

If the lung fails to re-expand fully (CXR shows a pneumothorax or hydropneumothorax), prolonged chest tube drainage may result in lung re-expansion in some cases, allowing pleurodesis.

Treatment options for malignant lung entrapment or failed pleurodesis

- *Pleurodesis* may be successful despite only partial lung re-expansion and should still be considered. It may be repeated if unsuccessful initially.
- *Repeated therapeutic pleural aspiration*
- *Thoracoscopy* enables the disruption of pleural adhesions and may have a role in facilitating pleurodesis in select patients with unexpandable lung.
- *Long-term indwelling pleural catheter* may be beneficial in patients with malignant lung entrapment and frequent accumulation of symptomatic effusions, and avoids the need for recurrent pleural aspiration. The most frequent complications are tumor seeding around the drain site and pleural space infection. The catheter can be inserted as an outpatient procedure. The procedure may need additional outpatient support, although most patients perform the drainage themselves after education.
- *Pleuroperitoneal shunts* are effective in patients with malignant lung entrapment or failed pleurodesis, in the absence of multiple locula-tions. Shunting of fluid may occur spontaneously, at high pressures, or may require manipulation of a percutaneous pump chamber, inserted at thoracoscopy or mini-thoracotomy. The main problem is shunt occlusion, which occurs in at least 10% of cases and necessitates shunt removal. Malignant spread may also occur.
- *Surgical parietal pleurectomy* may be performed as a VATS (video-assisted thorascopic surgery). The procedure is effective in the management of refractory malignant effusions. It may be useful in a minority of patients with good performance status and prognosis. It is not suitable for patients with heavily diseased visceral pleura and lung entrapment; consider it in patients who have failed pleurodesis. Pleurectomy should only be considered in those patients with an expected survival of more than 3 months.
- *Palliative care team* involvement should also be considered.

Parapneumonic effusion and empyema: definition and clinical features

Definition and pathophysiology

Pleural effusions occur in up to 57% of patients with pneumonia. An initial sterile exudate (uncomplicated parapneumonic effusion) may in some cases progress to a complicated parapneumonic effusion and eventually empyema (see Fig. 25.1).

Pleural infection may also occur in the absence of a preceding pneumonic illness and may be caused by penetrating trauma, esophageal rupture, or postoperatively.

Clinical features

Common

- Consider the diagnosis particularly in cases of "slow-to-respond" pneumonia or pleural effusion with fever, or in high-risk groups with nonspecific symptoms such as weight loss.
- Similar to clinical presentation of pneumonia: fever, sputum production, chest pain, breathlessness
- Anaerobic empyema may present less acutely, often with weight loss and without fever.

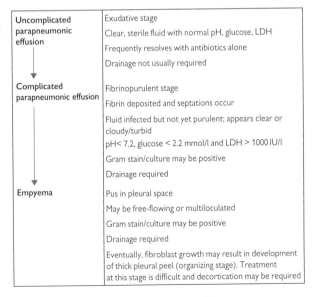

Uncomplicated parapneumonic effusion	Exudative stage
	Clear, sterile fluid with normal pH, glucose, LDH
	Frequently resolves with antibiotics alone
	Drainage not usually required
Complicated parapneumonic effusion	Fibrinopurulent stage
	Fibrin deposited and septations occur
	Fluid infected but not yet purulent; appears clear or cloudy/turbid
	pH< 7.2, glucose < 2.2 mmol/l and LDH > 1000 IU/l
	Gram stain/culture may be positive
	Drainage required
Empyema	Pus in pleural space
	May be free-flowing or multiloculated
	Gram stain/culture may be positive
	Drainage required
	Eventually, fibroblast growth may result in development of thick pleural peel (organizing stage). Treatment at this stage is difficult and decortication may be required

Figure 25.1 Progression of simple parapneumonic effusion to empyema.

Rare
- Empyema may spontaneously drain through the chest wall (*"empyema necessitates"*) or into the lung, leading to a bronchopleural fistula and severe pneumonia.
- History of atypical chest pain, severe vomiting, or esophageal instrumentation suggests possible underlying esophageal rupture (measure pleural fluid amylase).
- History of a recent sore throat may suggest Lemierre's syndrome (acute oropharyngeal infection with *Fusobacterium* species leads to septic thrombophlebitis of the internal jugular vein and subsequent metastatic infection and abscess formation, commonly in the lungs and pleura; consider ultrasound of internal jugular vein if suspected); see p. 235.

Risk factors
Risk factors for developing empyema include diabetes, alcohol abuse, gastroesophageal reflux, and intravenous drug abuse. Anaerobic infection is associated particularly with aspiration or poor dental hygiene. Empyema may rarely occur following bronchial obstruction from a tumor or foreign body. Some patients, however, have no apparent risk factors.

Differential diagnosis
Differential diagnosis includes malignancy and rheumatoid pleuritis.

Parapneumonic effusion and empyema: bacteriology and investigations

Bacteriology

Community-acquired infection (% of cases):
- *S. milleri* (28%)
- Anaerobes (19%)
- *S. pneumoniae* (14%)
- Staphylococci (12%)
- Other less common organisms include other streptococci, Enterobacteria, *H. influenza*, *Pseudomonas*, TB, and *Nocardia*. *Legionella* may very rarely cause empyema.

Hospital-acquired infection (% of cases):
- MRSA (27%)
- Staphylococci (22%)
- Enterobacteria (20%)
- Enterococcus (12%)
- Others include streptococci, *Pseudomonas*, and anaerobes.

Gram-negative organisms may occur in mixed growths with other gram-negatives or with anaerobes.

Investigations

Diagnostic pleural tap

This is essential if pleural infection is suspected. Frankly purulent or turbid/cloudy pleural fluid, organisms on pleural fluid Gram stain or culture, or pleural fluid pH <7.20 are all indications for chest tube drainage. 40% of pleural infections are culture-negative. Identification of anaerobes is improved following inoculation of blood culture bottles with pleural fluid at the bedside.

Ultrasound

Ultrasound typically shows echogenic effusion that may be septated. Very small effusions (<10 mm maximal thickness on ultrasound) probably do not require tapping and can be observed.

Contrast-enhanced CT

CT may be useful in supporting the diagnosis and visualizing distribution of fluid. Empyema is associated with pleural enhancement and increased attenuation of extrapleural subcostal fat. Displacement of adjacent lung by empyema may help to distinguish it from a parenchymal lung abscess.

Empyemas frequently appear lenticular and may exhibit the "split pleura" sign of enhancing, separated visceral and parietal pleura. Absence of pleural thickening on CT is unusual in empyema. CT may also sometimes identify a proximal endobronchial obstructing lesion.

Blood cultures

Blood cultures are positive in only 13% of cases, but in these cases they are often the only positive microbiology.

Bronchoscopy

This is indicated only if a bronchial obstructing lesion is suspected.

Parapneumonic effusion and empyema: management and outcome

Management

1. Antibiotics

All patients with pleural infection should be treated with antibiotics; refer to local hospital prescribing guidelines. Typical choices are as follows:

- *Community-acquired* empyema—second-generation cephalosporin (e.g., cefuroxime) plus metronidazole as anaerobic cover. Ciprofloxacin and clindamycin together may be appropriate. Add macrolide if *Legionella* is suspected
- *Hospital-acquired* empyema—cover gram-positive and gram-negative organisms and anaerobes. MRSA infection is common. Consult with microbiology team. One option is meropenem and vancomycin.

Rationalize with culture and sensitivity results (but note that anaerobes are frequently difficult to culture and may coexist with other organisms). Avoid aminoglycosides, which penetrate the pleural space poorly.

Switch to oral antibiotics when the patient is afebrile and improving clinically. Amoxicillin/clavulanate is a useful single agent with anaerobic coverage (not if penicillin allergic). Optimal duration of antibiotic treatment is unclear; antibiotics should be continued for up to 3 weeks.

2. Chest tube drainage (see Box 25.1)

> **Box 25.1 Indications for chest tube drainage**
>
> - Frankly purulent pleural fluid (definite)
> - Organisms on pleural fluid Gram stain or culture (probable)
> - Pleural fluid pH <7.20 (probable)

Consider earlier chest tube drainage in the elderly and patients with co-morbidity, and loculated effusions, as these are associated with a worse outcome.

Drain insertion should ideally be carried out under ultrasound or CT guidance, as effusions are frequently loculated. The ideal chest tube size remains subject to debate. Small (10–14 French), flexible tubes are more comfortable and have been demonstrated to be as effective as large drains in management of empyema. Usually apply suction (–20 cm water) and flush regularly (e.g., 30 mL normal saline every 6 hours) to prevent occlusion. Consider drain removal when clinical improvement occurs.

If there is no indication for drainage, give antibiotics and monitor closely. If patient is slow to improve or deteriorates, re-sample the effusion and consider chest drain.

3. Intrapleural fibrinolytics

Current evidence suggests that intrapleural fibrinolytics have no effect on mortality, need for surgery, or hospital stay, and routine use is not recommended in patients with empyema. Whether they are effective in the early fibrinolytic stage is unknown.

4. Nutritional support
Obtain dietitian review, consider supplementary nasogastric feeding.

5. Surgery
Consult with the thoracic surgeon should be obtained early. Surgical intervention should not be delayed if the patient is not responding appropriately despite tube drainage and treatment with antibiotics. Surgical techniques include the following:

Video-assisted thoracoscopic surgery (VATS)
VATS enables the breakdown of adhesions and drainage of residual collection, but it is frequently unsuccessful in chronic empyema with very thickened visceral pleura.

Thoracotomy and decortication
This entails removal of fibrinous and infected tissue from the pleural space, and is a major surgical procedure.

Open thoracic drainage
Resection of segments of several ribs adjacent to the empyema and insertion of a large-bore drain into the cavity is a more minor procedure that can be performed under local anesthesia, but results in an open chest wound for a long period (typically about 5 months).

Difficulties in management
Chest drainage ceases despite residual pleural collection
- Attempt to flush drain with sterile normal saline
- Ensure that drain is not kinked at skin insertion site or lying subcutaneously
- Consider CT to assess extent of residual collection and drain position
- Remove drain if persistently blocked
- Consider further image-guided chest drain(s), fibrinolytics, surgery

Failure to clinically improve despite antibiotics and chest drain
- Review microbiology results and ensure appropriate antibiotics
- CT to assess extent of residual collection and drain position
- Surgical referral
- Options if unfit for surgery:
  - Further image-guided small-bore drains into loculated effusions
  - Large-bore drain
  - Surgical rib resection and open drainage under local anesthesia.

Outcome
About 15% of patients require surgery. Empyema 1-year mortality is about 15%. Increased age, renal impairment, low serum albumin, hypotension, and hospital-acquired infection are associated with a poor outcome. CXR may remain abnormal despite successful treatment of empyema, with evidence of calcification or pleural scarring or thickening.

Further information
Davies CW, Gleeson FV, Davies RJ, et al. (2003). BTS guidelines for the management of pleural infection. Thorax **58**(Suppl. II):ii18–ii28.

Tuberculous pleural effusion

Definition and epidemiology

Tuberculous pleural effusion develops from a delayed hypersensitivity reaction to mycobacterial proteins released into the pleural space. It is a common manifestation of primary tuberculosis in regions with a high prevalence, affecting children and young adults; it may also be associated with reactivation of tuberculosis in older individuals. It may occur more commonly in the setting of HIV coinfection.

Rarely, tuberculosis may present as pseudochylothorax or tuberculous empyema.

Clinical features

- Clinical features are similar to those of pulmonary tuberculosis, i.e., fever, sweats, weight loss, and dyspnea, although it may present acutely with pleuritic chest pain and fever, mimicking pneumonia.
- Effusions are typically small to moderate in volume, although they can be massive.

Investigations

- Associated parenchymal infiltrate is on *CXR* in less than one-third of cases; CT scan shows a parenchymal lesion in 75% of cases.
- *Tuberculin skin tests* are positive in two-thirds of cases initially.
- *Pleural fluid* lymphocytosis, exudative effusion, pH is usually <7.40 and glucose is moderately decreased, mesothelial cells rare. Pleural fluid acid-fast bacilli (AFB) smears are positive in around 5%–10% of cases; pleural fluid cultures are positive in 25% of cases and take 2–6 weeks.
- Blind *Abrams pleural biopsy* alone has a sensitivity of 75%, but this increases to nearly 90% when histology and culture of both the fluid and biopsy are analyzed.
- *Thoracoscopic biopsies* have a sensitivity of nearly 100%.
- Measurement of *adenosine deaminase* (an enzyme released by macrophages after phagocytosis of mycobacteria) in pleural fluid may be of benefit in regions where tuberculosis is highly prevalent. A raised value is very sensitive for pleural tuberculosis, but is nonspecific and may also occur in empyema and malignancy.
- *PCR* for mycobacterial DNA in the pleural fluid may be useful diagnostically.
- *Induced sputum* for AFB may have a diagnostic role in high-risk patients with lymphocytic effusions, even in the absence of parenchymal disease on CXR.

Treatment and outcome

- Tuberculous pleural effusions resolve spontaneously in most cases, but two-thirds of untreated patients go on to develop pulmonary tuberculosis within 5 years, and so treatment is recommended.
- Treatment is the same as for pulmonary tuberculosis (p. 278).
- Pleural fluid volumes may increase during effective treatment, and therapeutic thoracentesis is often required.
- Steroids may result in more rapid resolution of symptoms and the effusion but do not appear to prevent pleural fibrosis.
- Pleural thickening is a common long-term consequence of tuberculous pleural effusion.

Other causes

Pleural effusion due to pulmonary embolism

- Fourth most common cause of pleural effusion in the United States
- Consider in all patients with undiagnosed pleural effusion, particularly if there is a history of pleuritic chest pain or of breathlessness/hypoxia out of proportion to the size of the effusion
- Frequently complicates other disease processes, e.g., occurs in one-fifth of patients with cardiac failure and pleural effusions
- Effusions are usually small (less than one-third of hemithorax) and unilateral.
- Pleural fluid analysis is nondiagnostic; appearance varies from clear to bloody, 80% are exudates and 20% are transudates. Bloodstained pleural fluid is not a contraindication to anticoagulation.
- Imaging investigations, such as CTPA of the chest, are required to make the diagnosis. These should be performed prior to thoracentesis if pulmonary embolism is strongly suspected.

Rheumatoid arthritis–associated pleural effusion

- Pulmonary changes may be the first manifestation of rheumatoid arthritis.
- Rheumatoid pleurisy is more common in men (70% are in men).
- Pleural fluid may be yellow-green, serous, turbid, or milky.
- May be unilateral or bilateral
- Pleural fluid glucose level is frequently low (<1.6 mmol/L), and progressively falls in chronic effusions.
- Pleural fluid pH is commonly reduced (~7.00).
- Pleural fluid LDH is usually >1000 IU/L.
- Low pleural fluid complement leveis (C4 <0.04 g/L) may also favor the diagnosis.
- Elevated pleural fluid rheumatoid factor titer is found, but it is not more diagnostically helpful than serum rheumatoid factor.
- Typically persist for 4 to 6 weeks; may progress to lung entrapment and cholesterol effusion
- Some patients with acute rheumatoid pleurisy may respond to steroids.

Hemothorax

- *Hemothorax* is defined as a pleural effusion with a hematocrit >50% of peripheral blood hematocrit.
- Causes include trauma, iatrogenic, malignancy, pulmonary infarction, benign asbestos-related pleural effusion, pneumonia, post-cardiac injury syndrome, pneumothorax, thoracic endometriosis, and aortic rupture.
- *Massive hemothorax* is defined as >1500 cm^3 of blood in hemithorax, and is most commonly due to trauma. Traumatic hemothorax generally requires a chest drain and sometimes thoracotomy. All cases should be discussed immediately with the cardiothoracic surgical team.
- Large volumes of residual blood in the pleural space will clot and may lead to pleural thickening, empyema or trapped lung. Tube drainage is difficult and thoracoscopy or thoracotomy with decortication is often needed. However, undrained cases can resolve without intervention.

Pleural effusion after coronary artery bypass grafting

Small, typically left-sided pleural effusions occur in most patients post-CABG, and most of them resolve spontaneously.

Larger (>25% of hemitorax) effusions can be subdivided:

- Pleural effusions occurring *within 30 days* of surgery. Classically bloody and eosinophilic exudate, with high LDH; probably related to postoperative bleeding into pleural space
- Pleural effusions *more than 30 days* after surgery. Typically clear and lymphocytic exudate; cause is unknown, perhaps immunological or a form of post-cardiac injury syndrome

The main symptom in each case is breathlessness; chest pain and fever are unusual.

Management consists of repeated therapeutic thoracentesis to alleviate breathlessness. Recurrent effusions after 1 year are uncommon and are due to trapped lung. Patients with post-cardiac injury syndrome may require steroids for resolution. Decortication is an option for symptomatic patients with trapped lung.

Differential diagnosis of early post-CABG pleural effusion includes pulmonary embolus, cardiac failure, pleural infection, post-cardiac injury syndrome, and chylothorax.

Pleural effusion following asbestos exposure

The main differential diagnosis is between benign asbestos pleural effusion (p. 348) and mesothelioma (pp. 352–3).

Pleural effusion in immunocompromised patients

Differential diagnosis includes cardiac failure and fluid overload, pulmonary embolism, parapneumonic or drug-related illness, PCP, other infections (fungal, *Nocardia*), or those related to the underlying disease (e.g., leukemic infiltrates, lymphoma, chylothorax, myeloma).

The most common causes of pleural effusion in HIV infection are Kaposi sarcoma, parapneumonic effusion, tuberculosis, PCP, and lymphoma.

Further reading

Heidecker J, Sahn SA (2006). The spectrum of pleural effusions after coronary artery bypass grafting surgery. *Clin Chest Med* **27**:267–283.

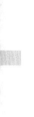

Asbestos and the lung

Asbestos

Asbestos consists of a family of naturally occurring hydrated silicate fibers that can be subdivided into two groups:

- Curly *serpentine* fibers, of which chrysotile (white) is the only representative. This fiber accounts for 95% of all asbestos used commercially worldwide.
- Straight, needle-like *amphiboles*, of which crocidolite (blue), amosite (brown), and anthophyllite have been used commercially. Tremolite and actinolite are found as contaminants of minerals such as chrysotile, talc and vermiculite.

While asbestos usage in developed countries is banned or restricted, the use of asbestos in developing countries continues to rise.

The pathogenicity of asbestos fibers varies in part because of their distinct morphology and physicochemical properties. The aspect ratio (width-to-length ratio) plays an important role. An aspect ratio of >1:8 confers an enhanced toxicity. In addition, lung clearance of amphibole fibers is slower than that of chrysotile.

Mechanisms of exposure

Occupational exposure accounts for the majority of cases of asbestos-related disease and includes the following:

- Mining, milling, and transport of asbestos
- Use of asbestos products, e.g., in construction and demolition, floor tiling, insulation, fireproofing, textiles, friction materials (brake linings), ship building, pipefitting, electrical repair, boiler fitting and lagging, carpentry, plumbing, and welding
- Remodeling or renovation in contaminated buildings

Para-occupational exposure may include the following:

- Relatives of asbestos workers exposed to "carry-home" asbestos in hair or clothes
- Community exposure due to mining of ore contaminated with asbestos, e.g., vermiculite mining in Libby, MT
- Local geological exposure from natural deposits, e.g., areas of central and southeast Turkey, northwest Greece, and Corsica
- Urban environment

There were more than 3000 commercial uses for asbestos. A complete occupational and environmental history is essential if asbestos-related lung disease is suspected. When taking an asbestos exposure history it is important to ask about job duties and work processes, as job titles alone are often uninformative. It is also important to consider all jobs a person has held because of the long period of time that passes between initial exposure to asbestos and development of disease (latency period).

Asbestos-related lung disease comprises:
- Benign asbestos-related pleural disease
  - Pleural plaques
  - Benign asbestos-related pleural effusion
  - Diffuse pleural thickening
  - Rounded atelectasis
- Asbestosis
- Mesothelioma
- Lung cancer (all cell types)

Other diseases linked to asbestos exposure include pericarditis, pericardial mesothelioma, and peritoneal mesothelioma. Head and neck cancers, gastrointestinal and kidney cancers, as well as leukemia and lymphoma have been associated with asbestos exposure, but the risk is much less than that for lung cancer and the data suggesting these associations are controversial.

Peak industrial asbestos use in the United States occurred in the 1960s and early 1970s. From 1940 through 1979, over 27,000,000 individuals had potential asbestos exposure at work, and asbestos-related disease is likely to remain common for at least the next 30 years. The incidence of mesothelioma in the United States has reached a plateau, but is forecast to peak in 2020 in other industrialized nations.

Benign asbestos-related pleural disease

Pleural plaques

- Most common manifestation of asbestos exposure
- Discrete areas of white or yellow thickening on the parietal pleura; may calcify
- Frequently bilateral and symmetrical; occur particularly on the posterolateral chest wall, over the mediastinal pleura, and on the dome of the diaphragm
- Develop 10–20 years after exposure; incidence increases with longer duration of exposure; found in up to 50% of asbestos-exposed workers, and may also occur after low-dose exposures
- Usually asymptomatic, therefore often recognized incidentally, although if extensive it may be associated with mild breathlessness due to pleural restriction
- Effect on pulmonary function is not common. Most studies have failed to demonstrate abnormal lung function, some studies have shown mild restriction in up to a third of the population studied, and other studies have described otherwise unexplained mild airways obstruction in some populations of asbestos workers with pleural plaques—the mechanism of this is unclear.
- HRCT is more sensitive than CXR in detecting pleural plaques; only 50%–80% of chest CT–detected plaques are seen on CXR. On CXR extra pleural fat can be mistaken for pleural plaque.
- Other potential causes especially for unilateral pleural plaques include previous hemothorax and empyema.
- There is no evidence that plaques are premalignant.

Benign asbestos-related pleural effusion

- Relatively early manifestation of asbestos pleural disease; usually occurs within 10 years of exposure
- Development is considered to be dose-dependent, although it can occur after minimal exposure.
- Typically small and unilateral, and may be asymptomatic or occasionally associated with pleuritic pain, fever, and dyspnea.
- Usually resolves spontaneously over a few months, although some cases recur
- The pleural effusion is an exudate, often bloodstained, with no characteristic findings on pleural fluid analysis.
- Diagnosis depends on a history of asbestos exposure and the exclusion of other causes, including mesothelioma.
- Benign asbestos pleurisy may precede the development of diffuse pleural thickening; there is no clear association with mesothelioma.
- Treat symptomatically, with pleural aspiration for breathlessness and NSAIDs for pain.

Diffuse pleural thickening (DPT)

- Consists of extensive fibrosis of the visceral pleura with areas of adhesion with the parietal pleura and consequent obliteration of the pleural space
- Unlike pleural plaques, its margins are ill defined and it may involve the costophrenic angles, apices, and interlobar fissures.
- Development appears to be dose related and may follow recurrent asbestos pleurisy.
- On CXR, it may be defined as a smooth, uninterrupted pleural opacity extending over at least a quarter of the chest wall, with or without obliteration of the costophrenic angles. On CT, the pleural density extends more than 8 cm craniocaudally and 5 cm laterally, and is more than 3 mm thick.
- Symptoms are relatively common and consist of exertional breathless-ness and chest pain, which can be chronic and severe.
- DPT may lead to significant restrictive pulmonary function impairment, especially if the costophrenic angle is obliterated; hypercapnic respiratory failure has been described.
- On rare occasions pleural biopsy may be required to distinguish it from mesothelioma.
- Treatment is difficult; decortication often fails to result in clinical or functional improvement.

Rounded atelectasis
(Also known as folded lung, Blesovsky syndrome, or shrinking pleuritis with atelectasis)

- Develops as contracting visceral pleural fibrosis ensnares and then twists the underlying lung, resulting in the distinctive radiological appearance of a rounded or oval pleural-based mass of 2.5–5 cm in diameter
- CT is often diagnostic, demonstrating a "comet tail" of vessels and bronchi converging toward the lesion, adjacent thickened pleura, and volume loss in the affected lobe.
- Rarely an atypical appearance may require biopsy to exclude malignant disease.
- Often asymptomatic, although breathlessness or dry cough may occur
- Usually stable or slowly progressive, and no specific treatment is required
- Surgical decortication may improve symptoms but frequently results in reduced lung volumes and is not generally recommended.

Further information

Becklake MR, Bagatin E, Neder JA (2007). Asbestos-related diseases of the lungs and pleura: uses, trends and management over the last century. *Int J Tuberc Lung Dis* **11**:356–369.

Asbestosis

Definition
The term *asbestosis* is sometimes used colloquially for any thoracic manifestation due to asbestos exposure. Strictly speaking it should only be used for the bilateral interstitial fibrosis of the lung parenchyma from asbestos inhalation.

Causes
Factors affecting disease development include the following:
- *Degree and length of asbestos exposure*—a clear dose–response relationship exists. It is usually seen in workers with many years of high exposure, although it may follow a very high exposure of short duration, resulting in a shorter latency period.
- *Susceptibility* is probably influenced by many factors including genetics, ethnic origin, immune function, and fiber clearance.

Latency period from first exposure to clinical disease is usually at least 15–20 years, and may be >40 years.

Clinical features
These include insidious onset of breathlessness, dry cough, and bibasilar late-inspiratory crackles, with clubbing in 40% of cases. Severe disease may lead to cor pulmonale, and progress to respiratory failure.

Differential diagnosis
Differential diagnosis includes other causes of interstitial pulmonary fibrosis, such as other pneumoconioses, pulmonary fibrosis due to metals, organic dust, drugs, infectious agents, collagen vascular disorders, and idiopathic pulmonary fibrosis (IPF).

Diagnostic evaluation
CXR
CXR shows a bilateral symmetrical reticulonodular pattern, primarily affecting the lower lobes peripherally, which may extend upward to involve the mid and upper zones. It may progress to honeycomb lung. Associated pleural thickening or plaques are seen in 90% of cases.
   CXR is insensitive to early disease; it may be normal in 15%–20% of symptomatic, biopsy-proven asbestosis.

HRCT
HRCT is more sensitive than CXR and is abnormal in 10%–30% of cases with a normal CXR. Features include basal ground-glass opacities (seen early in the disease), parenchymal bands, subpleural curvilinear lines and opacities, interlobular septal thickening (should be confirmed by prone imaging), and signs of fibrosis (traction bronchiectasis, loss of lobular architecture, honeycombing in advanced disease).

PFTs
PFTs are classically restrictive with reduced lung volumes and DLCO. On rare occasions obstructive or mixed patterns may also occur.

Histology
The gold standard is pathological demonstration of fibrosis (usual interstitial pneumonitis pattern) with demonstration of asbestos bodies on iron stain. In practice histology is rarely required since a diagnosis can be made on the basis of a history of significant asbestos exposure with appropriate delay between exposure and disease, and radiographic evidence of fibrosis.

Treatment
- No pharmacological treatment is of proven benefit.
- Supportive management, including supplementary oxygen as required, influenza and pneumococcal immunization, smoking cessation, prompt treatment of respiratory infections
- The lack of treatment options emphasizes the need for primary prevention, use of asbestos substitutes, engineering designs with no asbestos, or administrative controls.

Counseling
Written documentation of a diagnosis of a work-related illness may trigger the legal statute of limitations (i.e., the time frame in which the patient must file a legal claim for benefits). A patient with a diagnosis of asbestos-related lung disease should therefore be counseled that the disease may raise legal issues, which should be further explored with a knowledgeable lawyer.

Prognosis
Prognosis varies widely. After removal from exposure, progression occurs in 5%–40% of patients over 10 years; progression is faster following greater exposure. Fewer CXR opacities after exposure are associated with better prognosis. There is increased risk of developing lung cancer.

Mesothelioma: diagnosis

Definition
Mesothelioma is a malignant tumor of the pleura or peritoneum usually resulting from asbestos exposure.

Causes
Asbestos is the major single cause, and there is a history of occupational, para-occupational, or environmental asbestos exposure in up to 90% of cases. All types of asbestos can cause mesothelioma—amphibole fibers are the most potent, but chrysotile can also cause this cancer. The pleura is the most common site (80%–90%), followed by the peritoneum (<10%), the pericardium (<1%), and the tunica vaginalis testis (rare).

Mean latent interval between first exposure and diagnosis is around 40 years; cases with latency <15 years are rare. Mesothelioma is not dose related (unlike asbestosis or bronchogenic cancers), and there is no evidence for a threshold asbestos dose below which there is no risk, although the risk at low exposure levels is small. No significant association with smoking has been determined.

Other causes include non-asbestos fibers such as erionite, which is found in rocks in Cappadocia, Turkey—mesothelioma accounts for up to a quarter of all adult deaths in local villages. "Spontaneous" mesothelioma in children has been described.

Clinical features
- Chest pain (typically dull ache, "boring," diffuse, occasionally pleuritic), slowly progressive breathlessness, weight loss, fatigue. A small proportion of cases are asymptomatic.
- Pleural effusions occur in approximately 60% of patients. Consider mesothelioma in any patient with a pleural effusion or pleural thickening, particularly if chest pain is present.
- Rarely may present with persistent chest pain and a normal CXR
- Clubbing may occur but is rare.
- Chest wall invasion may be seen (especially at thoracentesis sites).
- Bilateral pleural involvement is unusual at presentation.
- Paraneoplastic syndromes are described, e.g., disseminated intravascular coagulation.

Differential diagnosis
This includes benign asbestos pleural effusion, diffuse pleural thickening, and adenocarcinoma involving the pleura.

Investigations
1. Pleural fluid
Aspiration typically reveals an exudate, often bloody. Cytological analysis rarely provides the diagnosis (sensitivity is 32%), although it may be useful in excluding other pathology, e.g., adenocarcinoma. No specific fluid characteristics or biomarkers are diagnostic for mesothelioma. Pleural fluid glucose and pH may be low in extensive tumors.

Mesothelioma may track through the chest wall along thoracocentesis sites; avoid repeated pleural aspiration if the diagnosis is suspected, and "tattoo" aspiration sites with indelible ink to guide subsequent prophylactic radiotherapy.

2. Imaging

CXR and CT features include the following:

- There are no pathognomonic radiological features.
- Moderate to large pleural effusion, usually with pleural nodularity and involvement of mediastinal pleura
- Pleural mass or thickening without free fluid
- Entrapment of lung resulting in small hemithorax on involved side
- Local invasion of chest wall, ribs, heart, mediastinum, hilar nodes, and diaphragm; transdiaphragmatic spread and invasion of contralateral pleura
- Associated pleural plaques or interstitial fibrosis in only a fifth of cases
- MRI and PET scanning can help confirm a diagnosis of pleural malignancy, but cannot help distinguish between mesothelioma and metastatic carcinoma.

3. Biopsy

The diagnosis should be confirmed histologically except when the patient is too ill or too frail for biopsy. Thoracoscopic biopsy of pleural masses has a high diagnostic yield and should be used in preference to blind closed pleural biopsy techniques. Early use of thoracoscopy may both provide a diagnosis and enable treatment of large effusions with talc pleurodesis, thereby avoiding repeated nondiagnostic procedures with attendant problems of needle-track spread.

Histological subtypes

- Epithelioid (around 50% of cases; may be confused with adenocarcinoma; better prognosis)
- Sarcomatoid (or fibrous) (around 10%)
- Mixed (biphasic)

A variety of stains may be useful in distinguishing mesothelioma from adenocarcinoma or benign pleural disease.

Staging

There is no widely accepted staging system. Proposed schemes include the stage I–IV scheme and TNM classification. The Butchart classification and the tumor–node–metastasis system developed by the International Mesothelioma Interest Groups are the most commonly used staging systems.

Poor prognostic features include transdiaphragmatic muscle invasion and involvement of mediastinal lymph nodes.

Further information

Ismail-Khan R, Robinson LA, Williams CC Jr, Garrett CR, Bepler G Simon GR (2006). Malignant pleural mesothelioma: a comprehensive review. *Cancer Control* **13**(4):255–263.

Mesothelioma: treatment and outcome

Treatment

Surgery

Currently there is no convincing published evidence demonstrating that surgery improves survival or quality of life. Extrapleural pneumonectomy is aggressive, results in removal of one lung with pleura, diaphragm, and pericardium. Perioperative mortality is 5%–7%.

If considered, it should be performed only in centers with experience, when there is a firm diagnosis of epithelioid mesothelioma, the patient is otherwise fit, and there is no radiological evidence of lymph node involvement. Avoid chemical pleurodesis in such cases.

Chemotherapy

Mesothelioma is poorly responsive to most chemotherapy agents. The only regimen that has shown some promise in extending survival is pemetrexed and cisplatin combined. In a large phase III trial, median survival was extended from 9.3 to 12.1 months.

Management of pleural effusions

Talc pleurodesis is the treatment of choice, and early pleurodesis is preferable to repeated pleural aspirations. This is most commonly achieved with thoracoscopy.

Pleurodesis is not possible if the lung does not re-expand following drainage of pleural fluid ("trapped lung"), and the resulting recurrent pleural effusions are difficult to manage. Indwelling pleural catheters allow fluid drainage without needle aspiration and can be useful in this situation. The value of pleuroperitoneal shunts remains uncertain.

Radiotherapy

Prophylactic radiotherapy greatly reduces chest wall invasion by tumor following pleural aspiration or biopsy; three daily fractions reduced the risk of tracking from 40% to 0 in a randomized study of 40 patients. Recurrence may follow delayed prophylactic radiotherapy, so it is usually administered within 4 weeks.

Palliative radiotherapy provides pain relief in a proportion of patients, but is less useful in the treatment of breathlessness.

New approaches

These include gene therapy, immunotherapy and trimodal therapy with extrapleural pneumonectomy and decortication followed by radiation and chemotherapy.

General management

Provide early supportive treatment with pain relief, nutritional support, supplemental oxygen if required, and counseling of the patient and family. A diagnosis of mesothelioma may raise legal issues, which should be further explored with a knowledgeable lawyer.

Ensure adequate analgesia; nerve blocks and cordotomy may be needed. Breathlessness may be multifactorial, e.g., pleural effusion, lung compression, chest wall restriction, pericardial involvement, pain, and anxiety.

Clinical course

Median survival is poor, varying from 8 to 14 months in different studies. Typically the disease progresses by local extension. Distant metastases are common (50% at autopsy) although occur late and are rarely clinically apparent.

Asbestos-related lung cancer

- An association between asbestos and an increased risk of lung cancer is well established.
- Every patient with lung cancer should be asked about asbestos exposure.
- Smoking and asbestos exposure confer a synergistic risk of lung cancer (a 60 times greater risk than that for non-asbestos-exposed never-smokers)
- The majority of cancers occur in patients with asbestosis.
- Clinical presentation, diagnostic evaluation, pathology, treatment, and prognosis of asbestos-related lung cancer do not differ from that of lung cancer due to other causes.

Sleep-related respiratory disorders

Introduction

Sleep-related respiratory disorders include several conditions: a) obstructive sleep apnea (OSA), b) central sleep apnea (CSA), c) Cheyne–Stokes respiration (CSR), d) obesity hypoventilation syndrome (OHS), and e) chronic alveolar hypoventilation syndromes.

Obstructive sleep apnea
OSA is defined by the absence (apnea) or reduction (hypopnea) of nasal and oral airflow, of at least 10 seconds in duration, which occurs despite continued efforts to breathe against an upper airway obstruction. A *hypopnea* is commonly defined by a reduction of airflow or amplitude of thoracoabdominal movement by at least 30% from baseline that is accompanied by oxygen desaturation of at least 4%.

The syndrome also includes *mixed* apneas that consists of an initial central apnea followed by an obstructive apnea/hypopnea, as well as *upper airway resistance syndrome*, which consists of repetitive sleep-related episodes of decreased inspiratory airflow secondary to increasing upper airway resistance, increased or constant respiratory effort, and arousals from sleep, but with no oxygen desaturation.

Central sleep apnea results from cessation or reduction of airflow secondary to absent or diminished respiratory effort.

Cheyne–Stokes respiration consists of periodic breathing with recurring periods central apneas or hypopneas separated by crescendo–decrescendo ventilation.

Obesity hypoventilation syndrome is characterized by the presence of hypercapnia ($PaCO_2$ >45 mmHg) during wakefulness associated with severe obesity (body mass index [BMI] $\geq$40 kg/m^2).

Chronic alveolar hypoventilation syndromes include disorders that are associated with ineffectual respiration and hypercapnia.

Obstructive sleep apnea: clinical features, pathophysiology, and consequences

The upper airway is a collapsible tube; its patency is maintained by the balance between the action of dilating muscles (e.g., genioglossus, geniohyoid, sternohyoid and tensor palatini) and forces that enhance upper airway collapse during sleep (e.g., negative intraluminal pressure).

Compared to normal individuals, the upper airways of patients with OSA are more vulnerable to collapse; the pressure at which upper airway collapse occurs (critical closing pressure, P_{Crit}) is less negative in patients with OSA. Upper airway obstruction occurs more commonly in the airspaces behind the tongue (retrolingual space) and behind the palate (retropalatal space).

Apneas and hypopneas are generally associated with episodic snoring, oxygen desaturation, and arousals. The latter, if frequent, can give rise to sleep fragmentation, and complaints of either excessive daytime sleepiness or insomnia.

Relative bradycardia occurs during respiratory events. This is followed by relative tachycardia following apnea termination. Paradoxical or "out-of-phase" motion of the ribcage and abdomen can be appreciated. Apneas and hypopneas typically occur more frequently, are longer in duration, and are associated with more pronounced oxygen desaturation during rapid eye movement (REM) sleep and during sleep in a supine position. Events occurring during REM sleep tend to be longer in duration and be associated with greater falls in oxygen saturation.

Pathophysiological mechanisms and adverse physiological effects are similar for obstructive apneas and obstructive hypopneas, and the two respiratory events are generally considered together when determining disease severity. The apnea-hypopnea index (AHI), or the number of apneas plus hypopneas per hour of sleep time, is often used to classify OSA into *mild* (5–15 events/hour), *moderate* (16–30 events/hour), or *severe* (>30 events/hour). Other factors that determine OSA severity include extent of oxygen desaturation, presence of respiratory event-related cardiac arrhythmias, and degree of daytime impairment.

The prevalence of OSA, if defined by an AHI of 5 or more, is estimated to be about 24% and 9% of middle-aged males and females, respectively. It affects men more commonly than women; among the latter, prevalence increases with menopause.

Risk factors for OSA include increasing age, male gender, excess body weight, positive family history, specific anatomic features (increased neck circumference (>17 inches in men, and >16 inches in women), nasal narrowing, macroglossia, adenotonsillar enlargement, low-lying palate, retro- or micrographia, medical and neurological disorders (untreated hypothyroidism, acromegaly, stroke, or neuromuscular conditions), and use of alcohol, muscle relaxants, anesthetics, and narcotic analgesics. African Americans, Mexican Americans, Asians, and Pacific Islanders may be at greater risk of developing OSA than Caucasians.

Consequences of untreated OSA consists of excessive daytime sleepiness; increased mortality; adverse physiological effects (decrease in SaO_2 and PaO_2, increase in $PaCO_2$, and increase in systemic and pulmonary artery pressure); sleep disturbance; systemic and pulmonary hypertension; ischemic coronary disease; congestive heart failure (CHF); cardiac arrhythmias (sinus arrhythmia, heart blocks, premature ventricular contractions, and recurrent atrial fibrillation after successful cardioversion); insulin resistance; gastroesophageal reflux; nocturia; erectile dysfunction; strokes; mood disorders; increased vehicular and work-related accidents; poor academic performance; and diminished quality of life.

Obstructive sleep apnea: evaluation

Assessment of patients with suspected OSA should start with a detailed sleep history. Patients may present with complaints of snoring, accounts of witnessed apneas, daytime sleepiness, repeated awakenings with gasping or dyspnea, morning headaches, dry mouth or throat sensation on awakening, or impaired cognition.

Behavioral disorders, including hyperactivity and attention deficit, may be observed in children with OSA. Less commonly, OSA may manifest with parasomnias (e.g., confusional arousals or sleep-related eating disorder). Questionnaires (e.g., Berlin or Epworth) may be useful in helping identify patients with OSA and the presence of associated daytime sleepiness.

Physical examination may reveal a large neck circumference, nasal septal deviation or turbinate hypertrophy, crowded posterior pharyngeal space, macroglossia, and retro- or micrognathia. Nonetheless, physical examination may be entirely normal.

However, clinical and physical examination features are neither sufficiently sensitive nor specific for the diagnosis of OSA. Therefore, a polysomnography (PSG) is routinely required to identify the presence and determine the severity of OSA. An attended overnight laboratory PSG with positive airway pressure (PAP) titration using either a full- or split-night protocol is recommended. Split-night studies consist of an initial diagnostic portion and a subsequent continuous positive airway pressure (CPAP) titration on the same night. In selected cases, particularly when laboratory testing is not readily available, portable home sleep testing is an acceptable alternative.

Multiple sleep latency testing may be used to assess the presence of hypersomnolence in patients whose sleepiness persists despite optimal PAP therapy to exclude other causes of hypersomnolence.

Patients with craniofacial anomalies, such as Crouzon, Apert, Pierre–Robin or Treacher–Collins syndrome, may require more extensive evaluation, including nasoendoscopy, lateral cephalometric views, or computed tomography, to determine the anatomic site(s) of upper airway narrowing.

Thyroid function tests should be considered in patients with a clinical history suggestive of hypothyroidism. Drug testing may be useful in patients with unexplained sleepiness.

Obstructive sleep apnea: therapy

Treatment is generally recommended for all patients with an AHI ≥15 per hour, or symptomatic patients (excessive sleepiness, insomnia, impaired cognition, mood disorder, hypertension, ischemic heart disease, or stroke) with an AHI of 5–30 per hour.

Therapy of OSA consists of optimal weight management; avoidance of alcohol, sedatives, and muscle relaxants; correction of precipitating factors, such as hypothyroidism, if present; avoidance of a supine sleep position (positional therapy) if respiratory events occur exclusively or predominantly during this position and if AHI is within normal limits during sleep in a lateral or prone sleep position; PAP therapy; oral devices; and/or upper airway surgery.

Positional therapy may be tried using a variety of techniques, such as sewing a pocket in the back of a well-fitted pajama top into which 3–4 tennis balls are placed, or sleeping with a backpack filled with a firm styrofoam pad. Long-term efficacy of positional therapy is not established.

Positive airway pressure therapy is the treatment of choice for patients with OSA. PAP functions as a pneumatic splint that increases airway pressure above P_{Crit} and maintains the patency of the vulnerable portions of the nasopharyngeal airway. PAP therapy includes CPAP, bilevel positive airway pressure (BPAP), automated positive airway pressure (APAP), adaptive servo ventilation (ASV), or noninvasive nighttime ventilation.

CPAP devices provide a constant pressure throughout the respiratory cycle. With BPAP, a higher pressure is provided during inspiration and a lower pressure during expiration.

APAP devices are able to automatically vary delivered pressures using device-specific diagnostic and therapeutic algorithms.

ASV devices generate three pressure levels, namely maximum and minimum inspiratory pressures, as well as an expiratory pressure. Salutary effects of PAP therapy for OSA include improvements in sleep quality, daytime alertness, cognitive function, cardiovascular parameters (hypertension), and mortality. Less than optimal PAP utilization is a significant problem in clinical practice.

Common reasons for noncompliance to therapy include perceived lack of efficacy, claustrophobia, aerophagia, mask discomfort, and rhinosinal dryness or pain. Addition of heated humidification and systematic educational program enhance adherence to PAP use.

BPAP may be considered for patients who complain of difficulty exhaling against a high fixed CPAP pressure, describe PAP-related gastric distention, or who have comorbid central hypoventilation, or obstructive or restrictive lung disease.

APAP is not recommended for patients with CHF, chronic obstructive pulmonary disease, daytime hypoxemia, respiratory failure from any cause, and obesity hypoventilation syndrome. There are no significant differences in PAP acceptance and use between CPAP, BPAP, or APAP.

Oral devices use mandibular advancers or tongue retainers to increase the dimensions of the upper airway by moving the mandible and/or tongue forward, and are indicated for treating mild to moderate OSA. Effectiveness of oral devices is influenced primarily by the degree of anterior displacement of the tongue. A repeat PSG is recommended once the device has been optimally adjusted to assess its therapeutic efficacy.

These devices should be avoided in patients who have a high resistance to nasal airflow, or with primarily central apnea. Mandibular repositioners are contraindicated in patients with inadequate or compromised dentition. Adverse consequences of oral devices include tooth pain, bite changes, and temporomandibular joint discomfort associated with mandibular repositioners, as well as excessive salivation.

Upper airway surgery consists of procedures designed to increase the nasal airspace (e.g., septoplasty or turbinate resection), retropalatal airspace (e.g., uvulopalatopharyngoplasty), retrolingual airspace (e.g., genioglossal advancement), or both the retrolingual and retrolingual airspace (e.g., maxillomandibular advancement).

Uvulopalatopharyngoplasty involves excision of the uvula, portions of the soft palate, and redundant pharyngeal tissue. Genioglossal advancement consists of a parasagittal mandibular osteotomy to create an anterior displacement of the genial tubercle of the mandible, to which the tongue is attached. With maxillomandibular osteotomy and advancement, there is anterior displacement of the maxilla by Le Fort maxillary osteotomy and of the mandible by sagittal split mandibular osteotomy.

In cases of severe, life-threatening OSA unresponsive to other types of therapies, a tracheostomy might be necessary. PSG should be repeated following upper airway surgery to determine its therapeutic efficacy.

Oxygen supplementation does not control obstructive apneas and hypopneas, and should not be used as sole therapy for OSA. Aside from topical nasal corticosteroids used as adjunct therapy for comorbid rhinitis, no pharmacological agent has been shown to be consistently effective for the treatment of OSA. Hormone replacement (e.g., thyroid for hypothyroidism, or medroxyprogesterone for postmenopausal women) has been shown in some studies to improve sleep-disordered breathing. Close monitoring of efficacy and safety is important when these agents are used.

Patients should be counseled to refrain from driving or engaging in potentially dangerous activities unless their OSA has been optimally treated and excessive sleepiness has resolved.

Modafinil, a wake-promoting agent, may be considered to treat persistent sleepiness in patients with OSA on effective PAP therapy and with no other identified cause of sleepiness.

Central sleep apnea

Clinical features of CSA include excessive sleepiness secondary to sleep fragmentation, insomnia, cognitive impairment, nocturnal dyspnea, and recurrent episodes of nocturnal hypoxemia and hypercapnia.

CSA can be either idiopathic (due to failure of ventilatory drive) or secondary to a medical or neurological disorder to or substance use (e.g., long-acting opioids). Secondary forms of CSA are more common than the idiopathic form.

CSA can also be classified according to the level of ventilation as hypercapnic or nonhypercapnic. Hypercapnic CSA is associated with diminished response to hypercapnia and daytime and sleep-related hypo-ventilation (high $PaCO_2$), and is due to neuromuscular disorders or neuro-logical disorders (affecting the brainstem).

In nonhypercapnic CSA there is an increased ventilatory response to hypercapnia with normal or low waking $PaCO_2$. It includes patients with idiopathic CSA, post-arousal CSA, or CHF, who sleep at high altitude, or during CPAP titration.

Treatment of OSA varies depending on the underlying cause of the disorder. Sleep-onset CSA not associated with insomnia and sleep dis-turbance requires no specific therapy. Possible therapies for CSA include oxygen supplementation (for some patients with nonhypercapnic forms of CSA), PAP therapy, nocturnal noninvasive ventilation, or judicious use of respiratory stimulants (e.g., acetazolamide for high-altitude periodic respiration, and theophylline for CSA related to CHF or immaturity in newborns).

Oxygen therapy should be closely monitored, particularly in patients with hypercapnic CSA, as it may result in worsening hypercapnia. Central nervous system depressant agents should be avoided in patients with hypercapnic forms of CSA.

Cheyne–Stokes respiration

Patients with CSR may be asymptomatic or may complain of excessive sleepiness, insomnia, and/or nocturnal dyspnea. CSR appears to be associated with a long circulation time and greater hypercapnic respiratory drive; the latter leads to "excessive" ventilation" with a fall in $PaCO_2$ below the apneic threshold.

CSR can develop in patients with CHF, strokes, and renal failure. In CHF, the risk of developing CSR is increased with a low ejection fraction, the presence of atrial fibrillation, age greater than 60 years, male gender, and low awake $PaCO_2$.

CSR typically occurs during the sleep–wake transition and non-rapid eye movement (NREM) stages 1 and 2 sleep, and usually resolves during slow-wave and REM sleep. CSR-related arousals occur at the peak of ventilation. Cycle length is related inversely to cardiac output and directly to circulation time.

Treatment consists of optimizing cardiac function, oxygen supplementation, and PAP therapy.

Obesity hypoventilation syndrome

Evaluation of patients with OHS may disclose the presence of periodic respiration, hypoxemia, hypercapnia, excessive sleepiness, insomnia, sleep fragmentation with frequent arousals, decreased attention or concentration, peripheral edema, and cyanosis. OSA is present in most cases of OHS.

Etiology of hypercapnia in OHS includes increased CO_2 production due to greater work of breathing, diminished ventilation and reduced hypercapnic and hypoxemic ventilatory responses. Complications of OHS include polycythemia, pulmonary hypertension, and cor pulmonale.

Therapy should include optimal weight management and noninvasive mechanical ventilation (e.g., BPAP therapy), with or without oxygen supplementation. Gastric surgery may be considered for patients with morbid obesity, as caloric restriction alone is ineffective in managing excess weight.

Chronic alveolar hypoventilation syndromes

Congenital central hypoventilation syndrome (CCHS)

CCHS is characterized by hypoventilation due to failure of autonomic respiratory control that is present from birth. Hypoventilation is most severe during NREM sleep. It can present during infancy with shallow breathing, episodic apnea, cyanosis, feeding difficulties, respiratory arrest or pulmonary hypertension.

Death is usually due to respiratory failure or cor pulmonale. Associated features include tumors of neural crest derivatives (e.g., neuroblastomas and ganglioneuromas), esophageal dysmotility, Hirschsprung disease, hypotension, decreased heart rate variability, strabismus, and seizures.

Mutations of the *PHOX2B* gene (autosomal dominant with incomplete penetrance) have been described.

Patients require either nocturnal or continuous ventilatory support (e.g., positive pressure ventilation, BPAP, negative-pressure ventilation, or phrenic nerve stimulators).

Lower airway obstruction (e.g., chronic obstructive pulmonary disease [COPD]), or *pulmonary* (e.g., interstitial lung disease), *chest wall* (e.g., severe kyphoscoliosis or diaphragm paralysis) or *neuromuscular* (e.g., post-polio syndrome, amyotrophic lateral sclerosis, or myopathies) disorders can lead to reduced ventilation, hypoxemia, and hypercapnia. If severe, they can predispose to polycythemia, pulmonary artery hypertension, or cor pulmonale.

Further reading

American Academy of Sleep Medicine (2005). *The International Classification of Sleep Disorders, Second Edition: Diagnostic and Coding Manual.* Westchester, IL: American Academy of Sleep Medicine.

Kushida CA, Littner MR, Hirshkowitz M, et al. (2006). Practice parameters for the use of continuous and bilevel positive airway pressure devices to treat adult patients with sleep-related breathing disorders. *Sleep* **29**(3):375–380.

Morgenthaler TI, Kapen S, Lee-Chiong T, et al. (2006). Practice parameters for the medical therapy of obstructive sleep apnea. *Sleep* **29**(8):1031–1035.

Standards of Practice Committee of the American Academy of Sleep Medicine (2002). Practice parameters for the use of auto-titrating continuous positive airway pressure devices for titrating pressures and treating adult patients with obstructive sleep apnea syndrome. An American Academy of Sleep Medicine report. *Sleep* **25**(2):143–147.

Young T, Palta M, Dempsey J, Skatrud J, Weber S, Badr S (1993). The occurrence of sleep-disordered breathing among middle-aged adults. *N Engl J Med* **328**(17):1230–1235.

Bronchiectasis

Epidemiology, pathophysiology, and causes

Definition

Bronchiectasis is irreversible abnormal dilatation of one or more bronchi, with chronic airway inflammation. Clinical consequences include cough and chronic sputum production, recurrent chest infections, and airflow obstruction.

Epidemiology

The exact prevalence of bronchiectasis is unknown, but in the United States, it has been estimated to be about 52 cases per 100,000 population, with an estimated total of more than 110,000 patients. It is more prevalent in older people, and about two-thirds of patients are women.

The prevalence of bronchiectasis resulting from acute infection is probably falling, due to vaccinations and the improved and earlier treatment of childhood infections. However, the advent of HRCT scanning may now lead to the diagnosis of more subtle (and possibly subclinical) disease. In some areas of the United States, nontuberculous mycobacterial infection is emerging as a significant cause of bronchiectasis.

Pathophysiology

An initial (usually infectious) insult is needed to damage the airways. Disordered anatomy leads to secretion stagnation and secondary infection, causing ongoing inflammation and further airway damage.

Major airways and bronchioles are involved, with mucosal edema, inflammation, and ulceration. Terminal bronchioles become obstructed with secretions, leading to volume loss. A chronic host inflammatory response ensues, with free radical formation and the production of neutrophil elastase, further contributing to the inflammatory process.

Bronchial neovascularization occurs with hypertrophy and tortuosity of the bronchial arteries (which are at systemic pressure), and may lead to intermittent hemoptysis.

Etiology

The causes of bronchiectasis are many and varied (see Table 28.1). In general, the etiology is either a one-off infectious insult or an underlying immune deficiency. The rationale behind determining the etiology of the condition is alteration in management, if, for example, the underlying cause is found to be cystic fibrosis (CF) or an immune deficiency.

The cause is idiopathic in as many as 50% of cases, and these are likely due to an (as yet unidentified) impairment in host defense.

An important cause to exclude, particularly in younger individuals, is CF (see p. 383). Even relatively mild bronchiectasis diagnosed in middle age can be due to CF. The diagnosis can alter management with

- Involvement of the multidisciplinary CF team
- Application of proven efficacious therapy
- Attention to other potential problems, e.g., gastrointestinal disease, sinus disease, diabetes

- Inheritance (relevant to the rest of the family)
- Fertility issues

Consider genotyping for CF if there is
- Predominantly upper lobe disease
- *Haemophilus influenzae* or *Pseudomonas aeruginosa* colonization
- Malnutrition ± malabsorption, diabetes
- Family history of CF or bronchiectasis
- Associated subfertility or infertility

A normal chloride sweat test does not exclude CF, as some mutations are associated with normal sweat chloride levels. The test is also difficult and subject to a number of technical errors. Only 90% of CF sufferers have a recognizable gene defect (there are over 1000 CFTR mutations).

Tabl e 28.1 Causes of bronchiectasis

Genetic	Cystic fibrosis
Congenital	Pulmonary sequestration
Postinfective	Tuberculosis
	Pertussis (if infection is in a localized area)
	Severe pneumonia
	Nontuberculous mycobacteria (NTM)—there is some debate as to whether the bronchiectasis seen in association with NTM (classically in elderly females) is caused by or secondarily infected by NTM
Immune deficiency	Primary—hypogammaglobulinemia
	Secondary—HIV, CLL, nephrotic syndrome
Mucociliary clearance abnormalities	
	Primary ciliary dyskinesia (PCD; see p. 630)
	Kartagener's syndrome
	Young's syndrome (bronchiectasis, sinusitis, azoo-spermia, i.e., clinical features identical to those of CF)
Toxic insults	Aspiration
	Inhalation (toxic gases, chemicals)
Mechanical insults	Foreign-body aspiration
	Extrinsic lymph node compression
	Endobronchial obstructing tumor
Immune-mediated	Allergic bronchopulmonary aspergillosis (ABPA)
	Rheumatoid arthritis
	Sjögren's syndrome, SLE
	Ulcerative colitis and Crohn's disease (see p. 582)
Miscellaneous	Yellow nail syndrome
	Marfan syndrome

Clinical features and diagnosis

Suspect bronchiectasis in a patient with recurrent episodes of bronchitis over several years prior to presentation.

Box 28.1 The clinical picture of bronchiectasis

Symptoms
- Cough
- Chronic sputum production (typically tenacious, purulent, and daily)
- Intermittent hemoptysis
- Dyspnea
- Intermittent pleuritic pain (usually in association with infections)
- Lethargy/malaise.

Signs
- Coarse inspiratory and expiratory crackles on auscultation
- Airflow obstruction with wheeze.

Diagnosis is usually made clinically, with high-resolution CT chest confirmation.

Investigations are aimed at
- Confirming the diagnosis
- Identifying a treatable underlying cause for the bronchiectasis (possible in about 40%)
- Optimizing management, to prevent exacerbations and further lung damage.

Essential investigations

CXR sensitivity is only 50%. It classically shows "ring shadows" and "tram-lines," indicating thickened airways, and the "gloved-finger" appearance, with consolidation around thickened and dilated airways.

HRCT chest is 97% sensitive in detecting disease. Expiratory scans may be useful to demonstrate postobstructive air trapping, indicative of small airways disease. Typically HRCT shows airway dilatation to the lung periphery, bronchial wall thickening, and airway appearing larger than its accompanying vessel (signet ring sign).

If a bronchiectasis is localized to a single lobe, CT is useful to determine whether a central obstructing lesion is present. Contiguous 3 mm slices are needed to exclude a central airway lesion if there is associated hemoptysis.

Symptoms correlate with wall thickening and mucous plugging on CT scan. Traction *bronchiectasis* seen in UIP is airway dilatation secondary to airway distortion, seen with chronic, severe interstitial fibrosis.

Sputum microbiology includes standard Gram stain, C & S (including for atypical organisms), acid-fast bacilli, and *Aspergillus*.

Pulmonary function tests with reversibility testing are required.

Second-line investigations

- *Immunoglobulins A, M, E, G* (including IgG subclasses if total IgG is low)
- *Aspergillus precipitins* (see p. 288)
- *CF genotyping* (see pp. 382–3)
- *Autoantibodies* (ANA, RF, dsDNA) if associated arthritis or connective tissue disease
- *Vaccination response* to tetanus, *Haemophilus influenzae*, and pneumococcal antibodies, *if underlying immunosuppression suspected*
- *Skin tests and radioallergosorbent test (RAST)* to identify specific sensitizers (usually *Aspergillus*)
- *Detailed immunological investigation* (including neutrophil and lymphocyte function studies)
- *Bronchoscopy* to exclude a foreign body if suggested by CT; obtain microbiological samples if there is an unusual clinical presentation or failure to respond to standard antibiotics
- *Nasal brushings/biopsy* (in tertiary center) to assess ciliary beat frequency with video microscopy
- *Blood testing for primary ciliary dyskinesia (PCD)* A new test detects mutations in the DNA/1 and DNAH5 genes, two ciliary outer dynein arm genes. Detection of two known deleterious mutations is diagnostic of PCD.
- α_1-*antitrypsin levels* if deficiency is suspected
- *Barium swallow or esophageal imaging* if recurrent aspiration is suspected
- *HIV testing*

General management

The main aims of management are the following:

- Treatment of any underlying medical condition
- Antimicrobial therapy to treat acute exacerbations, reduce bacterial load, and prevent secondary airway inflammation and damage
- Prevention of exacerbations and progression of underlying disease by physiotherapy. The options for airway clearance include
  - Postural or autogenic drainage
  - Active cycle of breathing technique. This involves breathing control with forced expiration (huffing) using variable thoracic expansion.
  - Cough augmentation, using flutter or acapella valves, cough insufflator, or high-frequency oscillation
  - Exercise regimes, which are important to prevent general deconditioning
  - The respiratory therapist is also vital during admission for exacerbations to help clear tenacious sputum.
- To give supportive treatment, treat associated airflow obstruction, optimize nutrition
- To refer for surgery if necessary for localized resection of affected area
- To refer for transplantation if indicated

Antimicrobial chemotherapy

- This may be intermittent for exacerbations only (for mild disease), or long term for more severe disease. Antibiotics may be oral, nebulized, or intravenous.
- Patients need a higher antibiotic dose for longer time period (usually 2 weeks minimum) than that for people without bronchiectasis.
- Regular sputum surveillance can identify the likely colonizing organism
- In vivo sensitivity may be different from in vitro sensitivity.
- Antibiotic treatment choice depends on the severity of underlying disease, results of sputum analysis, and previous antibiotic susceptibility pattern.
- Treatment response is usually assessed by a fall in sputum volume and change to mucoid from purulent or mucopurulent sputum, with an improvement in systemic symptoms, spirometry, and CRP.
- *Pseudomonas*-colonized patients have more frequent exacerbations, worse CT scan appearances, worse quality of life, and a faster decline in lung function.

Microbiology

Different bacteria may colonize the airways, and their attempted eradication and suppression is vital to the treatment of bronchiectasis. The most common organisms are as follows:

- *Haemophilus influenzae*
- *Moraxella catarrhalis*
- *Pseudomonas species*
- *Staphylococcus aureus*
- *Streptococcus pneumoniae*

In a sizable number of patients, no pathogen is isolated, underscoring the need for empiric therapy.

Exacerbation treatment

An exacerbation is usually a clinical diagnosis, with an increase in sputum volume, purulence, and tenacity. It may be associated with chest pain, hemoptysis, wheezing, and systemic upset—fevers, lethargy, and anorexia. The CRP may be elevated.

Treatment depends on the potential pathogens and resident flora. Nebulized bronchodilators and regular physiotherapy (as an in- or outpatient) may also be needed.

Exacerbation of mild bronchiectasis

- Antibiotics for exacerbations only (tailored to the colonizing organism)
- 2-week course of oral ciprofloxacin at 750 mg bid if *Pseudomonas aeruginosa* colonized
- If early relapse, with a return to purulent sputum within 6–8 weeks, consider long-term oral antibiotics, e.g., amoxicillin 500 mg bid or doxycycline 100 mg daily. There is, however, no proven efficacy.
- If treatment fails, change to appropriate intravenous antibiotics until there is clinical improvement.

Exacerbation of more severe bronchiectasis

Chronic suppressive or rotating antibiotics aim to prevent progression of disease, by reducing bacterial load and preventing ongoing inflammation, though clinical trial data establishing efficacy are lacking.

Antibiotics are usually given for at least 2 days after the sputum has cleared—often for 2 weeks.

If oral antibiotics fail, intravenous treatment is required. This may mean inpatient admission, or could involve long-line insertion, patient education in self-administration of intravenous antibiotics, and involvement of a home care team.

First isolate of Pseudomonas aeruginosa (see also p. 399)

Initial treatment is often aggressive with a 4- to 6-week course of oral ciprofloxacin 500–750 mg bid, and concurrent nebulized aminoglycoside, such as tobramycin, amikacin, or colistin.

If this fails and the patient still has *Pseudomonas* on sputum culture, give intravenous antibiotics, usually an aminoglycoside and antipseudomonal penicillin (minimum 2 weeks).

Consider long-term therapy with regular nebulized aminoglycoside to reduce levels of *Pseudomonas* and reduce subsequent exacerbations and airway inflammation.

Further management

- Self-management plan—patients need an individual plan for exacerbations, which usually involves having a supply of home antibiotics
- Treatment of associated airflow obstruction and wheeze with bronchodilators
- Anti-inflammatory: inhaled corticosteroids and macrolide antibiotics are promising but require further study. Chronic macrolide therapy should be avoided in patients with known or suspected NTM infection.
- Mucociliary clearance:
  - β_2 agonists may enhance clearance
  - N-acetylcysteine
  - Nebulized DNase (Dornase alpha)—although efficacious in CF, it is not effective and potentially deleterious non-CF bronchiectasis.
  - Hyperosmolar agents such as inhaled mannitol are being studied.
- Pneumococcal and annual influenza vaccinations
- Osteoporosis prophylaxis (if on long-term steroids)
- Reflux treatment if aspiration

Immunoglobulin replacement therapy
Patients found to have immunoglobulin deficiency should be referred to an immunologist for further assessment. Intravenous immunoglobulin replacement therapy is usually administered monthly

Surgery
This is the only potential curative treatment, with resection of a single chronically infected lobe occasionally being of benefit. It is less commonly needed these days, as the incidence of single-lobe disease related to previous severe childhood pneumonia is falling. Surgery may be indicated for life-threatening hemoptysis.

Transplant is most commonly performed for CF bronchiectasis, but referral may be warranted for severe, non-CF-related disease.

Complications of bronchiectasis
- Infective exacerbation
- Hemoptysis—small-volume hemoptysis (increasing during exacerbations) is common.
- Massive hemoptysis (usually from tortuous bronchial arteries around damaged lung, e.g., bulla) is a life-threatening emergency (see p. 31)
- Pneumothorax
- Respiratory failure
- Brain abscess (now very rare)
- Amyloidosis

Bronchiectasis and aspergillus

Allergic bronchopulmonary aspergillosis (ABPA)

This excessive immune response to the environmental fungus *Aspergillus* (most commonly *Fumigatus* species) may be the cause of bronchiectasis (suspect particularly if there is upper lobe disease), as mucus plugs become impacted in distal airways, causing airway damage and subsequent dilatation. See p. 288.

Aspergilloma

Aspergillus may colonize damaged airways with formation of a fungus ball (mycetoma) within a previously formed cavity. This is extremely difficult to treat, and most commonly causes hemoptysis. See p. 296.

Adult cystic fibrosis (CF)

General principles

Definition and pathophysiology

- CF is a multisystem disease, due to mutations in the gene encoding for the cystic fibrosis transmembrane conductance regulator (CFTR), a complex chloride channel.
- CFTR is important for regulating salt and water movement across epithelia. Clinically important expression of CFTR occurs in the sweat duct, airway, pancreatic duct, intestine, biliary tree, and vas deferens.
- Defects in CFTR formation or regulation result in dehydrated and viscous secretions.
- In the lungs, inflammation and obstruction of small airways initiates bronchiectasis, even in very young children. Subsequent infection with one or more pathogenic bacteria intensifies the inflammatory response. This in turn accelerates lung damage through increased obstruction, and thus worsening of bronchiectasis.
- In the pancreas, the exocrine ducts also become blocked by secretions, leading to pancreatic destruction and pancreatic exocrine insufficiency at birth. In adulthood, many patients will develop CF-related diabetes (CFRD).

Genetics

- Autosomal recessive
- Gene found on the long arm of chromosome 7
- Carrier frequency varies dramatically by ethnic groups, with the highest frequency generally found in association with European decent
- In the United States, incidence of a CFTR mutation is 1 in 25 in Caucasians, and the incidence of disease ranges from 1 in 3200 live births (Caucasians), to 1 in 15,000 (African Americans), to 1 in 31,000 (Asian Americans).
- More than 1500 specific mutations in the CFTR gene have been recorded to date.
- The most common mutation is ΔF508 and accounts for around 66% of CF alleles worldwide. This is a deletion of 3 nucleotides, resulting in the omission of a single amino acid, phenylalanine, at the 508 residue.
- Extensive mutational heterogeneity exists in the remaining one-third of all alleles, with certain alleles associated with specific ethnic populations.
- While the common ΔF508 mutation results in complete loss of CFTR expression, various other mutations result in only partial loss of expression or function.
- Patients with partial CFTR function may demonstrate a less severe clinical course. The relationship between a mild genotype and a mild phenotype is most apparent by the lack of pancreatic insufficiency in childhood.
- Non-CFTR "modifier" genes (such as TGF-β, mannose-binding lectin, and α_1-antitrypsin), as well as environmental factors probably further influence the clinical picture and account for phenotypic variation.

Screening

Newborn screening for CF has long been available, and by 2008, most states will require this test by law.

Screening is typically performed by the detection of elevated levels of immunoreactive trypsin from a neonatal heel-prick, using the same filter paper cards already obtained for tests like congenital hypothyroidism and phenylketonuria.

Diagnosis

The diagnosis of CF requires at least one compatible clinical finding, in combination with biochemical or genetic confirmation of a CFTR defect.

Patients are usually diagnosed with CF as neonates or children, with a median age of 6 months.

In addition to screening or a family history, classical features that lead to the diagnosis include meconium ileus, failure to thrive, malabsorption of protein and fat, rectal prolapse, chronic cough, electrolyte imbalance, nasal polyps and sinus disease, rectal prolapse, and acute or chronic respiratory symptoms or infections.

The sweat chloride test remains an important laboratory test, particularly in children. Typically, the diagnosis will ultimately be confirmed by the identification of two disease-causing CFTR mutations by genetic screens or *CFTR* sequencing.

Increasingly, patients are diagnosed with CF in adulthood. These patients nearly always have a "nonclassical" clinical presentation, usually without pancreatic insufficiency

The adult diagnosis of CF is typically associated with milder CFTR mutations, resulting in partial expression of the protein. Pulmonary manifestations are often quite typical for CF and can be severe, although delayed in progression, compared to the classic form of the disease.

Principles of disease management

Overview

- Whenever possible, CF patients should be cared for at an adult CF care center. There are 94 adult care centers accredited by the CF Foundation nationwide, and these can be located at www.cff.org.
- Comprehensive care is delivered via a multidisciplinary-team approach, consisting of physicians (usually including a pulmonologist), nurses with experience in CF care, respiratory therapists, dietitians, and social workers.
- The ongoing care of CF patients moves from the pediatric to adult program around the age of 18. This transition needs to be planned throughout childhood and adolescence, and marks the time when patients should take full responsibility for their care and treatment. Often, as patients enter college or become emancipated from their patients, there is a period when these young adults stop taking medications or performing physiotherapy, despite recognizing the need to do so.
- Incremental improvements in treatment strategies have led a to dramatic increase in survival for patients with CF. While in 1985 the median survival in the United States was only 25 years, in 2006 median survival exceeded 37 years. Approximately half of all CF patients in the United States are now over the age of 18 years, with the average age increasing each year. In the foreseeable future, CF will be increasingly viewed as a disease primarily of adulthood.

Management of CF lung disease

Assessment

The most useful objective assessment of the severity and progression of CF lung disease is FEV_1. Spirometry should be obtained at every visit (4 times yearly) in conjunction with oxygen saturation and physical exam. In addition, a complete microbiological assessment of sputum, including antibiotic susceptibility testing, needs to be performed regularly, preferably with each visit.

Multiple sputum samples are often required to fully appreciate the number of pathogens carried by each patient, as not every microorganism will be recovered in each sputum sample.

Airway clearance techniques

A cornerstone of CF treatment is effective clearance of sputum from the airways. In childhood, conventional chest physiotherapy (CPT), which incorporates hand percussion and postural drainage, is often administered by the parents. However, by adulthood, methods that can be performed without assistance are required.

An extensive variety of airway clearance methods are available, including high-frequency chest wall oscillation systems (i.e., The Vest), expiratory resistance devices (i.e., PEP valves), intrapulmonary percussive devices, flutter devices and methods of active cycle breathing, forced expiration, and autogenic drainage. Most adult CF patients have been exposed to various techniques in childhood and have a clear preference in modalities. Generally speaking, all techniques can be effective, and none are clearly superior.

Of primary importance is compliance with a method, often several times a day, over the entire life of the patient. The method(s) being used by each patient should be reviewed at each clinic visit by the care team, with a CF-trained respiratory therapist available to teach and review effective airway clearance techniques.

Often techniques that seemed ineffective when a patient was younger and had milder disease can prove to be useful when reintroduced later in life. In addition, aerobic exercise should be encouraged as an adjuvant to other sputum clearance techniques.

Recombinant DNase

Dornase alfa (Pulmozyme), is a nebulized enzyme that decreases sputum viscosity and improves airway clearance by cleaving the long strands of neutrophil DNA that accumulate through ongoing inflammation. In a variety of patient populations, administration of DNase has consistently demonstrated a modest improvement in FEV_1, and in several trials a reduction in frequency of pulmonary exacerbations was also noted.

It is well tolerated, and should be considered as part of the airway clearance strategy for all CF patients.

Hypertonic saline (3%–10%) may also serve to improve airway clearance, presumably through improved hydration of the mucous layer. In a randomized clinical trial with 1-year follow-up, a reduction in pulmonary exacerbations was noted. The compound can induce bronchospasm and should be pretreated with a bronchodilator. While a conclusive recommendation cannot yet be made for the optimal use of hypertonic saline, sufficient evidence exists to include hypertonic saline as a component of routine airway clearance.

Anti-inflammatory therapies

Ibuprofen

High-dose ibuprofen was one of the first drugs shown to slow the progression of mildly affected patients and helped to establish the principle of reducing inflammation as an important strategy in treating CF lung disease. Doses of ibuprofen required for this effect are very large (20–30 mg/kg, up to 1600 mg, bid), and a pharmacokinetic study is required to verify that a therapeutic blood level has been achieved.

Unfortunately, GI and renal toxicities of this therapy have greatly limited its use, especially in the adult population with more severe disease.

Inhaled steroids

Frequently, adult CF patients will have a component of reactive airway disease, and in some patients asthma-like symptoms are a predominate feature. Although few bronchodilators have been studied in the CF population, the full asthma armamentarium is often used to treat bronchospasm associated with CF. In particular, inhaled steroids and, to a lesser extent, cromolyn are widely used.

In many patients, short courses of systemic steroids seem to be of benefit, especially in the context of a pulmonary exacerbation, but long-term use in children and adolescents is generally avoided because of significant side effects, including growth impairment, osteoporosis, diabetes, and cataracts.

Chronic suppressive antibiotic therapy

Adult CF patients who have become infected with *P. aeruginosa* will not be able to clear this organism from the airways, even with aggressive treatment. However, a clear benefit has been demonstrated by keeping the burden of organisms at a minimum. Aerosolized tobramycin (TOBI) has been demonstrated to decrease the density of *P. aeruginosa* in sputum and produce significant and sustained improvement in FEV_1 as well as reduce the frequency of pulmonary exacerbations and hospitalizations.

Of obvious long-term concern is the emergence of increased antimicrobial resistance. However, by dosing the agent in 1-month intervals, followed by 1-month holidays, clinically important increases in the resistance to tobramycin have not been appreciated to date. Aerosolized tobramycin should be considered for all adult CF patients infected with *P. aeruginosa*. A wide range of other antibiotics have been delivered as an aerosol to CF patients, but none has clearly been established as beneficial in a large study.

More recently, the use of oral azithromycin has also been demonstrated to improve FEV_1 and decrease the frequency of pulmonary exacerbations in CF patients infected with *P. aeruginosa*. It is not entirely clear if this response is due to the antibiotic properties of azithromycin or to well-known anti-inflammatory effects of the macrolide group.

Immunization

Annual influenza vaccination is recommended, as well as the pneumococcal vaccination.

Lung transplantation

The role of transplantation in patients with CF is well established, and should be considered for all patients with advanced disease. Patients should be evaluated for transplantation when their FEV_1 is ≤30% predicted or FEV_1 >30% with rapid progression.

Patients who are listed for transplantation should be followed closely by both the CF team and the lung transplant team, with every effort made to optimize nutrition and maintain conditioning. In advanced CF lung disease, response to therapy diminishes, and often very intensive antibiotic treatment and frequent hospital admissions are required for these patients to survive to transplantation.

Patients must be given a realistic appraisal of the time they can expect to wait for transplantation, as the availability of appropriate organs can vary significantly between different transplant centers in different regions. Typically, bilateral cadaveric lung transplants are performed.

Five-year survival following transplantation is approximately 50%. Lung transplantation is associated with substantial morbidity and mortality, especially in CF patients. When presented with information concerning lung transplantation, many patients will opt not to pursue this option.

Respiratory support

Respiratory failure and cor pulmonale can occur with later-stage disease. Supplemental oxygen is often required, and in more advanced cases nocturnal noninvasive ventilation may be necessary. If support is needed for acute deterioration related to infection, with a major reversible component, noninvasive ventilation should be attempted initially, but the patient may progress to require intubation and mechanical ventilation. A significant percentage of CF patients requiring mechanical ventilation will not survive to extubation or lung transplantation.

Recent studies have shown that 1-year mortality after ICU admission is approximately 50% in CF patients, with mechanical ventilation serving as a predictor of poor outcome. The decision to proceed with mechanical ventilation can be difficult, and factors such as being on the transplant list may be relevant.

For patients receiving mechanical ventilation, end-of-life decisions are significantly more complicated. The CF team must be realistic in presenting options to patients and families, and needs to seek clear directives from patients with advanced disease who are near the end of life.

Other pulmonary disease

The majority of CF patients die during adulthood of respiratory failure. With progression of pulmonary disease, adults with CF are at a higher risk for serious respiratory complications that are a direct result of CF bronchiectasis.

Pneumothorax

The risk of spontaneous pneumothorax increases with age. The lifetime incidence of pneumothorax approaches 20% in CF patients and is associated with a poor prognosis.

While evidence-based guidelines are not available, in most centers there has been a high rate of failure and/or recurrence associated with observation alone, needle aspiration, and chest tube drainage. Ultimately, many patients will require pleurodesis, although this can result in increased complications at the time of lung transplantation.

Allergic bronchopulmonary aspergillosis (ABPA)

This condition is difficult to diagnose in CF, as the clinical signs and symptoms of ABPA are nearly identical to those associated with a CF pulmonary exacerbation. *Aspergillus fumigatus* is widely distributed in the environment, and frequently recovered in the sputum of adult CF patients. The reported incidence of ABPA in CF patients ranges from 1% to 15%.

Annual screening with serum IgE is recommended, and the diagnosis should be considered in the setting of unexpectedly rapid clinical deterioration that does not respond to typical CF treatment. A recent CF Foundation Consensus Conference (2003) recommended the following minimal diagnostic criteria:

• Acute or subacute clinical deterioration not attributable to another etiology
• Total serum IgE >500 IU/L
• Immediate cutaneous reactivity to *Aspergillus* or in vitro demonstration of IgE antibody to *A. fumigatus*
• One of the following: (a) precipitins to *A. fumigatus* or in vitro demonstration of IgE antibody to *A. fumigatus* or (b) new or recent abnormalities on chest radiograph or chest CT (infiltrates, mucous plugging, and/or bronchiectasis) that have not cleared with antibiotics and standard physiotherapy

Standard treatment recommendations include high-dose oral steroids with a prolonged taper in the setting of clinical improvement and decreasing serum IgE levels. Intensive physiotherapy is also an important part of the treatment regimen. Increasingly, there is support for the use of antifungal agents, such as itraconazole, as a steroid-sparing agent.

Nontuberculous mycobacteria (NTM)

Cultures positive for NTM occur in about 13% of CF patients, and an increase in prevalence is apparent in older CF cohorts. The clinical significance of NTM appears to vary among individual patients; in some cases the organism appears not to accelerate clinical decline.

Generally, "rapid-growing" species such as *M. abscesses* are considered more virulent than slow-growing species like *M. avium*. The organisms are widespread in the environment and sporadic detection is common.

In the absence of CF-specific diagnostic criteria, it has been proposed that the diagnosis requires three or more positive cultures for the organism, in the setting of a high-resolution CT scan that demonstrates at least two features of the disease. Especially in the setting of slow-growing species, unexpected clinical decline is an important factor in the decision to initiate treatment.

Antimycobacterial regimes and dosing have not been established for CF patients, thus clinicians typically use standard protocols. Treatment should be initiated with three agents to avoid selecting for resistant isolates. The duration of treatment is typically 12–18 months, with a goal of achieving consistently negative sputum cultures for a year prior to discontinuing therapy.

Response to treatment is extremely variable in CF patients and, frequently, clearing of the sputum for a sustained period is not achieved. Screening for NTM in the sputum should be performed at least once yearly, and more frequently in the setting of unexplained clinical decline.

CF "asthma"

Most adults with CF have some degree of reversible bronchoconstriction, and in some CF patients, asthma-like symptoms are a predominant feature. In addition, agents such as inhaled DNase, TOBI, and hypertonic saline have all been associated with increased bronchospasm. Many CF patients use a nebulized β-adrenergic agonist prior to CPT, and with symptomatic episodes of wheezing or chest tightness.

Small studies have shown encouraging responses to these agents, as well as anticholinergic bronchodilators such as ipratropium. In the absence of evidence-based recommendations, most CF centers treat reactive airway disease with the standard stepwise progression used with asthma: short-acting bronchodilator, inhaled corticosteroid, long-acting β_2 agonist, theophyllines (which may aid mucociliary clearance), leukotriene receptor antagonist (very limited evidence in CF), and oral steroids.

Hemoptysis

Small-volume hemoptysis is common, especially in the setting of a pulmonary exacerbation and with advanced disease. Nearly always, hemoptysis will resolve with antibiotic treatment and standard CPT. **Massive hemoptysis** (>240 mL in a 24-hour period, or 100 mL/day for several days) is rare, and usually reflects bronchial artery bleeding.

The prevalence of hemoptysis increases with age and advancing lung disease, and is statistically associated with the presence of *S. aureus* infection. Patients should be observed in the hospital.

Coagulation studies typically demonstrate an increase in protime secondary to vitamin K deficiency, thus vitamin K should be administered and agents such as NSAIDs, which interfere with platelet function, should be discontinued.

Patients may require blood transfusion or intubation to maintain the airway. In refractory cases, bronchial artery embolization should be attempted, and if unsuccessful, surgical resection should be considered.

Nonpulmonary disease

Nutritional management

Maintaining good nutrition is directly related to the patient's survival. Nutrition is more problematic as respiratory disease progresses, because of raised basal metabolic rate, increased work of breathing, ongoing inflammation, and infection.

The CF team should include a dietitian experienced with the disease. High-calorie and high-protein diets are encouraged. Patients may need dietary supplements or, if necessary, supplemental overnight feeding via nasogastric tube or gastrostomy. Perform weight and body mass index (BMI) measurements annually, with a goal of BMI >20 (>90% ideal body weight [IBW]).

Pancreatic insufficiency

Exocrine pancreatic insufficiency is present in 85%–90% of CF patients. The decision to treat a patient with enzyme supplements usually depends on the presence of steatorrhea, associated with weight loss, poor weight gain, abdominal discomfort, and fat-soluble vitamin deficiency.

The diagnosis can be confirmed with a 72-hour fecal fat collection. Typically, adults CF patients with pancreatic insufficiency will have been on enzyme replacement therapy since childhood.

Pancreatic enzyme supplements

These are typically capsules that contain varying amounts of lipase, protease, and amylase. Many different brands and preparations are available, and patients often express a clear preference for a particular formulation. Enzyme supplements should be given with meals and snacks, with dosing calculated on the basis of the amount of fat ingested with each meal.

Constant re-education is often required to optimize enzyme supplementation. Most enzyme preparations require a relatively neutral gastric pH, and many pancreatic insufficient CF patients have inadequate pancreatic secretion of bicarbonate.

Patients with a poor response to appropriate doses of enzymes should be treated with drugs that reduced gastric acid production as a first step.

Vitamins

Fat-soluble vitamins are not absorbed well in CF patients with pancreatic insufficiency. These patients require replacement of vitamins A, D, E, and K. Levels of vitamin A, D, and E should be checked annually, and a prolonged prothrombin time serves as evidence of vitamin K deficiency.

Gastrointestinal disease

Distal intestinal obstructive syndrome (DIOS)

DIOS represents a common cause of abdominal pain in CF patients. Excessively viscid intestinal contents (due to the CFTR mutation in the bowels) lead to abnormal digestive fluid secretion and recurrent episodes of intestinal obstruction in a subset of CF patients.

DIOS can occur spontaneously or be precipitated by dehydration and use of agents that reduce bowel motility (such as narcotics). The obstruction typically originates in the cecum and involves both the large and small intestines to varying degrees.

Common signs and symptoms include bloating, periumbilical and/or right lower-quadrant abdominal pain, palpable cecal mass, and decreased stool output. Abdominal radiographs typically reveal a right colon distended with bubbly-appearing intestinal contents, with increased stool throughout the remainder of the colon, and variable degrees of small-bowel dilation and air–fluid levels.

The most important aspect of management is to recognize the condition and initiate treatment as early as possible. Standard medical treatment includes correction of systemic dehydration with a large-volume polyethylene glycol (PEG) electrolyte solution. If the patient is not vomiting, the PEG solution can be administered orally or per nasogastric tube (NGT).

If the severity of obstruction is too great, large-volume enemas should be performed under fluoroscopic guidance with radiocontrast dye. The primary concern is the potential for the obstruction to progress to a loss of bowel integrity. An elevated WBC suggests this possibility, as well as alternative diagnoses such as appendicitis or *C. difficile* colitis.

On rare occasions, if evidence supports ischemic bowel, laparotomy is required to resect a nonviable section of bowel and relieve the intraluminal obstruction by irrigation.

Some adults with CF have experienced recurrent episodes of DIOS, and aggressive treatment is warranted at the first evidence of blockage. When the condition is mild, patients are relatively asymptomatic and relate symptoms only in response to direct questioning. Given the morbidity associated with this condition, preventive therapy with PEG solution on a scheduled basis is worthwhile in select patients.

Pancreatitis

Pancreatitis can occur in the 10%–15% of patients who are pancreatic sufficient. It usually presents as severe recurrent attacks or rarely as chronic abdominal pain. The approach to diagnosis and treatment is the same as that for the general population. One important clinical point is that as pancreatic functions wane, patients may have episodes of acute pancreatitis without elevations in amylase and lipase.

Liver and biliary disease

Approximately 24% of adult CF patients have evidence of hepatomegaly or persistently abnormal LFTs. Reduced bile production and deranged bile acid composition can lead sequentially to cholestasis, focal biliary cirrhosis, and multilobar cirrhosis. Less common are hepatic steatosis and hepatic congestion from cor pulmonale.

Recommended screening includes physical exam for evidence of hepatosplenomegaly at each visit, and yearly liver function tests (LFTs), with repeat testing if values are >1.5 normal. Patients with elevated LFTs for >6 months or values 3–5 times the upper limit of normal should undergo a complete workup for liver disease.

Medical treatment is administration of ursodeoxycholic acid, with aggressive replacement of fat-soluble vitamins. Treatment of portal hypertension and liver failure is the same as in the general population, with consideration of liver transplantation, especially in patients with relatively mild lung disease.

Given the relatively high prevalence and lack of effective treatment for CF liver disease, all patients should receive complete immunization series for both hepatitis A and B, and attempts should be made to limit potentially hepatotoxic medications and excessive ethanol use.

Metabolic disease

CF-related diabetes (CFRD)

CFRD is clearly an age-related complication of CF, thus is diagnosed with increased frequency as the median age of survival with CF increases. Pancreatic damage by CF causes decreased insulin secretion. It presents insidiously and nonspecifically, with weight loss or unexpected decline in lung function, and not with ketoacidosis.

Screening should include at least one random glucose measurement yearly. A value <126 mg/dL is normal, while a value >126 mg/dL should be followed by a fasting blood glucose (FBG). Two or more random glucose measurements >200 mg/dL or FBG >126 mg/dL are diagnostic for CFRD. Confirmation can be obtained by an oral glucose tolerance test, with a 2-hour value of >200 mg/dL considered diagnostic.

Treatment of CFRD is with insulin to control hyperglycemia. Patients are encouraged to continue a high-calorie and high-protein diet, although excessive intake of concentrated carbohydrates should be avoided.

Osteoporosis

Low bone mineral density (BMD) is common in adults with CF. The pathogenesis of low BMD involves both decreased levels of osteoblasts and increased levels of osteoclasts. Contributing factors include malabsorption of vitamin D and calcium, low BMI, decreased physical activity, delayed puberty and low growth factor levels, steroid use, and diabetes.

Screening is performed by dual energy X-ray absorptiometry (DEXA) and should be repeated every 2–5 years.

Treatment centers around aggressive normalization of calcium and vitamin D levels, in combination with weight-bearing exercises. Bisphosphonates have been used to treat CF-related osteoporosis, once normal calcium and vitamin D levels are achieved. A number of trials are underway to determine optimal treatment strategies.

Other organ systems
Arthropathy and CF vasculitis
Acute or subacute arthritis occurs in around 5% of patients with CF. It often responds to NSAIDs. Sometimes arthritis is associated with skin lesions, such as purpura or erythema nodosum. Up to 40% of cases may be ANCA positive.

Sinusitis and nasal polyps
Sinusitis can be very severe in association with CF, and persistent postnasal drip can worsen symptoms of brochospasm and airway obstruction. Aggressive treatment of acute and/or chronic sinusitis is very important, although CF-specific guidelines have not been developed.

Nasal polyps occur commonly, and can worsen nasal obstruction. Referral to an otolaryngologist with experience in CF-related sinus disease can be helpful in difficult cases. Sinus surgery, while usually of short-term benefit, must be applied judiciously, as CF sinus disease is a persistent problem for the life of the patient.

Fertility
Women with CF have normal reproductive anatomy. Previous opinions that women with CF have decreased fertility are now in question, as pregnancies are commonplace at most CF centers. Likely, historical difficulties with pregnancy were related mainly to poor nutrition and general health status.

Men are nearly always infertile due to failure of normal development or blockage of the vas deferens. Approximately 1%–2% of men with very mild disease are fertile. Testicular histology is normal, hence one option is microsurgical epididymal aspiration for sperm retrieval, followed by intracytoplasmic sperm injection (ICSI) into an oocyte, performed at larger fertility clinics.

Genetic counseling and screening should be offered to patients with CF, and their partners should be screened for the CFTR mutation. Generally speaking, pregnancies in women with CF are considered high risk, with very high rates of gestational diabetes, malnutrition, and exacerbations of pulmonary disease. Nevertheless, pregnancies appear not to significantly accelerate disease in most women with CF. Of greater concern is the long-term impact of the added work of motherhood superimposed on the increasing demands of caring for their own health.

Psychosocial support

Depression and anxiety are very common in the adult CF population, and should be treated aggressively when present. Whenever possible, psychologists or psychiatrists experienced with the psychological issues associated with progressive illness should work in close coordination with the CF team.

Social worker involvement is essential, as CF patients typically face formidable obstacles relating to health insurance, employment, disability benefits, and poverty as a result of medical bills and inability to work. Pretransplant psychological assessment is required.

Care of the dying CF patient

When all those concerned acknowledge that there are no further treatment options, the focus of care should be palliative, with an emphasis on symptom relief. This can be done at home or in the hospital.

Future developments

A cure for CF (at least in children) is theoretically possible via gene therapy to partially restore CFTR function in the airways. Although very promising in experimental models, this treatment has proven to be extremely difficult in patients, primarily due to the lack of a suitable vector for delivery of the gene into the airway epithelia.

Despite the lack of a cure, the incremental advances in airway clearance, anti-inflammatory and antibiotic therapies, nutrition, and other supportive treatments have together achieved an impressive increase in survival for CF patients. A wide array of promising therapies are currently undergoing clinical testing. Current information on new drug development can be found at the CF Foundation Web site, at: http://www.cff.org/research/DrugDevelopmentPipeline.

CF pulmonary exacerbation: etiology

Cough and sputum production as a result of chronic inflammation and infection are typical features of CF lung disease, even during periods of stable heath. Pulmonary exacerbations are episodic increases in these symptoms, which correlate with increased burden of infection and much worse airway inflammation.

Pulmonary exacerbations are a central feature of CF and represent the greatest periods of morbidity and mortality, along with the greatest health-care expenditures. Despite intense airway infection, systemic symptoms are remarkably mild. Exacerbations typically have a subacute onset, over days to weeks.

Diagnosis

Signs and symptoms of pulmonary exacerbations are relatively nonspecific (see Box 29.1). Patients generally experience fatigue, and worsening of respiratory symptoms. In particular, nearly all adults will report increased cough, increased sputum production, and sputum that is darker in color.

Examination and CXR can be unchanged from baseline, but FEV_1 is nearly always decreased. No standardized diagnostic criteria have been validated, but a definition in widespread use was proposed by the CF Foundation Clinical Practice Guideline, which recommends that at least 3 of the 11 signs and symptoms be present when compared to the most recent baseline visit.

> **Box 29.1 Typical signs and symptoms of a pulmonary exacerbation**
>
> - Increased cough
> - Increased sputum production
> - Fever
> - Weight loss
> - Absenteeism from school or work
> - Increased respiratory rate
> - Change in chest examination
> - Decreased exercise tolerance
> - Decreased spirometry (FEV_1)
> - Decreased SaO_2
> - Change in chest radiograph

Adults with CF have typically experienced many exacerbations during childhood. The most important criteria are symptom profile and the patient's subjective assessment that they are having an exacerbation.

Organisms

CF airway infections change over time. As the CF patient gets older, more organisms are acquired, and the organisms will become more resistant to antibiotics. Cultures from sputum should be obtained routinely, to direct antibiotic management during exacerbations.

Pseudomonas aeruginosa

P. aeruginosa is clinically the most important pathogen in CF lung disease. Over 80% of adults with CF are chronically infected, and acquisition of the organism is associated with an accelerated decrease in lung function and a more severe clinical course. *P. aeruginosa* rapidly adapts to the CF airway, developing a mucoid phenotype and resisting irradiation by forming a biofilm. In addition, the organism is capable of developing resistance to all antibiotics over time.

Successful treatment of a pulmonary exacerbation can achieve a >99.9% reduction in the burden of *P. aeruginosa* in the airway, resulting in a dramatic reduction in inflammation and resolution of symptoms. However, once chronic infection has occurred, eradication of *P. aeruginosa* from the CF lung is not expected.

Staphylococcus aureus

S. aureus is typically acquired earlier in life then *P. aeruginosa*. Many adults will have both *S. aureus* and *P. aeruginosa*. Both methicillin-sensitive and methicillin-resistant strains are common, and some individuals will have both. Often treatment is directed primarily toward *P. aeruginosa*, but in some individuals, additional antibiotics need to be used to specifically treat the *S. aureus* infection during a pulmonary exacerbation.

Other organisms

- *Stenotrophomonas maltophilia* is a gram-negative bacterium, often with multiple antibiotic resistance. It is usually considered less clinically significant then *P. aeruginosa* or *S. aureus*, but in some individuals clearly represents an important pathogen that can cause or contribute to a pulmonary exacerbation.
- *Burkholderia cepacia complex* There are at least 10 different strains, of *Burkholderia cepacia*. Some are associated with a worse clinical outcome and some are not. These organisms are resistant to many antibiotics. *B. cepacia* has been demonstrated to be highly transmissible in various CF centers. Thus, particular care should be taken to practice good infection control techniques when caring for patients with *B. cepacia*. **Cepacia syndrome** is a rare, systemic manifestation of *B. cepacia* infection in the airway. It is characterized by severe worsening of pulmonary infection, in association with septic shock, which can be rapidly fatal. This syndrome is caused by one strain, genomovar III, or *Burkholderia cenocepacia*. CF patients infected with this strain have worse outcomes with lung transplantation, and some transplant centers will not transplant CF patients with this specific strain.
- *Haemophilus influenzae* is one of the first pathogens cultured from the airways of infants with CF. In adults, it is rarely seen, and its significance is not known.
- *Nontuberculosis mycobacteria.* infections appear to be an age-related complication of CF, and may be associated with poor response to treatment of a pulmonary exacerbation.

CF pulmonary exacerbation: antibiotics

Antibiotic courses in patients with CF are longer and require higher doses than those in non-CF patients. The choice of antibiotics is based primarily on clinical response. However, in vitro resistance patterns from recent sputum culture results help to guide therapy. If *Pseudomonas* has previously been isolated, treatment of *P. aeruginosa* will be the primary focus of current antibiotic selection.

It is usually appropriate to give patients the same regimen they had during their last exacerbation, provided there was good clinical response.

In practice, antibiotic selection should be guided by the last sputum culture result.

Pseudomonas aeruginosa

Oral antibiotics

For patients with *P. aeruginosa* who have relatively mild disease and are not infected with a highly resistant strain, exacerbations may respond to a 2-week course of an oral quinolone (such as ciprofloxacin). This is administered concurrently with increased frequency of airway clearance treatments.

However, over time, CF strains of *P. aeruginosa* will acquire antibiotic resistance to these agents, and clinical response will diminish, forcing the use of other antimicrobial drugs.

IV antibiotics

These should be used when oral and nebulized treatments have previously failed. An aminoglycoside plus a fourth-generation cephalosporin is preferred, as they frequently have a synergistic effect when used in combination. Treatment should be for 14 days. Once-daily aminoglycoside dosing is used (up to 10 mg/kg) to achieve a high peak level (correlating to bacterial killing) and a low trough (correlating to reduced toxicity).

Adequate hydration is important prior to use of aminoglycosides to prevent renal toxicity.

First isolates of P. aeruginosa can frequently be eradicated by aggressive treatment with inhaled tobramycin (TOBI) for 4 weeks (see also Box 29.2). Clinical trials are underway to assess the efficacy of ciprofloxacin combined with inhaled tobramycin in this setting. All efforts should be made to clear *P. aeruginosa* from the airway at the time of initial infection, since once established, the infection cannot be eradicated, and acquisition of *P. aeruginosa* is clearly linked to accelerated decline in lung function.

Burkholderia cepacia

B. cepacia is characteristically resistant to a number of antipseudomonal antibiotics. Conventional IV therapy may be effective when combinations of three classes are used, such as a third-generation cephalosporin in combination with an aminoglycoside and a quinolone.

Staphylococcus aureus

S. aureus can be a significant pathogen causing exacerbations. If methicillin-sensitive, agents such as a first-generation cephalosporin or an anti-staphylococcal penicillin are preferred. If MRSA, vancomycin dosed with trough values >10 mg/L remains the first-line treatment. Some patients can be treated with linezolid, with close monitoring of platelet counts.

Box 29.2 General guidelines for tobramycin administration during CF pulmonary exacerbations

- Check serum creatinine at the start of course
- IV hydration prior to the first dose
- Once-daily dosing of tobramycin (10 mg/kg)
- Drug levels checked before and 1 hour after the third dose, and adjusted if necessary (satisfactory levels: before: <1 mg/L, 1 hour after: >20 mg/L)
- Check serum creatinine twice weekly throughout course
- If serum creatinine increases, administer additional IV hydration and consider holding dose(s) until baseline creatinine is achieved
- Any reports of tinnitus, dizziness, or balance problems suggest early ototoxicity. The aminoglycoside should be stopped and ENT referral made for middle ear testing.

Management of an exacerbation

Initial workup
- Spirometry with FEV$_1$
- Oxygen saturation
- CXR—usually unchanged, but will occasionally demonstrate lobar collapse, pneumothorax, or focal pneumonia
- Repeat sputum cultures for bacteria and AFBs
- Consider blood cultures if patient is febrile or systemically ill
- Complete blood count, chemistry panel, BUN and creatinine, and liver function tests

Treatment
- The appropriate antibiotic regimen is the most essential component of treatment.
- To allow for 2 weeks of IV antibiotics, placement of a peripherally inserted catheter (PICC) line is preferred.
- Patients who receive frequent courses of IV antibiotics or have experienced difficulties during PICC placement frequently need an indwelling port-a-cath that can be accessed when required.
- Often patients begin treatment in the hospital to allow for PICC line placement and adjustment of tobramycin dosage, as well as aggressive airway clearance. However, many exacerbations can be treated at home, with administration of IV antibiotic by the patient or family members.
- Often patients will require supplemental oxygen or an increased amount of oxygen if already using oxygen at home.
- Most patients will demonstrate bronchoconstriction and benefit from aggressive bronchodilator therapy.
- Some patients appear to benefit from a 2-week "burst" of systemic steroids.
- Patients should receive aggressive airway clearance.
- During an exacerbation, nutrition and good control of CF-related diabetes should be emphasized.

Monitoring
- Check tobramycin drug levels before and after the third dose.
- Check serum creatinine at least twice weekly, and follow up on any abnormal laboratory values from admission.
- Most patients should report subjective improvement after 1 week of treatment. If clinical progress seems slower then expected, review microbiological sensitivities from admission sputum cultures and consider adding or changing antibiotics if new pathogens or resistance patterns are detected.

Follow-up
- Patients should be evaluated following 2 weeks of antibiotic treatment.
- With effective antibiotic treatment, FEV_1 levels should rise to the preinfection level.
- Patients who have not reached their baseline should be continued on IV antibiotics for an additional week.
- Patients who do not satisfactorily respond to 3 weeks of treatment should be recultured, with consideration of other diagnoses or unusual organisms. Other combinations of antipseudomonal antibiotics can be tried, as laboratory sensitivities often do not correlate with clinical response in the setting of advanced lung disease, and coinfection by multiple strains of *P. aeruginosa* and other CF pathogens is common.

Seeing the patient with CF in the clinic

Routine visit

- The CF Foundation recommends that patients be seen every 3 months at an accredited CF care center.
- Check spirometry, weight, and oxygen saturation
- Review medications and airway clearance techniques
- Sputum culture
- Address declines in FEV_1 or weight if present
- Address specific issues relating to sinus disease, nutrition, and diabetes, as well as psychological and socioeconomic issues
- Patients may be offered the chance to participate in clinical trials (if ongoing at the center) and to participate in the CF Foundation registry, which provides a comprehensive assessment of the demographics, clinical care, and outcomes of CF patients in the United States.

At the annual review

- The CF Foundation recommends a more comprehensive evaluation on an annual basis.
- Check spirometry, weight, and oxygen saturation
- Review medications and airway clearance techniques
- Sputum culture including culture for AFBs
- Radiology
  - CXR
  - DEXA bone scan
- Laboratory tests
  - CBC, electrolytes, BUN and creatinine
  - PT
  - LFTs
  - Random glucose
  - Consider oral glucose tolerance test
  - HbA_{1c} if established diabetes
  - *Aspergillus* species RAST and precipitins
  - Fat-soluble vitamin levels A, D, E, and K, if available
- Airway clearance review with respiratory therapist
- Nutrition review with dietitian
  - Full assessment and review of dietary intake and enzyme and vitamin use
- CF nurse review
- Social work review
  - Full assessment of issues relating to insurance, disability, or employment, and planning for the future. In addition, the social worker screens for unaddressed psychological issues.
- Physician review
- Research coordinator review
  - Assess patient's interest in participating in ongoing or upcoming clinical trials

Lung transplantation

Background and current status

Human lung transplantation was first attempted in 1963, but it was not until two decades later that extended survival was achieved. Further refinements in patient selection, surgical technique, and postoperative care have since led to the successful application of lung transplantation in the treatment of a wide variety of advanced disorders of the airways, lung parenchyma, and pulmonary vasculature.

By 2006, over 26,000 lung and heart–lung procedures had been performed worldwide; approximately half of these were carried out in the United States. U.S. centers performed 1400 lung transplants in 2005, a 40% increase compared to annual activity for the previous 5 years.

Indications and patient selection

Underlying conditions (frequency noted in parentheses)
- COPD, including α_1-antitrypsin deficiency (46%)
- Idiopathic pulmonary fibrosis (19%)
- Cystic fibrosis (CF) (16%)
- Primary pulmonary hypertension (4%)
- Sarcoidosis (3%)
- Non-CF bronchiectasis (3%)
- Lymphangioleiomyomatosis (1%)
- Eisenmenger's syndrome and congenital cardiac disease (1%)
- Miscellaneous: Langerhans cell histiocytosis, lung disease related to collagen vascular disease, bronchoalveolar cell carcinoma (because recurrence of tumor in the donor lung is common, this is a controversial indication)

Indications

Referral for transplant assessment should be considered for patients who, despite maximal medical therapy, have severe, disabling, and progressive lung disease that poses a significant risk of death within the next several years (see also Box 30.1). Although estimation of a poor short-term prognosis should be the major impetus for referral, quality of life is an important secondary consideration.

Suggested age limits for candidates are 55 years for heart–lung, 60 years for bilateral lung, and 65 years for single lung transplantation. Some centers focus more on "functional" rather than "chronological" age.

> **Box 30.1 General referral criteria for lung transplantation**
>
> - Severe, progressive lung disease despite maximal medical therapy
> - Limited survival (high likelihood of death within several years)
> - No significant extrapulmonary organ dysfunction
> - Functionally disabled (NYHA class III–IV) but still ambulatory
> - Demonstrated compliance and ability to adhere to a complex medical regimen

Contraindications

Absolute

- Untreatable advanced dysfunction of a major extrapulmonary organ system. Coronary artery disease not amenable to angioplasty or bypass grafting, surgically uncorrectable congenital cardiac anomalies, and severe left ventricular dysfunction are absolute contraindications to lung transplantation but heart–lung transplantation may be considered in selected cases.
- Recent history of malignancy, except for cutaneous squamous cell and basal cell carcinoma. A period of disease-free remission sufficient to deem likelihood of recurrence to be extremely low is recommended. Use of lung transplantation as definitive treatment for active bronchoalveolar carcinoma localized to the lungs is controversial.

- Incurable chronic extrapulmonary infections, including human immunodeficiency virus (HIV) and hepatitis B. Some centers will accept patients with active hepatitis C if there is no clinical or laboratory evidence for significant hepatic dysfunction and liver biopsy does not demonstrate cirrhosis.
- Severe psychiatric illness that compromises the ability to comply with medical therapy
- Absence of a consistent or reliable social-support network
- Active or recent (6 months) substance addiction, including cigarette smoking

Relative

- Age older than 65 years. Post-transplant survival is lower for older patients, leading to the recommendation for an age cutoff. However, some programs will perform a transplant in patients over age 65 who are otherwise acceptable candidates without significant comorbidities.
- Critical or unstable clinical condition
- Poor functional status (e.g., minimally ambulatory or nonambulatory)
- Severe obesity (BMI exceeding 30 kg/m^2) or malnutrition
- Severe osteoporosis leading to chronic pain and functional limitation
- Mechanical ventilation (excluding noninvasive ventilation). Mechanically ventilated patients who are otherwise suitable candidates and who have not experienced superimposed complications (e.g., profound debility, infection) may be considered.
- Conditions leading to technical difficulties in explanting the native lung, e.g., aspergilloma with extensive pleural thickening, prior lobectomy, pleurodesis
- Active collagen vascular disease with significant extrapulmonary manifestations that could compromise the outcome of transplantation. Of particular concern is the presence of severe esophageal dysmotility and/or severe gastroesophageal reflux in patients with scleroderma, which predispose to aspiration and may lead to accelerated graft loss.
- Preoperative colonization of the airways with virulent or highly resistant organisms in patients with CF or non-CF bronchiectasis. Most centers exclude CF patients colonized with *Burkholderia cepacia* (especially genomovar III) because of a high risk of lethal post-transplant infections. In contrast, there are no definitive data to suggest that patients harboring pan-resistant *Pseudomonas aeruginosa* have inferior outcomes. Similarly, colonization with *Aspergillus* does not appear to compromise outcomes, and attempts to eradicate the organism preoperatively are not necessary.

Timing of referral and listing

The inherent risks of transplantation, including a 50% mortality rate by 5 years, dictate that this option be reserved for patients with advanced, life-threatening disease. Patients who have progressed to a stage of profound debility, however, are poor candidates at high risk for perioperative morbidity and mortality and for inferior functional recovery. Thus, patients should be listed during the "transplant window" when they are sufficiently ill to warrant the risks of transplantation but not so ill as to compromise the likelihood of a successful outcome.

In contrast to actual listing, which should occur when the patient is in imminent need of transplantation, early referral to a transplant center for initial evaluation is encouraged. This permits the transplant team to address factors that could compromise the suitability of the patient for future transplantation, such as obesity or malnutrition, debility, ongoing smoking, gastroesophageal reflux disease, or excessive steroid use. It also allows the team to educate the patient on the risks and benefits of transplantation and the commitment that the patient must make to the strict post-transplant medical regimen, rehabilitation, and preventive care.

Disease-specific guidelines for timely referral and listing of patients, based on available, albeit imprecise, prognostic indices, have been published and are listed below.

COPD
Referral
- BODE index >5

Transplantation
- BODE index of 7–10 *or* at least one of the following:
- History of hospitalization for exacerbation associated with acute hypercapnia (PCO_2 >50 mmHg)
- Pulmonary hypertension or cor pulmonale, despite oxygen therapy
- FEV_1 <20% predicted and either DLCO <20% or homogenous distribution of emphysema

Cystic fibrosis
Referral
- FEV_1 <30% predicted or a rapid decline in FEV_1 (particularly for females and those under age 18)
- Exacerbation of pulmonary disease requiring ICU admission
- Increasing frequency of exacerbations requiring antibiotic therapy
- Refractory and/or recurrent pneumothoraces
- Recurrent hemoptysis not controlled by embolization

Transplantation
- Oxygen-dependent respiratory failure
- Hypercapnia
- Pulmonary hypertension

Idiopathic pulmonary fibrosis and nonspecific interstitial pneumonia (NSIP)

Referral
- Histological or radiographic evidence of usual interstitial pneumonia irrespective of vital capacity
- Histological evidence of fibrotic NSIP

Transplantation
- Histological or radiographic evidence of UIP *and* any of the following:
  - DLCO <39% predicted
  - A 10% or greater decline in forced vital capacity (FVC) during 6 months of follow-up
  - Decrease in pulse oximetry below 88% during a 6-minute walk test
  - Honeycombing on HRCT (fibrosis score >2)
- Histological evidence of NSIP *and* any of the following:
  - DLCO <35% predicted
  - A 10% or greater decrement in FVC or 15% decrease in DLCO during 6 months of follow-up

Pulmonary arterial hypertension

Referral
- New York Heart Association (NYHA) class III or IV, irrespective of ongoing treatment
- Rapidly progressive disease

Transplantation
- Persistent NYHA class III or IV on maximal medical therapy
- Low (<350 meter) or declining 6-minute walk test
- Failing therapy with intravenous epoprostenol or equivalent
- Cardiac index <2 L/min/m^2
- Right atrial pressure >15 mmHg

Sarcoidosis

Referral
- NYHA class III or IV

Transplantation
Impairment in exercise tolerance (NYHA class III or IV) and any of the following:
- Hypoxemia at rest
- Pulmonary hypertension
- Right atrial pressure >15 mmHg

Surgical approaches

Single lung transplantation

- The most technically straightforward and expeditious procedure
- Maximizes use of limited donor pool, allowing two transplants to be performed from a single donor
- Remains the preferred procedure for patients with pulmonary fibrosis; also commonly used for older patients with COPD
- May occasionally result in progressive hyperinflation of the native lung and resultant crowding of the allograft when performed in patients with emphysema

Bilateral sequential lung transplantation

- Involves performance of sequential right and left single-lung procedures during a single operative session
- Cardiopulmonary bypass can often be avoided by ventilating the contralateral lung during implantation of each allograft
- The exclusive procedure for patients with CF and non-CF bronchiectasis, and the predominant procedure for patients with severe pulmonary hypertension (idiopathic and secondary forms)
- Increasingly used for patients with COPD, due to superior survival and functional outcomes compared to those with single lung transplantation in this patient population

Heart–lung transplantation

- Indicated principally for patients with Eisenmenger's syndrome and surgically uncorrectable cardiac anomalies. It is occasionally used for lung transplant candidates with concurrent severe left ventricular dysfunction or severe, uncorrectable coronary artery disease.
- Cor pulmonale is not in itself an indication, as right ventricular dysfunction resolves rapidly following lung transplantation alone.
- Only 33 heart–lung transplants were performed in the United States in 2005, compared to 1407 lung transplants.

Living donor bilobar transplantation

- Bilateral grafting of lower lobes from two living adult donors to replace lungs of child or small adult. CF patients are particularly well suited for this procedure because of their generally small stature.
- Typically reserved for patients with rapidly deteriorating status who are deemed unlikely to survive the wait for a cadaveric donor
- Survival and functional outcomes are commensurate with those of cadaveric transplantation.
- Appears to be safe for the donor; no deaths and only a 3% incidence of complications requiring surgical re-exploration among 273 donors in the largest reported series. Lobar donors experience an average decrement in vital capacity of 15%.
- Rarely performed. The new U.S. allocation system may further obviate the need for this procedure.

Organ allocation and donor–recipient matching

Until 2005, lung allocation in the United States was based on time accrued on the waiting list. In May 2005, a new system was put into place that prioritizes patients on the basis of "net transplant benefit" (the difference between predicted 1-year survival with and without transplantation). In other words, patients predicted to derive the greatest survival advantage from transplantation are afforded the highest priority.

Underlying diagnosis is a major determinant of the allocation score. The allocation system prioritizes patients with IPF and assigns relatively low scores to patients with COPD (reflecting the significant differences in natural history of these diseases).

Patients placed on mechanical ventilation are also given high lung allocation scores, providing a mechanism for more expeditious transplantation of patients with respiratory failure (assuming that they are otherwise suitable candidates)

Donor–recipient matching is based on ABO blood group compatibility, and size. Some centers also attempt to match CMV-negative candidates with CMV-negative donors.

HLA matching is not routinely performed. However, candidates identified through standard screening as having preformed circulating antibodies to foreign HLA antigens—arising from prior pregnancy, blood transfusions, or transplantation—require prospective donor–recipient cross-matching to ensure compatibility.

Routine post-transplant care

The usual stay in the hospital following transplantation is 2 weeks. Patients are typically required to attend an outpatient pulmonary rehabilitation program after discharge. Most centers also require patients to return frequently for office visits, blood work, and chest radiographs for the first several months.

Patients are instructed to monitor their lung function by handheld micropirometry on a daily basis and to contact the transplant center if they experience a sustained decline in spirometric parameters exceeding 10%.

Most transplant centers perform surveillance bronchoscopies with transbronchial lung biopsies several times throughout the first year to monitor for subclinical acute rejection and infection.

Patients are maintained on an immunosuppressive regimen consisting of a calcineurin inhibitor (cyclosporine or tacrolimus), an antiproliferative agent (azathioprine or mycophenolate mofetil), and prednisone. The use of calcineurin inhibitors requires frequent monitoring of blood levels and knowledge of interactions with other commonly used drugs (see Box 30.2). Some centers use rapamycin (sirolimus) in lieu of a calcineurin inhibitor or antiproliferative agent.

> **Box 30.2 Common interactions with the calcineurin inhibitors**
>
> *Agents that increase CI blood levels*
> - Calcium channel blockers: diltiazem, verapamil, nicardipine
> - Azole antifungal agents
> - Macrolides (except azithromycin)
> - Amiodarone
> - Grapefruit juice
>
> *Drugs that decrease CI blood levels*
> - Anticonvulsants: phenytoin, phenobarbital, carbamazepine
> - Rifampin, rifabutin
> - St. Johns Wort

Outcomes

Survival

According to the 2007 United Network for Organ Sharing (UNOS) annual report of U.S transplants, survival rates are 84% at 1 year, 68% at 3 years, and 53% at 5 years.

Infection and primary graft dysfunction are the major causes of death within the first year. Infection and bronchiolitis obliterans syndrome are the major causes of late deaths.

Risk factors for early mortality include an underlying diagnosis of idiopathic pulmonary arterial hypertension, IPF, or sarcoidosis; preoperative mechanical ventilation; and advanced recipient age (>60).

Among COPD patients under the age of 60, bilateral lung transplantation is associated with better survival than single lung transplantation. In contrast, no survival advantage is associated with the bilateral procedure in patients with pulmonary fibrosis.

Functional outcomes

Lung function usually normalizes after bilateral transplant and markedly improves following single lung transplant. In COPD, FEV_1 increases to 50%–60% of predicted value after single lung transplantation. Similarly, single lung transplantation for pulmonary fibrosis results in marked but incomplete improvement in lung volumes, with persistence of a mild restrictive pattern.

Arterial oxygenation rapidly normalizes. The vast majority of patients are weaned off of supplemental oxygen by hospital discharge.

Over 80% of recipients describe no functional limitations, with usual activities by 1 year following transplantation.

Peak exercise performance, as assessed by cardiopulmonary exercise testing, remains reduced, with maximum oxygen consumption in the range of 40%–60% predicted for both single and bilateral transplant recipients. Cardiac, ventilatory, and gas exchange parameters typically remain normal with exercise. The limitation in exercise performance appears to be due to skeletal muscle dysfunction caused by deconditioning, and the effects of calcineurin inhibitors on mitochondrial function.

Hemodynamics

Both single and bilateral lung transplantations lead to rapid normalization of pulmonary artery pressures in patients with preexistent pulmonary hypertension.

Right ventricular performance also normalizes, and right ventricular hypertrophy regresses. A threshold of right ventricular dysfunction, below which recovery will not occur, has not been defined.

Complications

Primary graft dysfunction (PGD)

PGD is characterized by pulmonary infiltrates and hypoxemia appearing within 72 hours of transplantation. Clinical severity ranges from very mild and transient edema to full-blown ARDS (i.e., grade 3 PGD, defined by a PaO_2/FiO_2 <200).

Other causes of early graft dysfunction need to be excluded, including aspiration, volume overload, pneumonia, hyperacute rejection, atelectasis, and pulmonary venous outflow obstruction. The underlying mechanism is presumed to be ischemia-reperfusion injury, but surgical trauma and lymphatic disruption may be contributing factors.

The incidence of severe (grade 3) PGD is approximately 10%.

Treatment is supportive (mechanical ventilation).

PGD has a high mortality rate (40% mortality at 30 days), and is the leading cause of perioperative deaths.

Airway complications

Anastomotic narrowing, due to granulation tissue, fibrotic stricture, or bronchomalacia, is the most common airway complication, with a reported frequency of 12%–25%. It typically occurs within several weeks following transplantation.

Presence of narrowing is suggested by localized wheeze, recurrent pneumonia, or suboptimal lung function. It is usually correctable with bronchoscopic interventions, such as balloon bronchoplasty, debridement, brachytherapy, and stenting, but may be a recurrent problem.

Major dehiscence of bronchial anastomosis is highly lethal but now rare. It can occasionally be treated successfully with placement of a bare metal stent.

Partial dehiscence is managed conservatively with a chest tube to evacuate pneumothorax. Reduce the steroid dose to promote healing.

Common infections

Bacterial

This is the most common cause of lower respiratory tract infections. Gram-negative organisms, particularly *Pseudomonas aeruginosa*, predominate.

Bacterial infection is common in first post-transplant month. It is also common as a late complication among recipients with bronchiolitis obliterans syndrome.

With the exception of patients colonized preoperatively with *Burkholderia cepacia*, recipients with CF are not at greater risk than other patients for bacterial lower respiratory tract infections.

CMV

CMV is the most common viral pathogen encountered post-transplant.

In the absence of prophylaxis, CMV-seronegative recipients who receive a lung from seropositive donors are at high risk for primary infections, which can be severe. Seropositive recipients are at risk for reactivation of latent, remotely acquired infection.

CMV infection is typically seen in the first 3 months in non-prophylaxed patients. Use of prophylactic antiviral therapy often delays the onset of infection until after therapy is completed. Infection may manifest as asymptomatic viremia, lead to a mononucleosis-like syndrome of fever and malaise, or cause organ-invasive disease (e.g., pneumonitis, gastritis).

Treatment of symptomatic disease consists of a 3-week course of intravenous ganciclovir.

Prophylactic administration of ganciclovir or valganciclovir is effective in decreasing frequency, delaying onset, and mitigating severity of CMV infections. Prophylaxis is administered to all CMV-negative recipients of CMV-positive organs. Most programs also administer prophylaxis to CMV-positive recipients.

Aspergillus

Aspergillus frequently colonizes the airways after lung transplant, but clinically apparent infection develops in only a small number of patients. *Aspergillus* infections of the airways occur early after transplantation, with an incidence of approximately 5%.

It is typically localized to the devitalized cartilage of the fresh bronchial anastomosis but may also cause more diffuse ulcerative bronchitis with pseudomembranes. It usually responds to treatment with oral azoles or inhaled amphotericin but may rarely lead to life-threatening hemoptysis due to erosion into the adjacent pulmonary artery. Patients with anastomotic infections are at increased risk for anastomotic strictures after healing of the infection.

Invasive aspergillosis occurs in approximately 5% of recipients, typically presenting as a single infiltrate or multiple nodular infiltrates, often with a rim of ground glass ("halo sign") or cavitation.

The treatment of choice is voriconazole. The dose of calcineurin inhibitor needs to be preemptively decreased and CI levels followed closely due to significant interactions with this agent. Amphotericin and caspofungin are alternative agents. Mortality rates of up to 60% have been reported despite treatment. The highest mortality is associated with disseminated infection.

Post-transplant lymphoproliferative disorder (PTLD)

The spectrum of abnormal B-cell-proliferative responses ranges from benign polyclonal hyperplasia to frank B-cell lymphomas. B-cell proliferation is driven by the Epstein–Barr virus (EBV).

Risk of PTLD is greatest in EBV-naïve recipients who develop primary infection from an EBV-positive donor. Incidence is greatest within the first post-transplant year, but can occur at any time throughout the post-transplant period.

Typically PTLD presents as one or multiple lung nodules, often accompanied by mediastinal adenopathy. The GI tract is another common site of involvement.

Rituximab, an anti-CD20 monoclonal antibody, has emerged as the treatment of choice. As an adjunct to treatment, the doses of immunosuppressive agents are reduced to permit partial restoration of native immunity to EBV.

Other malignancies

Bronchogenic carcinoma develops in 2%–4% of lung transplant recipients. Typically it arises in the native lung following single lung transplantation for COPD or IPF. Prior smoking is likely a more important risk factor than immunosuppression.

Squamous cell and basal cell carcinomas of the skin are the most common malignancies encountered following lung transplantation.

Drug toxicities

In addition to infectious complications related to global immunosuppression, the drugs used to prevent rejection have a number of potential toxicities that can cause significant morbidity.

Calcineurin inhibitors (tacrolimus, cyclosporine)
- Nephrotoxicity
- Metabolic: hyperglycemia, hyperkalemia, hypomagnesemia
- Neurological: tremor, headaches, seizures, posterior leukoencephalopathy
- Hypertension

Azathioprine
- Leukopenia, anemia, thrombocytopenia
- Hepatotoxicity
- Pancreatitis
- Nausea

Mycophenolate mofetil
- Leukopenia, anemia, thrombocytopenia
- Diarrhea

Rapamycin (sirolimus)
- Thrombocytopenia, anemia
- Hyperlipidemia
- Edema
- Pneumonitis

Prednisone
- Osteoporosis
- Hyperglycemia
- Cataracts
- Hypertension
- Weight gain
- Myopathy
- Mood lability, insomnia

Acute rejection

Approximately 50%–75% of recipients experience at least one episode of acute rejection within the first year. Beyond this time, risk of acute rejection diminishes to a low level.

Patients may be asymptomatic, or have symptoms of malaise, fever, dyspnea, cough, and hypoxemia.

CXR may be normal or show nonspecific infiltrates and/or pleural effusions. HRCT commonly demonstrates ground-glass opacities.

Acute rejection is often accompanied by fall in FEV_1 and/or FVC by >10%. Ideally, confirm the diagnosis histologically by transbronchial biopsy. The hallmark is presence of perivascular lymphocytic infiltrates, which may spill over into the adjacent interstitium.

Treatment is with a 3-day pulse of IV methylprednisolone (500–1000 mg/daily). The majority of patients respond quickly.

Chronic rejection

This is uncommon in the first 6 months after transplantation, but prevalence subsequently increases steadily, affecting approximately 50% of patients by 5 years. The major risk factor is a history of frequent or severe episodes of acute rejection. Nonimmune factors may also play a role, including prior primary graft dysfunction, viral respiratory tract infections, and aspiration.

Chronic rejection manifests histologically as bronchiolitis obliterans, a fibroproliferative process characterized by submucosal fibrosis and obliteration of the small airways. This leads to progressive and largely irreversible airflow obstruction. Onset is typically insidious with dyspnea, cough, and recurrent bouts of tracheobronchitis.

CXR is usually unrevealing. HRCT often shows evidence of air trapping and bronchiectasis. It is difficult to establish a histological diagnosis by transbronchial biopsy. Because of this, a surrogate diagnostic entity of *bronchiolitis obliterans syndrome* (BOS) is employed, based on demonstration of a decline in FEV_1 and exclusion of other causes.

Treatment has centered on augmentation of immunosuppression, but this appears to merely slow the rate of decline in lung function and increases the risk of opportunistic infections. Several small case series have suggested that azithromycin may be effective in some patients, presumably because of its anti-inflammatory rather than antimicrobial effects.

Prognosis is poor with a mortality rate of 40% within 2 years of diagnosis. Patients with early-onset BOS (<3 years after transplant) generally experience more rapid decline in lung function and higher mortality.

Retransplantation is the only definitive treatment for carefully selected candidates.

Recurrence of primary disease

Recurrence is documented in several diseases: sarcoidosis, lymphangioleiomyomatosis, giant cell interstitial pneumonitis, Langerhans cell histiocytosis, and bronchoalveolar cell carcinoma. Recurrence has also been described in a patient with α_1-antitrypsin deficiency who resumed smoking.

Further reading

Arcasoy SM, Kotloff RM (1999). Lung transplantation. *N Engl J Med* **340**: 1081–1091.

Glanville AR, Estenne M (2003). Indications, patient selection and timing of referral for lung transplantation. *Eur Respir J* **22**: 845–852.

Kotloff RM, Ahya VN (2004). Medical complications of lung transplantation. *Eur Respir J* **23**: 334–342.

Orens JB, Estenne M, et al. (2006). International guidelines for the selection of lung transplant candidates: 2006 update—a consensus report from the Pulmonary Scientific Council of the International Society for Heart and Lung Transplantation. *J Heart Lung Transplant* **25**:745–755.

Trulock EP (1997). Lung transplantation. *Am J Respir Crit Care Med* **155**: 789–818.

Pulmonary hypertension

Classification

Definition

Pulmonary hypertension is defined as a mean pulmonary artery pressure (PAP) >25 mmHg. See the WHO (2003) classification of pulmonary hypertension in Box 31.1

Box 31.1 WHO classification of pulmonary hypertension

1 Pulmonary arterial hypertension
- Idiopathic pulmonary arterial hypertension (IPAH, previously known as primary pulmonary hypertension)
- Familial pulmonary arterial hypertension (FPAH)
- Related to:
  - Collagen vascular disease
  - Congenital systemic to pulmonary shunts
  - Portal hypertension
  - HIV infection
  - Drugs and toxins: anorectic agents (fenfluramine, dexfenfluramine), rape seed oil, others
  - Very likely: amphetamine, L-tryptophan
  - Possible: meta-amphetamines, cocaine, chemotherapy agents
  - Other conditions (glycogen storage diseases, hemoglobinopathies, myeloproliferative disorders, hereditary hemorrhagic telangiectasia, splenectomy)
- Associated with significant venous or capillary involvement
  - Pulmonary veno-occlusive disease
  - Pulmonary capillary hemangiomatosis

2 Pulmonary venous hypertension
- Left-sided atrial or ventricular heart disease
- Left-sided valvular heart disease

3 Pulmonary hypertension associated with hypoxemia
- Chronic obstructive pulmonary disease
- Interstitial lung disease
- Sleep-disordered breathing
- Alveolar hypoventilation disorders
- Chronic high-altitude exposure

4 Pulmonary hypertension due to chronic thrombotic and/or embolic disease
- Thromboembolic obstruction of proximal pulmonary arteries
- Obstruction of distal pulmonary arteries
  - Pulmonary embolism (thrombus, tumor, ova, parasites, foreign material)
  - In situ thrombosis
  - Sickle cell disease

5 Pulmonary hypertension associated with miscellaneous disorders
- Inflammatory
  - Langerhans cell histiocytosis
  - Sarcoidosis
  - Other
- Extrinsic compression of the central pulmonary veins
  - Fibrosing mediastinitis
  - Lymphadenopathy or tumors

Idiopathic pulmonary arterial hypertension (IPAH)

Definition

Idiopathic pulmonary arterial hypertension (IPAH), formerly known as primary pulmonary hypertension (PPH), is a rare disease of uncertain etiology. The mean pulmonary artery pressure is >25 mmHg with a pulmonary capillary or left atrial pressure <15 mmHg. By definition there is no demonstrable cause. The presence of resting pulmonary hypertension is significant, as more than 70% of the vascular bed must be lost for the pulmonary arterial pressure to rise.

Epidemiology

The incidence of IPAH in Europe and the United States is 1–2 cases per million population per year. Although rare, it is important to diagnose, as it affects a relatively young age group and has an extremely poor outcome without treatment.

Pathophysiology

Vasoconstriction and thickening of peripheral "resistance" blood vessels, perhaps in association with in situ thrombosis, lead to a rise in pulmonary vascular resistance. This leads to further structural vessel changes, due to proliferation of vascular smooth muscle cells.

The mechanism for this is poorly understood, but the identification of the gene for familial PAH (which codes for BMPR2—bone morphogenetic protein receptor type II, a receptor in the transforming growth factor β (TGF-β) family) may provide important clues. It is hypothesized that defective signaling via this pathway may result in abnormal endothelial proliferation and cell growth in response to various insults, with an inability to terminate the proliferative response to injury.

Etiology

Sporadic IPAH

A number of risk factors have been identified for sporadic IPAH, and BMPR2 mutations may be present in up to 25% of cases. The identified risk factors for IPAH have in common an ability to damage the pulmonary endothelium, which may provoke an excessive proliferative response. In a proportion of patients, no risk factors are found.

Familial PAH

A familial predisposition is seen in 6%–10% of cases, where the disease is transmitted in an autosomal dominant fashion. Incomplete penetrance and genetic anticipation may exist, with presentation at a younger age in successive generations. The responsible gene has been localized to chromosome 2 (locus 2q 31–32). Abnormal cardiovascular responses to exercise have been demonstrated in asymptomatic carriers of BMPR2.

Prognosis

Prognosis is variable, depending on hemodynamic compromise and response to vasodilator therapy, with cardiac index and right atrial pressure being linked to prognosis. Untreated, the median survival from diagnosis in patients with IPAH is approximately 3 years.

Patients in New York Heart Association (NYHA) classes III and IV have a poorer prognosis than those in classes I and II. All patients are at risk of progressive right heart failure and sudden death.

IPAH: clinical features

The symptoms of IPAH are nonspecific, leading to a delay in diagnosis. The mean age at diagnosis is 36.

Presenting features

- Exertional breathlessness, due to the inability to increase cardiac output with exercise
- Chest pain (right heart angina)
- Syncope, due to a fall in blood pressure on exercise
- Palpitations
- Edema, or other signs of right-sided fluid overload.

Examination

Signs consistent with right heart fluid overload and right ventricular hypertrophy (RVH), including the following:

- Raised jugular venous pressure (JVP), with giant V waves
- Right ventricular heave and tapping apex beat
- Wide splitting of S2 with loud P2
- Murmur of tricuspid regurgitation
- Hepatomegaly
- Ascites
- Peripheral edema
- Hypoxia and exercise desaturation

Investigations

These are aimed at making a diagnosis of IPAH by excluding possible underlying causes for the pulmonary hypertension. The CXR and ECG are often abnormal.

- *CXR* may show enlarged pulmonary arteries and an enlarged cardiac silhouette, with pruning of peripheral vessels.
- *ECG* may indicate right-axis deviation and RVH
- *Arterial blood gas* may show hypoxia and hypocapnia, with a fall in oxygen saturation on exercise
- *Pulmonary function tests* The lung volumes may be normal, or show a mild restrictive or obstructive defect with a reduced TLCO.
- *HRCT chest* to exclude underlying lung disease
- *Ventilation-perfusion (V/Q) scanning/CTPA* to exclude chronic thromboembolic disease as a cause
- *Echocardiography* often shows right heart enlargement with paradoxical interventricular septum movement, and tricuspid regurgitation. Pericardial effusions may be present. The pulmonary artery pressure can be estimated from the tricuspid regurgitation jet, using Doppler techniques.
- *Right heart catheterization* to confirm the exact pulmonary artery pressure and cardiac output (with a Swan–Ganz catheter, by thermo-dilution), and to exclude an underlying shunt lesion. This is usually performed with vasodilator testing in a specialist center.
- *Selective pulmonary angiography* if the VQ scan or CTPA is inconclusive
- *Blood tests* Routine tests include autoantibodies (anti-centromere antibody, anti SCL-70, and RNP if connective tissue disease is suspected as a cause), HIV, TSH, thrombophilia screen, and serum ACE.

IPAH: general management

The diagnosis of IPAH is made when all other causes have been excluded. The management in this section applies to IPAH.

General management

Anticoagulation

All patients with pulmonary hypertension are at risk of venous thromboembolism and intrapulmonary thrombus because of sluggish pulmonary blood flow, dilated heart chambers, venous stasis, and an often sedentary lifestyle. Anticoagulation with warfarin should be considered in patients with IPAH in the absence of contraindications. Pulmonary embolism can have catastrophic effects in a patient who is already severely compromised.

Microscopic in situ thrombosis may also contribute to disease pathogenesis in IPAH. Two studies have suggested increased survival with warfarin in IPAH, which may reflect reversal of an underlying prothrombotic state, as well as the prevention of in situ thrombus formation.

There are no published data on the use of warfarin in associated (formerly known as secondary) pulmonary arterial hypertension (APAH).

Long-term oxygen

Hypoxemia is due to a combination of reduced cardiac output, ventilation/perfusion mismatching, and right–left shunting through a patent foramen ovale.

Diuretics and digoxin

Diuretics may be useful for the treatment of edema. Digoxin has been shown to improve cardiac output acutely in IPAH, though its longer-term effects are not known.

Immunization

Annual influenza and pneumococcal vaccination is recommended.

Contraception

Pregnancy is poorly tolerated in IPAH. Oral contraceptives may increase the risk of venous thromboembolism.

IPAH: vasodilator therapy

Impaired production of the vasodilators nitric oxide (NO) and prostacyclin, and overproduction of the vasoconstrictor endothelin by the pulmonary endothelium may contribute to the pathogenesis of IPAH. Acute **vasodilator responsiveness** is measured at right heart catheterization with incremental doses of a short-acting vasodilator such as inhaled NO, epoprostenol, or adenosine. Patients are defined as responders or nonresponders.

An acute "responder" has a significant reduction in mean pulmonary artery pressure (mPAP), with an unchanged or increased cardiac output and minimally changed systemic blood pressure. Perhaps only about 10% of patients are true responders.

Calcium channel blockers

Nifedipine, diltiazem, or amlodipine can be tried in patients with a positive acute vasodilator response (and normal right heart function). In appropriately selected patients, they can improve long-term survival. However, calcium channel blockers are unlikely to be beneficial (and may be harmful) in acute vasodilator challenge nonresponders.

Side effects include hypotension and edema, which may limit use.

Amlodipine has more selective vasodilating properties, and at doses of 2.5–5 mg daily may be useful in those intolerant of the other agents, or if right ventricular function is impaired.

Calcium antagonists should be titrated with careful monitoring.

Verapamil is not used, because of its negative inotropic effects.

Prostaglandin analogues

Prostaglandins are potent vasodilators. They inhibit platelet aggregation and have antiproliferative and cytoprotective properties.

Side effects include jaw pain, diarrhea, and arthralgias. Patients receiving prostanoid therapy intravenously may experience catheter-related complications including infection and thrombosis. Pump failure may also occur.

Prostaglandin therapy is expensive.

Epoprostenol (Flolan)

This potent vasodilator acts on receptors related to cAMP. It is a prostacyclin analogue (PGI_2). It probably has its effects as a pulmonary vasodilator and through vascular remodeling and platelet adhesion. It has been shown to improve exercise capacity and hemodynamics.

Long-term treatment improves survival in IPAH. It is inactive within the circulation after 5 minutes, and thus needs to be given by continuous intravenous infusion via a portable pump and central venous catheter.

Treprostinil is a prostacyclin analogue that can be given subcutaneously or intravenously.

Iloprost is a prostacyclin analogue approved for inhalational delivery in the United States.

Prostacyclin analogues have been shown in placebo-controlled trials to improve 6-minute walk distance and hemodynamics.

Intravenous prostaglandin (epoprostenol or treprostinil) therapy requires dose titration over time.

Endothelin receptor antagonists

Endothelin plasma levels are raised in patients with various forms of pulmonary hypertension.

Bosentan

Bosentan is an oral endothelin (ET) receptor A and B antagonist that is administered twice daily and improves 6-minute walk, increases cardiac output, and decreases pulmonary artery pressure and pulmonary vascular resistance compared to placebo.

Side effects include liver enzyme abnormalities (monthly liver function tests are required), fluid retention and edema, anemia, teratogenicity, and decreased efficacy of hormonal methods of birth control.

Ambrisentan

Ambrisentan is an oral ET receptor antagonist that is relatively selective for the ETA receptor, and improves 6-minute walk distance and hemodynamics. Ambrisentan may have less potential for hepatoxicity, but liver function tests still need to be monitored monthly. Other potential side effects include fluid retention, edema, and nasal congestion.

Nitric oxide and L-arginine

Endothelial production of NO is reduced in IPAH. A favorable acute pulmonary vascular response to inhaled NO predicts response to oral calcium antagonists.

Phosphodiesterase inhibitors

These prolong the vasodilatory effects of NO, and have historically been used for erectile dysfunction. An international, multicenter, randomized, and placebo-controlled trial of oral sildenafil in patients with PAH showed improvements in 6-minute walk distance and hemodynamics. Potential side effects include flushing, headache, dyspepsia, epistaxis, musculoskeletal aches and pains, and visual changes.

IPAH: surgical treatments, end-of-life care, and future developments

Surgical treatments

Atrial septostomy

Creation of a right–left shunt by balloon atrial septostomy aims to increase systemic blood flow, by bypassing the pulmonary circulation, particularly in patients with syncope or severe right heart failure. It is a palliative procedure and can be used for symptom control prior to transplantation, with the defect being closed at the time of transplant.

Arterial desaturation occurs following the procedure, but is normally offset by the increased cardiac output seen

Transplantation

Lung transplantation may improve survival and quality of life in patients with severe pulmonary hypertension refractory to advanced medical therapy. In those with preserved left ventricular function, a lung transplant is the procedure of choice. Return of normal right ventricular function often occurs after transplantation.

As for all diseases needing transplantation, timing of referral and operation is crucial, as organ availability is limited.

End-of-life care

Palliative care may be warranted to improve symptoms such as fatigue, breathlessness, abdominal bloating, nausea, and pain.

Future developments

Combination therapies are likely to be used more commonly in the future. A number of agents are currently being investigated, including vasoactive intestinal peptide (VIP), and drugs with antiproliferative effects, such as imatinib.

Associated pulmonary hypertension (APH): causes

The majority of patients with pulmonary hypertension seen by a pulmonary specialist will have associated pulmonary hypertension (APH), formerly known as secondary pulmonary hypertension (SPH), due to chronic hypoxic lung disease, such as COPD. In this case, the pulmonary hypertension is often an incidental finding in a patient with other chronic respiratory disease.

Chronic hypoxia

Chronic hypoxia causes pulmonary vasoconstriction due to changes in the pulmonary endothelium, including down-regulation of endothelial nitric oxide synthetase. COPD with pulmonary hypertension has a much poorer prognosis than COPD without pulmonary hypertension.

Chronic thromboembolic pulmonary hypertension

This is a potential cause of pulmonary hyptertension, due to incomplete clot resolution following treatment for an acute pulmonary embolic event. The pathogenesis is uncertain, with no consistent defect in fibrinolytic activity demonstrated. Antiphospholipid antibodies are present in 10%–20% of patients. The diagnosis is not usually made until advanced pulmonary hypertension is present.

Collagen vascular disease

Pulmonary hypertension develops in up to one-third of patients with scleroderma, and is most frequently seen as an isolated phenomenon in patients with limited cutaneous disease. It can also occur in association with interstitial lung disease and often has a poor prognosis.

Other connective tissue diseases, including rheumatoid arthritis and SLE, can also be associated with the development of pulmonary hypertension. There is an association with Raynaud's phenomenon, as well as a female predominance.

Drugs and toxins

Pulmonary hypertension can occur in association with drugs, e.g., anorectic agents such as fenfluramine or dexfenfluramine, cocaine, and amphetamines. The clinical syndrome can be indistinguishable from IPAH. A careful history must therefore be taken. The absolute risk for pulmonary hypertension with anorectic agents is 28 cases per million person-years of exposure. Pulmonary hypertension can develop within days of starting the drug.

HIV infection

Pulmonary hypertension is seen in up to 1 in 200 people who are HIV positive. It is hypothesized that HIV-infected macrophages release vasoactive cytokines that lead to endothelial damage and proliferation. Antiretroviral drugs may have a beneficial effect.

Congenital heart disease, valvular heart disease, and left ventricular systolic and diastolic dysfunction

Volume and pressure overload caused by left heart abnormalities (including mitral valve disease), constrictive pericarditis, and left-to-right intracardiac shunts, e.g., atrial and ventricular septal defects, can lead to the development of pulmonary hypertension. Left ventricular systolic and diastolic dysfunction are relatively common causes of pulmonary hypertension.

Portal hypertension

Portopulmonary hypertension, seen in patients with portal hypertension (of whatever cause), is probably due to failure of the liver to remove vasoactive substances from the portal circulation, with their resultant accumulation and presentation to the pulmonary arterial endothelium. Pulmonary hypertension can substantially increase the risk associated with liver transplantation.

Alveolar hypoventilation e.g., due to neuromuscular disease. Respiratory acidosis increases hypoxic vasoconstriction, thereby contributing to the development of pulmonary hypertension.

Associated pulmonary hypertension: management

The initial step in treatment is optimal management of the underlying lung or cardiac disease, with the addition of oxygen and diuretics.

Disease specific management

Chronic thromboembolic pulmonary hypertension

Pulmonary thromboendarterectomy should be considered in appropriately selected patients, including those with significant pulmonary hypertension and extensive proximally located thromboembolic disease, and without comorbidities that might substantially increase the operative risk.

Pulmonary thromboendarterectomy involves surgical removal of organized thrombotic material starting proximally and extending more distally. It is done on cardiopulmonary bypass, with periods of circulatory arrest.

The PAP usually falls within 48 hours of surgery. Operative mortality is <10% in experienced hands

Scleroderma

Patients with scleroderma should be screened for pulmonary hypertension, particularly in the presence of unexplained dyspnea or a decreasing diffusing capacity on pulmonary function testing. Treatment of PAH occurring in association with scleroderma is often challenging. Such patients may be even less likely to be vasoreactors and less responsive to calcium channel blockers than patients with IPAH.

Patients with scleroderma-associated pulmonary hypertension have been included in many of the clinical trials done in the field. Subgroup analyses are being conducted and published, looking at therapeutic response in this patient population. Patients with scleroderma-associated pulmonary hypertension may respond to treatment with an endothelin receptor antagonist, phosphodiesterase inhibitor, or prostanoid, but the clinical response tends to be less than that seen in IPAH.

Further information

Badesch DB, Abman SH, Simonneau G, Rubin LJ, McLaughlin VV (2007). Medical therapy for pulmonary arterial hypertension: updated ACCP evidence-based clinical practice guidelines. *Chest* **131**:1917–1928.

Badesch DB, Tapson VF, McGoon MD, et al. (2000). Continuous intravenous epoprostenol for pulmonary hypertension due to the scleroderma spectrum of disease. A randomized, controlled trial. *Ann Intern Med* **132**:425–434.

Barst RJ, Langleben D, Badesch D, et al. (2006).Treatment of pulmonary arterial hypertension with the selective endothelin-A receptor antagonist sitaxsentan. *J Am Coll Cardiol* **47**:2049–2056.

Barst RJ, Langleben D, Frost A, et al. (2004). Sitaxsentan therapy for pulmonary arterial hypertension. *Am J Respir Crit Care Med* **169**:441–447.

Barst RJ, Rubin LJ, Long WA, et al. (1996). A comparison of continuous intravenous epoprostenol (prostacyclin) with conventional therapy for primary pulmonary hypertension. The Primary Pulmonary Hypertension Study Group. *N Engl J Med* **334**:296–302.

Channick RN, Simonneau G, Sitbon O, et al. (2001). Effects of the dual endothelin-receptor antagonist bosentan in patients with pulmonary hypertension: a randomised placebo-controlled study. *Lancet* **358**:1119–1123.

Diagnosis and management of pulmonary arterial hypertension: ACCP evidence-based clinical practice guidelines. *Chest* 2004; **126**(1) Suppl.

Galie N, Badesch D, Oudiz R, et al. (2005). Ambrisentan therapy for pulmonary arterial hypertension. *J Am Coll Cardiol* **46**:529–535.

Galie N, Beghetti M, Gatzoulis MA, et al. (2006). Bosentan therapy in patients with Eisenmenger syndrome: a multicenter, double-blind, randomized, placebo-controlled study. *Circulation* **114**:48–54.

Galie N, Ghofrani HA, Torbicki A, et al. (2005). Sildenafil citrate therapy for pulmonary arterial hypertension. *N Engl J Med* **353**:2148–2157.

Hoeper MM, Schwarze M, Ehlerding S, et al. (2000). Long-term treatment of primary pulmonary hypertension with aerosolized iloprost, a prostacyclin analogue. *N Engl J Med* **342**:1866–1870.

McLaughlin VV, Oudiz RJ, Frost A, et al. (2006). Randomized study of adding inhaled iloprost to existing bosentan in pulmonary arterial hypertension. *Am J Respir Crit Care Med* **174**:1257–1263.

McLaughlin VV, Shillington A, Rich S (2002). Survival in primary pulmonary hypertension: the impact of epoprostenol therapy. *Circulation* **106**:1477–1482.

McLaughlin VV, Sitbon O, Badesch DB, et al. (2005). Survival with first-line bosentan in patients with primary pulmonary hypertension. *Eur Respir J* **25**:244–249.

Olschewski H, Simonneau G, Galie N, et al. (2002). Inhaled iloprost for severe pulmonary hypertension. *N Engl J Med* **347**:322–329.

Peacock A (1999). Primary pulmonary hypertension. *Thorax* **54**:1107.

Rubin LJ, Badesch DB, Barst RJ, et al. (2002). Bosentan therapy for pulmonary arterial hypertension. *N Engl J Med* **346**:896–903.

Simonneau G, Barst RJ, Galie N, et al. (2002). Continuous subcutaneous infusion of treprostinil, a prostacyclin analogue, in patients with pulmonary arterial hypertension: a double-blind, randomized, placebo-controlled trial. *Am J Respir Crit Care Med* **165**:800–804.

Sitbon O, Humbert M, Jais X, et al. (2005). Long-term response to calcium channel blockers in idiopathic pulmonary arterial hypertension. *Circulation* **111**:3105–3111.

Sitbon O, Humbert M, Nunes H, et al. (2002). Long-term intravenous epoprostenol infusion in primary pulmonary hypertension: prognostic factors and survival. *J Am Coll Cardiol* **40**:780–788.

Sitbon O, McLaughlin VV, Badesch DB, et al. (2005). Survival in patients with class III idiopathic pulmonary arterial hypertension treated with first-line oral bosentan compared with an historical cohort of patients started on intravenous epoprostenol. *Thorax* **60**:1025–1030.

Tapson VF, Gomberg-Maitland M, McLaughlin VV, et al. (2006). Safety and efficacy of IV treprostinil for pulmonary arterial hypertension: a prospective, multicenter, open-label, 12-week trial. *Chest* **129**:683–688.

Pulmonary thromboembolic disease

Epidemiology and pathophysiology

Definition

A *pulmonary embolism* (PE) is an obstruction of the pulmonary vascular tree, usually caused by thrombus from a distant site. *Venous thromboembolism* (VTE) refers to an embolus arising from a systemic vein.

Epidemiology

The annual incidence of VTE has been reported to be as high as 145 per 100,000 person-years, with a 3-month mortality rate of >15%.

It is estimated that there are 1.3 million cases of VTE per year in the United States. Only 1/3 of these are appropriately diagnosed.

PE accounts for up to 15% of all postoperative deaths. It is the most common cause of death following elective surgery, and is the most common cause of maternal death during pregnancy.

The recurrence of VTE after a single episode is as high as 30% at 10 years.

Pathophysiology

Venous thrombosis

Most patients with VTE have one or more components of Virchow's triad:

- Immobility results in venous stasis and leads to local accumulation of platelets and clotting factors.
- Endothelial damage causes activation of the clotting factors and thrombus formation.
- A hypercoagulable state can occur in patients with at-risk medical conditions (e.g., the acute-phase response, malignancy, and autoimmune disease) increasing the likelihood of VTE.

Venous thromboembolism

- 95% of thrombi that embolize to the pulmonary vasculature propagate proximally from the deep venous system of the lower limbs and pelvis prior to embolization.
- Clots that arise from the axillary–subclavian system usually occur in the setting of central venous catheters and/or malignancy, but can be idiopathic as well.
- A saddle PE is a massive thrombus that collects at the bifurcation of a main pulmonary artery resulting in hemodynamic compromise.
- Smaller thrombi are more common and travel distally to the subsegmental pulmonary vessels. Pleuritic chest pain is the end result of an infarct of the lung parenchyma.

Pulmonary physiological effects of PE

Acute pulmonary vascular occlusion results in V/Q mismatch from impaired gas exchange, and hypoxemia from right-to-left shunt if an intracardiac communication exists.

Hypoxemia triggers increased sympathetic tone, systemic vasoconstriction, and increased venous return, resulting in increased stroke volume. In the setting of a massive PE, however, cardiac output may decrease, causing systemic hypotension. Irritant receptors of the lungs cause a reflex hyperventilation.

Airway resistance may increase from bronchoconstriction, and pulmonary compliance may decrease from pulmonary edema, hemorrhage, or decreased surfactant.

Right ventricular dysfunction

Mortality related to acute PE is predominately due to right heart failure. The hemodynamic impact of an acute pulmonary embolic event depends on the balance of three main factors:

- Presence or absence of underlying cardiopulmonary disease
- Reduction of the cross-sectional area of the pulmonary vascular bed, determined by the size and location of the embolus
- Vasoconstriction of the pulmonary vascular bed, mediated by the release of neurohumoral substances from activated platelets on the surface of the embolism, such as thromboxane A_2 and serotonin

Important hemodynamic events that occur with clot burden include

- Increased pulmonary vascular resistance with increased pulmonary artery pressures (PAP)
- Increased right ventricular (RV) afterload, resulting in increased end diastolic pressure and RV dilatation and RV systolic dysfunction
- RV ischemia infarction, which occurs as a result of
  - RV wall tension causing RV systolic dysfunction due to increased RV O_2 demand. Decreased RV O_2 supply occurs in the setting of hypotension and is due to decreased coronary perfusion.
- Ventricular interdependence causes septal shift toward the left ventricle (LV), decreasing LV diastolic filling and end diastolic volume, ultimately resulting in decreased stroke volume and cardiac output.
- Decreased cardiac output worsens RV preload and may cause further RV ischemia.

The right ventricle is particularly prone to this chain of events because it is a thin-walled, low-pressure system, unaccustomed to large pressure changes. The RV dilates acutely in response to sudden increases in pulmonary vascular resistance. This dilatation can result in impingement of the interventricular septum on the LV, impairing its function.

Pulmonary artery pressure (PAP) begins to rise once 25%–30% of the vascular bed is occluded by emboli.

- Substantial elevation in mean PAP is seen in >50% obstruction of the arterial bed
- However, in an acute PE it is unlikely that PA systolic pressure will exceed 55 mmHg.
- In patients with a PAP of ≥55 mmHg, *chronic* thromboembolic disease, underlying previous pulmonary hypertension, or other causes of raised PAP should be entertained.

Further reading

Goldhaber SZ (2004). Seminar: pulmonary embolism. *Lancet* **363**:1295–1305.

Kreit, JW (2004). The impact of right ventricular dysfunction on the prognosis and therapy of normotensive patients with pulmonary embolism. *Chest* **125**:1539–1545.

McIntyre KM, Sasahara AA (1977). Clinical investigations: the ratio of pulmonary arterial pressure to pulmonary vascular obstruction. *Chest* **71**:692–697.

Piazza G, Goldhaber SZ (2005). The acutely decompensated right ventricle. *Chest* **128**:1836–1852.

Tapson VF (2004). Acute pulmonary embolism. *Cardiol Clin* **22**:353–365.

Etiology

Risk factors can be divided into major and minor factors (see Table 32.1). This division is important for an assessment of clinical probability.

Table 32.1 Risk factors for venous thromboembolism (VTE)

Major risk factors (relative risk x5–20)	
Surgery	Major abdominal or pelvic surgery
	Orthopedic surgery (especially lower limb)
	Postoperative intensive care
Obstetrics	Late pregnancy (higher incidence with multiple births)
	Cesarean section
	Preeclampsia
Malignancy	Pelvic or abdominal
	Metastatic or advanced
Lower-limb problems	Fracture or varicose veins
Reduced mobility	Hospitalization, institutional care
Previous proven VTE	
Minor risk factors (relative risk x2–4)	
Cardiovascular	Congenital heart disease
	Congestive cardiac failure
	Hypertension
	Central venous access
	Superficial venous thrombosis
Estrogens	Oral contraceptive pill (especially third-generation pills, containing higher estrogen)
	Hormone replacement therapy
Miscellaneous	Occult malignancy
	Neurological disability
	Thrombotic disorders
	Obesity
	Inflammatory bowel disease
	Nephrotic syndrome, dialysis
	Myeloprofilerative disorders
	Behçet's disease

Malignancy

The exact incidence of VTE in patients with occult cancer is unknown. When controlled for population, the tumors most commonly associated with VTE include pancreas, brain, ovary, and lung. The pathogenesis of the prothrombotic state is not clear.

Screening for malignancy in patients presenting with idiopathic VTE is not recommended unless clinically suspected. Patients should undergo age- and risk-appropriate screening.

Patients with VTE associated with underlying malignancy have a poor prognosis, as the malignancy is frequently associated with regional spread or distant metastases at diagnosis.

Low-molecular-weight heparin has been shown to be superior to oral vitamin K antagonists in the treatment of VTE associated with malignancy.

Thrombophilias

Thrombophilia describes an increased tendency toward VTE related to inherited or acquired disorders. As many as 50% of patients with their first unprovoked VTE have an identifiable inherited thrombophilia (i.e., antiphospholipid syndrome, antithrombin III deficiency, prothrombin gene G20210A mutation, factor V Leiden deficiency, hyperhomocysteinemia, or protein C or protein S deficiency).

Usually there are additional acquired risk factors that potentiate VTE (i.e., factor V Leiden deficiency *and* oral contraceptive use.)

Current recommendations do not advocate routine screening for thrombophilias, unless in specific circumstances.

Thrombophilia testing may be recommended in

- Patients with an unprovoked first VTE
- Patients with no history of cancer and recurrent venous thrombosis
- Age <50 with provoked VTE (i.e., oral contraceptive or hormone use)
- First VTE with a clear family history in first-degree relatives
- VTE related to pregnancy, trauma, or surgery
- VTE at an unusual site—cerebral, mesenteric, portal, or hepatic veins

There remains controversy as to the utility of screening for thrombophilia in unproved cases of VTE, as it is unclear that identification of its presence will alter management.

If the decision is made to screen for thrombophilias, one must consider timing in relation to the thrombotic event, as well as current therapy. Results can be influenced by the acute-phase reaction of VTE and concurrent anticoagulant treatment. Most thrombophilias, except those associated with factor V Leiden and prothrombin gene mutation, should be evaluated when the patient is no longer taking anticoagulants and the acute VTE event is passed.

Economy class syndrome

This is a rare cause of symptomatic venous thromboembolic disease associated with long-distance, sedentary travel. There are 27 cases per million passengers who travel.

Risk factors include age over age 40, female hormone use, varicose veins, obesity, previous VTE, limited mobility, and cancer.

There is a dose–response trend for both distance traveled and duration of travel. Substantial increases in risk were noted with flight distances traveled over 5000 km or flight time of more than 8 hours. A flight time of less than 6 hours rarely results in symptomatic PE.

Despite the term *economy class syndrome*, there are no studies that compare the rate of VTE in economy class versus that in first class.

Further reading

Goldhaber SZ (2004). Seminar: pulmonary embolism. *Lancet*; **363**:1295–1305.

Lee AY (2003). Epidemiology and management of venous thromboembolism in patients with cancer. *Thromb Res* **110**:167–172.

Lee AY, Levine MN, Baker RI, et al. (2003). Low-molecular-weight heparin versus a coumarin for the prevention of recurrent venous thromboembolism in patients with cancer. *N Engl J Med* **349**:146–153.

Philbrick JT, Shaumate R, Siadaty MS, Becker DM (2007). Air travel and venous thromboembolism: a systematic review. *J Gen Intern Med* **22**:107–114.

Simioni P, Tormene D, Spiezia L, et al. (2006). Inherited thrombophilia and venous thromboembolism. *Semin Thromb Hemost* **32**:700-708.

Clinical features

Presentation

Acute pulmonary embolism

Patients with VTE can present in a variety of ways. The history and physical exam are neither sensitive nor specific to the disease.

Symptoms can vary according to the cardiopulmonary reserve of the patient. Young, healthy patients may have more subtle findings Patients with concomitant illnesses may attribute symptoms to a previously encountered process (e.g., COPD exacerbation, MI).

The most common symptom is acute onset of dyspnea. Lightheadedness, anxiety, cough, and palpitations can also occur.

Emboli that cause pulmonary infarction can result in hemoptysis and chest pain.

Patients with large emboli or poor cardiopulmonary reserve can present with syncope or sudden death.

Chronic thromboembolic disease

Typically, chronic thromboembolic disease (CTED) presents with more insidious-onset breathlessness over weeks to months, due to the increasing load of recurrent small-volume clot. Dyspnea and tachypnea are common presenting features; these are absent in only 10% of patients.

Consider PE in the differential diagnosis of

- Unexplained shortness of breath
- Collapse, syncope, hypotension
- Hypoxemia
- New-onset atrial fibrillation
- Signs consistent with right heart failure
- Pleural effusion
- Sudden death

Examination of patient with suspected PE

Examination may be normal.

Constitutional

- Low-grade fever

Cardiac

- Tachycardia is the most common cardiac sign.
- Atrial fibrillation
- Classically, loud P_2 and splitting of the second heart sound, with a gallop rhythm or right-sided S_3 (acute right heart strain)
- Right heart failure—low cardiac output and raised JVP with reduced blood pressure and perfusion pressure. Jugular venous distension with prominent V waves due to tricuspid regurgitation may be noted in large pulmonary emboli.

Pulmonary
- Tachypnea is the most common pulmonary sign.
- Reduced chest movement (due to pleuritic chest pain)
- Pleural friction rub: inflamed pleural surfaces rub with respiration
- Wheezing, rales
- Hypoxia (with hypocapnea due to hyperventilation, and an increased A–a gradient). **Note:** PaO_2 may be in the normal range in young, healthy individuals with cardiac reserve.

Lower extremity
- Signs of DVT are not always present—pain with dorsiflexion of foot (Homan's sign), pain, erythema, warmth, and swelling

Further reading

Goldhaber SZ (2004). Seminar: pulmonary embolism. *Lancet* **363**:1295–1305.
Goldhaber SZ, Visani L, De Rosa M (1999). Acute pulmonary embolism: clinical outcomes in the International Cooperative Pulmonary Embolism Registry (ICOPER). *Lancet* **353**:1386–1389.
Tapson VF (2004). Acute pulmonary embolism. *Cardiol Clin* **22**,:353–365.

Diagnosis of acute pulmonary embolism

The diagnosis of a pulmonary embolism can be difficult and involves a clinical assessment of probability. Such an evaluation involves the consideration of risk factors, clinical presentation, and clinical signs. Diagnostic testing that may add weight to clinical suspicion can then be performed. The estimation of the pretest clinical probability of PE is of vital importance in interpreting the diagnostic modalities performed.

Pretest clinical probability scoring systems

The *Modified **Wells score*** is an objective clinical assessment strategy used to estimate the probability that a patient has a PE (shown in Box 32.1). Clinical assessment should be performed prior to imaging.

D-dimer testing

D-dimer testing has an important role in diagnosing and excluding PE, and should be used with a pretest clinical probability scoring method such as the Wells[1] or Geneva[2] scores.

Plasma D-dimer is generated as a result of endogenous fibrinolysis. The fibrin produced in a patient with a PE is degraded into cross-linked derivatives (D-dimers) via circulating plasmin. It is important to note that other disease states can produce an elevated D-dimer level—neoplasia, disseminated intravascular coagulation (DIC), sepsis, infection, myocardial infarction, postoperative states, and second- and third-trimester pregnancies. Levels also increase linearly with age and may not be accurate in the elderly.

Recent studies have utilized assays such as the whole-blood agglutination (SimpliRED) or ELISA (VIDAS) (see Table 32.2). Epidemiological characteristics and interpretation of the results depend on the prevalence of VTE in the population evaluated and the assay itself. They are rarely in the normal range in cases of acute VTE. These assays are not valid as a stand-alone screening test for VTE as they have poor specificity.

Box 32.1 Modified Wells score

Clinical characteristics	*Score*
Heart rate >100 beats/minute	3.0
Immobilization in the previous 4 weeks	1.5
Surgery in the previous 4 weeks	1.5
Previously objectively diagnosed DT or PE	1.5
Hemoptysis	1.0
Malignancy (current or treatment within the last 6 months)	1.0
PE as likely as, or more likely than, an alternative diagnosis	3.0

Score	**Probability of PE**
≤4	Unlikely
>4	Likely

Data adapted from: Wells et al. (2000). *Thromb Haemost* **83**:416–420.

Table 32.2 Predictive values of SimpliRED and ELISA

Parameter	SimpliRED	ELISA (VIDAS)
Test type	Qualitative (positive/negative)	Quantitative (numerical)
Sensitivity	60%–100%	96%–100%
Specificity	68%–94%	34%–100%
Negative predictive value	82%–99.5%	88%–100%

The above ranges of data are compiled from the articles listed in the section Further reading.

SimpliRED has a high sensitivity and moderate specificity.
- The relatively high specificity allows for a reduction in further diagnostic testing, in a low-risk population.

ELISA (VIDAS) has an even greater sensitivity but lower specificity.
- Typical cutoff values for a negative test are <500 ng/mL.
- Due to risk of false-negative results, patients with a negative ELISA and a high-probability clinical score require further evaluation.

The negative predictive value (NPV) depends on the prevalence of VTE in a given population; as the prevalence increases, the NPV decreases.
- The NPV of a low-risk Wells Score (patients with a low prevalence of PE) and negative SimpliRED is ≥99%.
- However, in a population with a prevalence of >5% PE, SimpliRED may not safely exclude PE.

Box 32.2 D-dimer test interpretation

- A positive D-dimer result requires further investigation
- A negative D-dimer test reliably excludes PE in patients with a low or intermediate pre-test clinical probability with a NPV of 99.5% and 93.9% respectively (SimpliRED). These patients do not need further imaging.
- In patients with a high pre-test probability a negative d-dimer may not safely rule out VTE, and further studies should be obtained.
- The D-dimer becomes less useful the longer the period spent in hospital (i.e. increasing false positives), due to clot formation at venipuncture sites, venous stasis due to bed rest, concomitant medical issues, etc.

---

1 Wells PS, Anderson DR,, Rodger M, et al. (2000). Derivation of a simple clinical model to categorize patients' probability of pulmonary embolism: increasing the models utility with the SimpliRED D-dimer. *Thromb Haemost* **83**:416–420.
2 Wicki J, Perrier A, Perneger TV, Bounamaeux A, Junod AF (2000). Predicting adverse outcome in patients with acute pulmonary embolism: a risk score. *Thromb Haemost* **83**:548–552.

Further reading

Kelly J, Hunt BJ (2002). Commentary: role of D-dimers in diagnosis of venous thromboembolism. *Lancet* **359**:456–458.

Kelly J, Rudd A, Lewis RR, et al. (2002). Plasma D-dimers in the diagnosis of venous thromboembolism. *Arch Intern Med* **162**:747–756.

Michiels JJ, Gadisseur A, van der Planken M, et al. (2006). Different accuracies of rapid enzyme-linked immunosorbent, turbidimetric and agglutination D-dimer assays for thrombosis exclusion: impact on diagnostic work-ups of outpatients with suspected deep vein thrombosis and pulmonary embolism. *Semin Thromb Hemost* **32**:678–693.

van Belle A, Büller HR, Huisman EV, et al.; Christopher Study Investigators (2006). Effectiveness of managing suspected pulmonary embolism using an algorithm combining clinical probability, D-dimer testing, and computed tomography. *JAMA* **295**:172–179.

van de Graaf F, van den Borne H, van der Kolk M, et al. (2000). Exclusion of deep venous thrombosis with D-dimer testing. *Thromb Haemost* **83**:191–198.

Wells PS, Anderson DR,, Rodger M, et al. (2000). Derivation of a simple clinical model to categorize patients' probability of pulmonary embolism: increasing the models utility with the SimpliRED D-dimer. *Thromb Haemost* **83**:416–420.

Wells PS, Anderson DR, Rodger M, et al. (2001). Excluding pulmonary embolism at the bedside without diagnostic imaging: management of patients with suspected pulmonary embolism presenting to the emergency department by using a simple clinical model and D-dimer. *Ann Intern Med* **135**:98–107.

Diagnostic studies

Often in medicine the clinician must weigh the risks and benefits of performing a diagnostic test. Even exams with low direct risk to the patient may have significant clinical repercussions. Before ordering a diagnostic test for a suspected PE, it is imperative to assess the clinical probability of PE. Other considerations include the availability of diagnostic tests at a particular institution and the risk of exposure to contrast and radiation.

After determining the patient's pretest probability for PE, the physician can choose appropriate diagnostic studies to aid in the decision-making process regarding admission, further testing, and potential treatment. One-quarter to one-third of patients with suspected PE are eventually diagnosed with PE.

Initial studies

An ECG and CXR are often performed when evaluating a patient with chest or respiratory complaints, or with significant physical findings. These tests are not adequate to diagnose or exclude PE, but may note nonspecific abnormalities.

ECG

ECG can be used to rule out other processes (ST elevation MI or pericardial disease). In patients with PE an ECG is often abnormal (tachycardia, ST- or T-wave changes); however, up to 25% of patients with acute PE have normal ECGs.

In cases of large embolic burden, evidence of right heart strain and pulmonary hypertension may occur, manifested as T-wave inversion in V_{1-4} or RBBB. Although helpful in the diagnosis of acute cor pulmonale, the $S_1Q_3T_3$ pattern is uncommon. New-onset atrial fibrillation is also not common but may suggest the diagnosis.

CXR

CXR may be helpful in ruling out other disease processes. Infrequently seen findings include
- *Hampton's hump*, a wedge-shaped infarct in the lung periphery
- *Westermark's sign*, focal oligemia in the area of embolized lung

Additional findings may include cardiac enlargement, effusion, elevated hemidiaphragm, pulmonary artery enlargement, atelectasis, or infiltrate.

Laboratory studies
- *D-dimer* is useful for risk stratification and can be used to exclude VTE in the appropriate clinical scenario.
- *Arterial blood gas* is of limited diagnostic utility in patients with suspected PE. Studies comparing patients evaluated for PE showed no statistically significant difference in ABG values between those with and those without PE. Results may be normal, especially in the young and healthy, or there may be evidence of hypoxia, hypocapnia due to hyperventilation, or an increased A–a gradient.

Chest imaging

Contrast-enhanced single-row or multidetector helical CT pulmonary angiogram (CTPA) is frequently recommended as an initial imaging technique in suspected PE. Previously, the sensitivity of a single-slice detector varied between 60% and 100%. However, the use of multirow detectors has improved sensitivity to 90%–100%, as demonstrated in a number of outcome studies.

Another benefit of CTPA is that it can suggest an alternative diagnosis for the patient's symptoms.

According to the Christopher Study Investigators, a simple algorithm with dichotomous clinical decision rule (Modified Wells), D-dimer testing, and single-row or multidetector CT scan is sufficient to exclude PE, with subsequent total incidence of VTE at 3 months of 1.3%.

Isotope lung scanning (ventilation/perfusion or V/Q scan) (see Table 32.3) may be useful as a first-line imaging investigation in patients with a normal CXR and with no concurrent cardiopulmonary disease, in whom a negative scan would reliably exclude a PE. Scans are reported as low, intermediate, or high probability and must be interpreted in light of the pretest clinical probability score.

Further imaging (such as CTPA or digital subtraction angiography) is necessary for results in which
• The scan is indeterminate
• There is discordant lung scan and clinical probability

Other diagnostic imaging techniques and strategies

When diagnostic tests such as CTPA or V/Q scan are unavailable or non-diagnostic or cannot be performed, other imaging studies may be used to rule out the diagnosis of PE. In addition, a combination approach to imaging may enhance the predictive value of a single study.

Pulmonary angiography (digital subtraction angiography) (DSA)

DSA remains the gold standard for diagnosis of PE; however, as multidetector CTPA becomes more sensitive, the usefulness of DSA to diagnose acute PE is being questioned. It is now in limited use because of the need for specialized equipment and expertise, its expense, and potential complications.

Table 32.3 Clinical significance of V/Q scan report

Scan results	Pretest clinical probability	Outcome
Normal		PE excluded
Low	Low	PE excluded
High	High	PE diagnosed
Any other		Need further imaging

Lower extremity ultrasound

Compression ultrasonography is now the imaging test of choice to diagnose DVT. The sensitivity of detecting DVT in the proximal veins (above the popliteal fossa) is 97%, whereas the sensitivity to image a clot below the popliteal fossa is only 73%.

Twenty percent of symptomatic patients have clot below the knee, and in this group only 20%–30% propagate proximally. Around 70%–80% of patients with proven PE have a proximal DVT.

Leg imaging can be used as an alternative to lung imaging in those with clinical signs of DVT and PE. In patients with suspected DVT alone, it is safe to withhold anticoagulation with a single negative leg ultrasound. It is unclear if these data can be extrapolated to patients with suspected PE. These patients require further evaluation.

Use of serial ultrasound to search for DVT has not been shown to be cost-effective after an initial negative ultrasound; only 1%–2% of these patients develop proximal DVT.

Computed tomographic venography (CTV)

CTV can be combined with CTPA for evaluation of PE. In the PIOPED II study by Stein et al.,[11] CTV added to CTPA significantly increased the sensitivity for detection of VTE from 83% to 90%, with a similar specificity of 95% for both.

Risk stratification

Once a diagnosis of PE has been made, risk stratification can aid in establishing appropriate initial treatment and planning long-term management.

Biomarkers

The studies performed using biomarkers in PE patients are observational. They can be used to identify patients at high risk of mortality who may benefit from more intense monitoring or interventions. No management studies have shown a mortality benefit to acting on this information.

Brain natriuretic peptide (BNP)

High BNP levels indicate myocardial dilation. Studies have evaluated N-terminal-proBNP (wider spectrum of values) and BNP (more precise values) in assessment of VTE. BNP has a NPV and low positive predictive value (PPV), and can identify low-risk PE patients when levels are low.

1 Stein PD, Fowler SE, Goodman LR,, et al. (2006), Multidetector computed tomography for acute pulmonary embolism (PIOPED II). *N Engl J Med* **354**:2317–2327.

Troponin

Troponin levels have also been studied as a means of risk stratification in pulmonary embolism. Elevation of troponin (either I or T) can reflect RV strain, RV micro-infarction, and myocardial cell damage.

Imaging

Echocardiography

Transthoracic echocardiography is generally not useful for the diagnosis of PE, as it lacks adequate sensitivity and specificity. Echocardiography is useful in risk stratification of patients with known PE, however.

Patients with significant clot burden may show RV enlargement, hypokinesis, abnormal septal shift, tricuspid regurgitation, and pulmonary hypertension. The presence of RV dysfunction in patients with PE increases the relative risk of death 6-fold over that of patients with normal RV function after PE. Retrospective analysis showed that 31% of patients with submassive PE (SBP >90) had RV dysfunction; 10% developed cardiogenic shock within 24 hours and 5% of the hypotensive patients died.

Transesophageal echocardiography may aid in diagnosis and localization of clot in main pulmonary arteries, but it is technically challenging.

CTPA

RV enlargement is determined by evaluating a coronal slice of the heart and measuring the distance from the maximal outer wall to the IV septum, with massive PE defined as an RV–LV ratio of 1.5. The degree of RV dilatation is related to proximity and size of PE, with more RV dysfunction in proximal than in distal PE.

Combined approach

- Patients with normal troponin and RV function at lowest risk of death
- Patients with RV dysfunction with increased troponin had 10-fold increased in-hospital adverse outcomes and 20% mortality
- Patients with RV dysfunction and increased NTpro-BNP have 12-fold increased in-hospital death and adverse outcomes

Further reading

Goldhaber SZ (1998). Pulmonary embolism. *N Engl J Med* **339**:93–104.

Goldhaber SZ (2002). Echocardiography in the management of pulmonary embolism. *Ann Intern Med* **136**:691–700.

Goldhaber SZ (2004). Seminar: pulmonary embolism. *Lancet* **363**:1295–305.

PIOPED Investigators (1990) Value of the ventilation/perfusion scan in acute pulmonary embolism: Results of the prospective investigation of pulmonary embolism diagnosis (PIOPED). *JAMA* **263**:2753–2759.

Reid JH, Murchison (1998). Acute right ventricular dilatation: a new helical ct sign of massive pulmonary embolism. *Clin Radiol* **53**:694–698.

Rodger MA, Carrier M, Jones GN, et al. (2000). Diagnostic value of arterial blood gas measurement in suspected pulmonary embolism. *Am J Respir Crit Care Med* **162**:2105-2108.

Scarvelis D, Wells PS (2006). Diagnosis and treatment of deep-vein thrombosis. *CMAJ* **175**: 1087–1092.

Tapson VF (2004). Acute Pulmonary Embolism. *Cardiology clinics* **22**, 353–65.

van Belle A, Büller HR, Huisman EV, et al.; Christopher Study Investigators (2006). Effectiveness of managing suspected pulmonary embolism using an algorithm combining clinical probability, D-dimer testing, and computed tomography. *JAMA* **295**:172–179.

Management

Anticoagulation

Empiric therapy is often appropriate while awaiting results of diagnostic testing, especially for high-probability patients or if testing cannot be performed in a timely fashion.

Low molecular-weight heparin (LMWH)

Per randomized controlled trials and current ATS guidelines, weight-based doses for treatment of PE are as effective as unfractionated IV heparin. Patients with massive PE (see Box 32.3) were excluded from these trials, and safety of use in this population is unclear. There is usually no need to follow Xa levels during treatment.

Unfractionated heparin (uFH)

This is the treatment of choice for massive PE (there is a faster onset of action with bolus) and renal dysfunction, since LMWH is excreted by the kidneys. uFH can be discontinued quickly, especially in the setting of bleeding (it has a short $t_{1/2}$). uFH has a higher association with heparin-induced thrombocytopenia (HIT) than LMWH.

Oral anticoagulation

Once PE is proven and the patient has been on a heparin derivative for at least 24 hours, treatment with a vitamin K antagonist (VKA) can be initiated. Many experts recommend overlap with LMWH or uFH to prevent paradoxical hypercoagulable state (protein C–deficient patients). Target INR is 2.0–3.0 (treat with heparin for 5 days when overlapping).

VKAs are contraindicated in certain populations and conditions, such as pregnancy. Risk versus benefit must be considered for patients in whom there is high risk of bleed or high risk of falls or trauma.

Duration of warfarin anticoagulation

- First episode of PE due to a transient risk factor (i.e., central venous catheter or orthopedic surgery): VKA for at least 3 months
- First episode of idiopathic PE: VKA for 6–12 months; consider indefinite treatment
- PE due to malignancy: LMWH for first 3–6 months, then consider indefinite anticoagulation with VKA or treatment until malignancy resolves
- First episode of PE due to hypercoagulable state, either positive antiphospholipid antibody alone or combination of the two (i.e., factor V Leiden + prothrombin gene mutation 20210A): 12 months of VKA, and consider indefinite treatment
- First episode of PE due to a single hypercoagulable state (i.e., protein C or S, or factor V Leiden or prothrombin gene mutation or homocysteinemia or high factor VIII or deficiency of antithrombin): treatment with VKA for 6–12 months and consider indefinite treatment
- Recurrent PE (2 or more episodes): indefinite treatment
- Goal INR is 2–3: no benefit to higher- or lower-intensity treatment

Side effects
- The risk of bleeding increases with age and concurrent illness.
- There is a higher bleeding rate with concomitant aspirin use and a previous gastrointestinal bleed.
- Risk of bleeding relates to duration and intensity of anticoagulation.
- When treating indefinitely reassess risk–benefit of continued treatment

---

Box 32.3 Management of acute massive PE

Acute massive PE, defined by systemic arterial hypotension, has a mortality of up to 52%, 90 days after diagnosis.
1. Oxygenation either via non-rebreather or intubation if necessary
2. IV access. Send baseline labs. Perform ECG and CXR
3. Analgesia if needed; consider IV opiates
4. Management of cardiogenic shock—consider fluids to correct hypovolemia and then vasoactive medications (dopamine or norepinephrine) to improve blood pressure. There are no human trials comparing pressors in acute PE.
5. Start IV heparin unless active GI bleeding or intracerebral hemorrhage:
   a. Use a weight-based algorithm
   b. Adjust infusion rate until APTT is 1.5–2.5× control. Check APTT 4–6 hours after initial bolus and 6–10 hours after any dose change. When APTT is in the therapeutic range, check it daily.
6. Investigation to confirm PE depends on the clinical state of the patient. Ideally, perform a CT scan if there are no contraindications to contrast dye, and try not to delay more than 1 hour. It may be unwise to move a sick patient for imaging. If they have circulatory collapse and PE is the *most likely* cause, treatment should be prioritized. Aortic dissection, cardiac tamponade, and acute MI may mimic PE—rule out these clinical entities.
7. Assess risk stratification for the patient with urgent echocardiogram and biomarkers.
8. Consider thrombolysis if there is massive PE or the patient is hypotensive (if there are no contraindications such as active GI bleeding or intracerebral hemorrhage):
   a. Alteplase 100 mg over 2 hours given peripherally
   b. Or streptokinase 250,000 units in 20 minutes with 100,000 units/hr for 24 hours (plus hydrocortisone to prevent further circulatory instability)

Thrombolysis

There is emerging evidence to support the use of thrombolytics in certain subgroups of patients with PE. The risk—benefit analysis of this treatment must always be carefully considered. The patient population generally targeted is those with hemodynamically unstable PE and a low risk of bleeding.

There are several thrombolytics (alteplase, streptokinase, and urokinase) that have been used in the treatment of PE. These drugs act to convert plasminogen to plasmin, which cleaves fibrin, causing clot lysis. The goal of thrombolytics in acute PE is improved pulmonary perfusion and RV function. The American College of Chest Physicians (ACCP) guidelines do not recommend catheter-directed thrombolysis. There is a lack of controlled studies in this area.

Massive PE

Massive PE is defined as cardiogenic shock with SBP <90 mmHg. Patients with massive PE and RV dysfunction are at significant risk of death. There are no large prospective, randomized controlled trials showing efficacy of thrombolysis in patients with cardiogenic shock secondary to PE.

A single-center study of 8 patients (study stopped early) randomized to streptokinase and heparin versus heparin alone showed survival benefit in the group receiving thrombolytics.

A retrospective review of 2392 patients with PE from the International Cooperative Pulmonary Embolism Registry (ICOPER) database showed no mortality benefit or decrease in recurrent PE with thrombolytic therapy at 90 days.

Regardless of these results, experts generally recommend thrombolysis for patients with hemodynamic instability related to PE. The prognosis is very poor in this patient population and the risk benefit—ratio favors use of thrombolytics.

Non-massive PE

This is a controversial topic; use of thrombolytics is variable among clinicians. Konstantinides et al. showed that there may be evidence supporting the use of IV alteplase in addition to IV heparin for treatment of hemodynamically stable submassive PE in association with pulmonary hypertension or right ventricular dysfunction. There was no mortality benefit with use of thrombolytics at 30 days; however, a significant benefit was shown in decreasing escalation of care (use of mechanical ventilation, vasopressors or thrombolysis).

Inclusion criteria for thrombolysis for submassive PE

It is controversial whether these patients should receive thrombolysis.
- Acute PE (diagnosed by CT pulmonary angiography or V/Q scan) and
- Right ventricular dysfunction on echocardiogram (right ventricular enlargement and loss of inferior vena cava (IVC) collapse on inspiration without left ventricular dysfunction or mitral valve disease) *or*
- Pulmonary artery hypertension (tricuspid regurgitant jet velocity >2.8 m/second) *or*
- New electrocardiographic signs of right ventricular strain *or*

- Precapillary pulmonary hypertension on right heart catheterization (mean PAP >25 mmHg at rest, pulmonary capillary wedge pressure [PCWP] <18 mmHg)

Relative Contraindications for thrombolysis

- Age >80
- Recent major trauma within 10 days
- Neurological event (TIA, CVA, neurosurgery, or head trauma) within preceding 6 months
- GI bleeding within preceding 3 months
- Uncontrolled hypertension
- Known bleeding disorders

Embolectomy

This is rarely performed for acute PE. Embolectomy is used when conservative measures for treatment of PE have failed and thrombolysis is contraindicated or has failed. The ACCP recommends that patients fulfill the following criteria before embolectomy is pursued:

- Massive PE
- Hemodynamic instability (shock) despite efforts to resuscitate the patient and use of anticoagulation
- Failure of thrombolytic therapy or contraindication to its use

Operative mortality is variable and depends on the site where the procedure is performed. Access to a regional center that performs surgical embolectomy may be a limitation.

IVC filter placement

This intervention is used to prevent lower-extremity thrombi from embolizing to the pulmonary vasculature. The filters are usually placed via the internal jugular or femoral vein into the IVC. Their use increases the incidence of lower-extremity DVT formation at 1 year. Anticoagulation should be resumed (if possible) shortly after placement of the filter.

IVC filters may, however, be indicated in

- Acute VTE in patients with an absolute contraindication to anticoagulation
- Recurrent VTE despite adequate anticoagulation

Filters are sometimes placed in the setting of a massive PE (presence of right ventricular dysfunction or pulmonary hypertension) or in patients with preexisting pulmonary hypertension and RV dysfunction when further embolization may be lethal.

Temporary (retrievable) filters are being used more commonly. They can be removed after the risk of an embolic event has decreased and can be placed in patients with transient risks for anticoagulation. Initial recommendations stated that these filters should be retrieved within 4–6 weeks of placement to improve the success of retrieval without complications. Reports of successful retrieval at later time points are surfacing.

Scenarios in which retrievable IVC filters may be considered include

- Recent major surgery
- Temporary risk of major bleeding
- Trauma with significant orthopedic injury

Further reading

Büller HR, Agnelli G, Hull RD, et al. (2004). Antithrombotic therapy for venous thromboembolic disease: the seventh ACCP conference on antithrombotic and thrombolytic therapy. *Chest* **126**(Suppl.):401S–428S.

The Columbus Investigators (1997). Low-molecular-weight heparin in the treatment of patients with venous thromboembolism. *N Engl J Med* **337**:657–662.

Goldhaber SZ (2004). Seminar: pulmonary embolism. *Lancet* **363**:1295–1305.

Jerjes-Sanchez C, Ramirez-Rivera A, de Lourdes Garcia M, et al. (1995). Streptokinase and heparin versus heparin alone in massive pulmonary embolism: a randomized controlled trial. *J Thromb Thrombol* **2**:227–229.

Konstantinides S, Geibel A, Heusel G, et al. (2002). Heparin plus alteplase compared to heparin alone in patients with submassisve pulmonary embolism. *N Engl J Med* **347**:1143–1150.

Kucher N, Rossi E, De Rosa M, Goldhaber SZ (2006) Massive pulmonary embolism. *Circulation* **113**:577–582.

Lee AY, Levine MN, Baker RI, et al. (2003). Low-molecular-weight heparin versus a coumarin for the prevention of recurrent venous thromboembolism in patients with cancer. *N Engl J Med* **349**:146–153.

Tapson VF (2004). Acute pulmonary embolism. *Cardiol Clin* **22**:353–365.

Special considerations

Pregnancy and thromboembolic disease

- More pulmonary emboli occur during pregnancy than after delivery. Fatal PE is one of the most common causes of maternal death in pregnancy (1/100,000 pregnancies).
- Risk of PE in pregnancy is greater with increasing maternal (>35 years) and gestational age, mode of delivery (C-section more than vaginal delivery), multiparity, prolonged bed rest, current infection, inherited or acquired thrombophilia, and personal or family history of VTE.
- The physiological changes of pregnancy can often be confused with PE, as many patients have symptoms of dyspnea during pregnancy.
- 90% of DVTs occur in the left leg, as the gravid uterus compresses the left iliac veins.
- A low serum D-dimer level has a high negative predictive value in pregnancy, but an elevated D-dimer value is of limited utility as it is often elevated in normal pregnancy.
- There are no prospective randomized, controlled clinical trials addressing the risk of radiation to the fetus with CTPA or V/Q scan.
- Experts agree that an undiagnosed PE or inappropriate anticoagulation outweighs the risk incurred from imaging in most scenarios. Decisions regarding diagnostic algorithms and treatment must be decided on a case-by-case basis. The availability of LMWH has improved treatment options in this patient population.
- Warfarin is teratogenic (class X), thus its use is contraindicated during pregnancy. It can be safely used in breast-feeding mothers.
- In those with antenatal thromboembolic disease, LMWH is used over uFH because of its decreased association with osteoporosis, heparin-induced thrombocytopenia, and ease of use.
- As the time of delivery approaches, LMWH is discontinued and uFH initiated, as it is easier to monitor and to reverse. It is unclear whether heparin should be stopped or the dose reduced at the time of delivery.
- For patients diagnosed with PE during pregnancy, the duration of anti-coagulation depends on the underlying cause of VTE (see Pregnancy and thromboembolic disease).

Thromboembolic disease and oral contraceptive pills, HRT

- Oral contraceptive pills (OCP), pregnancy, and hormone replacement therapy (HRT) increase the risk of VTE.
- Risk of fatal PE is twice as high among those taking third-generation pills compared to risk with first- or second-generation pills, and risk increases among cigarette smokers and increased age.
- A previous history of DVT or PE is an absolute contraindication to OCP use.
- Relative contraindications include a strong family history of VTE and inherited prothrombotic states.
- Meta-analyses show a relative risk of VTE of 2.1 in HRT users (highest in the first year of use).

Flight prophylaxis for thromboembolic disease

As previously noted, there is an increased risk of VTE in individuals who travel long distances or for prolonged periods of time (>5000 km or >8 hours flight duration)

Those individuals at highest risk include those who have had previous VTE, recent surgery, or trauma, have active malignancy or chronic disease, use estrogen, are obese or at advanced age, or have thrombophilia.

The ACCP guidelines on prophylaxis for VTE are as follows:
- The general population without extra risk factors for VTE should avoid constrictive clothing around the waist and lower extremities, avoid dehydration, and do frequent calf stretches.
- Those with additional risk factors should employ these general strategies and may need active prophylaxis consisting of compression stockings (providing a pressure of 15–30 mmHg at the ankle) or a single dose of LMWH.
- Use of aspirin is not recommended.

Further reading

Geerts WH, Pineo GF, Heit JA, et al. (2004) Prevention of venous thromboembolism: the seventh ACCP Conference on Antithrombotic and Thrombolytic Therapy. *Chest* **126**:338S–400S.

Goldhaber SZ (2004). Seminar: pulmonary embolism. *Lancet* **363**:1295–1305.

Kher A, Bauersachs R, Nielsen JD (2007). The management of thrombosis in pregnancy: role of low-molecular-weight heparin. *Thromb Haemost* **97**:505–513.

Philbrick JT, Shaumate R, Siadaty MS, Becker DM (2007). Air travel and venous thromboembolism: a systematic review. *J Gen Intern Med* **22**:107–114.

Scarsbrook AF, Bradley KM, Gleeson FV (2007). Perfusion scintigraphy: diagnostic utility in pregnant women with suspected pulmonary embolic disease. *Eur Radiol* **17**:2554–2560.

Tapson VF (2004). Acute pulmonary embolism. *Cardiol Clin* **22**:353–365.

Rare causes of embolic disease

Air embolism is defined as air within the arterial or venous circulation. Small amounts of air can be tolerated, but large amounts can occlude the vasculature and cause mechanical obstruction and death. This is a rare occurrence.

Causes
Neck vein cannulation, intrauterine manipulations (such as illegal abortion procedures in which a frothy liquid is passed under pressure into the uterus), bronchial trauma, or barotraumas can lead to air embolism. Air in the left ventricle causes impairment to venous filling and subsequent poor coronary perfusion as air enters the coronary arteries. Air in the right ventricle or pulmonary artery impedes RV cardiac output and raises right-sided filling pressures.

Diagnosis
The diagnosis of air embolism requires a high clinical suspicion and is usually suggested by the clinical scenario (recent placement or discontinuation of central venous access, etc.). Clinical signs are not specific but can include dizziness, loss of consciousness, and convulsions. Air may be seen in the retinal arteries or from transected vessels.

Venous air emboli may cause raised venous pressure, cyanosis, hypotension, tachycardia, syncope, and a "mill-wheel" murmur over the precordium.

Treatment
Patients should lie in the left lateral decubitus position, with the head down and feet up (Trendelenburg). This position traps air in the apex of the ventricle. From here it can be aspirated via thoracotomy or catheter-guided aspiration, or potentially reabsorbed.

Amniotic fluid embolism
This condition is estimated to occur in 1 out of 25,000–80,000 live births. It is the third most common cause of maternal death, and the most common cause of death in the immediate postpartum period. Usually catastrophic, 80% of women die, 20%–50% of them in the first hour.

An anaphylactic-type response to amniotic fluid entering the circulation is seen. Amniotic fluid enters circulation because of torn fetal membranes, which can occur in Cesarean section, uterine or cervical trauma, or uterine rupture. It has a thromboplastic effect, causing disseminated intravascular coagulation and thrombi to form in pulmonary vessels.

Not all women react in this way to amniotic fluid. It is more common in older, multiparous mothers who have had short tumultuous labor, often involving uterine stimulants.

Clinically amniotic fluid embolism presents with sudden-onset respiratory distress, hypoxia, bronchospasm, cyanosis, cardiovascular collapse, pulmonary edema, convulsions, coma, and cardiac arrest. Coagulopathy with intractable uterine bleeding and uterine atony is seen.

Diagnosis is clinical. Fetal debris or cells can be identified in blood sampled from the maternal pulmonary artery, but this is not pathognomonic.

Treatment is supportive while the thrombi clear from the maternal lungs. Maintain the circulation with fluids and ionotropes. Respiratory support with oxygen and ventilation may be needed. Correct coagulopathy with fresh frozen plasma and packed cells. Control placental bleeding.

Fat embolism

Fat embolism occurs especially with lower limb fractures of the pelvis and femur. It is more common in fractures that have not been immobilized. It can also occur after prosthetic joint replacement, cardiac massage, liver trauma, burns, bone marrow transplant, rapid high-altitude decompression, and liposuction. It presents 24–72 hours post-fracture. Marrow fat enters the circulation and lodges in the lungs, causing mechanical obstruction.

Classically fat embolism presents with hypoxia, coagulopathy with transient petechial rash on the neck, axillae, and skin folds, and neurological disturbance, such as confusion, disorientation, or sometimes coma. Stable patients may deteriorate with low-grade fever, petechial rash, hypoxia, and confusion. Jaundice and renal dysfunction are possible.

Diagnosis is usually made clinically in a patient with a lower limb fracture presenting with tachypnea and hypoxia. Fat globules can be identified in the urine. CXR shows bilateral alveolar infiltrates. ARDS can develop.

Treatment is with early immobilization of fracture, fluid replacement, oxygen, and supportive care.

Septic and tumor emboli are also causes of embolic disease.

Future developments

Subsegmental pulmonary emboli

Although rare findings, the ability of multidetector row CT scans to visualize smaller pulmonary arteries at the subsegmental level has raised questions about the clinical significance of these findings. It is unclear whether subsegmental defects represent pathological thrombi, flow artifacts, or a physiological function of the lungs to filter debris. Further studies are needed to investigate the significance of these findings and determine if anticoagulation is necessary.

Ximelagatran

This is a novel oral, direct thrombin inhibitor with a wide therapeutic range that does not need anticoagulation monitoring. It results in liver function abnormalities in up to 6% of patients and thus requires LFT monitoring. It is now licensed in some European countries, but there are concerns about toxicity.

PIOPED III

Prospective Investigation of Pulmonary Embolism Diagnosis (PIOPED) III investigators are currently planning a trial to assess the utility of gadolinium-enhanced magnetic resonance angiography (MRA) in the diagnosis of pulmonary embolism.

Sarcoidosis

Etiology and pathology

Definition

- *Sarcoidosis* is a multisystem inflammatory disorder of unknown cause.
- It is characterized by noncaseating granulomata and CD4 Th1-biased T-cell response in affected organs.
- It commonly involves the respiratory system, but can affect nearly all organs.
- 50%–60% of people have spontaneous remissions; others may develop chronic progressive disease.

Etiology

Incidence varies with population studies, from 5 to 100/100,000, according to geographic distribution. It is more common among African Americans, West Indians, and the Irish. Commonly presenting between 20 and 40 years of age, sarcoidosis is unusual in children and the elderly. It is typically a more aggressive disease in Black populations than in Caucasians, especially with skin disease, peripheral lymphadenopathy, bone marrow, and liver involvement.

Environmental factors such as moldy environment and insecticides may be associated with sarcoidosis. Other studies suggest infections such as Propiniobacter acnes or mycobacteria may be the trigger for disease.

Genetics

Familial and ethnic clustering of cases suggest a genetic predisposition. A genome-wide scan for susceptibility genes in familial sarcoidosis has been performed, pointing to a locus on chromosome 6, which includes the genes for HLA. HLA-DRB1*1101 is associated with susceptibility of disease in Blacks and Whites. HLA DRB1*0301 and DQB1*0201 have been associated with a good prognosis.

Pathology

Sarcoidosis is caused by an immunological response:

- Unknown antigenic stimulus triggers CD4 (helper) T-cell activation and expansion. This response is exaggerated and Th1 biased, with resultant interferon-γ and IL-2 production from these T cells.
- There is concomitant macrophage activation and immune granuloma formation, which is enhanced by interferon-γ.
- Granulomas cause increased local fibroblast stimulation and, hence, fibrosis (see Box 33.1 for differential diagnosis of granuloma).
- Metabolic activity of macrophages causes raised angiotensin-converting enzyme (ACE) levels in serum, lung tissue, and bronchoalveolar fluid. Increase in T-cell activity causes B-lymphocyte stimulation, which can cause raised serum immunoglobulins and immune complexes.
- In most patients, the response resolves over 2–5 years.

Delayed-type hypersensitivity reactions are depressed in sarcoidosis. This is thought to be due to the migration of lymphocytes to the active compartment (lungs), with resultant peripheral blood lymphopenia and a decreased response to tuberculin. This is not clinically significant.

Sarcoid-like reactions are reported in association with malignancy in HIV patients starting on antiretroviral therapy, and in patients receiving A-interferon therapy (very rare). These conditions do not usually require specific therapy.

Box 33.1 Differential diagnosis of granuloma on lung biopsy

- Sarcoidosis
- Specific exposures
  - Berylliosis
  - Hypersensitivity pneumonitis
  - Pneumoconiosis, e.g., silicosis
  - Medication reaction, e.g., α-interferon therapy
- Infections
  - Tuberculosis
  - Tertiary syphilis
  - Brucellosis
  - Fungal infections—coccidioidomycosis
  - Schistosomiasis
  - Cat scratch fever
  - Leprosy
- Vasculitis
  - Wegener's granulomatosis
  - Giant cell arteritis
  - Polyarteritis nodosa
  - Takayasu's arteritis
- Autoimmune mediated
  - De Quervain's thyroiditis
  - Crohn's disease
  - Primary biliary cirrhosis
- Immunodeficiency
  - Hypogammaglobulinemia
  - HIV on HARRT
- Malignancy
  - Lymphoma
- Miscellaneous
  - Granulomatous orchitis
  - Langerhans' cell histiocytosis

Further information

Grunewald J, Eklund A (2007). Sex-specific manifestations of Lofgren's syndrome. *Am J Respir Crit Care Med* **175**:40–44.

Newman LS, Rose CS, Bresnitz EA, et al. (2004). A case control etiologic study of sarcoidosis: environmental and occupational risk factors. *Am J Respir Crit Care Med* **170**:1324–1330.

Rossman MD, Thompson B, Frederick M, et al. (2003). HLA-DRB1*1101: a significant risk factor for sarcoidosis in blacks and whites. *Am J Hum Genet* **73**:720–735.

Schürmann M, Lympany PA, Reichel P, et al. (2000). Familial sarcoidosis is linked to the major histocompatability complex region. *Am J Respir Crit Care Med* **162**: 8 61–864.

Chest disease: clinical features

More than 90% of patients with sarcoidosis have thoracic involvement, with an abnormal CXR. Pulmonary sarcoidosis can be an incidental CXR finding.

Clinical features

There are probably at least two distinct clinical courses.

Löfgren's syndrome

This mild, acute disease is usually nonprogressive. It presents with fever, bilateral hilar lymphadenopathy, erythema nodosum, and arthralgia.

Löfgren's syndrome occurs particularly among Caucasians. It has a good prognosis and resolves completely and spontaneously in 80% of patients within 1–2 years. A minority may develop chronic disease.

Persistent progressive infiltrative lung disease (see Table 33.1)

Hilar/mediastinal lymphadenopathy

This condition may be asymptomatic or cause cough or chest pain. It is often bilateral and symmetrical, but can be unilateral and asymmetrical. Lymphadenopathy can be associated with systemic symptoms of malaise and arthralgia, which are helped by treatment with nonsteroidal anti-inflammatory drugs. The disease has a benign course.

It is important to exclude other causes of lymphadenopathy such as TB and lymphoma (see Box 33.2); HRCT and lymph node aspirate or biopsy may be needed.

In stage I disease, 85% of patients resolve spontaneously over 2 years, and 15% develop lung infiltrates. The average time for bilateral hilar lymphadenopathy resolution is 8 months. No systemic therapy is required in asymptomatic patients.

Interstitial lung involvement

This form may be asymptomatic or cause morbidity and mortality, with dyspnea, cough, chest ache, or frank pain and malaise. There are pulmonary infiltrates on CXR.

The lungs can return to normal over time, or disease can progress to fibrosis and respiratory failure. Lung function tests may be normal or show a restrictive defect with reduced diffusing capacity.

Differential diagnosis includes other interstitial lung disease, malignancy, and infection.

Table 33.1 Radiological classification of thoracic sarcoidosis

Stage 0	Normal
Stage I	Hilar lymphadenopathy
Stage II	Hilar lymphadenopathy and parenchymal infiltrate
Stage III	Parenchymal infiltrate
Stage IV	Fibrosis

Seeing a patient with possible sarcoidosis in the clinic

- Make diagnosis—clinically, HRCT ± histology
- Assess extent, severity, and presence of extrapulmonary involvement—CXR, PFT, ECG, eyes, rash, renal function, serum calcium, liver function, immunoglobulins, and ACE (the latter two can be raised in active sarcoidosis)
- Is it stable or progressive? Check CXR, pulmonary function test (PFT) (vital capacity [VC] and DLCO), oximetry, ACE, BUN and creatinine (if there is renal involvement)
- Treatment?

Box 33.2 Differential diagnosis of bilateral hilar lymphadenopathy on CXR

- Sarcoidosis
- Berylliosis
- Tuberculosis
- Coccidioidomycosis and histoplasmosis
- Lymphoma
- Leukemia
- Hypogammaglobulinemia and recurrent infections

Further information

Judson MA, Baughman RP, Thompson BW, et al. (2003). Two year prognosis of sarcoidosis: the ACCESS experience. *Sarcoidosis Vasc Diffuse Lung Dis* **20**:204–211.

Chest disease: management

Diagnosis is based on a characteristic clinical picture, plus:
• Histological evidence of noncaseating granuloma in any tissue
• Characteristic picture on imaging (thoracic HRCT scan or gallium scan)
• Lymphocytosis on bronchoalveolar lavage (BAL)

Other diseases capable of producing a similar clinical and histological picture, particularly tuberculosis and lymphoma, should be excluded.

Investigations

HRCT

HRCT shows micronodules in a subpleural and bronchovascular distribution. There is also fissural nodularity and bronchial distortion. Irregular linear opacities, ground-glass shadowing related to bronchovascular bundles, and nodular or ill-defined shadows are also apparent.

Air-trapping due to small-airway granulomata is common. Endobronchial disease occurs in 55%. Honeycomb lung may be evident. Hilar and mediastinal lymphadenopathy is seen.

Bronchoscopy (transbronchial biopsy, bronchial biopsy, or BAL)

Bronchoscopy may not be necessary if there is no diagnostic doubt clinically and radiologically. A positive yield of bronchial biopsy is 41%–57%; it is higher if abnormal mucosa is visible. A positive yield of transbronchial biopsy is 40%–90%.

BAL in sarcoidosis generally shows a CD4:CD8 ratio of >3.5. If this test is not available, a lymphocytosis of $>2 \times 10^5$ cells/mL supports the diagnosis but is not diagnostic. (Lymphocytosis can also be seen in UIP, COP, hypersensitivity pneumonitis, and smokers.)

Others

• **Mediastinoscopy** for central or paratracheal nodes or open lung biopsy: 90% positive yield. May be necessary to exclude lymphoma
• **Biopsy other affected areas** such as skin, liver, etc., if indicated, as these may be easier to biopsy to make a diagnosis
• **Mantoux test** may show minimal reaction or grade 0 in sarcoid (peripheral cutaneous anergy to tuberculin due to migration of T cells to active sites of disease). Thus a positive Mantoux test makes sarcoidosis less likely as a diagnosis, although it does not necessarily make tuberculosis more likely as the diagnosis.
• **Kveim test** is no longer generally available because of the risks of transmissible diseases. It involved injecting homogenized splenic tissue from a patient with sarcoidosis to see if a granulomatous reaction occurred.

Monitoring disease

There is no single measurement to assess all the aspects of patients with sarcoidosis. Clinical examination and serial measurements are key.

- **PFT** DLCO provides the most sensitive measurement of change, although a properly performed VC is probably adequate for clinical purposes. It may improve with steroids.
- **CXR** may improve with time or treatment.
- **ACE** levels increased in up to 80% of patients with acute sarcoidosis. Levels become normal as disease resolves. An elevated level indicates persistent disease, although corticosteroids suppress ACE levels, so when steroids are stopped, levels usually increase, unrelated to sarcoidosis activity. This is not a specific test. False positives include TB. Lymphoma is associated with a low level.
- **Calcium** may rise with active sarcoidosis or in the summer months. This may cause renal impairment, so BUN and creatinine should also be checked.
- **BAL** is not performed routinely to assess progress of sarcoidosis, but changes in proportions of cells seen in lavage would indicate improvement. Increased neutrophils in BAL are associated wth fibrotic pulmonary disease,
- **PET** scan may be positive in areas of disease activity. PET is not reliable for studying the brain or heart. There are limited studies of serial data.
- **Gallium scan** is rarely used now, as it is nonspecific and expensive. Areas of active inflammation are positive, with a classic "panda" pattern. Positive areas soon become negative with steroid use. The gallium scan is bowel and liver positive, so disease cannot be charted in these areas.

General management

Most patients with pulmonary sarcoidosis do not require treatment (but see Box 33.3). Asymptomatic CXR infiltrates are usually monitored.

> **Box 33.3 Indications for drug treatment**
>
> - Increasing symptoms, deteriorating PFTs, and worsening CXR infiltrates
> - Cardiac sarcoidosis
> - Neurosarcoidosis
> - Sight-threatening ocular sarcoidosis
> - Hypercalcemia
> - Lupus pernio
> - Splenic, hepatic, or renal sarcoidosis.

Starting drug treatment

- When required, treatment is usually initiated with corticosteroids.
- Give high doses, such as 40 mg prednisone/day, to control active disease. Patients rarely need more than 40 mg/day. Usually give this high dose for 4 weeks and then reduce it if there has been a response
- **Maintenance dose** of around 5–15 mg, to control symptoms. Leave patient on this dose for a few months and then slowly reduce steroid dose further. Maintain on low dose of prednisone (5–7.5 mg/day or alternate days) for a prolonged period of 6–12 months to consolidate resolution before considering complete withdrawal
- Some patients, especially those with progressive pulmonary sarcoidosis, may require longer treatment
- **Relapses** often occur when treatment is stopped and may require the reintroduction of steroids or an increase of steroid dose. Duration and dose of steroids are dictated by the site and response to treatment.
- Avoid futile high-dose steroid treatment for end-stage disease, such as honeycomb lung.
- If steroid treatment fails or sarcoidosis is life threatening, other immunosuppressive regimes may be indicated. Pulsed high-dose intravenous methylprednisolone and cyclophosphamide are options for refractory sarcoidosis. Infliximab is also sometimes very effective.
- In cases where prolonged immunosuppression is required or if corticosteroid side effects cannot be tolerated, other immunosuppressive drugs should be considered. Possibilities include azathioprine and methotrexate. There is more information on methotrexate than azathioprine in treating sarcoidosis.
- Patients who have troublesome symptoms related to sarcoidosis, such as arthralgia, skin disease, fever, sweats, ocular symptoms, and systemic symptoms such as fatigue, may require symptomatic corticosteroid treatment. Lower initial doses such as 20 mg/day are likely sufficient to gain symptomatic control, and doses can then be reduced.
- Prescribe gastric and bone protection with steroids when necessary.

Extrathoracic disease

Extrathoracic disease varies according to ethnic origin and gender of the patient.

Systemic symptoms are common, such as fever, sweats, loss of appetite, weight loss, fatigue, malaise, chest pain, dyspnea, and cough. Polyarthralgia often affects the knees, ankles, wrists, and elbows and can be improved by NSAID treatment. Fatigue is a common problem.

Hypercalcemia

Granulomas convert vitamin D_3 to active 1,25 dihydroxycholecalciferol, causing enhanced calcium absorption from the intestine. Sunlight also increases levels of vitamin D and calcium. High calcium levels may cause systemic effects and are often associated with renal damage and hypercalciuria. Hypercalcemia is more common in Caucasians and in men.

Treatment

Steroids are given, often at low dose once the calcium level is controlled. Decrease dose when the calcium level is satisfactory.

Some patients may only need steroids during the summer months. Hydroxychloroquine can also be used.

Skin

25% of patients have skin involvement. This is more common in women.
- *Erythema nodosum* consists of raised papules, nodules, or plaques, usually on shins. It has a tender, indurated, or bruised appearance. Papules are firm and often have a shiny appearance. Nodular change of different tattoo colors is recognized and characteristic of sarcoidosis. Sarcoid tissue may arise in old scars or cause scar hypertrophy.
- *Lupus pernio* is a bluish tinge that occurs on the nose, cheeks, and ears. It is associated with chronic disease.

Diagnosis

Sarcoidosis affecting the skin is usually easily biopsied.

Treatment

Treat initially with topical preparations. Treat lupus pernio with systemic steroids. Hydroxychloroquine or MTX may be necessary. The role of long-term tetracyclines for cutaneous sarcoidosis is under investigation.

Eye

Eye involvement is common, occurring in over 25% of cases, especially women and African Americans.
- *Uveitis (acute or chronic), episcleritis, scleritis, glaucoma, conjunctivitis, and retinal involvement* can occur. It may be asymptomatic or cause painful, red eye with photophobia, lacrimation, and blurred vision. The pupil is irregular or constricted. Untreated, it can cause visual impairment.
- *Lacrimal involvement* in sarcoidosis produces keratoconjunctivitis sicca— dry eye with diminished tear secretion, causing painful, red eyes. Treat with artificial tears.

Diagnosis

Assessment is made by an ophthalmologist with slit-lamp examination for all patients. Mild asymptomatic eye involvement is common. Conjunctival biopsy may be needed with no evidence of sarcoid features elsewhere.

Treatment

Local steroids are commonly used if there is no other indication for systemic steroids. However, if there is no response, systemic steroids should be used. Methotrexate is commonly used for chronic disease.

Heart

Cardiac sarcoidosis occurs in 5% of patients with pulmonary disease. Postmortem studies show cardiac sarcoidosis being present in 25% of patients, so it is often undiagnosed.

Patients may present with chest pain or, more commonly, have conduction defects on ECG. These may be benign and asymptomatic, like first-degree heart block, but more significant arrhythmias can occur, the first indication of which may be sudden death.

Myocardial granulomata can occur in any part of the heart. Commonly they occur in the interventricular septum, where they can affect nodal and conducting tissue.

The left ventricular wall can be affected, with fibrosis causing reduced compliance and contractile difficulties, leading to cardiac failure. Aneurysms can form, and pericarditis can occur.

Valvular dysfunction due to infiltration of the papillary muscles is rare. The clinical course can be uncertain.

Diagnosis

The echocardiogram may show signs of cardiomyopathy, usually restrictive. MRI, technetium scan, or gallium scan show nonsegmental fixed defects. Biopsy is diagnostic but can be difficult, as sarcoidosis is patchy; it is not recommended in general. ECG and a 24-hour Holter monitor may be helpful in investigation. PET scanning can be useful.

Treatment

Cardiac sarcoidosis must be treated with systemic steroids 20–40 mg prednisolone/day, which improve symptoms and ECG and echocardiographic features. Dosage should be slowly reduced, although intractable arrhythmias may need continued high dosage. The patient may need other immunosuppressants. Use Holter monitoring to look for arrhythmias.

A pacemaker and defibrillator should be considered in patients with significant arrythmias, independent of use of systemic therapy for the sarcoidosis. Heart transplant may be necessary.

In clinic

Consider performing a screening ECG on all patients with sarcoidosis. Use Holter monitoring on all symptomatic patients.

Kidney

Renal involvement occurs in up to a third of patients with sarcoidosis. Rarely patients can present with renal failure, obstructive uropathy, nephrolithiasis, or a urinary tract disorder. Nephrocalcinosis is a common cause of chronic renal failure. Renal involvement is often associated with hypercalcemia or other manifestations of sarcoidosis.

Diagnosis

Renal biopsy with granulomata found in the interstitium confirms the diagnosis, but this is rarely needed in this context. Search for pulmonary sarcoidosis.

Treatment

Give steroids ± hydroxychloroquine for hypercalcemia.

CNS

The CNS is involved in 4%–18% of sarcoidosis patients. Any part of the peripheral or central nervous system can be affected, presenting as a peripheral nerve or cranial nerve lesion. Most common is lower motor neuron facial nerve palsy, with optic nerve involvement being the next most common feature.

Mononeuritis multiplex is recognized. It may be less specific, with psychiatric features. Hypothalamic granulomata may cause diabetes insipidus, appetite disturbance, or hypersomnolence.

Diagnosis

Diagnosis is difficult, but may be made easier if there is another sign of systemic sarcoidosis, e.g., bilateral hilar lymphadenopathy. Lumbar puncture may show a raised CSF ACE and an increased lymphocyte count. Confirm with biopsy if possible, of cerebral or meningeal tissue, if there is no pulmonary involvement.

Treatment

These conditions must be treated with steroids, but are often quite resistant to treatment. Further immunosuppressants may be required.

Musculoskeletal

Arthralgia is common in sarcoidosis, but arthritis is unusual. Arthralgia commonly affects the ankles and feet, but also the hands, wrists, and elbows. Subacute, proximal myopathy can occur, as well as bone cysts, especially of terminal phalanges. The latter show little response to systemic steroids.

Diagnosis

Granuloma is seen on muscle biopsy.

Treatment

Give NSAIDs; steroids may be necessary.

GI

Sixty percent of liver biopsies on patients with sarcoidosis show granuloma, which is frequently asymptomatic. Hepatomegaly is unusual, but can result in portal fibrosis and cirrhosis. LFTs are suggestive if findings are 3 times the normal levels, especially alkaline phosphatase or γGT.

Diagnosis
Biopsy is required.

Treatment
Give steroids for symptomatic disease, including hyperbilirubinemia. These may reduce the size of the liver and improve LFTs.

Hematological

Splenomegaly can occur and may be massive, causing abdominal discomfort. Massive spleen may occasionally require splenectomy to avoid rupture. Associated anemia, neutropenia, and thrombocytopenia can occur. Lymphopenia is often seen.

ENT

Nasal or laryngeal granuloma is found, along with sinus invasion. There is parotid and other salivary gland enlargement, as well as dry mouth.

Rarely is sarcoidosis associated with breast disease or ovarian or testicular masses.

Further information

American Thoracic Society/European Respiratory Society/World Association of Sarcoidosis and Other Granulomatous Disorders statement on sarcoidosis. *Eur Respir J* 1999; **14:** 735–737.

Baughman RP, Drent M, Kavuru M, et al. (2006). Infliximab therapy in patients with chronic sarcoidosis and pulmonary involvement. *Am J Respir Crit Care Med* **174**:795–802.

Baughman RP, Lower EE (2005). Therapy for sarcoidosis. *Eur Respir Mon* **32**:301–315.

Paramothayan S, Jones PW (2002). Corticosteroid therapy in pulmonary sarcoidosis: a systematic review. *JAMA* **287**:1301–1307.

Idiopathic interstitial pneumonias

Overview

Definition

The *idiopathic interstitial pneumonias* (IIPs) comprise a group of diffuse lung diseases of unknown etiology that primarily involve the *pulmonary interstitium*—the area between the alveolar epithelium and capillary endothelium—as well as the septal and bronchovascular tissues that make up the fibrous framework of the lung. While primarily interstitial processes, the airways, vasculature, and alveolar airspaces may all be involved. The underlying pathological process is one of varying degrees of inflammation and fibrosis.

The terminology used to describe the IIPs may be confusing; these conditions have been subject to much classification and reclassification, reflecting the lack of understanding of their underlying etiology and pathogenesis. Idiopathic pulmonary fibrosis (IPF) is the most common IIP. The other IIPs are distinct disease entities with differing prognoses and are rare.

Diagnosis

Diagnosis is made from a combination of clinical features (see Table 34.1), HRCT, and histological patterns—they are distinguished from other causes of diffuse lung disease by the absence of an alternative cause of disease, i.e., are idiopathic (see Chapter 5). Histopathologic patterns are the strongest predictors of outcome and form the basis for the current classification of IIPs.

Surgical lung biopsy is recommended for most cases of suspected IIP when a definitive diagnosis is required, with the exception of patients exhibiting typical clinical and HRCT features of IPF.

Transbronchial biopsies have a limited role because of the patchy distribution of the IIPs, although biopsies may be useful in the exclusion of other causes of diffuse lung disease (e.g., sarcoidosis).

Treatment

The optimal treatment of many of the IIPs is poorly defined, and there is a general lack of supportive data from randomized, controlled trials. Steroids and immunosuppression constitute the mainstay of treatment, but these can have significant side effects and are often ineffective.

The conditions currently included within the classification of idiopathic interstitial pneumonias, together with their key clinical, imaging, and histological features and prognosis, are presented in Table 34.1 and discussed in detail in the remainder of this chapter. They are listed in order of frequency.

Further information

American Thoracic Society/European Respiratory Society International Multidisciplinary Consensus Classification of the Idiopathic Interstitial Pneumonias. *Am J Respir Crit Care Med* 2002; **165**:277–304.

Table 34.1 Idiopathic interstitial pneumonias: summary of key features

Idiopathic pulmonary fibrosis (IPF)	*Onset* is over years *HRCT* shows fibrosis, honeycombing, minimal ground-glass, subpleural, and basal distribution *Histology* shows areas of interstitial fibrosis (including foci of proliferating fibroblasts) interspersed with normal lung (temporal and spatial heterogeneity), minimal inflammation *Prognosis* is poor
Nonspecific interstitial pneumonia (NSIP)	*Onset* is over months–years *HRCT* shows diffuse ground-glass, fine reticulation, minimal honeycombing *Histology* shows varying degrees of inflammation and fibrosis, more uniform appearance than UIP *Prognosis* is variable
Cryptogenic organizing pneumonia (COP) (Idiopathic bronchiolitis obliterans organizing pneumonia [BOOP])	*Onset* is over weeks to months *HRCT* shows areas of consolidation; basal, subpleural, and peribronchial predominance *Histology* shows alveolar spaces "plugged" with granulation tissue, ± extension into bronchioles *Prognosis* is generally good
Acute interstitial pneumonia (AIP)	Many similarities to ARDS *Onset* is over days *HRCT* shows diffuse ground-glass and patchy consolidation *Histology* shows diffuse alveolar damage: interstitial edema, intra-alveolar hyaline membranes, followed by fibroblast proliferation and interstitial fibrosis *Prognosis* is poor
Respiratory bronchiolitis –associated interstitial lung disease (RB-ILD)	Occurs in smokers *Onset* is over years Symptoms are usually mild *HRCT* shows centrilobular nodules, ground-glass, thick-walled airways *Histology* shows pigmented macrophages in bronchioles *Prognosis* is good
Desquamative interstitial pneumonia (DIP)	Occurs in smokers *Onset* is over weeks–months *HRCT* shows ground-glass appearance *Histology* shows pigmented macrophages in alveolar air spaces, temporally uniform appearance *Prognosis* is good
Lymphoid interstitial pneumonia (LIP)	*Onset* is over years *HRCT* shows ground-glass appearance, often reticulation and perivascular cysts *Histology* shows diffuse interstitial lymphoid infiltrates *Prognosis* is variable

Idiopathic pulmonary fibrosis (IPF): diagnosis

Definition

IPF is an IIP characterized histologically by the presence of a UIP histopathologic pattern on surgical lung biopsy. However, the pathologic pattern of UIP is not unique to IPF and may occur in the context of other diseases of known cause (see Pathophysiology, below).

Epidemiology

Prevalence figures vary from 6 to 14 per 100,000, although prevalence may be 175/100,000 in patients >75 years old. IPF is slightly more common in males. Mean age at presentation is 67. A familial form is well described but rare.

Pathophysiology

The development of fibrosis was previously thought to reflect a response to chronic inflammation resulting from an unknown initial injury. This key role of inflammation in the pathogenesis of UIP has been questioned, however, in part because of observations that inflammation is not a major feature on pathologic specimens and responses to "anti-inflammatory" treatment with steroids are often poor.

An alternative theory is that repeated lung injury leads to abnormal wound healing and fibrosis. This concept of fibrosis without inflammation has been demonstrated in animal models and other human diseases. The nature of the lung injury remains unknown.

Cytokine production (e.g., plasminogen activator inhibitors, matrix metalloproteinases, transforming growth factor β) by alveolar epithelial cells may play an important role in the development of fibrosis. Host genetic factors are also likely to be important in modifying the wound-healing response.

Clinical features

- Typically presents with gradual-onset exertional breathlessness and cough; average of 9–24 months of symptoms prior to presentation
- 5% of patients are said to be asymptomatic
- Arthralgia occurs in about 20%
- Fine basal, late inspiratory crackles
- Clubbing may occur
- Cyanosis and cor pulmonale occur in severe disease.

Investigations

Blood tests

Look for mildly raised ESR and CRP. Positive rheumatoid factor (RF) and/or ANA may occur at low titers in the absence of associated connective tissue disease.

PFTs

Typically PFTs reveal a restrictive pattern with reduced vital capacity and diffusing capacity. Smokers may exhibit a coexisting obstructive defect. Oxygen saturations are frequently reduced, particularly on exertion.

CXR

CXR shows peripheral and basal reticular shadowing that may extend to other zones, sometimes with honeycombing. Rarely CXR may be normal.

HRCT

HRCT features include bilateral, peripheral, and subpleural reticulation, with honeycombing, traction bronchiectasis, architectural distortion, and minimal or no ground-glass change. Features are predominantly basal initially, and more extensive later in the disease course.

The extent of disease on CT correlates with physiological impairment and prognosis. Predominant ground-glass appearance suggests an IIP other than UIP.

BAL

Typically BAL shows neutrophilia, sometimes mild eosinophilia. Marked eosinophilia (>20%) or lymphocytosis (>50%) should raise the possibility of an alternative diagnosis.

Lung biopsy (surgical lung biopsy via VATS or thoracotomy) is indicated if the diagnosis is in doubt.

Histology

The usual interstitial pneumonia (UIP) pattern of fibrosing interstitial pneumonia is characterized by temporal and spatial heterogeneity: patches of active fibroblast foci are interspersed with honeycombing and architectural distortion (reflecting chronic scarring) and areas of normal lung. Interstitial inflammation is minimal.

This histopathologic pattern is not solely restricted to IPF and, when found, additional potential clinical diagnoses should be considered, including asbestosis, connective tissue disease, drug reactions, and hypersensitivity pneumonitis, among others.

Diagnosis

Diagnosis can be confidently made in most cases on the basis of clinical and HRCT findings. Lung biopsy is not generally required in patients with typical clinical and HRCT features of UIP, but should be considered in the presence of unusual clinical or radiographic features (e.g., predominant ground-glass appearance, nodules, consolidation, upper lobe involvement on HRCT, or features in a young patient).

When required, a surgical lung biopsy (VATS or thoracotomy) should be obtained. Transbronchial biopsies can only very rarely provide a specific diagnosis.

Differential diagnosis

- Left ventricular failure
- Asbestosis (may mimic IPF clinically, radiologically, and histologically; occupational history and presence of pleural plaques may suggest this diagnosis)
- Connective tissue disease (may mimic IPF clinically, radiologically, and histologically and precede extrapulmonary manifestations of disease)
- Chronic hypersensitivity pneumonitis (suggested by typically upper to mid-zone predominance, micronodules, ground-glass features, areas of reduced attenuation)
- Drug-induced lung disease

Prognosis

Prognosis is poor. Some patients decline rapidly, others remain stable or decline slowly over years. However, several studies have demonstrated a median survival of 2.5–3.5 years.

Improved survival may be associated with young age, less advanced disease, female gender, and absence of advanced fibrosis and honeycombing on HRCT. Death is commonly due to respiratory failure and/or infection. Risk of developing lung cancer is increased.

Causes of acute deterioration in patients with previously stable IPF

- Acute exacerbation of IPF—mechanism is poorly understood; biopsy often shows diffuse alveolar damage
- Pneumothorax—collapsed lung is often relatively resistant to re-expansion, making treatment difficult
- Infection (especially if immunocompromised), e.g., PCP
- Pulmonary embolism
- Acute deterioration may also occur postoperatively following major surgery, e.g., cardiac or orthopedic—the reasons for this are unclear.

IPF: management

There is currently no evidence from well-controlled trials that any drug treatment improves survival or quality of life. Therefore, the decision to treat should be approached with all available information reviewed with the patient. Specific drug treatment may not be indicated or appropriate in all patients.

The following types of management should be considered for all patients with IPF.

Supportive treatment

Consider use of home oxygen if the patient is limited by breathlessness and in respiratory failure. Use of oxygen during exercise may improve exercise tolerance. Encourage participation in a pulmonary rehabilitation program if there are no contraindications.

Cough may be troublesome—consider a treatment trial of modest doses of oral corticosteroids.

Lung transplantation

Because successful lung transplantation is the only therapy shown to prolong survival in patients with IPF, for the eligible patient, referral for consideration of transplantation is appropriate even early in the disease course. Single-lung transplantation results in an 80% survival rate at 1 year and 55% at 3 years.

Conventional drug treatments

Oral corticosteroids

Prior to the recent reclassification of IIPs, studies suggested that oral corticosteroids might improve lung function (in around 20%–30% of patients) and symptoms (in around 50%). However, these studies probably included patients with conditions other than IPF that are associated with a better treatment response and prognosis (e.g., NSIP).

Significant side effects may affect at least a quarter of patients (e.g., hyperglycemia necessitating insulin, osteoporosis, myopathy, peptic ulcer disease, cataracts, raised intraocular pressure, psychosis). Consider prophylaxis against PCP.

Azathioprine in combination with corticosteroids may improve survival, though this is unproven. Data supporting this approach may reflect studies undertaken on individuals with IIPs other than UIP. Potential side effects include liver, hematologic, and systemic abnormalities. Use of azathioprine alone has not been investigated.

N-acetyl cysteine (NAC) has been studied with the combination of azathioprine and corticosteroids and appears to be associated with a slower rate of physiologic progression and fewer side effects compared to azathioprine and corticosteroids alone. However, azathioprine and corticosteroids alone have yet to be proved beneficial.

Cyclophosphamide does not appear to improve survival, and side effects are common.

Initial assessment and decision to treat

On presentation, all patients should have full clinical assessment, pulmonary function tests, and HRCT chest. In general, decisions regarding treatment are based on patient preference, severity of disease at baseline and rate of progression of symptoms, and changes in pulmonary function.

Specific treatment options include supportive therapy alone, lung transplantation, conventional drug therapy with corticosteroids, azathioprine, and NAC. Available off-label medications with a potential or theoretic benefit and enrollment in a treatment trial can also be useful.

Further information

American Thoracic Society/European Respiratory Society (2000). International Consensus Statement Idiopathic Pulmonary Fibrosis: Diagnosis and Treatment. *Am J Respir Crit Care Med* **161**:646–664.
Demedts M, Behr J, Buhl R, et al.; IFIGENIA Study Group (2005). High-dose acetyl cysteine in idiopathic pulmonary fibrosis. *N Engl J Med* **353**:2229–2242.

Nonspecific interstitial pneumonia (NSIP)

Definition
NSIP is an IIP with a surgical lung biopsy pattern of NSIP. The histopathologic pattern of NSIP may be seen in the setting of an IIP or in association with other systemic conditions, most notably, connective tissue diseases and hypersensitivity pneumonitis.

Epidemiology
Typically, NSIP affects younger patients than those with IPF; the age of onset is 40–50 years.

Clinical features
There are few specific clinical features that help distinguish NSIP from other IIPs. Described features include the following:
- Breathlessness, cough
- Weight loss.
- Onset is gradual or subacute; typical symptom duration before diagnosis varies from 0.5 to 3 years.
- Crackles at lung bases, later more extensive
- Clubbing occurs in a small proportion of patients.

Investigations
- **HRCT** frequently shows diffuse, symmetrical ground-glass change, with or without reticulation and traction bronchiectasis. The confluent and homogeneous appearance contrasts with the patchy, heterogeneous distribution seen in UIP. Honeycombing is rare.
- **PFTs** typically indicate a restrictive pattern and decreased diffusing capacity. Desaturation on exertion is common.
- **BAL** lymphocytosis is common.
- *Lung biopsy*
- Investigations to exclude underlying disease (see Differential diagnosis, below).

Histology
The nonspecific pneumonia (NSIP) pattern has variable features, ranging from a predominantly "cellular" pattern (mild–moderate interstitial inflammation, no fibrosis) to a "fibrotic" pattern (interstitial fibrosis, more homogeneous appearance than in UIP, and lack of fibroblast foci or honeycombing, lung architecture may be relatively preserved). Features of both NSIP and UIP are sometimes seen on biopsies from the same individual—in such cases, the prognosis is dictated by the presence of UIP.

When this histopathologic pattern is found, it should prompt consideration of multiple clinical diagnoses, including hypersensitivity pneumonitis, connective tissue disease, and drug reactions, among others.

Diagnosis

Clinical and HRCT features are suggestive, but surgical lung biopsy is required for a definitive diagnosis. Consider the presence of associated diseases (Differential diagnosis, below).

Differential diagnosis

- Connective tissue disease (NSIP may be the first manifestation of disease)
- Hypersensitivity pneumonitis
- Drug-induced lung disease
- Infection
- Immunodeficiency (including HIV, after bone marrow transplant, chemotherapy)

Management

Treatment is with corticosteroids (see p. 700 for examples). Additional immunosuppressive agents may be considered in patients who fail to respond to corticosteroids alone (see pp. 698–725).

Prognosis

Prognosis is variable. Patients with NSIP have a generally better prognosis and greater response to steroids than that of patients with IPF. Most patients improve or remain stable on treatment. The "cellular" pattern on biopsy is associated with a good prognosis. Disease progression to death does occur.

Cryptogenic organizing pneumonia (COP)

COP was formerly known as bronchiolitis obliterans organizing pneumonia (BOOP).

Definition

COP is an IIP characterized by the presence of organizing pneumonia on surgical lung biopsy. Use of the term *BOOP* is no longer recommended, as it erroneously suggests a primary airways disease and is easily confused with bronchiolitis obliterans, a distinct disease entity. In addition to the "cryptogenic" form, the pathologic pattern of organizing pneumonia may also occur in the context of other diseases (see below).

Epidemiology

COP is more common in nonsmokers. Mean age of onset is 55 years, although COP can occur at any age. It affects males and females equally.

Clinical features

- Typically short (<3 month) history of breathlessness and dry cough, often with malaise, fevers, weight loss, and myalgia. COP often presents as a chest infection that is slow to resolve, after several courses of antibiotics.
- Breathlessness is usually mild, although a minority of patients experience severe breathlessness and rapid onset of respiratory failure and sometimes death.
- Examination may be normal or reveal crackles. Clubbing is absent.

Investigations

- **Blood tests** show raised CRP and ESR, and a mild neutrophilia
- **PFTs** Mild–moderate restrictive pattern is typical, but mild airways obstruction may also be seen in smokers. Mild hypoxemia is common.
- **CXR** classically shows patchy consolidation, sometimes with nodular shadowing. May present as a solitary mass on CXR
- **HRCT** shows areas of consolidation with air bronchograms, sometimes with associated ground-glass opacities or small nodules. Often basal, subpleural, and peribronchial. May migrate spontaneously. Reticulation may suggest poor response to treatment.
- **TBB** often confirms the diagnosis, but the relatively small tissue samples may not effectively exclude associated diseases. TBB may be adequate in patients with typical clinical and HRCT features who are subsequently followed closely. Surgical lung biopsy is required for a definitive diagnosis.
- **BAL** if performed, shows lymphocytosis, neutrophilia, and eosinophilia.

Histology

- An organizing pneumonia pattern is seen, consisting of alveolar spaces "plugged" with granulation tissue (fibrin, collagen-containing fibroblasts, often with inflammatory cells), sometimes with extension up into the bronchiolar lumen. The pattern is patchy, with lack of architectural distortion. Examine for evidence of an underlying cause, e.g., infection and vasculitis. This histopathologic pattern is not solely restricted to COP and, when found, other potential clinical diagnoses should be considered, including:

- Infection (including pneumonia, lung abscess, bronchiectasis)
- Drug reaction or radiotherapy
- Connective tissue disease (particularly myositis, rheumatoid arthritis, Sjögren's syndrome)
- Diffuse alveolar damage
- Hypersensitivity pneumonitis
- Eosinophilic pneumonia
- Inflammatory bowel disease
- Post-bone marrow transplant
- Lung malignancy or airways obstruction
- Pulmonary infarction.

Diagnosiss

Diagnosis is usually made on the basis of clinical and HRCT features and transbronchial biopsy. Surgical lung biopsy may be required in atypical cases or if an underlying disease is suspected. Remember that the histological finding of organizing pneumonia is nonspecific, so search for secondary causes (see list above). Lung cancers may be surrounded by patches of organizing pneumonia, and biopsy of these areas in patients with a solitary lung mass may give misleading results.

Differential diagnosis

- Infective consolidation
- Connective tissue disease, vasculitis
- Lymphoma, alveolar cell carcinoma
- Lung cancer (when COP presents as lung mass).

Management

Corticosteroids are the mainstay of treatment. Optimal dose and duration are unknown. Slowly taper over several months. Additional treatment with azathioprine or cyclophosphamide may be considered in patients with minimal response to steroids.

Prognosis

Prognosis is generally good. Most patients respond to steroids and improve within a week of starting treatment. Consider an alternative diagnosis (e.g., lymphoma) if there is no improvement on steroid doses >25 mg/day. Relapse may occur with the tapering of the steroid dose, and treatment courses of 6–12 months are usually required. A minority of patients improve spontaneously. Lack of steroid response and progressive respiratory failure and death are rare but well documented.

Further information

Cordier J-F (2000). Organising pneumonia. *Thorax* **55**:318–328.

Acute interstitial pneumonia (AIP)

Definition
AIP is a rapidly progressive form of IIP characterized histologically by diffuse alveolar damage (DAD). It was formerly known as Hamman–Rich syndrome, and is considered an idiopathic form of ARDS. The pathologic pattern of DAD is not restricted to AIP and also occurs in the context of ARDS, as well as in other disorders (see Differential diagnosis, p. 495).

Epidemiology
Occurrence is poorly described. Mean age of onset is 50, but AIP may occur at any age. Patients are often previously healthy.

Clinical features
- Often preceded by "viral-type" illness, with systemic symptoms, e.g., fevers, tiredness, myalgia, arthralgia
- Rapid onset (over days) of breathlessness; usually presents <3 weeks after symptom onset
- Widespread crackles on examination

Investigations
- *CXR* shows bilateral diffuse airspace shadowing with air bronchograms, progressing to widespread reticulation and ground-glass features; often spares costophrenic angles, heart borders, and hila
- *HRCT* shows bilateral diffuse ground-glass and patchy airspace consolidation in early stages; later traction bronchiectasis, cystic change, reticulation
- *PFTs* reveal a restrictive defect with a reduced diffusing capacity. Often there is profound hypoxia and respiratory failure.
- *BAL* reveals an increased number of total cells and red blood cells. BAL is nondiagnostic, but may be useful in excluding infection.
- *Lung biopsy* is required for a definitive diagnosis. Transbronchial biopsy may rarely be diagnostic; the risk of pneumothorax is higher in mechanically ventilated patients (about 10%), although serious complications are rare. Surgical lung biopsy is otherwise required.

Histology shows a diffuse alveolar-damage pattern: hyaline membranes, edema, interstitial inflammation, and alveolar septal thickening, progressing to organizing fibrosis and sometimes honeycombing. This histopathologic pattern is not restricted to AIP and, when found, other potential clinical diagnoses should be considered, including the causes of ARDS, connective tissue disease, and an accelerated decline of IPF, among others.

Diagnosis is based on a lung biopsy pattern of DAD and exclusion of other explanations.

Differential diagnosis
- ARDS (ARDS is of known cause, whereas AIP is idiopathic; often they are otherwise indistinguishable on clinical and histological grounds)
- Accelerated decline of IPF (with diffuse alveolar damage on biopsy)
- Connective tissue disease (causing diffuse alveolar damage)
- Diffuse infection (community-acquired pneumonia, PCP, CMV)
- Drug-induced lung disease
- Acute hypersensitivity pneumonitis
- Acute eosinophilic pneumonia
- Cardiogenic pulmonary edema
- Pulmonary hemorrhage/vasculitis

Management
No treatment has been demonstrated to be of benefit. In practice, treat infection (including consideration of unusual organisms) and consider steroids (often given at high dose, e.g., intravenous methyl-prednisolone). Provide high-flow oxygen.

ICU admission and mechanical ventilatory support are usually required.

Prognosis
Overall mortality is at least 50%, although it is difficult to predict in individuals. Survivors may stabilize, develop chronic, progressive interstitial lung disease, or experience recurrent exacerbations.

Respiratory bronchiolitis–associated interstitial lung disease (RB-ILD)

Definition
Respiratory bronchiolitis is a pathologic term referring to the accumulation of bronchiolar pigmented macrophages in cigarette smokers; it is asymptomatic in nearly all cases. A minority of smokers with respiratory bronchiolitis, however, develop a clinically identifiable form of interstitial lung disease known as respiratory bronchiolitis–associated interstitial lung disease (RB-ILD).

Epidemiology
RB-ILD invariably occurs in current or previous smokers, typically with >30 pack-years. Male–female incidence is 2:1. The usual age of onset is 30–40 years.

Clinical features
- Usually mild breathlessness and cough
- Small proportion have severe dyspnea and respiratory failure
- Often crackles on examination.

Investigations
- *PFTs* often show a restrictive or combined obstructive and restrictive picture, with mildly impaired diffusing capacity.
- *CXR* shows thick-walled bronchi, reticular or ground-glass change; it may be normal.
- *HRCT* shows centrilobular nodules, ground-glass change, thick-walled airways, often with associated centrilobular emphysema
- *BAL* typically reveals increased total cell numbers with pigmented alveolar macrophages.

Histology
A respiratory bronchiolitis pattern is seen, with the accumulation of pigmented brown macrophages in terminal bronchioles. There is patchy, bronchiolocentric distribution. These findings are frequently seen as an incidental finding in smokers, thus the diagnosis of RB-ILD requires consideration of clinical and imaging features in conjunction with histology.

Management
Smoking cessation is the mainstay of treatment. Corticosteroids are occasionally used, with uncertain benefit.

Prognosis
Prognosis is generally good, although there are limited available data. Patients who refrain from smoking tend to improve. Progression to severe fibrosis is not documented.

Desquamative interstitial pneumonia (DIP)

Definition
DIP is an IIP that occurs in smokers and is associated with the pathologic pattern of desquamative interstitial pneumonia: abundant pigmented macrophages located diffusely throughout alveolar airspaces. It may represent a more extensive form of RB-ILD, in which macrophages are restricted to peribronchiolar regions.

Epidemiology
DIP is very rare. The majority of patients are smokers. It typically occurs at age 30–50.

Clinical features
Onset of breathlessness and cough over weeks to months is typical. Clubbing is common.

Investigations
- *PFTs* Mild restrictive pattern is common, sometimes with reduced diffusing capacity
- *CXR* may be normal, or may demonstrate reticular or ground-glass pattern, particularly affecting lower zones
- *HRCT* Ground glass is seen in all cases, typically with lower-zone or peripheral predominance. Reticulation and honeycombing may be present, although they tend to be mild.
- *BAL* shows an increase in pigmented macrophages.

Histology
A DIP pattern is seen, consisting of a diffuse accumulation of pigmented macrophages in alveolar air spaces. Changes are uniform.

Diagnosis
Clinical and HRCT features are nonspecific, and surgical lung biopsy is required for a definitive diagnosis.

Management
Smoking cessation is required, though universal improvement cannot be assured. Corticosteroids are often used, although their efficacy has not been studied.

Prognosis
Survival is 70% after 10 years. Improvement in ground-glass features on HRCT may correlate with response to treatment.
  A fluctuating course with remissions and relapses may occur.

Lymphoid interstitial pneumonia (LIP)

Definition
LIP is an IIP characterized by the presence of an LIP pattern: diffuse lymphoid infiltrates and lymphoid hyperplasia on surgical lung biopsy. It was previously considered a precursor to pulmonary lymphoma, and difficult to distinguish from lymphoma histologically. It is now considered a distinct entity and is thought to only very rarely undergo neoplastic transformation.

Epidemiology
LIP is very rare, occurring more commonly in women. It may occur at any age.

Clinical features
Gradual-onset breathlessness and cough occur over several years. Fever and weight loss may occur. Crackles may be heard on examination.

Investigations
- *Blood tests* Mild anemia may occur; a poly- or monoclonal increase in serum immunoglobulins is common.
- *CXR* shows lower-zone alveolar shadowing or diffuse honeycombing.
- *HRCT* shows predominant ground-glass change, often with reticulation and nodules. Unusual perivascular cystic change is often seen.
- *BAL* shows nonclonal lymphocytosis.
- Investigations to identify underlying cause (see Histology, below)

Histology
An LIP pattern is found, with diffuse interstitial lymphoid infiltrates, predominantly involving alveolar septa, sometimes with lymphoid hyperplasia or honeycombing. Cellular NSIP, follicular bronchiolitis, and lymphoma may give similar appearances. This histopathologic pattern is not solely restricted to LIP and, when found, other potential clinical diagnoses associated with diffuse lymphoid hyperplasia should be considered.

Differential diagnosis
- Idiopathic
- Connective tissue disease—particularly Sjögren's syndrome, also rheumatoid arthritis, SLE, among others
- Immunodeficiency, e.g., HIV
- Infection, e.g., PCP, hepatitis B

Management
Steroids are frequently used and often appear to improve symptoms.

Prognosis
Progression to extensive fibrosis occurs in around one-third of patients.

Hypersensitivity pneumonitis

Causes

Definition

Hypersensitivity pneumonitis (HP) is a group of diffuse parenchymal lung diseases caused by inhalation of organic or inorganic antigens (e.g., bacteria, fungi, protozoa, animal or insect protein, and chemicals) to which an individual has been previously sensitized. HP (previously termed extrinsic allergic alveolitis) is often divided into acute, subacute, and chronic forms based on the time course of presentation and the intensity of antigen exposure.

Acute HP often follows a short period of exposure to a high concentration of antigen, and is usually reversible. Subacute and chronic HP typically follows a period of chronic exposure to a low antigen dose and is less reversible.

Epidemiology

The exact prevalence is unknown and depends on various factors such as geography, local customs, season, occupation, pets, and other risk factors. Bird fancier's lung occurs in 20–20,000 per 100,000. From 6% to 21% of pigeon breeders and 0.4% to 9% of farmers may develop HP. An estimated 1% of workers exposed to diisocyanate vapor or aerosol develop HP.

Nonsmokers are more commonly affected by HP (the mechanism is unclear; it may reflect inhibition of alveolar macrophage or interference with cellar immunity or cytokine production). HP occurs less frequently in the pediatric population. Active smokers appear to have some protection from the development of HP.

Causes

Many different antigens have been reported to cause HP, ranging from the relatively common (bird fancier's lung and farmer's lung in the United States; summer-house HP in Japan) to the more unusual and exotic (shell lung, from proteins on mollusk shells; pituitary snuff-taker's disease; sericulturist's lung, from silk worm larvae proteins; sax lung, from yeast on saxophone mouthpieces). Important examples are listed in Table 35.1.

Pathophysiology

Pathogenesis of HP is not fully understood and may involve T-cell-mediated immunity and granuloma formation (type IV hypersensitivity) and less likely antibody–antigen immune complex formation (type III hypersensitivity). HP has also been shown to involve major histocompatibility complex (MHC, especially class II), chemokines (e.g., CXCL10), and cytokines (e.g., TNF-α).

It is not an atopic disease, and is not characterized by a rise in tissue eosinophils or IgE (type I hypersensitivity). This may in part be due to the small particle size of offending antigens, which tend to be deposited more distally in the airspaces than the larger particles associated with asthma. The disease likely occurs in patients predisposed to an immune reaction and who are exposed to an offending antigen.

Lung histology specimens typically reveal an airway-centered interstitial inflammatory infiltrate (cellular interstitial pneumonia), with granulomata, and organizing pneumonia.

Acute HP may involve interstitial and alveolar inflammation involving lymphocytes (mainly CD8+ T cells), neutrophils, mast cells, and macrophages that initially involve the bronchioles and later spread diffusely throughout the lung parenchyma.

Subacute HP characteristically involves noncaseating granulomata, which typically are ill defined and single (in contrast to sarcoidosis, in which granulomata are well defined and grouped subpleurally or near bronchi).

Chronic HP can present histologically as organizing pneumonia (OP), fibrotic or cellular nonspecific interstitial pneumonitis (NSIP), or usual interstitial pneumonitis (UIP). Often the pathology is characterized by interstitial fibrosis with thickening of the alveolar septae, and absence of or few granulomata and airways involvement, particularly if antigen exposure has ceased.

Table 35.1 Causes of hypersensitivity pneumonitis

Antigen	Sources	Diseases
Organisms		
Thermophilic actinomycetes (*Micropolyspora faeni, Thermoactinomyces vulgaris*), *Aspergillus* spp.	Soil; moldy hay; sugarcane; compost; mushrooms; contaminated water in humidifiers and air conditioners	Farmer's lung; bagassosis; compost lung; mushroom worker's lung;; humidifier lung
Aspergillus clavatus	Moldy barley	Malt worker's lung
Trichosporon cutaneum	House dust	Summer-house HP (Japan)
Cladosporium spp.	Ceiling mold	Hot-tub lung
Animal protein		
Bird proteins	Bloom on bird feathers and droppings	Bird fancier's lung
Rat proteins	Rat droppings	Rat lung
Chemical		
Toluene diisocyanate	Paints	Isocyanate HP

Diagnosis

Clinical features

Acute HP

- Symptoms present abruptly and include breathlessness, dry cough, chest tightness. Systemic symptoms (fever, chills, arthralgia, myalgia, frontal headache) occur 4–8 hours after intense or intermittent exposure to antigen. Respiratory failure with significant hypoxia can be seen with an intense exposure.
- Examination: bibasilar crackles and squeaks on auscultation, fever
- In the absence of ongoing exposure, symptoms resolve spontaneously within 1–3 days or can progress (subacute HP).

Subacute and chronic HP

- Progressive exertional breathlessness, cough with mucoid sputum, sometimes systemic symptoms (weight loss, fatigue, myalgia) over the course of months to years. A history of preceding acute episodes may not be present.
- Examination: tachypnea, diffuse crackles and squeaks on auscultation, clubbing (rare); cor pulmonale may develop in late disease

Investigations

Imaging: acute HP

- **CXR** is normal in up to 20%–48% of cases. Diffuse (1–3 mm) micronodules or infiltrates, sometimes ground-glass change, and apical sparing can be seen.
- **HRCT** shows patchy or diffuse ground-glass change and poorly defined nodules. There are areas of increased lucency (enhanced on expiratory HRCT) due to air trapping from bronchiolar involvement.
- Both CXR and HRCT appearances may quickly normalize following removal from antigen exposure.

Imaging: subacute and chronic HP

- **CXR** typically shows upper- and mid-zone reticulation. CXR can be normal in subacute HP.
- **HRCT** in subacute HP shows diffuse, well-defined, centrilobular nodules, ground-glass change, and increased lucency from air trapping. Chronic HP may mimic UIP and present with honeycombing as well as cysts. Lymphadenopathy can be seen in about 50% of patients with HP, however, the lymph nodes are typically <15 mm.

PFTs

Typically a restrictive pattern with reduced DLCO and lung volumes is found. Mild obstruction is also sometimes observed, which may be secondary to bronchitis or hyperreactive airways. There is no direct correlation between the severity of HP and that of PFT results.

ABG

Hypoxia may occur, which is worsened with exercise. The A–a gradient is increased, and PCO_2 can be decreased or normal.

Blood

Acute HP can be associated with neutrophilia, but not eosinophilia. Inflammatory markers are often increased. LDH may be a marker of disease activity. Polyclonal hypergammaglobulinemia can occur in chronic HP.

Serum antibody (IgG) precipitin results are presented either as an ELISA or as a number of precipitin lines, referring to the number of different epitopes an individual responds to such as molds, dust, and animal antigens. Precipitins to organic antigens are found in 90% of patients, but are also present in up to 30–40% of asymptomatic farmers and 40%–50% of pigeon breeders. Precipitin levels often fall in the absence of ongoing antigen exposure. The test has low sensitivity and specificity and, while not diagnostic, can be useful in assessing exposure.

BAL can help evaluate the stage of disease and the amount of exposure to the associated antigen. In the first 24 hours, there are increased lymphocytes (>40%), neutrophils (>5%), eosinophils (>5%), and mast cells (>1%). After 2–7 days, there are increased lymphocytes, plasma cells, and mast cells.

After a week, the BAL normalizes, except for a persistent lymphocytosis mostly consisting of CD8+ T cells. A CD4+/CD8+ ratio <1 can be seen and may be suggestive of those patients less likely to progress to fibrosis. Immunoglobulins IgG, IgA, and IgM may also be increase. Hyaluronic acid and procollagen 3 N-terminal peptide levels can be increased in farmer's lung.

Transbronchial or surgical lung biopsy may be required in cases of diagnostic uncertainty. TBB may provide insufficient tissue for adequate histological analysis.

Inhalation antigen challenge is still investigational and should only be considered in those with a negative workup with continued suspicion of HP secondary to a specific antigen. It entails reintroducing a presumed antigen in aerosolized form to evaluate for signs and symptoms.

The induced response may be acute or delayed. Therefore, the patient should be hospitalized for at least 24 hours for observation. Change in symptoms, exam findings, PaO_2, BAL, CXR, FVC, and DLCO indicate a positive result.

Diagnosis

Diagnosis is based on the combination of history of antigen exposure and typical clinical and HRCT features. The most diagnostically useful clinical features are onset of symptoms 4–8 hours after exposure, history of recurrent episodes of symptoms, weight loss, and finding of crackles on examination.

An absence of serum precipitins is very unusual but described. Atypical presentations require further investigation to support the diagnosis, such as BAL lymphocytosis or characteristic histological features on lung biopsy.

Differential diagnosis

- Atypical pneumonia
- Idiopathic interstitial pneumonias (particularly UIP and COP)
- Sarcoidosis
- Vasculitis
- Occupational asthma (e.g., from isocyanates)
- Drug-induced lung disease (including pesticides)
- Organic dust toxic syndrome (follows very high levels of exposure to agricultural dusts, symptoms are transient, benign course)
- Silo-filler's disease (variable respiratory manifestations after exposure to nitrogen dioxide in silos; from mild bronchitis to fatal bronchospasm)
- Tuberculosis
- Chronic bronchitis

Management

Management

Management of HP centers on antigen avoidance, which is frequently difficult. If complete removal from the antigen is unrealistic (e.g., farmers), measures to reduce exposure may be of benefit (such as respiratory protection with high-performance, positive-pressure masks; avoidance of particularly heavy exposure; improved ventilation and use of air filters; drying of hay prior to storage).

When treatment is required, corticosteroids are frequently used, although there is a lack of randomized, controlled evidence to support this. Steroids can be considered in severe acute cases as well as in subacute and chronic cases. A typical regimen is prednisone 40–60 mg daily for up to a month, and then a slowly reduced dose over several months to 10–15 mg/day, which is continued until clinical and functional resolution occurs. Inhaled steroids may be of some benefit, especially in those with hyperreactive airways.

Prognosis

Prognosis is highly variable. Prognosis is usually excellent after removal from antigen exposure in acute HP, although progression to respiratory failure and death may very rarely occur after short-term exposures of very high intensity. Recurrent episodes of acute HP do not necessarily progress to chronic HP and fibrosis, and chronic HP may develop in the absence of previous acute HP episodes.

Development of chronic HP may eventually lead to cor pulmonale and death, although this is variable and many patients do not exhibit disease progression despite chronic exposure. Persistent, low-dose exposure (e.g., birds within the home) may be more likely to progress to the chronic, fibrotic form of HP than intermittent high-dose exposure (e.g., pigeon breeders with cooped birds), which predisposes more to episodes of acute HP. Chronic, fibrotic HP has been shown to have as high as a 25% mortality rate over 5 years.

Prognosis is worse in smokers and in those with significant fibrosis, honeycombing, and clubbing. Those with cellular NSIP and organizing pneumonia in chronic HP tend to have a better prognosis.

Further information

Costabel U, du Bois RM, Egan JJ (eds.) (2007). Diffuse parenchyma lung disease. *Prog Respir Res* Basel: Karger, Vol. 36, pp. 139–147.

Schwarz MI, King TE, Raghu G (2003). Approach to the evaluation and diagnosis of interstitial lung disease. In King TE, Schwarz MI (eds.). *Interstitial Lung Disease*. Ontario, Canada: BC Decker; pp. 1–30.

Selman M, Estrada A, Navarro C (n.d.). Hypersensitivity pneumonitis. Lesson 14, Volume 17 in PCCU Education Series online at: http://www.chestnet.org

Bronchiolitis and related disorders

Pathophysiology and causes

Definition and epidemiology

Bronchioles are small airways of diameter <2 mm, lined by bronchial epithelium and with no cartilage in their walls. Terminal bronchioles lead to alveoli. Considerable numbers of bronchioles need to be affected by disease before a patient experiences symptomatic airway obstruction from increased airway resistance.

Diseases that affect bronchioles can be categorized as follows:
- Disease processes predominantly affecting the bronchioles (primary bronchiolar disorders)
- Disease processes predominantly affecting the lung parenchyma (e.g., cryptogenic organizing pneumonia [COP]) or large airways (e.g., bronchiectasis) with associated bronchiolar involvement

Pathophysiology

Pathophysiology is unclear but likely varies with different forms of bronchiolar disorders. There is probably an initial injury to the epithelium of the bronchioles with subsequent inflammation and fibrosis. A broad spectrum of bronchiolar injury patterns is encountered, varying widely, as does its severity. Whether bronchiolar disease becomes clinically manifest or not probably depends on the underlying cause, extent, and severity of bronchiolar injury, and premorbid status. Recognizable histopathological patterns of bronchiolitis are as follows (see Box 36.1).

Respiratory bronchiolitis

The distinctive feature is the prominent accumulation of pigmented macrophages in the lumen of respiratory bronchioles and the adjacent alveoli. Most cases are related to cigarette smoking or other inhalational exposures that trigger an inflammatory reaction in the bronchioles.

Acute bronchiolitis

This form is histologically characterized by intense acute and chronic inflammation of small bronchioles with associated epithelial necrosis and sloughing. Respiratory syncytial virus is the most common etiologic agent but other viral and nonviral infections can cause a similar injury pattern.

Constrictive bronchiolitis

This pattern comprises a broad spectrum of changes ranging from bronchiolar inflammation to peribronchiolar fibrosis and ultimately complete cicatrization of the bronchiole lumen, with associated epithelial necrosis and sloughing. It can be associated with a wide variety of causes including lung or bone marrow transplant rejection, infections, connective tissue diseases, inhalational injuries, drugs, inflammatory bowel disease, microcarcinoid tumorlets, diffuse idiopathic neuroendocrine cell hyperplasia, and paraneoplastic pemphigus. At times the cause may be unidentifiable, i.e., cryptogenic constrictive bronchiolitis.

Follicular bronchiolitis

Characterized histopathologically by the presence of hyperplastic lymphoid follicles with reactive germinal centers distributed along bronchioles (bronchiolocentric), this bronchiolitis can be associated with chronic infections or inflammation of the airways (e.g., cystic fibrosis, bronchiectasis, or chronic aspiration), connective tissue diseases, and immunodeficiency syndromes, including AIDS.

Diffuse panbronchiolitis

This is characterized histopathologically by bronchiolocentric infiltration of lymphocytes, plasma cells, and foamy macrophages at the level of the respiratory bronchioles. It is of unknown cause and described mainly in Asia, particularly in Japanese adults.

Mineral dust airway disease

In this disease there is deposition of inhaled dust around small airways, primarily respiratory bronchioles, with increased fibrous tissue in the walls of the bronchioles with luminal narrowing. It may occur with inhalation of a number of inorganic dusts, including asbestos, iron oxide, aluminum oxide, talc, mica, silica, silicate, and coal. It is generally not associated with respiratory symptoms.

Other unusual forms of bronchiolitis include diffuse-aspiration bronchiolitis, usually from recurrent, occult aspiration, and lymphocytic bronchiolitis associated with the nylon flocking process.

In practice, these are the most common situations in which a diagnosis of bronchiolitis is encountered:

- Smokers (respiratory bronchiolitis)
- Acute viral bronchiolitis
- Post-lung transplant (constrictive or obliterative bronchiolitis)
- Post-bone marrow transplant (constrictive or obliterative bronchiolitis)
- Connective tissue diseases (constrictive or obliterative bronchiolitis)

Several interstitial lung diseases and large-airway diseases (see Box 36.1) can involve bronchioles with varying degrees of inflammation and scarring. Respiratory bronchiolitis-associated interstitial lung disease, desquamative interstitial pneumonia, and pulmonary Langerhans cell histiocytosis occurring in adults are usually forms of smoking-related interstitial lung disease and can manifest bronchiolar injury related to smoking exposure. Histological evidence of a cellular bronchiolitis is seen in more than half of the cases of hypersensitivity pneumonitis.

Organizing pneumonia (also called bronchiolitis obliterans organizing pneumonia, or BOOP) is a histopathological pattern characterized by polypoid intraluminal plugs of granulation tissue within alveolar ducts and spaces with varying degrees of involvement in the bronchioles. It is a nonspecific reparative reaction and may be seen in a variety of clinical contexts, including connective tissue diseases, eosinophilic lung diseases, vasculitis, aspiration or toxic inhalants, drugs, radiation therapy, infections, allograft recipients, inflammatory bowel diseases, and many others. When a cause cannot be identified, the term *cryptogenic organizing pneumonia* (COP) is used. Bronchiolitis can also be seen in cases of sarcoidosis and idiopathic pulmonary fibrosis.

Bronchial abnormalities are found in large-airway diseases (bronchiectasis, chronic bronchitis, cystic fibrosis) and include variable degrees of inflammation in the wall and lumen of bronchioles, smooth muscle hypertrophy, and mucostasis.

Box 36.1 Classification of bronchiolitis and related disorders

Primary bronchiolar disorders
- Respiratory bronchiolitis
- Acute bronchiolitis
- Constrictive bronchiolitis (obliterative bronchiolitis, bronchiolitis obliterans)
- Follicular bronchiolitis
- Diffuse panbronchiolitis
- Mineral dust airway disease
- Other primary bronchiolar variants.

Bronchiolar involvement in interstitial lung diseases
- Respiratory bronchiolitis–associated interstitial lung disease or desquamative interstitial pneumonia
- Organizing pneumonia (bronchiolitis obliterans organizing pneumonia [BOOP], proliferative bronchiolitis)
- Hypersensitivity pneumonitis
- Other interstitial lung diseases, e.g., pulmonary Langerhans cell histiocytosis, sarcoidosis, idiopathic pulmonary fibrosis

Bronchiolar involvement in large-airway diseases
- Chronic bronchitis
- Bronchiectasis
- Asthma

Management

Clinical features

Clinical presentation will depend on the underlying cause, form, and severity of bronchiolar disease. Symptoms, when present, generally consist of dyspnea and/or cough. The mode of onset can be acute, as in acute bronchiolitis, but is more commonly insidious in other forms of bronchiolitis such as constrictive bronchiolitis or interstitial lung diseases with bronchiolar involvement.

The clinical context, such as smoking history, respiratory infections, lung transplant, connective tissue disease, or a history of environmental or drug exposure, provides important clues in the diagnostic evaluation.

Investigations

PFTs

Obstructive defect is found with most forms of primary bronchiolar disorders. Restrictive defect is usually seen if bronchiolar disease is a component of an underlying interstitial lung disease such as COP.

CXR

CXR can be normal, or may show hyperinflation, especially with constrictive bronchiolitis, or diffuse infiltrates with COP and other interstitial lung diseases.

HRCT

HRCT is essential in evaluating most cases of suspected bronchiolar disease. Expiratory views may be added to look for air trapping. Normal bronchioles are too small to be seen on HRCT; diseased bronchioles with thickened walls due to inflammation and dilatation may be visualized and are sometimes associated with the "tree-in-bud" appearance. Indirect signs of bronchiolar disease may include hyperinflation, air trapping with a mosaic pattern, and subsegmental atelectasis.

CT is also useful to assess for signs of underlying interstitial lung disease or large-airway disease such as bronchiectasis. Clinical context and HRCT features may suffice to yield a likely diagnosis.

Bronchoscopy can occasionally yield diagnostic features via biopsy or bronchoalveolar lavage.

Open or thoracoscopic lung biopsy may be required to make a definitive diagnosis.

Management

- Treatment varies widely depending on the underlying cause or disorder.
- Respiratory bronchiolitis is caused by smoking in most cases; treatment is with smoking cessation.
- Most patients with acute viral bronchiolitis can be managed with supportive care. Bronchodilators, epinephrine, and corticosteroids have been commonly used but are of questionable efficacy.
- Azithromycin therapy has been beneficial for some patients with constrictive bronchiolitis associated with lung transplantation (bronchiolitis obliterans syndrome). Constrictive bronchiolitis occurring in other contexts, e.g., connective tissue diseases, have generally not responded to corticosteroid or immunosuppressive therapy.
- Treatment of follicular bronchiolitis generally consists of corticosteroids and azathioprine as well as management of the underlying disorder.
- Long-term macrolide therapy, e.g., erythromycin 200–600 mg/day, improves symptoms, lung function, and mortality rates in those with diffuse panbronchiolitis.
- Bronchiolitis associated with underlying interstitial lung disease or large-airway disease is managed by treating the underlying disease.

Further information

Ryu JH, Myers JL, Swensen SJ (2003). Bronchiolar disorders. *Am J Respir Crit Care Med* **168**:1277–1292.

Eosinophilic lung disease

Introduction

Definition

Classically, *eosinophilic lung disease* is defined as the presence of peripheral and/or tissue eosinophilia plus the presence of radiographic pulmonary infiltrates. More broadly, one may consider any disease with peripheral and/or tissue eosinophilia plus pulmonary impairment as defined by physiologic, radiological, or gas exchange abnormalities to be an eosinophilic lung disease. It should be remembered that eosinophilic lung disease is not a disease per se, but rather a clinically useful paradigm in which the presence of eosinophilia generates a specific and limited differential diagnosis.

- Normal circulating eosinophil counts are below 400/mm^3 (0–8% of peripheral white blood cell count)
- The pathologic finding of eosinophilic pneumonia (eosinophil-rich infiltrates throughout the lung parenchyma) can be seen in a broad array of eosinophilic lung diseases, including chronic eosinophilic pneumonia, acute eosinophilic pneumonia, Churg–Strauss vasculitis, hypereosinophilic syndromes, and drug reactions.

Differential diagnosis of eosinophilic lung disease

The differential diagnosis is usually divided into primary disorders and secondary disorders (see Box 37.1). Primary disorders may be further subdivided into organ-specific diseases and systemic diseases. Secondary disorders are much more common than primary disorders.

Box 37.1 Differential diagnosis of eosinophilic lung disease

Primary disorders—lung-limited
- Chronic eosinophilic pneumonia
- Acute eosinophilic pneumonia

Primary disorders—systemic
- Churg–Strauss vasculitis
- Hypereosinophilic syndromes and eosinophilic leukemias

Secondary disorders
- Infection
  - Parasitic
  - Other (fungal, *Pneumocystis*, bacterial, mycobacterial)
- Drugs and medications
  - Antibiotics
  - NSAIDs
  - Other
- Asthma and atopy
  - Allergic bronchopulmonary mycosis (ABPM)
- Primary malignancy with eosinophilia
  - Leukemias and lymphomas
  - Other

Eosinophilic lung disease: secondary disorders

Asthma, atopy, and ABPM

Asthma and other atopic diseases may be accompanied by peripheral and/or airway eosinophilia.

ABPM (allergic bronchopulmonary mycosis)

ABPM is caused by an allergic or immune response to fungus, most commonly (but not exclusively) *Aspergillus fumigatus*.

ABPM is defined by the presence of the following:

- Asthma (often severe and/or steroid-requiring)
- Eosinophilia
- Elevated IgE
- Central (proximal) bronchiectasis
- Fleeting and/or migratory infiltrates
- **Positive skin-prick test**, precipitating antibodies (precipitins), or elevated specific IgE to **Aspergillus or other fungal species**

Treatment commonly requires steroids. Antifungal agents may provide additional benefit.

Infection

Parasitic infections will often prominently feature eosinophilia. A travel history and the presence of GI and constitutional symptoms may suggest parasitic infection.

Simple pulmonary eosinophilia (Löffler's syndrome)

- Generally caused by immune response to the larvae of *Ascaris lumbricoides*
- Symptoms include cough, malaise, anorexia, rhinitis, night sweats, low-grade fever, wheezing, and dyspnea.
- Sputum may contain eosinophils and/or larvae.
- *Strongyloides, Ancylostoma* and *Necator* may cause similar disease.

Tropical pulmonary eosinophilia

- Caused by the immune response to migrating larvae of the filarial worms *Wucheria bancrofti* and *Brugia malayi*
- Insidious onset of cough, wheeze, sputum, dyspnea, and chest pain, with associated fever, weight loss, and fatigue
- Prominent peripheral eosinophilia and elevated IgE

Other

- Other parasites causing eosinophilia include *Toxocara, Schistosoma, Paragonimus, Loa loa, Trichomonas, Dirofilaria,* and *Clonorchis.*
- Nonparasitic infections, including protozoal infections, fungal infections, mycobacterial infections, and, less commonly, bacterial infections, may also present with eosinophilia and lung disease

Drug-induced pulmonary eosinophilia

- Pulmonary symptoms and/or infiltrates usually develop within hours to days of starting the drug and resolve within a week of stopping it.
- Illness ranges from asymptomatic to severe, and may include cough, dyspnea, fever, hypoxia, wheezing, rash, and/or infiltrates.
- Implicated drugs include penicillins, cephalosporins, tetracyclines, sulfa agents, nitrofurantoin, carbamazepine, isoniazid, L-tryptophan, NSAIDs, cocaine, ACE inhibitors, phenytoin, and sulfonamides.

Eosinophilic lung disease: primary disorders, lung-limited

Chronic eosinophilic pneumonia

- Idiopathic
- Insidious onset over weeks to months
- Symptoms may include cough, dyspnea on exertion or exercise intolerance, wheezing, and constitutional symptoms.
- **Imaging studies commonly demonstrate airspace disease that is often misdiagnosed as pneumonia.** While the "classic" radiographic description of CEP is peripheral, dense opacities with ill-defined margins that suggest the photographic negative of pulmonary edema, this is seen in only a minority of patients.
- **BAL** eosinophil count is elevated (>25%)
- **Blood** eosinophilia is common but not required for diagnosis.
- **Pathology** demonstrates eosinophilic pneumonia.
- **Treatment** is with oral corticosteroids and improvement is usually relatively brisk (weeks). Slow steroid taper over 6–12 months is recommended, as relapses are common when steroids are abruptly stopped.

Acute eosinophilic pneumonia

- Idiopathic
- Rare
- Acute onset with fulminant, hypoxemic respiratory failure over a period of days
- Peripheral eosinophilia is uncommon
- BAL eosinophils >25%
- Interstitial or alveolar CXR infiltrates
- Often misdiagnosed as pneumonia or ARDS
- Prompt response to intravenous steroids
- As a rule, does not recur after resolution

Eosinophilic lung disease: primary disorders, systemic

Churg–Strauss vasculitis (see p. 570)

- Characteristic triad of severe asthma, peripheral eosinophilia, and small-vessel vasculitis
- Eosinophilic pneumonia may commonly be seen.
- Manifestations may include life-threatening cardiac (conduction blocks, cardiomyopathy, coronary arteritis) and GI (perforation, infarction, hemorrhage) disease
- Other common features may include arthralgias, arthritis, myalgias, fever, fatigue, malaise, mononeuritis multiplex, asymmetric polyneuropathy, cutaneous vasculitis, sinusitis, and rhinitis.
- ANCA (predominantly p-ANCA) and/or anti-myeloperoxidase ELISA positive in 50%–75% of cases
- Most cases have radiographic abnormalities, most commonly fleeting infiltrates, but an array of abnormalities have been described.
- Treatment consists of steroids and immunosuppression.

Hypereosinophilic syndrome (HES)

- Classically, defined as >1500 cells/mm^3 for >6 months, negative workup for known causes of eosinophilia plus end-organ damage
- More recently, specific cytogenetic and molecular abnormalities have been defined, allowing for accurate classification and targeted therapy of HES.
- Commonly associated with high-grade, peripheral eosinophilia that is difficult to control with oral corticosteroids
- Symptoms may vary depending on the subtype of HES.
- Constitutional symptoms are common—fever, weight loss, night sweats, fatigue, malaise, and pruritus.
- **Pulmonary involvement** may present with cough, dyspnea, interstitial infiltrates, eosinophilic pneumonia, and pleural effusions.
- **Cardiovascular involvement** with myocarditis, endocardial fibrosis, restrictive cardiomyopathy, and mural thrombus formation causes considerable morbidity and mortality.
- Skin, vascular, central and peripheral nervous system, gastrointestinal, reticuloendothelial, renal, articular, and muscular involvement may all be seen.
- **Diagnosis** generally requires bone marrow biopsy.
- **FIP1-L1-PDGFR-α fusion protein** may be seen in up to 50% of patients with myeloproliferative subtype HES. This fusion protein–positive subgroup is generally responsive to therapy with imatinib.
- For patients who do not fall within the imatinib-responsive subgroup, initial therapy is with high-dose steroids, which produces improvement in about 50% of cases. Other therapeutic options include hydroxyurea, interferon-α, or a conventional immunosuppressive agent.
- The role of anti-IL-5 monoclonal antibodies remains under investigation, as do a number of other targeted biological therapies.

Pneumocnioses

Overview and causative mineral dusts

Pneumoconioses are non-neoplastic pulmonary diseases caused by the reaction of the lung to the inhalation of mineral dusts (see Table 38.1 and Box 38.1). Asthma, chronic bronchitis, and emphysema may also develop as a result of these dust exposures, but are not considered pneumoconioses.

The risk of developing a specific pneumoconiosis is dependent on the

- Physical and chemical properties of the particles
- Intensity and duration of exposure
- Individual's susceptibility. *Susceptibility* reflects a balance between airway anatomy and innate clearance mechanisms, and genetic predisposition toward specific immune responses leading to inflammation and fibrosis.

Inhaled particles of dust size <5 μm reach the terminal airways and alveoli and settle on the epithelial lining. From here they are slowly cleared by macrophages or alveolar cells. They may pass into the lymphatic system, be cleared via the airway, or remain in the alveolus.

The dust particles can lead to an inflammatory reaction within the lung (alveolitis), resulting in characteristic radiological abnormalities, as well as alterations in pulmonary structure and function.

Regulatory standards for exposure to hazardous dusts exist, but are generally based on average exposures across an 8-hour work period and do not guarantee that any given air sample is within the exposure limit. Consequently, pneumoconioses continue to occur even in developed nations, usually in smaller industries that may be unaware of potential hazards. They remain an important public health problem in many low- and middle-income countries without strict industrial exposure regulations.

The pneumoconioses discussed in this chapter include coal-worker's pneumoconiosis, silicosis, and berylliosis. Asbestos-related diseases are discussed separately in Chapter 26.

Table 38.1 Examples of mineral dusts implicated in pneumoconiosis

Mineral dust	Disease	Examples of exposure
Coal dust	Simple pneumoconiosis, silicosis, Caplan's syndrome	Coal mining, especially hard coal (anthracite)
Silica	Silicosis (acute, accelerated, chronic) Progressive massive fibrosis	Foundry work, sandblasting, stone cutting, hard-rock mining, ceramics
Asbestos	Asbestosis Benign asbestos-related pleural disease Mesothelioma Lung cancer	Mining, milling, and fabrication. Installation and removal of insulation
Beryllium	Acute berylliosis Chronic beryllium disease	Workers in nuclear and aerospace industry, mining, fabrication of electrical and electronic equipment, ceramics
Iron oxide, iron fume (commonly contains silica)	Siderosis, silicosis	Arc-welding, metal polishers
Barium sulfate (barite)	Baritosis, silicosis/mixed-dust fibrosis (if barite is contaminated with silica)	Mining
Cobalt (combined with tungsten carbide)	Hard-metal lung disease	Maintenance and sharpening of carbide-tipped tools, diamond tooling, armored plate production (tanks, naval ships)
Aluminum metal	Pulmonary fibrosis	Fireworks manufacturing.
Aluminum oxide	Pulmonary fibrosis (possibly due to concurrent exposure to silica)	Abrasives manufacturing and processing.
Aluminum silicates	Mixed-dust fibrosis (due to concurrent silica or asbestos exposure)	Kaolin (china clay) mining, ceramics manufacturing

Note: the above list is not exhaustive. Many dust exposures in the work environment consist of mixed-dust exposures (e.g., coal mine dust consists of mainly carbon, but also trace metals and silica). Detailed information regarding the exact nature of the exposure is crucial to determining the disease and its cause.

Box 38.1 Types of mineral-dust exposure

Nonfibrous mineral dusts
- Crystalline silica
- Coal dust (peat, lignite, sub-bituminous, bituminous, anthracite)
- Mixed mineral dusts containing quartz silica: slate, kaolin, talc, non-fibrous clays

Fibrous mineral dusts
- Asbestos
- Other mineral fibers

Metal dusts and fumes
- Iron, aluminum, beryllium, cobalt

The *Work-Related Lung Disease (eWoRLD) Surveillance System* is produced by the National Institute for Occupational Safety and Health (NIOSH). It presents up-to-date summary tables, graphs, and figures of occupationally related respiratory disease surveillance data on the pneumoconioses, occupational asthma and other airways diseases, and several other respiratory conditions. For many of these diseases, selected data on related exposures are also presented.

Further information
www.cdc.gov/niosh/topics/surveillance/ORDS/default.html

Coal-workers' pneumoconiosis

It was recognized many years ago that coal miners had higher levels of respiratory disease than those in the general population. Coal miners may be affected by any or all of the following:

- Chronic bronchitis
- Emphysema
- Coal workers' pneumoconiosis (simple and complicated, or progressive massive fibrosis)
- Caplan's syndrome (pulmonary rheumatoid nodules associated with coal workers' pneumoconiosis)
- Silicosis
- Tuberculosis

It has been difficult to establish the independent effects of coal dust because of the high smoking rates among miners. However, it is now thought that coal dust contributes to the emphysema and chronic bronchitis caused by smoking, because

- Miners have an increased prevalence of cough, sputum, and decreased FEV_1 compared to that in non-miners. The risk of cough increases with increasing dust exposure.
- FEV_1 declines in proportion to the amount of dust exposure.
- In smokers, the response to dust is probably different from that of nonsmokers, with worse disease at a given level of exposure.

There are two types of coal-workers' pneumoconiosis:

- Simple pneumoconiosis, which can progress to
- Complicated pneumoconiosis, also known as progressive massive fibrosis (PMF).

These are common diseases among coal miners who work in poorly ventilated conditions. Risk of pneumoconiosis increases with total lung dust burden and higher rank (carbon content) of coal. The latter may be due to greater relative surface area, higher surface free radicals, and greater silica content in high-grade than in low-grade coal.

Pathology

Simple pneumoconiosis

Coal dust is inhaled into the alveolus and engulfed by macrophages. With increasing dust burden, macrophages release reactive oxygen species, triggering the release of cytokines (interleukins, tumor necrosis factor) responsible for the processes of inflammation and fibrosis. This leads to the development of *coal macules,* small nonpalpable lesions distributed initially in the upper lobes, although lower lobes may be involved as well. They consist of an aggregation of dust, dust-laden macrophages, and fibroblasts with irregular collagen fibrosis around respiratory bronchioles.

The macules may enlarge to form *coal nodules,* palpable lesions that also contains reticulin fibers and irregular collagen fibrosis. Proteases are also released and, with time, contribute to the weakening and dilation of the respiratory bronchiole to create an area of focal emphysema. Focal emphysema in combination with the coal macule is the typical lesion of coal workers' pneumoconiosis.

PMF

PMF occurs on this background, but with aggregation of the fibrotic nodules to form larger lesions, 2–10 cm in diameter. Macroscopically, these are bulky, irregular, black tissue masses usually in the posterior upper lobes or apical lower lobes. The central area of these nodules may be necrotic due to ischemic necrosis or mycobacterial infection.

It is not understood what causes the progression of small nodules to PMF. Possible factors include total coal dust burden, proportion of inhaled silica, individual immunological factors, and whether mycobacteria are present.

Clinical features

Simple pneumoconiosis is usually asymptomatic and without clinical signs. Diagnosis is based on typical chest radiograph findings in a patient with an appropriate exposure history. Symptoms of cough and sputum production are likely due to dust-induced chronic bronchitis.

Progressive massive fibrosis is usually associated with cough productive of mucoid or blackened sputum (melanoptysis, due to rupture of a cavitating PMF lesion into an airway), and exertional dyspnea. Severe cases may in time lead to the development of cor pulmonale. Abnormal breath sounds may be heard if PMF lesions impinge on airways.

The presence of rheumatoid arthritis or subcutaneous nodules raises the possibility of Caplan's syndrome. The presence of crackles or clubbing suggests an alternative infectious or malignant etiology, or another interstitial lung disease.

Caplan's syndrome

Miners with seropositive rheumatoid arthritis or positive serum rheumatoid factor can develop large, well-defined nodules. These occur on a background of simple pneumoconiosis and in those with a relatively low coal dust exposure. They may be multiple and may cavitate. They cause no significant functional impairment and have no malignant potential.

Investigations

CXR

In *simple pneumoconiosis* there is nodular shadowing, with nodules of varying size, up to 10 mm, particularly in the upper and middle zones. Pneumoconiosis can be graded according to the number of different-sized nodules: p = <1.5 mm, q = 1.5–3 mm, and r = 3–10 mm. Nodule numbers increase with increasing dust inhalation and usually stop forming when the miner has left the work environment.

PMF is diagnosed when one or more opacities of >1 cm diameter are present, on a background of simple pneumoconiosis. These lesions are often located in the upper lobes and enlarge, becoming increasingly radiodense and clearly demarcated with time. They may distort the adjacent lung and cause emphysema. The lesions may continue to progress once the patient is out of the work environment

HRCT

HRCT of *simple pneumoconiosis* shows parenchymal nodules 1–10 mm in size, with upper-zone predominance. In *PMF*, nodules of >1 cm are seen, with irregular borders and associated parenchymal distortion and emphysema. Larger lesions may have cavitation and necrosis. They may also have areas of calcification.

PFTs

There is poor correlation of PFT abnormalities with presence of nodules on imaging. Early disease may show normal PFTs. With disease progression there may be a restrictive pattern with reduced DLCO, or a mixed obstructive–restrictive pattern due to emphysematous changes around the coal macule.

PMF shows severe and rapidly progressive mixed obstructive–restrictive defect with reduced DLCO.

Management

This entails minimization of dust exposure with improved mine ventilation, water spraying at points of dust generation, provision of respirators, and monitoring of dust levels. Miners should have periodic radiographic and spirometric surveillance, and should be moved to a less dusty work area if they show signs of pneumoconiosis, to prevent the development of PMF.

All dust exposure should be prevented when PMF is detected. Advice and support for smoking cessation should be offered. Management is also focused on diagnosis and treatment of complications such as rheumatoid arthritis and mycobacterial infection, as well as assistance with pulmonary disability that may occur with advanced disease.

Miners with signs of coal workers' pneumoconiosis are entitled to industrial injury benefits from the Federal Black Lung Benefits Act.

Silicosis

This is a fibrotic lung disease caused by the. prolonged inhalation and retention of, and lung reaction to, silicon dioxide (silica) particles.

- Duration of exposure is on the order of decades for chronic silicosis, but is shorter for accelerated (<10 years) and acute (months) silicosis.
- Disease may first present and progress well after exposure has ceased.
- Usually small (1–3 mm) upper-zone rounded opacities. Occasionally these may not be visible on chest radiography. Opacities larger than 1 cm define PMF.
- The pattern of disease (acute, accelerated, chronic) depends on the intensity, duration, and size and surface characteristics of silica particles, as well as individual susceptibility factors.

Silica is present mostly as crystalline quartz, which is mined and quarried and used in industries such as ceramics, brick-making, stone masonry, and sandblasting. Small workplaces with less well-known uses of silica and lack of awareness of its hazards may pose risk to workers, even in developed nations with industrial exposure standards.

Pathology

Quartz is the usual form of crystalline silica causing silicosis. Silica may be directly cytotoxic to pulmonary cells and stimulate generation of reactive oxygen species and inflammatory cytokine and chemokines from macrophages. Polymorphonuclear cells and macrophages are then recruited, and phagocytic oxidant species are generated, leading to tissue damage. Silica also stimulates secretion of fibrogenic factors from macrophages and alveolar epithelial cells, leading to collagen synthesis and fibrosis.

The hallmark lesion of silicosis is the *silicotic nodule*, a cell- and dust-free lesion consisting of concentrically arranged collagen fibers, with a more peripheral zone of random fibers and dust-laden macrophages. Nodules first involve the hilar lymph nodes and may calcify or erode the airway. The lung parenchyma is subsequently involved, usually the upper lobes. With time, the nodules may enlarge and, in a small number of cases, become confluent, leading to progressive massive fibrosis.

Clinicopathological types of silicosis

Chronic silicosis occurs with lower dust concentrations than those seen in acute or accelerated silicosis. The disease may be marked by breathlessness or be asymptomatic. Symptoms may also be due to complications such as PMF, mycobacterial disease, lung cancer, or airways disease due to either dust exposures or cigarette use.

CXR

Small, rounded opacities in the upper and mid-zone (nodules) are present, measuring between 3 and 5 mm in diameter. They are initially indistinct but become clearer with time. Enlargement and calcification of hilar lymph nodes (egg shell calcification) may occur before parenchymal lesions develop. Nodules continue to develop with continued exposure and may develop after exposure ceases. Nodules can calcify and coalesce, leading to PMF. Over time, these coalescing lesions contract and leave hypertranslucent zones at their margins.

Mycobacterial disease should always be considered in the setting of changing lesions, particularly those that cavitate. Lung cancer is also a diagnostic consideration in this setting.

PFTs

No consistent profile exists, because of the variety of clinical and pathological manifestations and frequent coexistence of bronchitis and emphysema. Spirometry usually reflects airflow limitation due to occupational exposure or cigarette smoking. Total lung capacity and DLCO may be reduced in advanced disease. Changes are more marked and progression is more rapid in accelerated and acute forms of silicosis.

Acute silicosis is caused by intense exposure to fine dusts, such as those produced by sandblasting. It may become apparent in workers within a few months of starting work. Rapid deterioration over several months occurs. Treatment is often ineffective.

- *Clinically* there is dry cough, dyspnea, chest tightness, fatigue, and weight loss. Rapid deterioration occurs over a few weeks. Fine crepitations are heard over the lower zones bilaterally. Cyanosis and respiratory failure develop, often complicated by mycobacterial infection.
- *CXR* shows diffuse airspace and interstitial disease in middle and lower lobes.
- *Pathology* Interstitial inflammation is adjacent to alveolar spaces filled with a proteinaceous fluid rich in surfactant, similar to that found in alveolar proteinosis. Silica particles may be identified in bronchoalveolar lavage (BAL) fluid.

Accelerated silicosis

Changes are similar to those of chronic silicosis, but are more intense, involve a greater amount of lung tissue, and occur after a shorter, more intense silica exposure over a 5- to 10-year period. Nodules are more cellular than fibrotic. Dry cough and gradual onset of shortness of breath, often with progression to respiratory failure and death, can occur. Cavitation and mycobacterial infection are not uncommon.

Silicotuberculosis

There is an increased risk of mycobacterial infection in people with silicosis as well as those exposed to silica without evidence of silicosis. Risk is increased even after exposure ceases. Silica depresses macrophage clearance of mycobacteria and may alter cell-mediated immunity and serum immunoglobulin levels.

Mycobacterial infection can be difficult to diagnose, because of multiple preexisting CXR nodules. Cavitation may occur, *which does not occur with silicosis alone.*

New radiographic opacities, as well as frank symptoms of hemoptysis, fever, and weight loss should prompt examination of a sputum sample induced by hypertonic saline examination and BAL.

Management

Primary prevention of silicosis is by monitoring and minimizing dust levels. National silicosis elimination programs exist in many countries, under the guidance of the ILO/WHO global silicosis elimination campaign. Early detection of cases of silicosis and tuberculosis through monitoring of current and formerly exposed workers is crucial.

There is no evidence of benefit for anti-inflammatory therapies for chronic silicosis. Whole-lung lavage, steroid use, and treatment of mycobacterial infection are the therapeutic considerations in acute and accelerated silicosis.

Disability benefits are available from the Department of Social Security.

Berylliosis

Beryllium is a light, strong industrial metal. It is usually alloyed with copper, aluminum, nickel, and magnesium, and has favorable characteristics for use in the manufacturing of high-technology products, including electronics, aerospace, nuclear weapons, nonsparking tools, high-technology ceramics, and dental prostheses.

While cases of acute beryllium disease are now rare, cases of chronic beryllium disease continue to occur, as the current occupational exposure standards were not based on direct data on beryllium dose–response relations. There is a variable latency period between exposure and granuloma formation, and no clear association between magnitude of exposure and disease incidence. Two types of disease are known, acute and chronic.

Acute beryllium disease

Inhalational exposure to high concentrations of beryllium dust or fumes can cause acute tracheitis, bronchitis, and alveolitis. There may be widespread airway and pulmonary edema, causing chest pain, dyspnea, dry cough, cyanosis, and inspiratory crackles or rhonchi on auscultation. Myalgias, anorexia, and fever may also occur.

CXR may be normal, show bilateral infiltrates, or fulminant pulmonary edema. Mild disease may be self-limiting, but severe disease is usually fatal. Removal from exposure is the most important therapeutic maneuver. Corticosteroids may prevent progression, but their efficacy has not been proven. The patient is often left with residual pulmonary impairment, with potential for progression to chronic beryllium disease.

Chronic beryllium disease (CBD)

CBD is a granulomatous disease affecting primarily the lungs and lymphatics, although the skin, liver, heart, and other organs may be affected. CBD usually occurs on average 6–10 years after exposure has ceased, although latency may range from 2 months to 30 years.

The disease is clinically, radiographically, and histopathologically indistinguishable from sarcoidosis. It has also been diagnosed in people with seemingly minimal exposure, such as security guards and secretaries working in plants where beryllium is used, as well as spouses of beryllium workers.

Inhalation of beryllium or the exposure of a skin abrasion to beryllium causes sensitization in 2%–19% of exposed individuals, with higher prevalences observed in those with higher exposures. A CD4+ T-cell-mediated immune response develops, with the production of predominantly Th-1 inflammatory cytokines, leading to granulomatous inflammation. Following a variable latency after exposure, noncaseating granulomas may occur in the lungs or skin as in sarcoidosis.

There is a genetic predisposition to the development of beryllium sensitization and disease that is HLA mediated (HLA-DPB1(Glu69)).

Clinical features of chronic beryllium disease
- *Symptoms* include nonproductive cough, fatigue, and gradual onset of exertional dyspnea as well as atypical chest pain. Night sweats, weight loss, fevers, chills, arthralgias, and myalgias may be seen.
- *Signs* include scattered bibasilar crackles and wheezes in early disease. Crackles are more prominent with progressive disease, and lymphadenopathy may develop. Digital clubbing, cyanosis, and right heart failure may occur in advanced cases. Subcutaneous tender skin nodules can develop if beryllium penetrates the skin or enters an open cut.

Investigations

CXR

CXR is usually normal in early disease. Diffuse, bilateral, small opacities mainly in the middle and upper lung fields develop subsequently, and these may progress to interstitial fibrosis over time. Bilateral hilar adenopathy similar to sarcoidosis may occur. The chest radiograph is far less sensitive than HRCT for detecting changes consistent with CBD.

HRCT

Small nodules and septal lines are the most common abnormalities. The nodules are usually distributed along bronchovascular bundles and interlobular septae. Associated ground-glass attenuation may be seen. Traction bronchiectasis and honeycombing may occur in advanced cases. HRCT may not show evidence of CBD in up to 25% of cases identified by screening.

Blood BeLPT

This is performed in only a few specialized laboratories. The patient's mononuclear cells from blood or BAL fluid are cultured in the presence and absence of beryllium salts at varying concentrations.

Cell proliferation is measured by incorporation of tritiated thymidine in dividing cells. The cellular immune response is then quantified and reported as a stimulation index, which is the ratio of counts per minute of radioactivity in the cells stimulated by beryllium salts divided by the counts per minute in the unstimulated cells. An abnormal test result should be confirmed with repeat testing, as a single abnormal blood BeLPT is usually insufficient to establish that a person is sensitized to beryllium.

BAL

BAL testing can show an elevated total white blood cell count with a predominance of CD4+ T lymphocytes. BeLPT can be performed on BAL cells, although results may be inconclusive in smokers.

PFTs

There is no classic pattern, and normal function may be seen. An obstructive pattern, restrictive pattern, mixed pattern, or isolated decrease in DLCO may be seen. In many patients, disease may progress from an obstructive to a mixed to a purely restrictive pattern with progression.

Cardiopulmonary exercise testing

This is a more sensitive test for detection of physiological abnormalities in CBD. Gas exchange and ventilatory abnormalities may be seen in patients with CBD, including an elevated Vd/Vt ratio, abnormal reduction in PaO_2, and abnormal widening of the A–a gradient. Sensitivity of testing is improved with the use of an indwelling arterial catheter.

Pathology

Noncaseating granuloma is found that is indistinguishable from sarcoidosis. Tuberculosis and fungal infection should be ruled out by means of appropriate staining and culture methods.

Management

There is no cure for CBD. Exposure should be minimized for sensitized patients and eliminated for patients with CBD, although it is not known whether this affects the natural history of the disease. Corticosteroids may prevent disease progression, although evidence for their benefit is based on large clinical case series, and not randomized trials.

Indications for treatment include progressive symptoms with objective evidence of decline on pulmonary function testing and worsening gas exchange abnormalities on cardiopulmonary exercise testing. Evidence of pulmonary hypertension or cor pulmonale secondary to CBD is also an indication for treatment.

Treatment is usually life-long, as disease relapses when steroids are withdrawn. Prednisone is administered in doses similar to that given for pulmonary sarcoidosis (0.5 mg/kg), tapered after 3–6 months to the lowest effective dose.

Prognosis

Clinical course is variable. Some individuals remain clinically stable, although many experience progressive symptoms and physiological abnormalities, with a subset experiencing a rapidly progressive course, developing respiratory failure within a few years of diagnosis. Mortality rates range from 5% to 38% and depend on the type of exposure. A small number of subjects may spontaneously improve after exposure ceases.

Differential diagnosis

• Sarcoidosis
• Tuberculosis.
• Fungal infection
• Hypersensitivity pneumonitis

In the clinic

- Obtain from patients with suspected sarcoidosis a detailed occupational history, and specifically ask whether they may have been exposed to beryllium.
- If previous beryllium exposure is likely, arrange for the patient to have a blood beryllium lymphocyte proliferation test (blood BeLPT).
- If the blood BeLPT is abnormal, repeat the test to confirm the result. Two or more abnormal blood BeLPT results require further evaluation, including PFTs, cardiopulmonary exercise testing, and bronchoscopy to perform a beryllium lymphocyte proliferation test on BAL fluid, and transbronchial biopsies to assess for granulomatous inflammation.
- Monitor PFTs, cardiopulmonary exercise test, and CXR to assess disease response or progression. Repeat bronchoscopy should be performed to definitively rule out progression from beryllium sensitization to disease if the patient has progressive symptoms or physiological deterioration.

Rheumatoid arthritis (RA)

- RA is characterized by symmetrical, peripheral arthropathy.
- Pulmonary disease is more common in men.
- Smoking is a significant risk factor for ILD.
- Pneumonia is the terminal event in 15%–20% of patients with RA.
- There are multiple pulmonary manifestations of RA.

Pleuritis

This is usually mild. It occurs in up to 30% of RA patients, but is probably present in a greater proportion of patients with available histology.

Pleural effusion

Pleural effusion is usually asymptomatic. It can be large. Fluid is typically a lymphocytic exudate with exquisitely low glucose and low pH. Other causes for effusion, such as empyema or malignancy, must be excluded. If it is problematic (e.g., large and associated with dyspnea), patients may require drainage and steroids (see p. 342).

Pulmonary fibrosis

Minor pulmonary fibrosis is found in up to 60% of patients in lung biopsy studies; symptomatic disease is not as common. It tends to occur in patients who have severe and perhaps multisystem disease. It is more common in men.

- Presentation: progressive dyspnea
- Examination: bibasilar crackles
- PFTs show restriction and impaired diffusion.
- Radiological and histological results are similar to those for the idiopathic interstitial pneumonias (IIP), with a usual interstitial pneumonia (UIP) pattern seen far more commonly than a nonspecific interstitial pneumonia (NSIP) pattern.
- If treatment is given, the regimen usually includes glucocorticoids, usually in combination with an immunomodulatory agent.

Acute interstitial pneumonia-like reaction

Patients present with rapidly progressive dyspnea, new or worsening radiographic opacities, and impaired oxygenation. This can be the initial presentation of RA-related ILD, or it can occur on a background of chronic fibrosis. Treatment usually involves high-dose glucocorticoids, usually in combination with an immunomodulatory agent.

Pulmonary nodules

Pulmonary nodules occur in <5% of patients with RA. They are usually found incidentally on CXR. They seem to only occur in seropositive disease and in patients with nodules elsewhere, such as on the elbows or fingers. They may be more common in patients taking methotrexate.

Single or multiple nodules may occur, and they occasionally cavitate. They can cause hemoptysis or rarely pneumothorax, but they are most often entirely asymptomatic.

The main differential diagnosis is lung cancer. Follow up with CT to ensure they are of stable size. Biopsy may be needed to exclude malignancy.

Bronchiectasis

This condition is often subtle with minimal clinical features, but it may be found in 30% of patients with RA. Diagnosis is made on HRCT.

Treatment is based on symptoms; when necessary, implement standard approaches to therapy for bronchiectasis of unknown cause (e.g., sputum drainage, antibiotics).

Organizing pneumonia

Clinical features may include fever, dyspnea, hypoxemia, leukocytosis, elevated acute inflammatory markers, multifocal consolidation, and lack of responsive to antibiotics. Organizing pneumonia can be disease related or drug induced. It is confirmed by transbronchial or, far more definitively, surgical lung biopsy, showing alveoli filled with plugs of loose connective tissue and a variable inflammatory infiltrate.

Often there is a dramatic response to steroids. These patients may need long-term immunosuppression.

Obliterative bronchiolitis

This condition is rare in general, but among the CTDs occurs most commonly in RA. The histological pattern is called constrictive bronchiolitis, and involves the terminal bronchioles, which are progressively obliterated by connective tissue infiltrating within the confines of the elastic lamina.

- May present with dyspnea, hyperinflated chest, and diminished breath sounds or inspiratory squeaks
- PFTs: irreversible obstructive pattern
- CXR: hyperinflation without infiltrates
- HRCT: mosaic pattern of attenuation that is accentuated on expiratory imaging
- Histology: constrictive bronchiolitis; patchy process of progressive bronchiolar narrowing by infiltrating connective tissue internal to the elastic lamina

Some advocate a trial of high-dose oral steroids with or without an immunomodulatory agent. Most patients are also treated with a macrolide antibiotic, to take advantage of its putative anti-inflammatory and antifibrotic properties.

The course is quite variable, but progression is the rule. It may be rapidly progressive.

Vasculitis and rarely pulmonary hemorrhage occur in the setting of RA.

Cricoarytenoid arthritis

In studies using fiber-optic laryngoscopy and HRCT to detect it, this type of arthritis is seen in up to 75% of subjects with RA, but it is only rarely symptomatic. It is unrelated to lung fibrosis. It can cause sore throat, hoarse voice, or upper airways obstruction with stridor and may predispose to aspiration. Flow-volume loop may be abnormal. In the worst cases, tracheostomy may be required.

Caplan's syndrome

Caplan's syndrome consists of rheumatoid arthritis, single or multiple chest nodules, and coal-workers' pneumoconiosis.

Systemic lupus erythematosus (SLE)

- SLE is a multi-organ autoimmune disease (see Box 39.2 for classification), mainly affecting women.
- Double-stranded DNA antibodies are present.
- One can also get a drug-induced lupus syndrome, which improves when the drug is stopped (see Box 39.2)
- Pulmonary disease is often seen and may be a presenting feature of the disease. Pleural disease is the most common pulmonary manifestation.

Pleural disease

Pleural disease is often asymptomatic, but patients may have pain due to pleuritis. Pleural effusions occur in up to 50% of patients. These are often unilateral, but can be bilateral. They are exudative and can be hemorrhagic. Other causes of effusion, such as empyema or malignancy, need to be excluded.

If symptomatic, patients may need NSAID treatment. For more refractory cases, a 2-week course of oral glucocorticoids appears beneficial.

Atelectasis is usually associated with pleurisy or effusion.

Infectious pneumonia

For reasons that are poorly understood, patients with SLE are at high risk for developing bacterial pneumonia.

Diffuse lung disease

According to autopsy studies, diffuse lung disease may occur in up to 70% of SLE patients. It is usually mild and asymptomatic. Radiologically, it most often appears as an NSIP or UIP pattern. Perhaps 5% develop progressive ILD. PFTs show restrictive defect with reduced DLCO.

Treatment is based on the severity and course but is usually similar to that used for RA-related ILD.

Acute lupus pneumonitis

This is the same entity as the acute interstitial pneumonia-like reaction in RA. This rare, life-threatening illness has a mortality rate of >50%. Patients have fever, dyspnea, cough, diffuse radiographic opacities, and hypoxemia. Histology shows diffuse alveolar damage without capillaritis or hemorrhage.

Treatment is with high-dose glucocorticoids and immunomodulatory drugs. The acute form can progress to chronic interstitial pneumonitis.

Obliterative bronchiolitis is rare in SLE.

Organizing pneumonia is the same as in RA.

Pulmonary hypertension is not uncommon in SLE and is associated with Raynaud's phenomenon. Pulmonary emboli must be considered as a cause, especially in those with antiphospholipid antibodies. Treatment is as for primary pulmonary hypertension.

Pulmonary emboli are most common in the 20%–30% of SLE patients with antiphospholipid antibodies.

Shrinking lung syndrome

In this syndrome, dyspnea is caused by reduced lung volumes and poor respiratory reserve. The underlying reason for this is unclear, but it may be diaphragmatic muscle weakness. Small lungs appear on PA chest radiograph. CT shows normal lung parenchyma. Lung function tests indicate restricton. Symptoms may improve with oral glucocorticoids.

Alveolar hemorrhage

This condition is rare, but life threatening. It can be associated with glomerulonephritis. It is marked by acute onset of dyspnea with new radiographic opacities. Hemoptysis need not be present. Declining hematocrit is found. Diagnosis is confirmed when increasingly or persistently bloody return is noted in serial aliquots of bronchoalveolar lavage fluid.

Treat with high-dose steroids and cyclophosphamide. Plasmapheresis may be helpful.

Box 39.2 Criteria of the American College of Rheumatology for classification of SLE

SLE is confirmed if four or more criteria are present, serially or simultaneously, during any interval:

- Malar rash
- Discoid rash
- Photosensitivity
- Oral ulcers
- Arthritis
- Serositis: pleuritis or pericarditis
- Renal disorder: proteinuria >0.5 g/24 hours or 3+ persistently, or cellular casts
- Neurological disorder: seizures, or psychosis (having excluded drugs or other causes)
- Hematological disorder: hemolytic anemia, leukopenia (<4.0 × 10^9/L on two or more occasions), lymphopenia (1.5 × 10^9/L on two or more occasions), or thrombocytopenia (<100 × 10^9/L)
- Immunological disorder: elevated anti-dsDNA antibody, anti-Sm antibody, positive finding of antiphospholipid antibodies
- Elevated antinuclear antibody (in the absence of drugs known to be associated with drug-induced lupus)

Drug-induced lupus: causative drugs include the following:
- Isoniazid
- Procainamide
- Hydralazine
- Minocycline
- Penicillamine
- Anticonvulsants
- Sulfonamides

Further information

Swigris JJ, Fischer A, Gillis J, et al. (2008). Pulmonary and thrombotic manifestations of systemic lupus erythematosus. *Chest* **133**:271–280.

Polymyositis and dermatomyositis

These are two separate disorders:
- *Polymyositis* (PM) is an inflammatory myopathy, causing symmetrical proximal muscle weakness.
- *Dermatomyositis* (DM) is an inflammatory myopathy with a characteristic rash.

Creatine kinase levels are elevated up to 50 times the normal levels; however, there is a subset of patients who do not have muscle involvement. Antinuclear and myositis-specific (e.g., anti-Jo-1, PL-7, PL-12) antibodies are positive. Dermatomyositis may be associated with an underlying malignancy, but this is less common when the Jo-1 (or other myositis-specific) antibody is present. Diffuse parenchymal lung disease is the most common pulmonary manifestation of PM/DM.

See Box 39.3 for diagnostic criteria for PM and DM.

Interstitial lung disease

This occurs in 20%–30%. Patients present with dyspnea.
- HRCT: The most characteristic pattern is bilateral lower-lobe volume loss with reticular abnormality, ground-glass opacities, and patchy consolidation in the extreme bases and tracking along bronchovascular bundles.
- Histology: Often a mixed pattern of NSIP and organizing pneumonia
- Lung involvement is frequently associated with antisynthetase antibodies (e.g., anti-Jo-1, PL-7, PL-12).
- Therapy usually involves oral glucocorticoids and an immunomodulatory agent (e.g., cyclophosphamide).

Ventilatory failure is due to intercostal and diaphragmatic muscle weakness.

Pulmonary hypertension is secondary to lung disease.

Pulmonary vasculitis is rare.

Aspiration pneumonia occurs in 20% of patients and is associated with a marked increase in mortality. It is caused by dysphagia and pharyngeal muscle weakness.

Box 39.3 Criteria for diagnosis of polymyositis and dermatomyositis

- Symmetrical proximal muscle weakness developing over weeks or months
- Elevated serum muscle enzymes, creatine kinase, and aldolase
- Typical electromyographic (EMG) findings
  - Myopathic potentials (low amplitude, short duration, polyphasic)
  - Fibrillation
  - Complex repetitive discharges
  - Typical muscle biopsy findings—endomysial inflammation
- Dermatological features of dermatomyositis
  - Gottron's papules and patches, involving fingers, elbows, knees, and medial malleoli
  - Heliotrope rash around the eyes
  - Erythematous rash around the back, shoulders, upper chest and face (shawl distribution)

Systemic sclerosis

This disease affects women more than men (4:1), and often presents in the fifth decade. It is a clinical diagnosis and there are separable phenotypes.

Limited cutaneous

This type accounts for 60% of systemic sclerosis cases. Patients often have long-standing Raynaud's, and develop non-pitting edema of the fingers, which become "sausage-shaped." After a few weeks to months, they develop thickened, shiny skin but limited to the face, upper extremities distal to the elbows, and lower extremities distal to the knee.

These patients may develop microstomia, digital and facial telangectasias, intradermal and subcutaneous calcification, and esophageal dysmotility (74%). Many develop pulmonary fibrosis (26%), pulmonary hypertension (21%), cardiac disease (9%), and renal disease (8%), but less commonly than in diffuse cutaneous disease. The term CREST is reserved only for patients with limited cutaneous systemic sclerosis, anti-centromere antibodies, Raynaud's phenomenon, sclerodactyly, and telangiectasias.

Diffuse cutaneous

This abrupt-onset disease is characterized by widespread symmetrical itchy, painful swelling of the fingers, arms, feet, legs, and face, often in association with constitutional symptoms. There is subcutaneous edema, which is replaced by tight, shiny skin, bound to underlying structures, within a few months. Cutaneous thickening occurs, as well as hypo- or hyperpigmentation. Raynaud's phenomenon is present, as well as skin sclerosis on the trunk and upper arms, arthropathy, renal disease (18%), pulmonary fibrosis (41%), pulmonary hypertension (17%), and cardiac disease (12%), and GI disease (68%).

Systemic sclerosis sine scleroderma

Vascular or fibrotic visceral features without scleroderma occur. Patients may or may not have Raynaud's phenomenon. They may develop interstitial lung disease, esophagitis, arrhythmias, malabsorption, pseudo-obstruction, pulmonary hypertension, or renal failure. This type accounts for <2% of cases.

Systemic sclerosis pulmonary disease (either ILD or pulmonary hypertension) is the most common cause of death in patients with systemic sclerosis.

The extent of skin disease is useful for disease categorization, but the autoantibody profile is more useful for determining which patients are at greatest risk for developing specific pulmonary manifestations. For example, among patients with anti-centromere antibodies, progressive pulmonary fibrosis occurs in only about 5%, but they are at great risk for developing pulmonary hypertension. Patients with Scl-70 antibodies (regardless of the extent of skin involvement) are at risk for developing progressive pulmonary fibrosis.

Pulmonary fibrosis is seen at postmortem in up to 75% of patients.
- Presentation: dyspnea and a history of Raynaud's phenomenon
- Examination: signs of systemic sclerosis, fine bibasal crackles
- PFTs: restrictive ventilatory defect and reduced DLCO
- Radiography: fibrotic NSIP is most common radiographic and histological pattern
- Treatment: for progressive disease, oral glucocorticoids combined with an immunomodulatory agent

Pulmonary hypertension may be isolated or secondary to ILD. Isolated pulmonary hypertension is associated with anti-centromere antibodies. It is pathologically similar to idiopathic pulmonary arterial hypertension. Subintimal cell proliferation, endothelial hyperplasia, and the obliteration of small intrapulmonary vessels occur.
- Presentation: dyspnea, signs of right ventricular hypertrophy, and right heart failure
- Diagnosis: pulmonary artery pressures estimated by transthoracic echocardiography and confirmed by right heart catheterization
- Treatment: is as for primary pulmonary hypertension.

Chest wall limitation may occur and is due to scleroderma over the chest ("hide-bound chest")

Aspiration pneumonia is due to esophageal dysmotility.

Sjögren's syndrome

This syndrome consists of lymphocytic inflammation and destruction, primarily of the salivary and lacrimal glands, causing keratoconjunctivitis sicca (dry eyes) and/or xerostomia (dry mouth).

Pulmonary involvement occurs in about 25% of patients, and airways and interstitial disease are most common.

Airways inflammation results in bronchial hyperresponsiveness, chronic bronchitis, bronchiectasis, or cellular or obliterative bronchiolitis.

Dry cough is due to atrophy of mucus glands in the trachea and bronchi and lymphoplasmocytic infiltrate (xerotrachea). There may be a higher incidence of chest infections. Treatment is with nebulized saline and physiotherapy.

Organizing pneumonia is rare.

Diffuse lung disease produces cough and dyspnea with crackles on examination. PFTs show a restrictive defect. Radiographic and histological patterns include lymphoid interstitial pneumonia (LIP) in particular or NSIP or UIP patterns.

Lymphoma is unusual, but is 40 times more common in Sjögren's syndrome, especially in patients with high levels of immunoglobulins, autoantibodies, and cryoglobulins. It is usually B-cell lymphoma, and can mimic organizing pneumonia.

Ankylosing spondylitis

This chronic, inflammatory disease causes spinal ankylosis with sacroiliac joint involvement. Ninety percent of Caucasian patients are HLA B27 positive.

Pulmonary fibrosis occurs in 2% of patients, especially those with advanced disease. Remarkably, it is confined to the upper lobe. Patients may develop cysts or cavities and become colonized with *Aspergillus*, which can require treatment.

Pleural involvement reflects pleuritis and apical pleural thickening.

Restrictive defect is due to a fixed deformity of the thorax.

Vasculitis and the lung

Classification

The vasculitides are rare conditions with nonspecific clinical features similar to those seen in multiple other diseases (e.g., infection, drug reaction, malignancy) and a high, untreated mortality rate. The combination makes the diagnosis difficult but crucially important.

The primary pathologic finding in vasculitis is inflammation and necrosis of blood vessels. The clinical features of the disease are dictated by the vessel size, its anatomic location and the relative contribution of vessel necrosis, scarring, and active inflammation.

Suspect a diagnosis of vasculitis with the following clinical scenarios:
- Diffuse alveolar hemorrhage
- Acute glomerulonephritis
- Pulmonary–renal syndromes
- Deforming or ulcerating upper airway lesions
- Nodular or cavitating lesions on chest radiography
- Palpable purpura
- Mononeuritis multiplex
- Evidence of multisystem disease

Classification of the vasculitides (Table 40.1) is dictated by clinical features, the size of the affected vessels, and the findings on serum anti-nuclear cytoplasmic antibody (ANCA) testing (see Box 40.1).

The small vessel vasculitides are the most common to involve the lung (see Table 40.1). Arterioles, capillaries, and venules can all be affected. Inflammatory cell infiltration and subsequent fibrinoid necrosis cause vessel wall destruction. For example, when the pulmonary capillaries are involved (pulmonary capillaritis) a marked neutrophilic infiltration of the interstitium occurs, the capillaries are damaged, allowing red blood cells to enter the alveolus. Thus, alveolar hemorrhage is a feature of many of the small vessel vasculitides.

Further information

Frankel SK, Cosgrove GP, Fischer A, Meehan RT, Brown KK (2006). Update on the diagnosis and management of pulmonary vasculitis. *Chest* **129**:452–465.

Table 40.1 Classification of vasculitis, based on Chapel Hill International Consensus (1992)

Primary vasculitis	Lung involvement	ANCA positivity
Small vessel		
Wegener's granulomatosis	70%–95%	c-ANCA in 75%, p-ANCA in 15%
Churg–Strauss syndrome	>95%	p-ANCA in 45%–70%
Microscopic polyangiitis	10%–30%	p-ANCA in 50%–70%
Goodpasture's disease	Frequent	p-ANCA in 10%–20%
Medium-size vessel		
Polyarteritis nodosa	Rare	Negative
Large vessel		
Giant cell arteritis	Rare	Negative
Takayasu arteritis	Frequent	Negative

Box 40.1 ANCA testing and vasculitis

Anti-neutrophil cytoplasmic antibodies (ANCA) react with cytoplasmic granule enzymes in neutrophils and stain them in one of three ways:
- Diffusely cytoplasmic pattern, or **c-ANCA**
- Perinuclear pattern, or **p-ANCA**.
- Atypical pattern (neither c- nor p-ANCA patterns)

These autoantibodies may have a direct role in pathogenesis as well as being disease markers.

ANCA have multiple, but two major, specificities:
- Antiproteinase 3 antibodies (anti-PR3), associated with c-ANCA pattern
- Antimyeloperoxidase antibodies (anti-MPO), associated with p-ANCA pattern

c-ANCA (anti-PR3) targets proteinase 3 and is most often associated with Wegener's granulomatosis (75% of cases are c-ANCA positive).

p-ANCA (anti-MPO) targets myeloperoxidase and has a wider range of disease associations, including other vasculitides and autoimmune diseases, HIV, lung cancer, and pulmonary emboli.

Wegener's granulomatosis: presentation and diagnosis

Definition and epidemiology

Wegener's granulomatosis is an ANCA-associated necrotizing granulomatous vasculitis affecting small and medium-size vessels, especially in the upper and lower respiratory tract and kidneys.

- Unknown cause
- Male = female
- 3/100,000, 80%–97% Caucasian
- Occurs at any age, but most common between 40 and 55 years

Clinical features

ENT

In 90% of cases, upper airways involvement is the first presenting sign. Nasal congestion and epistaxis occur, with inflamed, crusty, ulcerated nasal mucosa. There is nasal septum perforation (a late sign is a saddle nose deformity). Sinusitis is common and may be painful. Patients may have otitis media, as well as subglottic stenosis, causing upper airway obstruction, dyspnea, voice change, and cough. Abnormal flow-volume loops are seen.

Lung

The lungs are affected in 85%–90% of patients. Hemoptysis, cough, and dyspnea occur. There may be pleuritic chest pain.

Kidney

The kidneys are affected in 50%–90% of patients, with hematuria, proteinuria, and red cell casts. Only 10% have renal impairment initially, but up to 90% will have involvement during their disease course. Characteristic progressive deterioration of renal function, often occult, occurs.

Systemic

Fever and weight loss are present.

Other organ systems (skin, eyes, joints, CNS)

Vasculitic skin rash with granulomatous involvement occurs in 46% of patients. They may also have muscle and joint pains, along with conjunctivitis, scleritis, proptosis, eye pain, and visual loss. Mononeuritis multiplex and CNS disease can also occur.

Investigations

Consider the following investigations:

- **CXR** to look for cavitating pulmonary nodules, consolidation, or pulmonary infiltrates, alveolar hemorrhage, parenchymal distortion, large and small airway disease, pleural effusion, bronchiectasis. Can look like neoplasm, infection, or fluid overload
- **HRCT** of chest
- **Oxygen saturations**
- **CBC, urinalysis, CRP, ESR**

- *Serum ANCA*, especially c-ANCA, is sensitive and fairly specific. It is present in 90% of patients with generalized active Wegener's and in 60% with limited disease. p-ANCA is positive in 5%–10% of patients. Combining serum ANCA with specific immunoassays for antibodies to PR3 and MPO increases sensitivity and specificity for Wegener's to over 90%. However, **ANCA can be negative in active disease, especially in disease confined to the upper and/or lower respiratory tract (limited disease)**. ANCA levels should not be used in isolation to determine the level of disease activity or treatment.
- *Urine dipstick and microscopy* for proteinuria and red cell casts
- *Pulmonary function tests, including spirometry with a flow-volume loop to look for subglottic stenosis*
- *Image sinuses* Bony destruction increases the likelihood of Wegener's
- *Bronchoscopy* may show inflammation, ulceration, scarring, and stenosis of the larynx, trachea (subglottic stenosis), and bronchi. BAL is neutrophilic, with eosinophils and lymphocytes. Transbronchial biopsy is unlikely to be diagnostic.
- *Biopsy*
  - *Respiratory tract and nose*—granulomatous inflammation in association with medium- and small-vessel necrotizing vasculitis and surrounding inflammation. Nasal biopsies are most often nonspecific and unlikely to be diagnostic.
  - *Renal biopsy*—focal segmental or diffuse necrotizing glomerulonephritis may be seen. Pauci-immune and granulomata rare. Not specific for Wegener's
  - *Skin biopsy*—leukocytoclastic vasculitis is a common finding

Diagnosis

The clinical scenario, ANCA results, and biopsy findings from an affected organ are key to the diagnosis. Strongly suggestive clinical findings combined with high-titer c-ANCA and anti-proteinase 3 (PR3) antibodies are highly suggestive of Wegener's and may occasionally be adequate for diagnosis when competing diagnoses have been excluded.

Biopsy should be performed at a site that is both clinically affected and easily and safely biopsied. It may be nasal, lung (open or thoracoscopic), skin, or renal. The disease may be patchy, requiring repeat biopsy if the first is negative. Surgical lung biopsy provides the highest likelihood of a definitive diagnosis.

Differential diagnosis

This includes malignancy, TB, sarcoidosis, allergic bronchopulmonary aspergillosis, Goodpasture's disease (anti-glomerular basement membrane disease with pulmonary hemorrhage and nephritis), SLE, microscopic polyangiitis, connective tissue disease, and disseminated infection.

Wegener's granulomatosis: management

Involve the appropriate consultants (i.e., nephrology) early and create a multidisciplinary team to share care of the patient. Stratify disease severity by means of the EUVAS grading of disease severity (see Table 40.2).

Use an initial induction remission regimen followed by a maintenance regimen. The goal is to control active inflammation and prevent irreversible tissue damage.

Table 40.2 EUVAS grading of disease severity and first-line treatment options

Disease classification	Constitutional symptoms	Threatened organ function	Treatment options
Active disease			*Induction regimen*
Limited	No	No	Corticosteroids OR methotrexate OR azathioprine
Early generalized	Yes	No	Cyclophosphamide + corticosteroids OR Methotrexate + corticosteroids
Active generalized	Yes	Yes	Cyclophosphamide + corticosteroids
Severe	Yes	Yes*	Cyclophosphamide + corticosteroids + plasma exchange
Refractory	Yes	Yes	Consider trial of an investigational agent or referral to tertiary center (see text)
Disease remission			*Maintenance regimen*
Remission	No	No	Azathioprine + corticosteroids

Severe disease includes severe renal failure (creatinine >5.7 mg/dL), diffuse alveolar hemorrhage, or other life-threatening organ failure such as severe cardiac, central nervous system, or gastrointestinal disease.

The standard regimen for active generalized disease is as follows:
- Oral corticosteroids decreased over approximately 6 months
- Combined with cyclophosphamide orally until remission (generally 3–6 months), then switch to azathioprine for maintenance therapy
- There is good evidence that this regime gives improvement in 90% of patients.
- Immunosuppression is generally recommended for at least 1 year.
- Relapses will occur in up to 50% of patients. Retreatment with the standard regimen is the initial approach.

For patients with rapidly progressive renal failure or severe alveolar hemorrhage:
- Plasma exchange or plasmapheresis has been shown to be more effective than corticosteroids alone.
- Dialysis for renal failure

PCP prophylaxis with trimethoprim-sulfamethoxazole is strongly recommended. There is some evidence that trimethoprim-sulfamethoxazole may help prevent relapse of disease, although the reasons for this are not clear. It may be due to the suppression of *Staphylococcus aureus*.

Bone protection should be considered.

Routine and clinically indicated monitoring should be performed looking for evidence of disease activity, medication toxicity, and infection. Testing should include medication-specific monitoring plus consideration of the following: CBC, urinalysis and measures of renal function, CRP, LFT, ANCA, and chest imaging.

Prognosis

Limited disease with pulmonary and/or upper airway but no renal involvement has a better prognosis. However, this can progress over time to *generalized disease*, with classical destructive sinusitis, nephritis, and vasculitis and strong c-ANCA positivity, and is associated with higher mortality. Untreated, 80% of people with extensive Wegener's granulomatosis will die in 1 year.

Further information

Langford C, Hoffman G (1999). Wegener's granulomatosis. Rare diseases 3, *Thorax* **54**:629–663.

Microscopic polyangiitis

Microscopic polyangiitis is an ANCA-associated small vessel vasculitis that universally affects the kidney and variably affects the lung. It may be difficult to distinguish from Wegener's. It is managed in the same way (see Table 40.2).

- **Incidence** Male = female, mean age 50, mainly Caucasians
- **Kidneys** are the main organ affected, by a small vessel necrotizing vasculitis. It presents as rapidly progressive glomerulonephritis (RPGN), with proteinuria, and hematuria. Renal biopsy shows focal segmental glomerulonephritis with fibrinoid necrosis and sparse immune deposits.
- **Pulmonary involvement** occurs in 30%–50% of patients, primarily with alveolar hemorrhage.
- **p-ANCA** positive in 50%–75%, c-ANCA in 10%–15%

Treatment is with immunosuppression: steroids and cyclophosphamide (see Table 40.2).

Goodpasture's disease

Definition and epidemiology

Goodpasture's disease (also known as anti-glomerular basement membrane [anti-GBM] disease) is the classic pulmonary–renal syndrome. A primary immune complex–mediated vasculitis, it is defined as the combination of RPGN, alveolar hemorrhage, and anti-GBM antibody formation, though the clinical presentation varies. The antibodies are directed against a glycoprotein epitope on type IV collagen.

- Important differential diagnosis of pulmonary–renal syndrome
- Annual incidence of 1 case per million
- Male–female ratio = 2–9:1
- Most common at age 20–30 years
- Second peak occurs when women in their late 60s are affected by glomerulonephritis alone
- Cause is unknown. Often a preceding viral infection. Smokers are at greater significantly greater risk of alveolar hemorrhage.
- HLA DR2 association in over 70%

Clinical features

- Hemoptysis in 80%–90%—much more common in smokers
- Cough, dyspnea, fatigue, and weakness
- Examination: inspiratory crackles are common.

Investigations

- Serum electrolytes show renal disturbance and, often, renal failure.
- *CBC* shows iron-deficiency anemia.
- *Urine dip and microscopy* Hematuria, proteinuria, granular and typically red blood cell casts. Occasionally, macroscopic hematuria
- *Anti-GBM* and autoantibody screen
- *Coexisting ANCA (usually p-ANCA) is identified in 25% of patients.*
- *Chest radiography* shows diffuse bilateral patchy airspace shadowing in mid and lower zones. May see air bronchograms
- *PFTs* indicate restrictive defect with raised DlCO if alveolar hemorrhage is present.

Diagnosis

Renal biopsy usually shows diffuse crescentic glomerulonephritis. Linear IgG deposition on the basement membranes of alveoli and glomeruli are detected by immunofluorescence. Lung biopsy shows active intra-alveolar hemorrhage with collections of hemosiderin-laden macrophages.

Differential diagnosis includes Wegener's granulomatosis and other pulmonary renal syndromes.

Management

- Involve the renal team early and share care of the patient.
- Plasma exchange is indicated to remove circulating antibody.
- Corticosteroids and cyclophosphamide are indicated to minimize ongoing antibody production.
- Renal failure usually requires dialysis. Renal function may not improve and renal transplant is only an option if anti-GBM antibody levels become low.
- Recurrence is uncommon once disease is controlled. It usually responds to further immunosuppression. Residual defects in PFTs are frequent.

Prognosis

Rapidly progressive alveolar hemorrhage and renal failure are usually fatal if not treated.

Churg–Strauss syndrome

Definition and epidemiology

Churg–Strauss syndrome is an ANCA-associated small vessel vasculitis with a presentation generally distinct from Wegener's granulomatosis. A triad of asthma, blood eosinophilia, and a necrotizing vasculitis affecting small and medium-sized vessels is seen, often in association with an eosinophilic granulomatous inflammation of the respiratory tract.

- Rare, 2.4 per million population, but 64 per million of an asthmatic population
- Middle-aged adults
- Male–female ratio is 2:1
- Unknown cause. Development of Churg–Strauss syndrome in severe asthmatics on leukotriene antagonists appears to be related to their decreased steroid requirement "unmasking" Churg–Strauss syndrome.

Clinical features

A diagnosis of Churg–Strauss syndrome can be made if 4 of the following 6 criteria are present:

- Asthma is essentially universal and may have been present for years. Often it has maturity onset, is difficult to control, and is associated with rhinitis and nasal polyps.
- Blood eosinophilia of >10%
- Vasculitic neuropathy, such as mononeuritis multiplex (occurs in >50%)
- Pulmonary infiltrates
- Sinus disease (20%–70%)
- Extravascular eosinophils on biopsy findings
- Patient may also may have
  - Cardiac involvement (30%–50%) conduction delay, cardiac failure, cardiomyopathy, coronary artery inflammation, pericardial effusion
  - Gastrointestinal involvement (30%–60%) with eosinophilic infiltration of mesenteric vessels causing GI disturbance or hemorrhage
  - Alveolar hemorrhage
  - Renal involvement, uncommon but may be seen in about10% of patients;
  - Skin nodules and purpura
  - Myalgia and arthralgia
  - Fever and weight loss.

The typical pattern of disease has three phases: with a prodromal phase of rhinitis, sinusitis, and asthma, the development of blood and tissue eosinophilia (e.g., eosinophilic pneumonia), and a final systemic vasculitic phase. The asthma precedes the vasculitis, often by years (mean 8 years).

Investigations

- **CXR** shows fleeting peripheral pulmonary infiltrates and bilateral multifocal consolidation.
- **HRCT** shows ground-glass inflammation, pulmonary nodules, bronchial wall thickening, or alveolar hemorrhage.
- **Bronchoscopy** BAL reveals marked eosinophilia.

- *Pathology* Extravascular tissue eosinophilia, necrotizing angiitis, granulomata
- *Serum markers* for peripheral blood eosinophilia. p-ANCA and anti-MPO are positive in two-thirds of patients.

Diagnosis

Diagnosis is predominantly clinical. Pathological confirmation of eosinophilic tissue infiltration or vasculitis is desirable. Biopsy the easiest site affected, such as skin, or by open or thorascopic lung biopsy.

Differential diagnosis

Other causes of eosinophilic syndromes include allergic bronchopulmonary aspergillosis, drug and parasitic causes of eosinophilic pneumonias, and hypereosinophilic syndrome.

Management

Management depends on the severity of disease at presentation (see Table 40.2).
- Treatment is aimed at reversing organ damage and reducing the relapse rate (see Table 40.2).
- *If isolated pulmonary disease*, oral corticosteroids until disease is in remission, then slowly decrease over 1 year, with increases if symptoms recur
- *With significant organ dysfunction such as cardiac or GI disease, alveolar hemorrhage, relapse, or life-threatening situations* pulsed methyl prednisolone IV for 3 days, followed by high-dose oral steroids, with cyclophosphamide
- Plasma exchange is of no benefit.
- *To maintain remission*, corticosteroids and one other immunosuppressant drug are usually required. Cyclophosphamide is often changed to azathioprine after 4–6 months.
- Prophylactic trimethoprim-sulfamethoxazole should be given; consider bone protection for steroids.
- *Follow up* regular clinical evaluation with checks of CBC, eosinophil count, and CXR.

Prognosis

The prognosis is good for isolated pulmonary disease. The asthma often persists despite good control of vasculitis, and can be severe and difficult to control.

Poor prognosis is associated with cardiac disease and severe gastrointestinal disease, causing bleeding, perforation or necrosis, renal disease, and CNS involvement. Untreated, the 5-year survival rate is 25%. Cardiac disease is the main cause of death.

Further information

Noth I, Strek ME, Leff AR (2003). Churg–Strauss syndrome. *Lancet* **361**:587–594.
The European Vasculitis Study Group: www.vasculitis.org

Rare pulmonary vasculitic diseases

Polyarteritis nodosa
- Lung involvement is rare.
- Clinically similar to microscopic polyangiitis, but affecting medium-sized vessels
- May exist as an "overlap" disorder with ANCA-associated vasculitides
- Sometimes associated with previous hepatitis B or rarely hepatitis C infection, which alters the treatment regimen.

Takayasu's arteritis
- Predominantly young women are affected, often Asian.
- Vasculitis affecting the aorta and its major branches. Large- and medium-sized pulmonary vessels are affected, but involvement is usually clinically silent. Pulmonary artery stenosis and occlusion are common, occasionally with mild pulmonary hypertension.
- **Presents** with fevers and weight loss. Patients are noted to have absent peripheral pulses, arterial bruits, and discrepancies in extremity blood pressure.
- **Diagnosis** is made by angiography.
- **Treatment** Corticosteroids may reduce symptoms, but do not affect mortality. Angioplasty and surgical procedures may reduce the vascular complications. Spontaneous remissions may occur.

Giant cell arteritis
- Most common form of systemic vasculitis, affects large- and medium-sized vessels
- 24 cases per 100,000. Predominantly elderly females
- **Present with** nonspecific symptoms of fever and weight loss, also headache, scalp tenderness, and jaw pain. Amaurosis fugax and visual loss are due to optic neuritis.
- **Pulmonary complications** occur in 9%–25% of cases. They are relatively clinically mild, with cough, sore throat, and hoarseness. Pulmonary function tests and CXR are generally normal.
- **Diagnosis** High ESR, temporal artery biopsy showing panarteritis and giant cell formation
- **Treatment** Good response to oral steroids. Continue for 1–2 years.

Gastrointestinal disease and the lung

Hepatic hydrothorax

Hepatic hydrothorax involves transdiaphragmatic migration of large amounts of ascites fluid in cirrhotic patients in the absence of cardiopulmonary disease.

Prevalence is 4%–12% of patients with cirrhosis and is not associated with a specific etiology of cirrhosis. The condition is found on the right two-thirds of the time, but can be seen on the left only or bilaterally.

Unlike the pleural cavity, a patient can hold approximately 10 L of ascites before symptoms become evident, whereas 1 L of pleural fluid may cause symptoms.

Pathophysiology

It is likely that defects in the diaphragm, particularly fenestrations in the tendinous portion on the right, permit passage of ascites fluid from the abdomen into the pleural space. Anatomic thinning related to congenital factors or increased intra-abdominal pressures result in small diaphragmatic ruptures. Negative pleural pressure produces a one-way valve and draws in fluid from the abdomen. Once the absorptive capacity of the pleura is exceeded, fluid accumulates in the pleural space.

Pleural effusion in the absence of ascites has been described. This is dependent on an imbalance of pleural fluid absorption and hepatic fluid production—if the rate of pleural fluid absorption is high, no peritoneal fluid will accumulate.

Diagnosis

Diagnosis requires high clinical suspicion in patients with a history of cirrhosis and right-sided pleural effusion in the presence of ascites, although exceptions have been noted.

Thoracentesis demonstrates a serous transudate with a low nucleated cell count (mostly monocytes), pH <7.40, a glucose level similar to serum glucose, and a protein level higher than that for ascitic fluid.

VATS (video assisted thoracoscopic surgery) can be used to visualize flaws in the diaphragm (although not routinely done for this purpose).

Management

Initial management requires salt restriction and diuresis (although prolonged use can lead to intravascular volume depletion and renal failure). Patients are considered *refractory* if there is no response to these initial steps. One-third of patients with hepatic hydrothorax respond to medical treatment temporarily.

Paracentesis and thoracentesis can be performed for temporary relief of symptoms; it is usually best to remove ascitic fluid first, then pleural fluid. Serial thoracenteses are generally not recommended due to the inherent risk of repeated procedures.

Pleural drainage with a chest tube can lead to protein, fluid, and electrolyte imbalances; pleural sclerosis also is not helpful as fluid accumulates rapidly and does not permit adequate apposition of pleural surfaces. Treatment of the underlying cause is the best option (if possible).

Further reading

Roussos A, Philippou N, Mantzaris GJ, et al (2007). Hepatic hydrothorax: pathophysiology, diagnosis, and management. *J Gastroenterol Hepatol* **22**:1388–1393.

Hepatopulmonary syndrome

Hepatopulmonary syndrome (HPS) consists of the triad of
- Chronic liver disease or portal hypertension
- Intrapulmonary vascular vasodilatation
- Widened A–a gradient on room air (>15 mmHg) with or without arterial hypoxemia (PaO_2 <70 mmHg)

Pathophysiology

Patients with HPS exhibit a variable degree of hepatic dysfunction, cirrhosis, or portal hypertension; HPS does not correlate with severity of liver disease. The pathogenic hallmark of HPS is microvascular dilatation of precapillary arterioles due to excessive production of nitric oxide (NO). The exact mechanism of increased endogenous NO and relationship to liver disease is unknown.

Presentation

Progressive dyspnea and cyanosis occur. Examination may reveal clubbing and telangectasias, with associated stigmata of chronic liver disease. Classically, patients may complain of platypnea (dyspnea when positioned upright, improved when supine) and orthodeoxia may be noted (hypoxemia worsened when upright), both caused by preferential perfusion of dilated basal pulmonary vasculature producing V/Q mismatching. Spider angiomata, clubbing, and distal cyanosis may also be noted.

Diagnosis

Making of a diagnosis of HPS can be difficult. The clinical criteria are not specific, and there is no consensus on defining diagnostic criteria.

ABG

Perform an ABG, as O_2 saturation by oximetry may not be accurate in liver disease. Calculate an A–a gradient and determine if the patient is hypoxemic on room air.

Platypnea and orthodeoxia can be seen in other lung diseases, but in the presence of liver disease is suggestive of HPS. Hypoxia is poorly reversed with 100% oxygen, due to pulmonary shunting.

Contrast-enhanced echocardiogram

Agitated saline is intravenously injected, producing bubbles that are normally seen only in the right heart and subsequently filtered by the pulmonary vascular bed. An intracardiac shunt may display bubbles in the left ventricle early (within 3 cardiac cycles); if later (after 3 cycles), an intrapulmonary shunt may be present. It is unclear if the size of the shunt reflects the degree of gas exchange abnormalities.

Pulmonary technetium-99 perfusion scan

This scan assesses shunt fraction and can be used to determine contribution of HPS in a patient with intrapulmonary vasodilatation and cardiopulmonary disease. Normally, technetium-radiolabeled albumin is trapped in the pulmonary capillary bed. In the presence of intrapulmonary or cardiac shunts, there is significant uptake of radiolabeled albumin in other organs such as the brain or spleen. A shunt index fraction of >20% indicates severe hepatopulmonary syndrome.

CT chest can identify pulmonary microvascular dilatations and can rule out other comorbid pulmonary disease.

PFTs usually show decreased DLCO.

Treatment

Oxygen is the mainstay of therapy for patients with PaO_2 <60 mmHg at rest or with exercise. There are no randomized trials that prove the efficacy of oxygen therapy. However, based on the benefits of O_2 therapy in other hypoxemic pulmonary conditions, it is thought to be helpful.

There are no effective medical therapies to treat HPS.

The mainstay of treatment is liver transplantation, which improves postoperative gas exchange in >85% of patients. The effect is not always immediate, and hypoxemia may take months to 1 year to show improvement. Severe preoperative hypoxemia (PaO_2 <50 mmHg) is associated with increased mortality post-transplant.

Complications include increased risk of hepatic ischemia, pulmonary hypertension, cerebral embolic hemorrhage, and prolonged mechanical ventilation due to postoperative deoxygenation.

The efficacy of transjugular intrahepatic portosystemic shunt (TIPS) is unclear at this time.

Coil embolization can be tried in cases with large anatomic intrapulmonary shunts. This should preferentially shunt blood from dilated vessels to areas of the lung that do not, thus decreasing the amount of deoxygenated blood in the arterial circulation.

Prognosis

Prognosis is poor. In a prospective study comparing patients with cirrhosis and those with HPS, the median survival was 40.8 months versus 10.6 months, respectively. Deaths were related to hepatic dysfunction and portal hypertension and correlated with the degree of hypoxemia.

Further reading

Mandell MS (2006). The diagnosis and treatment of hepatopulmonary syndrome. *Clin Liver Dis* **10**:387–405.
Palma DT, Fallon MB (2006). The hepatopulmonary syndrome. *J Hepatol* **45**:617–625.

Portopulmonary hypertension (POPH)

Definition

POPH is pulmonary artery hypertension (PAH) occurring in association with portal hypertension. It occurs in an estimated 2%–5% of patients with cirrhosis and is present in around 16% of those referred for liver transplantation. The mechanism is unclear, but probably relates to a hyperdynamic circulation, high cardiac output, cytokine release, and possible pulmonary emboli.

POPH can be defined as follows:

- Elevated mean pulmonary artery pressure (>25 mmHg at rest, >30 mmHg during exercise)
- Increased pulmonary vascular resistance due to pulmonary vasoconstriction and obliterative vascular remodeling (>240 dyne s^{-1} cm^{-5}) similar to that of pulmonary arterial hypertension
- Normal pulmonary artery occlusion pressure (PAOP) <15 mmHg

Presentation

Early in the disease process patients may be asymptomatic or have symptoms related to portal hypertension. The most common symptom is dyspnea on exertion. However, in patients with liver disease, dyspnea is a nonspecific symptom that can be attributed to other processes such as cardiomyopathy, hepatic hydrothorax, tense ascites causing a restrictive lung pattern, or parenchymal lung disease.

Additional complaints can include fatigue, palpitations, hemoptysis, and orthopnea. Later in the disease course, patients may present with syncope or chest pain, which are ominous signs.

On physical exam there may be signs of stigmata of chronic liver disease, including jaundice, ascites, and spider telangiectasias. Progression of the disease leads to volume overload and right-sided cardiac dysfunction, with raised JVP and pedal edema as well as increased P2 with a widely split S2, RV heave, and pulmonary and/or tricuspid regurgitation. It is usually diagnosed 4–7 years after the diagnosis of portal hypertension.

Diagnosis

- **Hypoxia** is mild to moderate on blood gases and not as pronounced, as in patients with hepatopulmonary syndrome. A decreased carbon dioxide level <30 mmHg in a patient with portal hypertension may indicate the presence of PAH. There may also be an increased A–a difference.
- **CXR** may be normal or show prominent pulmonary arteries and an enlarged right heart.
- **ECG** may show right atrial enlargement, right ventricular hypertrophy (RVH), right bundle branch block (RBBB), right axis deviation (RAD), or sinus tachycardia.
- **PFTs** may display decreased DLCO and can exclude airflow obstruction.

Echocardiography is the main screening test. Findings suggestive of POPH are as follows:

- Increased tricuspid peak regurgitant (TR) jet velocity
- Pulmonic valve insufficiency
- Paradoxical septal motion
- RVH and dilatation
- Increased right ventricular systolic pressure (RVSP)

Patients with RVSP >50 mmHg should undergo right heart catheterization (RHC), although no consensus exists regarding the degree of transthoracic echocardiogram (TTE) findings and referral for RHC.

Right heart catheterization is the gold standard for diagnosis and provides a multitude of hemodynamic measurements to aid in the diagnosis of POPH.

- One-third of patients with RVSP >50 mmHg have normal pulmonary vascular resistance (PVR) on RHC. This may represent an overestimation of the TR jet on TTE due to hyperdynamic state (increased cardiac output [CO] with decreased systemic vascular resistance).
- PVR = [(mPAP – PAOP)/CO] × 80
- Vasodilator response can be performed using NO. A positive response is a decrease in mPAP and PVR >20% without an increase in CO. The goal of testing is to determine the severity of disease and response to therapy. It is not used to determine responsiveness to calcium channel blockers (CCB), as is used in pulmonary hypertension. The use of CCBs in POPH is contraindicated, as it may increase the hepatic venous pressure gradient.

Treatment

There are no large randomized, controlled clinical trials evaluating long-term medical management in patients with POPH. Therapy should be initiated when the patient is symptomatic, mPAP is >35 mmHg, and PVR is increased.

Treatment of volume overload with diuretics is beneficial. Anticoagulation is not advised due to the risk of variceal bleeding. Avoid beta-blockers, as they may worsen pulmonary hemodynamics and exercise tolerance. Epoprostenol (continuous IV) has been studied and decreases mPAP and PVR, but it is unclear if a survival benefit is offered.

Oral agents used for PAH, such as endothelin antagoinists and sildenafil, may be beneficial in the treatment of POPH; however, larger studies to evaluate efficacy, safety, and mortality benefit need to be performed.

Liver transplantation can be performed in select patients with POPH. Patients with POPH are at increased perioperative and long-term morbidity and mortality. These findings correlate with the degree of mPAP and PVR elevation.

After RHC is performed, an mPAP ≥50 mmHg is a contraindication to liver transplantation. However in patients with mPAP ≤35 mmHg and PVR <240 dyne s^{-1} cm^{-5} can undergo liver transplantation. Those with mPAP between 35 and 50 mmHg and a PVR >250 dyne s^{-1} cm^{-5} are at higher risk and should be treated with vasodilator therapy prior to liver transplantation. Like HPS, symptoms after liver transplantation may take months to years to resolve.

Prognosis

Prognosis is poor and survival is shorter compared to patients with idiopathic PAH. Survival of patients with POPH at 1, 2, and 5 years has been demonstrated to be 71%, 58%, and 44%, respectively (regardless of liver transplantation).

Further reading

Golbin JM, Krowka MJ (2007). Portopulmonary hypertension. *Clin Chest Med* **20**:203–218.

Inflammatory bowel disease, celiac disease, and pancreatitis

Inflammatory bowel disease (IBD)

Extraintestinal manifestations of IBD can be articular (arthropathy), dermatologic (pyoderma gangrenosum, erythema nodosum), ophthalmological (episcleritis, anterior uveitis), and hepatic (pericholangitis, fatty liver) and can involve the respiratory system (see Box 41.1). Prior studies have shown that 40%–50% of patients with IBD have respiratory complaints (wheeze, productive or nonproductive cough or breathlessness) presumed due to IBD.

The prevalence of pulmonary involvement related to IBD is not known. This disease entity is likely underreported for multiple reasons: lack of knowledge, respiratory symptoms that can occur years after IBD has been treated (medically or after colectomy) and GI symptoms have resolved, and symptomatic patients with a normal chest X-ray not undergoing further diagnostic studies.

The GI manifestations of IBD usually predate the pulmonary symptoms, although there are exceptions. Pulmonary involvement is more common in ulcerative colitis (UC) than Crohn's disease.

Clinical manifestations

Patients can develop a variety of clinical syndromes. Typically this is organized according to site of involvement.

Box 41.1 Pulmonary manifestations of IBD

Airway
- Upper airway—obstruction, subglottic stenosis
- Large airways—Bronchiectasis, acute or chronic bronchitis, chronic bronchial suppuration
- Small airways—bronchiolitis, diffuse panbronchiolitis obliterans

Parenchymal
- Organizing pneumonia (BOOP)
- Necrobiotic nodules
- ILD
- Pulmonary infiltrates and peripheral eosinophilia

Serositis
- Pleural disease—pleuritis, pleural effusion, pleuropericarditis
- Pericardial disease—pericarditis, myocarditis

Vascular
- Pulmonary embolism

Diagnostic studies

Symptomatic patients should undergo further evaluation with high-resolution CT (HRCT) and pulmonary function testing (PFT). Abnormalities seen on HRCT may include air-trapping, ground-glass opacities, peripheral reticular opacities, and cysts.

Asymptomatic patients with IBD have a mildly decreased DLCO on PFTs when compared to normal controls. DLCO levels decrease significantly during periods of active GI inflammation. Patients may also display evidence of airflow obstruction, although no significant difference was found in FEV_1 in IBD versus control groups.

Some investigators have identified small airways dysfunction as a potential etiology of obstruction. Hyperinflation can also be seen and may correlate with disease activity, as indicated by elevated functional residual capacity (FRC) and residual volume (RV).

A methacholine challenge can demonstrate bronchial hyperreactivity. Bronchoscopy with bronchoalveolar lavage (BAL) may reveal alveolar lymphocytosis in asymptomatic patients.

Treatment

Before initiating treatment for IBD-related pulmonary disease, the patient should first undergo evaluation for a pulmonary infection (send cultures and start antibiotics) and drug-induced lung disease. Drugs used in the treatment of IBD may also cause lung disease, such as sulfasalazine (alveolitis), mesalazine, or infliximab (both cause pulmonary infiltrates and eosinophilia; infliximab induces reactivation of latent TB).

Upper airway lesions can be treated with laser ablation of inflammatory tissue and usually respond to steroids. Inhaled steroids can be used for large airway treatment and systemic steroids may benefit patients with bronchiectasis and sputum production (not responsive to inhaled steroids). Other medications, such as azathioprine and cyclophosphamide, have been used.

Celiac disease

Celiac disease may be associated with pulmonary fibrosis, causing restrictive defect. Patients may be at increased risk of asthma, bird fancier's lung, and hemosiderosis, as well as for lymphoma and GI tract malignancy.

Pancreatitis

Acute pancreatitis is frequently associated with exudative pleural effusion. Raised amylase in the pleural fluid is suggestive. Adult respiratory distress syndrome (ARDS) may develop, which requires supportive care and mechanical ventilation

Further reading

Black H, Mendoza M, Murin S (2007). Thoracic manifestations of inflammatory bowel disease. *Chest* **131**:524–532.
Sharma S, Eschun G (2007). Pulmonary manifestations of IBD. *J Respir Dis* **28**:227–234.

Acute respiratory distress syndrome (ARDS)

Pathophysiology and diagnosis

Definition and epidemiology

ARDS is a common form of lung injury characterized by disruption of the alveolar–capillary membrane leading to accumulation of proteinaceous pulmonary edema and coincident hypoxemia. Since the initial description of ARDS in 1967, investigators initially used a variety of different diagnostic criteria to define ARDS. In 1994, the European–American Consensus Conference (AECC) developed diagnostic criteria for the definition of ARDS that have been universally adopted:

- Bilateral opacities on the chest radiograph that are consistent with pulmonary edema
- PaO_2/FiO_2 <200 mmHg
- Not due to clinical left ventricular failure or associated with a wedge pressure of over 18 mmHg (non-cardiogenic)

The AECC also recognized that ARDS is a spectrum of disease and defined a milder form of ARDS, called acute lung injury (ALI), which is differentiated from ARDS by a PaO_2/FiO_2 <300 mmHg. In the United States there are approximately 190,000 cases of ARDS/ALI annually.

Although ARDS develops in critically ill patients with a variety of illnesses, the most common predisposing conditions include sepsis, pneumonia, trauma, and aspiration of gastric contents. These four diagnoses account for up to 85% of cases. Other less common causes of ARDS include the following:

- Blood transfusion, or other plasma-containing blood products
- Drug overdose, e.g., tricyclic antidepressants, opiates, cocaine, aspirin
- Acute pancreatitis
- Near drowning
- Following upper airway obstruction; mechanism unclear
- Smoke inhalation
- After bone marrow transplantation, as bone marrow recovers

Clinical features

The manifestations of ARDS are variable and depend on the predisposing illness, severity of lung injury, and presence of nonpulmonary organ dysfunction. Most patients will complain of dyspnea and have increased work of breathing due to the reduction in lung compliance. Subsequently, patients will develop rapidly worsening hypoxemia, requiring escalating amounts of supplemental oxygen. Intubation and mechanical ventilation are nearly always required.

Many biochemical abnormalities are present in these patients, as ARDS is the pulmonary manifestation of a more systemic process called the multiple organ dysfunction syndrome (MODS). However, there is no laboratory abnormality or serological marker specifically associated with ARDS. The chest radiograph in ARDS patients will reveal bilateral infiltrates that are consistent with pulmonary edema but they can be very mild. While these infiltrates may appear to be homogeneous on chest radiograph, CT scanning demonstrates a more heterogeneous and patchy pattern.

ARDS usually develops hours to days after the onset of the predisposing condition. In general, most patients (85%) will develop ARDS within 3 days, and almost all patients will develop ARDS within 7 days after the development of the predisposing condition.

Differential diagnosis

The possibility of ARDS should be considered in any patient with acute hypoxemic respiratory failure. Left ventricular failure may be excluded on clinical grounds or by echocardiography, but confident exclusion requires the placement of a pulmonary artery catheter.

In the absence of an obvious predisposing condition such as sepsis or trauma, other causes of diffuse acute parenchymal lung diseases should be considered, including acute eosinophilic pneumonia, bronchiolitis obliterans organizing pneumonia (BOOP), acute interstitial pneumonia, bronchoalveolar cell carcinoma, and pulmonary alveolar proteinosis.

Diffuse alveolar infiltrates and hypoxemia may also be related to alveolar hemorrhage that can occur in Goodpasture's disease, Wegener's granulomatosis, and SLE. Clues will include a drop in hemoglobin, blood in the airways and pulmonary secretions, and other clinical features of one of these disorders. When other causes of acute respiratory failure with diffuse infiltrates cannot be excluded, it may be appropriate to perform a bronchoalveolar lavage and transbronchial biopsy or, if necessary, a surgical lung biopsy.

Pathophysiology

Inflammatory damage occurs in the alveoli and lung capillary endothelium, either by locally produced proinflammatory mediators or those remotely produced and arriving via the pulmonary artery. This leads to loss of the integrity of the alveolar–capillary barrier, with transudation of protein-rich pulmonary edema fluid.

Type I cells (comprising 90% of the alveolar epithelium) are the most easily damaged, allowing increased entry of fluid into the alveoli and decreased clearance of fluid from the alveolar space. Type II cells are less easily damaged but serve multiple roles, including surfactant production, ion transport, and proliferation and differentiation into type I cells after injury. Their damage leads to decreased surfactant production and decreased compliance.

This cellular dysfunction and damage lead to the following:

- Gross impairment of V/Q matching with shunting, causing arterial hypoxia and very large A–a gradients. There are usually enough remaining functioning alveoli such that a degree of hyperventilation maintains CO_2 clearance; thus hypercapnia is infrequently a problem.
- Pulmonary hypertension
- Reduced compliance (stiff lungs), due to loss of functioning alveoli (alveolar collapse, filled with fluid and protein), and hyperinflation of remaining alveoli to their limits of distension
- Interference with the normal repair processes of the lung, leading to the fibrosis seen in later stages of ARDS

Management and complications

Management

The essential aspects of management of patients with ARDS are to treat the precipitating cause, provide best supportive care, and avoid further complications.

There have been great advances in the mechanical-ventilatory strategy for patients with ARDS. The use of high tidal volumes and thus higher plateau pressures is associated with various forms of barotrauma including pneumothorax, pneumomediastinum, subcutaneous emphysema, air embolism, and primary alveolar damage. Therefore, low tidal volume ventilation (6 mL/kg ideal body weight) should be used in all patients with ARDS. The use of low tidal volumes may result in a reduction in minute ventilation and subsequently an elevated $PaCO_2$.

Positive end expiratory pressure (PEEP) is usually required to maintain an adequate level of oxygenation. However, the use of high levels of PEEP does not improve outcome but may be helpful in patients that are difficult to oxygenate.

Prone positioning can also be used to improve oxygenatation but is not associated with a reduction in mortality.

There are no specific medical therapies that are effective for patients with ARDS. However, the use of a conservative fluid strategy, keeping the central venous pressure (CVP) as low as possible, will decrease the length of time that patients require mechanical ventilation. Based on the results of several studies, the use of corticosteroids or nitric oxide is not recommended for ARDS.

Patients with ARDS should receive diligent supportive care to decrease the risk of developing a variety of common complications.

Complications of ARDS include the following:
- Nosocomial infections occur in about half of patients.
- Myopathy associated with long-term neuromuscular blockade, high steroid doses, and poor glycemic control
- Nonspecific problems of venous thromboembolism, GI hemorrhage, and inadequate nutrition are common in these ICU patients.

Prognosis has improved over the last 20 years, probably due to improvements in supportive care and mechanical-ventilation strategies. Factors that influence mortality rate include age (higher rate >65 years), the presence of chronic liver disease, and development of multiple-organ dysfunction. Measurement of physiological dead space has also been demonstrated to correlate with outcome.

Early deaths are usually due to the precipitating condition, and later deaths secondary to complications. Over half of patients will survive with varying residual lung damage, although pulmonary function tests often show only minor restrictive abnormalities (and reduced DLCO), indicating the considerable capacity of the lung to recover. Patients who survive ARDS may also have problems with neuromuscular function, post-traumatic stress disorder, and depression.

Upper airway diseases

Acute upper airway obstruction

Presentation

Sudden respiratory distress occurs along with cyanosis and aphonia. Airway obstruction can occur at any level within the airway.

Partial airway obstruction leads to noisy breathing, with stridor, gurgling, or snoring.

Complete airway obstruction is associated with distress and marked respiratory effort, with paradoxical chest and abdominal movement ("see-saw breathing"), and use of accessory muscles of respiration. This may be followed by collapse with loss of consciousness, and progress to cardiorespiratory arrest.

Look for chest and abdominal movements and listen and feel for airflow at the nose and mouth.

Causes

- Pharyngeal occlusion by tongue and other muscles, secondary to loss of muscle tone. This may be secondary to drugs, alcohol, a neurological event, or cardiorespiratory arrest.
- Vomitus or blood
- Inhaled foreign body, which may also cause laryngeal spasm
- Laryngeal obstruction due to edema from burns, inflammation, or anaphylaxis
- Excessive bronchial secretions, mucosal edema; bronchospasm may cause airway obstruction below the larynx
- Infection, such as epiglottitis
- Any cause of chronic airway obstruction, such as an airway tumor or extrinsic compression due to tumor or lymphadenopathy

Management

This is a life-threatening medical emergency. Call for help early if you are not an expert in airway management.

1. Open the airway with backward head tilt, chin lift, and forward jaw thrust. In cases of trauma, do not tilt the head, but perform a jaw thrust only.
2. If unsuccessful at restoring normal respiration, visually inspect the mouth for obvious occlusion and remove it with a finger sweep. Leave well-fitting dentures in place.
3. If there is a witnessed history of choking, consider performing the Heimlich maneuver to dislodge the object (firm and rapid pressure applied beneath the diaphragm in an upward movement), or directly visualize the airway with a laryngoscope and use forceps to remove the object, or with bronchoscope and the use of biopsy forceps.
4. If the patient is breathing, consider inserting an airway to maintain patency—oropharyngeal or nasopharyngeal. Maintain oxygenation, using a mask with reservoir bag, delivering 10–15 L/minute. If there is no spontaneous respiratory effort, insert a laryngeal mask or endotracheal tube and deliver oxygen via self-inflating bag with supplemental oxygen 10 L/minute and reservoir bag. If the patient is not breathing and cannot be ventilated, a cricothyroidotomy may be necessary (pp. 760–1).
5. Suction secretions

6. Maintain circulation with cardiac compression, if necessary.
7. Seek definitive treatment for the cause of airway obstruction, as appropriate.

Heliox

Helium–oxygen mixtures have been used for patients with airway obstruction, often due to tumor compression or invasion. Helium has a lower density than that of nitrogen and can improve ventilation rapidly when used with oxygen. It can be used as an interim measure until more definitive management is available, such as radiotherapy, or to allow time for radiotherapy to take effect. The evidence relating to its use is mainly with case studies, and no randomized control trials have been performed.

Nebulized adrenaline may also be helpful in upper airway obstruction, especially laryngeal edema. This is only a stabilizing measure until definitive treatment is available.

Anaphylaxis

Causes

Anaphylaxis is an IgE-mediated type 1 hypersensitivity reaction to allergen. Histamine release causes the clinical syndrome. Typical allergens include bee or wasp sting, peanuts, fish, drugs, foods, latex, contrast media, muscle relaxants, and anesthetic agents.

Presentation

There is varying severity of the following:
- Angioedema
- Urticaria
- Dyspnea
- Wheeze
- Stridor
- Hypotension
- Arrhythmias
- Also rhinitis, abdominal pain, vomiting, diarrhea, and sense of impending doom

The patient may have had previous episodes of severe allergic-type reactions.

Management

This can be a life-threatening medical emergency. Call for help early.
- Remove likely allergen
- Cardiopulmonary resuscitation if necessary
- *Airway and breathing:* Administer high-flow oxygen through on-rebreathable mask. If airway obstruction is present, consider tracheal intubation. Airway swelling may make this difficult and cricothyroidotomy may need to be performed (see pp. 760–1).
- *Circulation:* Give adrenaline (epinephrine) IM. Repeat after 5 minutes if there is no improvement or with deterioration.
- In those with profound shock and immediately life-threatening anaphylaxis, such as during anesthesia, or those with no pulse, IV adrenaline can be given slowly. Stop as soon as there is a response. This can be hazardous and needs cardiac monitoring.
- Give IV fluids if hypotension persists: 1–2 L rapidly infused
- Antihistamines
- Consider IV corticosteroidsw
- Consider nebulized salbutamol or adrenaline for bronchospasm
- On discharge, provide an Epipen (IM self-administered adrenaline) and advice on future episodes. Provide medic alert bracelet and card.
- Consider an immunology referral if the allergen is unknown.

Future developments

Allergen immunotherapy aiming to desensitize patients to the allergen would be useful in those who cannot avoid allergen exposure. Small amounts of the allergen are injected, usually weekly, with slowly increasing dose strengths until the maximum dose of the allergen is administered, which can take up to 12 months. The mechanism for this unknown, but is probably related to increased IgG binding to the allergen, falling allergen-specific IgE levels, and a decreased amount of circulating inflammatory cytokines.

Allergen immunotherapy can protect against anaphylaxis for 3–5 years. It is effective for dust; grass, tree, and weed pollen; mold spores; latex; and insect venom as well as some animal allergens.

Side effects of administration include anaphylaxis, bronchoconstriction, and local reaction. Some centers may not perform immunotherapy in people with chronic asthma because of the risk of death.

Anti-IgE therapy (omalizumab) contains a new IgG highly humanized monoclonal antibody to human IgE that binds to IgE, preventing its binding to mast cells and basophils and preventing severe allergic reactions. Studies have shown its utility in asthmatics with significant environmental atopy who are unable to be controlled with inhaled corticosteroids alone and require frequent oral steroid therapy.

Further information

Abramson M, Puy R, et al. (2003). Allergen immunotherapy for asthma. *Cochrane Database Syst Rev* **4**:CD001186.

American Heart Association (2007). *Advanced Cardiovascular Life Support Provider Manual.* Dallas, TX: American Heart Association.

Upper respiratory tract infections 1

Acute upper respiratory tract infections (URTI) include rhinitis, pharyngitis, tonsillitis, and sinusitis.

Acute rhinitis

Nasal congestion occurs along with rhinorrhea, mild malaise, and sneezing. Rhinitis is most commonly due to viral infection (the common cold).

Topical decongestants may be useful. There is no evidence for the use of antibiotics or antihistamines.

Candidiasis

Oral candida infection is common in those who have received antibiotics, are immunosuppressed, or on oral or inhaled steroids. It is seen as white plaque-like lesions on the tongue and pharyngeal mucosa. Treat with oral antifungal lozenges, and with oral hygiene.

Severe infection can be debilitating, leading to difficulties with eating, especially in the elderly. Exclude underlying immunocompromised state (e.g. HIV, leukemia) in those with persisting infection despite treatment.

Acute epiglottitis (supraglottitis)

This infection is mainly localized to the epiglottis and surrounding supraglottic structures. It is more common in children than adults. A mortality of up to 7% is reported in adults, which is due to upper airways obstruction from grossly edematous upper airway tissue.

- *Haemophilus influenza*, streptococci, and staphylococci are primary causative organisms.
- Acute epiglottitis typically presents with a sore throat and dysphagia. Inspiratory stridor is less common, but it can also present with acute upper airway obstruction and CXR infiltrates consistent with pulmonary edema (due to high negative intrathoracic pressure).
- The patient may need airway protection with an endotracheal tube or tracheostomy; early consultation with ENT/anesthesia is advisable.
- In severe infection, epiglottic swabs may be of diagnostic use, but beware of precipitating airway obstruction. Treat with third-generation cephalosporin, macrolides, or quinolones for 2 weeks (to cover β-lactam-producing *H. influenzae*). Change to amoxicillin if the patient is sensitive.

Sinusitis

The sinuses are normally sterile. The paranasal sinuses communicate with the nose and are therefore susceptible to infection from this route. All the sinuses drain by means of the mucociliary escalator. Blockage of free sinus drainage is a predisposing factor for bacterial infection. Sinusitis is a common cause of persistent cough. Dental infection may lead to maxillary sinusitis, by direct spread.

Acute sinusitis complicates 1 in 200 upper URTIs and usually presents with fever and sinus pain, which is worse on leaning forward. Respiratory viral infection interrupts normal defenses of the mucosal lining, producing mucous exudates, with secondary bacterial infection.

S. pneumoniae and *H. influenzae* are the most common pathogens. *S. aureus* and *S. pyogenes* are also causes, with *Pseudomonas* seen in cystic fibrosis. Mixed infections with anaerobes are seen in 10%. Specific diagnostic tests are not usually needed.

Chronic sinusitis, by definition, is present for >3 months. The ciliated epithelial sinus lining is replaced by thickened stratified squamous lining, with absent cilia, due to repeated infection. Anaerobic infection is more common. Fungal infection is more common in atopic people with nasal polyps. Sinus mycetoma is a rare complication in neutropenic patients, diabetics, and the immunocompromised.

Sinusitis presents with frontal headache (frontal sinusitis), maxillary pain, pain over the bridge of the nose (ethmoidal sinusitis), retro-orbital headache (sphenoidal sinusitis), with purulent nasal discharge and blockage. A systemic granulomatous vasculitis may mimic the symptoms of sinusitis.

Investigations are not usually warranted, but a sinus radiograph may show an air–fluid level, with thickened mucosal lining or sinus opacification. CT is more sensitive but not usually warranted unless surgical intervention is planned or malignant disease is suspected.

Treatment

Treatment is with analgesia, topical decongestants, and antibiotics if mucopurulent discharge and other constitutional symptoms suggest a severe bacterial infection (amoxicillin is first line). Consider macrolides or quinolone antibiotics for patients with refractory or recurrent infections.

Surgery may be warranted for prolonged infection, an anatomical abnormality, or other complications, e.g., if infection has spread to the cranial cavity or orbit. Spreading infection is uncommon if there has been prior antibiotic treatment.

Upper respiratory tract infections 2

Acute pharyngitis and tonsillitis

Most (80%–90%) cases are caused by viruses, most commonly adenoviruses, coronaviruses, rhinoviruses, and influenza viruses. Group B streptococci, *Streptococcus pneumoniae*, and *Haemophilus influenzae* may cause secondary infection. Mycoplasma and chlamydia are seen less commonly.

Pharyngitis and tonsillitis present with a sore throat, which is usually self-limiting. It may be associated with fever, malaise, lymphadenopathy, conjunctivitis, headache, nausea, and vomiting. Infectious mononucleosis (EBV) is associated with pharyngitis in 80% of cases.

Diagnose with the Paul Bunnell test for heterophile antibodies, and atypical mononuclear cells in peripheral blood. Specific EBV antibody detection kits are available.

- Coxsackie A and herpes simplex cause "herpangina syndrome" with ulcerating vesicles on the tonsils and palate.
- CMV can also cause pharyngitis associated with lymphadenopathy and splenomegaly.
- Lemierre's syndrome (jugular vein suppurative thrombophlebitis) is a rare anaerobic pharyngeal infection.

Other causative agents

- *Corynebacterium diptheriae* in unvaccinated populations. A pharyngeal membrane may form, with systemic symptoms, and "bull neck" from cervical lymphadenopathy. There is low-grade fever, with a relatively high pulse rate. Treat urgently with diphtheria antitoxin.
- Vincent's angina is anaerobic infection in those with poor mouth hygiene. It is caused by gram-negative *Borrelia vincenti* and other anaerobic infections. Treat with penicillin.
- Group A streptococcus may cause dysphagia due to pharyngotonsillar edema.

Treatment

Treatment is supportive, and antistreptococcal antibiotics should be considered. There is no evidence that antibiotics reduce the duration of symptoms, but they may reduce complications of bacterial suprainfections (e.g., sinusitis, peritonsillar abcess, and rheumatic fever).

Oral penicillin is the first-line treatment (or a macrolide if the patient is penicillin allergic). Amoxicillin can cause a rash in infectious mononucleosis and so should be avoided. Throat swabs for group A streptococcus may be helpful in directing treatment.

Complications of untreated infection include peritonsillar abscess, retropharyngeal abscess, and cervical abscess. Treat with appropriate antibiotics. Surgical drainage is occasionally required.

Laryngitis

This is usually part of a generalized upper respiratory tract infection. *M. catarrhalis* is the causative agent in up to 50% of patients. It may cause a hoarse voice or aphonia.

Other causes include inhaled steroids, occupational exposure to inhaled chemicals, and gastroesophageal reflux disease. If a hoarse voice persists in a smoker, a laryngeal or lung cancer (with recurrent laryngeal nerve involvement) must be excluded. Other causes include tuberculous infection, HSV, CMV, diphtheria, fungal infections, and actinomycosis.

Treatment

Usually no specific treatment is required, as the illness is typically self-limiting.

Acute bronchitis, tracheitis, and tracheobronchitis

Inflammation due to infection can occur in any part of the tracheobronchial tree, and is termed *tracheitis, tracheobronchitis,* or *bronchitis* depending on the anatomical site. It usually follows viral infection, especially of the common cold type, and is more common during influenza epidemics. Secondary bacterial infection is common, with *H. influenza* and *S. pneumoniae* being most common. There is increased prevalence in the winter months.

Patients present with a productive cough, small-volume streaky hemoptysis, and fever. Breathlessness and hypoxia are uncommon unless there is coexistent cardiorespiratory disease or a concomitant pneumonia. Retrosternal chest pain is common in tracheitis. Examination is often normal.

Diagnosis

Diagnosis is made usually on the basis of the history. A persisting cough, especially in a smoker, may warrant further investigation.

Treatment

Treatment is usually symptomatic, particularly in the previously well. Use antibiotics for persistent cough productive of mucopurulent sputum or if there is coexistent cardiopulmonary disease. Macrolide antibiotics or fluoroquinolones are the drugs of choice in this setting.

Further information

Aboussouan LS, Stoller JK (1994). Diagnosis and management of upper airway obstruction. *Clin Chest Med* **15**(1):35–53.

Brook I (2007). Bacterial infection and antibiotic treatment in chronic rhinosinusitis. *Clin Allergy Immunol* **20**:147–162.

Chang TW, Wu PC, Hsu CL, Hung AF (2007). Anti-IgE antibodies for the treatment of IgE-mediated allergic diseases. *Adv Immunol* **93**: 63–119.

Hamilos DL (2007). Approach to the evaluation and medical management of chronic rhinosinusitis. *Clin Allergy Immunol* **20**:299–320.

Masood A, Moumoulidis I, Panesar J (2007). Acute rhinosinusitis in adults: an update on current management. *Postgrad Med J* **83**(980): 402–408.

Rosenfeld RM, Andes D, Bhattacharyya N, et al. (2007). Clinical practice guideline: adult sinusitis. *Otolaryngol Head Neck Surg* **137**(3 Suppl.):S1–S31.

Siempos II, Dimopoulos G, Korbila IP, Manta K, Falagas ME (2007). Macrolides, quinolones and amoxicillin/clavulanate for chronic bronchitis: a meta-analysis. *Eur Respir J* **29**(6):1127–1137.

Hyperventilation syndrome

Definition

Hyperventilation is an abnormal increase in alveolar ventilation in excess of carbon dioxide production, necessarily associated with a fall in the partial pressure of arterial CO_2. Occurring in the setting of metabolic acidosis, significant metabolic stress, hypoxia, or primary pulmonary disease, it is understood to be a compensatory reaction.

By less well-understood mechanisms, hyperventilation is also associated with heart failure, sepsis or systemic inflammatory response syndrome (SIRS), drug effect as with early salicylate toxicity or progesterone therapy, hepatic failure, hyperthyroidism, pregnancy, and central nervous system lesions including malignancies and stroke.

Emotional stresses such as anxiety, fear, or pain can cause psychogenic hyperventilation. "Idiopathic" hyperventilation is likely a psychogenic variant without a clear emotional precipitant. The latter two, psychogenic and idiopathic, can be termed the *hyperventilation syndrome*.

Pathophysiology

Ventilation is under complex control from central drive, peripheral chemoreceptors and behavioral variables, and is still incompletely understood.

In the hyperventilation syndrome, a psychogenic stress drives behavioral modification of the breathing cycle. The consequent diminution of arterial carbon dioxide increases blood pH, resulting in a rightward shift of the oxygen–hemoglobin dissociation with hemoglobin favoring the oxy-state for any given PaO_2. This results in mild tissue hypoxia, causes cellular shifts of Ca, K, phosphorus, and other electrolytes, and can cause cerebral vasoconstriction. These effects produce the common clinical manifestations of carpal-pedal spasms, paresthesias, and light-headedness, and can potentiate feelings of anxiety.

Clinical features

- Dyspnea and tachypnea at rest, which may improve with exercise (i.e., become appropriate to the level of exertion rather than worsen as with a primary pulmonary or cardiac disease)
- Paresthesias, carpal-pedal spasm, light-headedness
- Palpitation and chest pain
- This syndrome can overlap and share characteristics with panic attacks.
- Presence of emotional stress

Diagnosis

The diagnosis is one of exclusion, and the impetus is on the clinician to search for and exclude a physiologic stress. Accordingly, the following conditions need to be excluded from the differential diagnosis.

Differential diagnosis

- Hypoxia
- Other significant pulmonary disease (e.g., asthma, COPD, interstitial disease, pulmonary hypertension, etc.). Often this needs to be investigated with routine CXR, CT scanning, full pulmonary function testing, and, if still unclear, provocative testing for bronchial reactivity and exercise testing.

- Acidosis
- Pulmonary embolus
- Significant cardiac disease, including ischemia and heart failure
- Hyperthyroidism
- Liver disease
- Pregnancy

Management

There are no controlled trials to guide the management of psychogenic hyperventilation. Similar to the diagnostic framework, treatment is predicated on treating any potential physiological contributors first, then addressing the emotional precipitant if possible. Pain should be adequately treated, excessive emotional stimuli removed, and calming measures introduced (e.g., family to calm a child).

Cognitive-behavioral therapy may be useful. Careful explanation and, occasionally, controlled breathing with a coach can be effective in halting an acute attack.

Use of a rebreathing device, e.g., paper bag, will prevent effective ventilation by increasing ambient CO_2, impairing CO_2 exchange, which depends on a concentration gradient, increasing $PaCO_2$, and preventing alkalosis, but has other obvious dangers and cannot be recommended.

Anxiolysis, particularly with benzodiazepines, is effective in decreasing respiratory drive. However, if the patient is misdiagnosed with the hyperventilation syndrome, benzodiazepines may unmask the true pathology by interfering with a previously appropriate compensation. They should, therefore, be used with some caution, and failure to respond should always prompt a reconsideration of an underlying disorder.

Prognosis

There are few physiological repercussions of the hyperventilation syndrome. Light-headedness, syncope, and seizures can occur as a result of cerebral vasospasm. Coronary vasospasm can cause infarction, and alkalosis can promote cardiac arrhythmias.

A theoretical danger exists at the cessation of hyperventilation: significant hypocapnia from hyperventilation, especially when prolonged, can blunt central respiratory drive to a point where hypoxia can occur prior to the correction of the CO_2 and restoration of normal ventilation. This sequence has been postulated in the deaths of freedivers who volitionally hyperventilate prior to diving.

Although there are potential complications, significant consequences are rarely reported and the prognosis is good.

Further reading

Mason RJ, Murray JF, Nadel AF, Broaddus VC (2005). *Murray and Nadel'sTextbook of Respiratory Medicine*. fourth edition. New York: Elsevier, p. 2082.

Unusual conditions

Alveolar microlithiasis

This is a rare interstitial lung disease of unknown etiology, characterized by the accumulation of numerous, diffuse, calcified microliths (calcium and phosphate hydroxyapatite bodies) in the alveolar space. There is no identifiable abnormality of calcium metabolism. Microliths are occasionally identified in the sputum.

At postmortem the lungs are heavy and rock hard, often needing a saw to cut them. Fewer than 200 cases are reported.

Clinical features
- Typically presents in young adults, most commonly in the third and fourth decades of life
- May be an incidental CXR finding in asymptomatic patients
- Familial tendency—probable autosomal recessive inheritance
- Equal sex distribution in sporadic cases, 2:1 female preponderance in familial cases
- Usually slowly progressive, with progressive breathlessness, hypoxia, respiratory failure, and death
- CXR and chest CT show fine micronodular lung calcification, predominantly basally or around the hila. It may produce complete radiographic opacification. There is no associated lymph node enlargement. Progressive lung infiltration causes restriction of lung movement and impairs gas exchange, leading to progressive respiratory failure.

Treatment
- There is no effective medical treatment.
- Lung transplantation has been successful.

Pulmonary alveolar proteinosis (PAP): pathophysiology and clinical features

Pulmonary alveolar proteinosis (PAP) is a rare alveolar filling disorder that presents in mid-adulthood.

Pathophysiology

PAP is due to failure of alveolar macrophages to clear surfactant proteins, leading to the filling of alveoli lipoproteinaceous material. Abnormalities in granulocyte macrophage colony–stimulating factor (GM-CSF) function appear to play a major role in the disease, as defects in GM-CSF signaling have been identified in animal models of PAP. Because of the common presence of antibodies to GM-CSF in adults, it is thought that the adult human disease has an autoimmune basis. These antibodies inhibit GM-CSF activity and alter normal alveolar macrophage function, leading to abnormalities of surfactant homeostasis.

Congenital disease is thought to be due to mutations in surfactant gene proteins, particularly surfactant protein B. Other mechanisms for surfactant accumulation have also been identified:

- *Heavy dust exposure* leads to surfactant hypersecretion, which exceeds the lungs' normal clearance mechanism. Animal models have shown that this condition leads to the accumulation of lipid-laden macrophages, which break down to release surfactant.
- *Amphiphilic drugs*, e.g., amiodarone, chlorphenetermine
- *Lymphoma, leukemia, and immunosuppression:* The mechanism is uncertain, but it is thought that the lipoprotein may be generated from degenerating alveolar cells.

Disorders with an appearance similar to alveolar proteinosis include endogenous lipoid pneumonia resulting from bronchial obstruction, and have been described in surfactant-secreting bronchoalveolar cell carcinomas.

Histology

The alveoli are filled with a granular acellular, eosinophilic PAS (periodic acid–Schiff) positive deposit. Cholesterol clefts and large foamy macrophages may also be seen. The alveolar architecture is usually well preserved. Surfactant protein can be identified using immunohistochemistry. Electron microscopy shows multiple osmiophilic bodies consistent with denatured surfactant.

Epidemiology

- Presents at ages 30–50 (case reports in children and the elderly)
- Male-to-female ratio of 2.4:1
- Increased is incidence in smokers.
- Familial cases have been reported.

Clinical features

- Typically presents with breathlessness and a nonproductive cough. Examination may be normal, or crackles may be heard on auscultation. Clubbing occurs in one-quarter of patients.
- May present with infection
- Median duration of symptoms before diagnosis is 7 months.
- Opportunistic infection is a major complication, most commonly *Nocardia* species, fungi, and mycobacteria. This occurs from impaired macrophage function and impaired host defense, due to surfactant accumulation.

PAP: diagnosis and treatment

Diagnosis

Diagnosis is usually made on the basis of a characteristic CT appearance, although other tests may also be useful.

- Raised serum LDH
- **ABGs:** Hypoxia and increased alveolar–arterial (A–a) gradient
- **PFTs** show restrictive defect, with reduced lung volumes and diffusing capacity.
- **CXR** shows bilateral consolidation with thickened interlobular septa. The pattern is variable, and in up to 50% may be perihilar (bat's-wing appearance).
- **CT** appearance is highly suggestive of the diagnosis, with airspace shadowing in a geographic distribution alternating with areas of normal lung, the so-called crazy-paving pattern. This CT appearance is not unique to alveolar proteinosis, but is also seen in lipoid pneumonia and bronchoalveolar cell carcinoma, among others.
- **BAL** reveals milky washings. Identification of antibodies to GM-CSF in BAL washings may be diagnostic but is a test not generally available. Cytological examination shows a granular extracellular deposit with foamy macrophages and cellular debris.
- **Transbronchial/open lung biopsies** are occasionally needed if the CT is not characteristic, or atypical clinical or radiographic features are present.

Treatment

The mainstay of therapy remains repeated therapeutic whole-lung lavage, which should be performed at a specialist center. Although there are no randomized controlled trials of this treatment, there is evidence of efficacy with improvements in symptoms, physiology, and radiology.

- The indication for whole-lung lavage is usually breathlessness limiting activities of daily living
- The procedure is done under general anesthesia with 100% oxygen, and one-lung ventilation using a double-lumen tube. Repeated warm-saline lavage using a closed circuit should continue until the bronchial washing returns are clear—this may take up to 40 L lavage. One or both lungs may be treated at a time.
- The response is variable—some patients need only one treatment, others may need multiple treatments, and about 10% fail to respond.
- Whole-lung lavage may be done on bypass if the patient is too hypoxic to tolerate single-lung ventilation.
- Characteristic milky lavage fluid is obtained.

Granulocyte colony-stimulating factor (subcutaneous injections) appears to be an alternative treatment option in subjects less severely ill, with response rates of about 50%. Inhaled GMCSF therapy is also being studied.

There is no benefit from treatment with steroids, and they may exacerbate opportunistic infections.

Prognosis with whole-lung lavage is generally good. Spontaneous remission occurs in one-third of patients, one-third remain stable, and one-third progress to respiratory failure and death.

There are reports of progression to pulmonary fibrosis (which may be a coincidental occurrence).

Further information

Juvet SC, Hwang D, Waddell TK, Downey GP (2008). Rare lung disease II: pulmonary alveolar proteinosis. *Can Respir J* **15**(4):203–210.

Seymour JF, Presneill JJ (2002). Pulmonary alveolar proteinosis: progress in the first 44 years. *Am J Respir Crit Care Med* **166**:215–235.

Amyloidosis: pathophysiology and classification

Definition

Amyloidosis is the extracellular deposition of low-molecular-weight protein molecules as insoluble fibrils. More than 20 such proteins have been described in different diseases and circumstances.

Pathophysiology

The disease is one of abnormal protein folding, and classified by the origin of the precursor proteins that form the amyloid. For example, AL amyloid forms from the light chains of immunoglobulins.

In familial forms, genetic missense mutations produce abnormal folding of the protein. Little is known of the specific genetic and environmental factors that lead to the development of this abnormal folding.

Despite their differing origins, these protein molecules are misfolded in ways that are very similar to each other: in the classic β-pleated sheet structure, fibrils form in an ordered fashion, with uniformity of fibril structure within the sheet. Substitutions of particular amino acids at specific positions in the light-chain variable region lead to destabilization of the light chains, increasing the chance of fibrillogenesis.

In certain models, this abnormal folding can be initiated by the addition of "amyloid-enhancing factor," rather like the initiation of crystal formation in a supersaturated solution. Amyloid deposits accumulate in the extracellular space, disrupting normal tissue architecture and leading to organ dysfunction, both directly, and by space-occupying effects. The fibrils may be directly cytotoxic (possibly by promoting apoptosis).

The classification of amyloid is largely based on the origin of the amyloid protein and shown in Box 45.1.

Epidemiology

The epidemiology of the disease is difficult to define accurately, as the disease is often un- or misdiagnosed. The age-adjusted incidence is estimated to be 5.1 to 12.8 per million person-years.

Future developments

Anti-amyloid drugs are under investigation, including drugs to stabilize the amyloid precursor proteins in their normal configuration and enhance fibril degradation.

Box 45.1 Classification of amyloidosis

Primary/light-chain amyloid (AL)

AL is from immunoglobulin light-chain fragments (λ or κ), usually monoclonal due to a plasma cell dyscrasia (a lymphoproliferative disorder)

- 1 in 5000 deaths due to this type of amyloid
- Median survival is 6–15 months.
- Myeloma is present in 20%, and a subtle monoclonal gammopathy in 70% (MGUS).
- Systemic form is due to circulating monoclonal light chains, widespread organ involvement, particularly heart, liver, and kidneys
- Localized amyloid production by local clonal B cells. Hence heterogeneous organ involvement is seen, commonly in the upper respiratory tract, orbit, and urogenital and gastrointestinal systems—virtually any organ (except the brain) can be involved.

Secondary amyloid (AA)

- A complication of chronic disease with ongoing or recurring inflammation, e.g., rheumatoid arthritis or chronic infections
- The fibrils are fragments of an acute-phase reactant, serum amyloid A.
- Commonly there is renal, hepatic, and lower GI involvement, rarely neurological, lung, and cardiac involvement.
- Median survival is 5 years.
- Only a small number of patients with chronic inflammation will develop AA amyloidosis, and the time period for the development of the disease is quite variable.

Other forms

- *Dialysis-related* (DA), due to fibrils derived from β_2-microglobulin that accumulate in dialysis patients
- *Inherited amyloidosis*, e.g., due to abnormal pre-albumin (transthyretin, TTR), damaging neural and cardiac tissue
- *Organ-specific amyloid*, such as Alzheimer's disease, plaques of the beta protein derived from the larger amyloid precursor protein (APP). Protein is presumed to be generated locally.

Further information

Comenzo RL (2006). Amyloidosis. *Curr Treat Options Oncol* **7**(3):225–236.
Falk RH, Raymond L, et al. (1997). Systemic amyloidosis. *N Engl J Med* **337**:898–908.

Online support and discussion group for patients: www.acor.org/amyloid.html

Amyloidosis: lung involvement

Clinically significant respiratory tract disease is almost always AL in type, though the presence of a strong family history or chronic inflammatory disease may suggest other types.

Laryngeal amyloid

Amyloid causes up to 1% of benign laryngeal disease. It may present as discrete nodules or diffuse infiltration, and is usually localized, though can be a rare manifestation of systemic (AL) amyloid. Deposits are seen most commonly in the supraglottic larynx (presenting with hoarse voice or stridor).

Patients may present with choking and exertional dyspnea that can be progressive.

Tracheobronchial amyloid

This type is rare. Macroscopically it is either diffusely infiltrative or tumor-like. It is associated with tracheobronchopathia osteoplastica (a disorder characterized by the deposition of calcified submucosal airway nodules). It presents after the fifth decade with dyspnea, cough, and rarely hemoptysis. Airway narrowing can lead to atelectasis or recurrent pneumonia; solitary nodules may lead to investigation for presumed lung cancer. Symptomatic disease is usually localized.

Parenchymal amyloid

This is the most frequently diagnosed amyloid respiratory disease. It is usually divided into nodular (solitary or multiple pulmonary nodules, usually localized AL amyloid) and diffuse (alveolar septal, usually a manifestation of systemic AL amyloid) types.

Nodules are usually peripheral and subpleural. They may be bilateral, and are more common in the lower lobes, ranging in diameter from 0.4 to 15 cm. They may cavitate or calcify.

In either disorder, clinical signs are nondiagnostic, and PFTs may show a restrictive defect with reduced diffusing capacity. The differential diagnosis usually includes pulmonary fibrosis. Cardiac amyloid may coexist, and attributing the relative contribution to the symptoms of the pulmonary and cardiac disease can be difficult.

Median survival with clinically overt lung disease is about 16 months (similar to that of systemic amyloid).

Mediastinal and hilar amyloidosis are rarely associated with pulmonary amyloidosis, and their diagnosis should lead to a search for a systemic cause of amyloid. Amyloid lymphadenopathy can also represent localized AL deposition in association with B-cell lymphoma.

Other

There are rare reports of the following:
• Ventilatory failure due to diaphragm or other respiratory muscle involvement
• Sleep apnea from macroglossia due to amyloid
• Exudative pleural effusions

Clinical features

- Dyspnea and cough
- May be an incidental finding on routine chest radiography
- Consider the diagnosis particularly in patients with odd upper airway symptoms and parenchymal disease, or those with unexplained CHF or nephrotic syndrome.

Diagnosis

Histological conformation is required.

Histology

Transbronchial biopsy or occasionally open or VATS biopsy (more likely if the investigation is for solitary pulmonary nodule) is used. Congo red stain producing apple-green birefringence in crossed polarized light is the gold standard. Positive histology must lead to immunohistochemistry to determine the fibril type.

I^{123}-labeled scintigraphy

Radiolabeled serum amyloid P (SAP) localizes to amyloid deposits in proportion to the quantity of amyloid present, therefore allowing identification of the distribution and burden of disease. It is most sensitive for solid-organ disease, though in lung disease it is useful for determining the extent of disease in other organs. It is expensive and carries an infectious risk, as the SAP component is currently obtained from blood donors.

HRCT identifies nodules or parenchymal disease.

Laryngoscopy and bronchoscopy may be needed to obtain samples for histology, depending on the clinical presentation.

PFTs are used to assess effect on pulmonary physiology. They may show a reduced diffusing capacity and a restrictive pattern. Tracheobronchial involvement may lead to abnormal flow-volume loops due to upper airway obstruction.

Systemic disease

- CBC, biochemistry, and urinalysis
- Investigate for underlying blood cell dyscrasia, e.g., myeloma, Waldenstrom's macroglobulinemia (bone marrow examination, and search for urine and serum monoclonal protein by immunofixation—the clonal proliferation underlying systemic AL amyloid is usually very subtle, and its identification may be difficult)
- Echocardiogram for associated cardiac involvement (when CHF is present, survival is 4–6 months)
- Thyroid and adrenal functions are impaired in up to 10%.

Treatment

There are limited clinical trials for guiding management of respiratory tract amyloid. Management decisions are thus often made empirically.

- No treatment may be needed.
- Local measures may be warranted for endobronchial disease, e.g., symptomatic laryngeal disease—endoscopic excision, laser evaporation (useful for small recurrent lesions), stenting. Steroids have no effect on laryngeal amyloid.
- Tracheobronchial amyloid—management depends on symptoms and treatment may involve repeated endoscopic resection, laser therapy, and surgical resection. Repeated endoscopic procedures are thought to be safer than open surgery.
- Chemotherapy may be warranted for diffuse parenchymal amyloid if there is objectively measurable disease (prednisolone and melphalan, to suppress the underlying blood cell dyscrasia). More intensive chemotherapy has a better clinical response, but there are few trials.

Further information

Lachmann HJ, Hawkins PN (2006). Amyloidosis and the lung. *Chronic Respir Dis* **3**(4):203–214.

Idiopathic pulmonary hemosiderosis

This is a rare disease of undetermined etiology, characterized by otherwise unexplained recurrent episodes of alveolar hemorrhage, usually leading to iron deficiency anemia.

Pathophysiology

Recurrent bleeding occurs within the alveolar space. No antibodies have been identified, although serum IgA levels are sometimes raised. Vasculitis is not seen.

Because alveolar hemorrhage is associated with a wide variety of immune-mediated disorders (including primary and secondary vasculitis, thyrotoxicosis, celiac disease, and autoimmune hemolytic anemia), an autoimmune mechanism may be operative in at least some cases. With recurrent alveolar hemorrhage, the alveolar blood provokes a mild fibrotic reaction, with the development of diffuse pulmonary fibrosis.

Iron turnover studies show that the accompanying iron-deficient anemia is due to loss of iron into the lung through hemorrhage.

Etiology

Etiology is uncertain, but likely to be multifactorial. Possible associations include toxins (epidemiological studies in rural Greece) and premature birth.

Epidemiology

The disease has an equal sex incidence in childhood, with twice as many men clinically affected in adulthood.

Most patients present in childhood, with 85% of cases having onset of symptoms before age 16. The actual prevalence is unknown, but a Swedish childhood cohort study in the 1960s described an incidence of 0.24 per million children.

Clinical features

The clinical course is variable and ranges from continuous low-level bleeding to massive alveolar hemorrhage. The latter may be fatal but is, fortunately, rare.

• Continuous mild pulmonary hemorrhage leads to a chronic nonproductive cough with hemoptysis, malaise, lethargy, and failure to thrive in children.
• Iron deficiency anemia is common, as are positive fecal occult blood tests (due to swallowed blood).
• Generalized lymphadenopathy and hepatosplenomegaly are recognized.
• With an acute bleed, cough and hemoptysis may worsen, and dyspnea, chest tightness, and pyrexia may develop.
• Chronic bleeding leads to chronic disabling dyspnea, chronic anemia, and clubbing (in 25%). Cor pulmonale secondary to pulmonary fibrosis and hypoxemia may develop.

Examination may be normal. Clubbing, basal crepitations, and cor pulmonale are all recognized, depending on the severity of the resulting lung disease.

Investigations

The diagnosis is one of exclusion, with no evidence of other organ involvement. The main differential diagnosis is Goodpasture's syndrome, Wegener's granulomatosis, SLE, and microscopic polyarteritis.

Histology

A definitive diagnosis requires a surgical lung biopsy. The alveolar space and interstitium contain hemosiderin-laden macrophages, with variable degrees of interstitial fibrosis and degeneration of alveolar, interstitial, and vascular elastic fibers, depending on the chronicity of the condition. Vasculitis should be specifically sought out, but is not identified. Electron microscopy shows damage to the endothelial and basement membranes, but no consistent or diagnostic features have been recognized.

- **Blood tests** show microcytic, hypochromic anemia, with low iron levels. ANCA, dsDNA, and anti-GBM antibodies should be negative.
- **CXR** may show transient patchy infiltrates, which worsen during an acute bleed. The apices are usually spared. Progressive disease leads to the development of reticulonodular infiltrates and a ground-glass-appearance that is typically perihilar or in the lower zones. Hilar lymphadenopathy may be seen.
- **CT:** The changes seen are fairly nonspecific, showing a diffuse bilateral infiltrate, with patchy ground-glass change.
- **PFTs:** DlCO is transiently elevated during bleeding episodes (≥130% is abnormal), but this is only useful acutely. A restrictive defect with a reduced DlCO may develop with chronic disease.
- **BAL samples** identify alveolar hemorrhage and contain hemosiderin-laden macrophages.

Management

There is no specific treatment.

- Steroids and immunosuppressive drugs may be of benefit during acute bleeding episodes, but do not appear to affect the long-term outcome. There are no published data to guide the optimal timing of treatment during the course of disease.
- The iron deficiency anemia responds to replacement therapy, and blood transfusion may be needed in severe bleeds.

Prognosis

The prognosis is very variable, with some patients showing spontaneous remission. The duration of disease in the literature ranges from death within days following an acute severe illness to survival with cor pulmonale associated with chronic disease after 20 years.

Pulmonary Langerhans cell histiocytosis (PLCH)

Definition

Pulmonary Langerhans cell histiocytosis (PLCH; previously termed pulmonary histiocytosis X or pulmonary eosinophilic granuloma) is a rare condition characterized by infiltration of the lung with histiocytes (Langerhans cells).

Pulmonary LCH overlaps with a number of other conditions with similar pathological findings but diverse clinical features. These range from localized infiltration of a single organ (e.g., eosinophilic granuloma of bone) to systemic diseases affecting multiple organs (Letterer–Siwe disease, a multiorgan disease affecting infants and the elderly, associated with poor prognosis; also Hand–Schueller–Christian syndrome).

Although the isolated pulmonary form most commonly presents to chest physicians, pulmonary manifestations also commonly occur in the systemic forms of the disease.

Epidemiology

Pulmonary LCH is rare, tending to affect young adults aged 20–40 years. The vast majority of cases occur in current smokers, usually heavy smokers. It may be more common in men, who tend to present at a younger age than women.

Pathogenesis

Langerhans cells are involved in antigen presentation, and are characterized by the presence of well-demarcated cytoplasmic organelles called Birbeck granules on electron microscopy. The Langerhans cells seen in LCH appear to be monoclonal, although it is unclear if this represents a true neoplastic process.

The antigen stimulus for activating Langerhans cells in the lung is unknown, although cigarette smoke is a possible candidate. Langerhans cells accumulate in bronchiolar walls and subsequently enlarge and invade adjacent structures. This results in the radiological appearance of nodules that at first cavitate and then become cystic.

Clinical features

Typically there is exertional breathlessness and cough, sometimes with systemic symptoms (e.g., fever, weight loss). Pneumothorax occurs in at least 10% of patients and may be the presenting feature. Rib lesions may also give rise to chest pain. Around 25% of patients are asymptomatic. Examination may be normal.

Investigations

- *CXR* typically shows diffuse reticulonodular shadowing, sometimes with cystic change; there is upper and middle lobe predominance. Costophrenic angles are classically spared. CXR may be normal.
- *HRCT* shows diffuse centrilobular nodules, sometimes with cavitation, and thin-and thick-walled cystic lesions, reflecting lesions of varying age. These are interspersed with normal lung. Upper and middle lobe

predominance; costophrenic angles are typically spared. Purely nodular or purely cystic appearances may occur. Unusual manifestations such as single nodules or large airways involvement are also described.

- **PFTs** are variable, ranging from normal to obstructive, restrictive or mixed patterns. Reduced diffusing capacity and exertional hypoxia are common.
- **TBB** may yield diagnostic material, although is generally nondiagnostic. The risk of pneumothorax is unknown, although it may be increased. Surgical lung biopsy is diagnostic.
- **BAL:** Increased total cell counts and pigmented macrophages simply reflect cigarette smoking. Use of antibodies (e.g., OKT6) to detect Langerhans cells in BAL fluid is limited by poor sensitivity.
- **Extrathoracic tissue biopsy** of other involved sites (e.g., bone) may be diagnostic.

Diagnosis

Diagnosis is usually based on the combination of clinical and HRCT findings: typically a young adult smoker with cysts and nodules on HRCT. Confirmation by surgical lung biopsy may be considered in atypical presentations, such as the finding of solely nodular or cystic disease on HRCT.

The appearance of purely cystic disease on HRCT may be confused with emphysema or lymphangioleiomyomatosis (where cysts are present uniformly in all regions of lung, including the costophrenic angles).

Associations

- Severe pulmonary hypertension may be seen in the absence of significant parenchymal lung involvement; direct involvement of pulmonary vessels has been described.
- Manifestations of systemic LCH, particularly diabetes insipidus from pituitary disease, skin involvement, lytic bony lesions, and rarely cardiac or gastrointestinal disease
- Lymphoma may precede, complicate, or coexist with pulmonary LCH.
- Lung cancer is more common, probably as a result of cigarette smoking.

Management

Treatment other than smoking cessation is often not required. Oral corticosteroids may be tried in symptomatic disease, although there is little evidence to support their use. Lung transplantation should be considered in patients with severe respiratory failure or pulmonary hypertension. Disease may recur in transplanted lungs. Experimental treatments such as the use of IL-2 and anti-TNF-α may be of benefit in the systemic forms of LCH seen in children.

Prognosis is variable. A minority of patients deteriorate rapidly with respiratory failure and death within months. Overall life expectancy is reduced, with median survival 12–13 years from diagnosis. Death is most commonly due to respiratory failure. Poor prognostic factors include reduced FEV_1, increased residual volume, and reduced diffusing capacity.

Further information

Sundar KM, Gosselin MV, Chung HL, Cahill BC (2003). Pulmonary Langerhans cell histiocytosis. *Chest* **123**:1673–183.

Lymphangioleiomyomatosis (LAM): clinical features

Definition and etiology

This rare disorder is characterized by abnormal proliferation of smooth muscle cells, affecting women of child-bearing age. Diagnosis is usually made in the patients' 30s, although the diagnosis has been made in women in their late 60s.

- Incidence of 1 in 1.1 million population
- Unknown cause
- Not hereditary
- 40% of adult women with tuberous sclerosis (TS) (learning difficulties, seizures, facial angiofibromas, autosomal dominant inheritance) develop pulmonary changes identical to those of LAM.
- Rare cases have been described in men.

Pathology

There is abnormal proliferation of atypical smooth muscle cells (LAM cells) throughout the lung, airways, blood vessels, and lymphatics. Nodular infiltration is initially subtle. Progressive growth causes lymphatic and airway obstruction, leading to cyst formation throughout the lungs.

Clinical features

Common

- Secondary pneumothorax (in two-thirds of patients; occurs due to parenchymal cysts; recurrence is common)
- Dyspnea (in 42%)
- Cough (in 20%)
- Hemoptysis (in 14%)
- Chylothorax (in 12%, thoracic duct leakage as a result of lymphatic obstruction by LAM cells, may be bilateral)

Less common

- Pleural effusion
- Chest pain
- Pulmonary hemorrhage (due to blocked blood vessels and increased intraluminal pressure)

Other organs affected

Kidney

Angiomyolipoma, a benign tumor, occurs in 50% of LAM patients. Usually diagnosed on CT, these are mostly small and single, but can be multiple and large. Smaller tumors are usually asymptomatic, but larger ones can cause flank pain and bleeding into the renal tract. Treatment options include tumor resection or endovascular embolization. Nephrectomy is not usually required. Screening for these lesions is important, as it allows careful treatment planning in case they become symptomatic.

Abdomen

Lymphadenopathy is due to lymphatic blockage. This occurs in one-third of patients and is usually asymptomatic.

Pelvis

Lymphangioleiomyomas are cystic lymphatic masses that enlarge during the day and cause fullness and bloating.

Chylous ascites can occur in the absence of chylothorax.

Skin

Cutaneous swellings are likely due to localized edema.

Examination may be normal. There may be crackles or signs of pleural effusion. Palpable abdominal masses rarely present.

Investigations

- **PFTs** may be normal or show a predominantly obstructive pattern. They are rarely restrictive. There is decreased DLCO, with a normal or increased TLC.
- **CXR** may be normal. Lungs may appear hyperinflated, with reticular shadowing and septal lines due to obstructed lymphatics. There may also be a diffuse interstitial infiltrate.
- **HRCT** shows a characteristic appearance, with multiple cysts throughout the lung of varying size, which are usually small (<1 cm) and thin-walled. The adjoining lung parenchyma is normal. There may be pleural effusions.

LAM: diagnosis and management

Diagnosis

Consider LAM in young or middle-aged women with
- Sponteous pneumothorax, especially those with preexisting dyspnea or hemoptysis
- Cystic lung disease, airflow obstruction, or chylous pleural effusions
- Angiomyolipomas or other retroperitoneal tumors
- Tuberous sclerosis and respiratory symptoms

The disease is easily missed in its early stages. The diagnosis can be made on characteristic CT appearances or with open lung biopsy. Transbronchial biopsies are generally not diagnostic. Large retroperitoneal abdominal lymph nodes can also be biopsied.

Management

- There are no controlled trials of treatment
- The course of LAM is variable. Treatment should be aimed at those who are symptomatic and declining.
- *Diet:* A low-fat diet with medium-chain triglyceride supplementation may prevent chylothorax recurrence, but there is no strong evidence for this. The diet is difficult to adhere to.
- *Bronchodilators* may improve airflow obstruction.
- *Hormonal manipulation* with progesterone, Tamoxifen and oophrectomy, have been tried, with little data supporting their use.
- *Avoid estrogens*, i.e., the oral contraceptive pill and hormone replacement therapy.
- *Contraception:* An increase in symptoms and accelerated disease decline have been reported to occur in pregnancy. Use the progesterone-only pill.
- *Pleural aspiration* when required for pleural effusions. For recurrent effusions or chylothoraces, thoracic-duct ligation or pleurectomy may be effective. Pleurodesis can be performed, but this is relatively contraindicated if future lung transplant is an option.
- *Pneumothoraces:* Advise regarding flying and diving, as these activities may increase their risk of development. Surgical pleurodesis may be necessary with recurrent pneumothoraces.
- *Transplant:* Single or double lung, or heart–lung. LAM can recur in the transplanted lung.
- *Smoking cessation,* as active smoking accelerates the rate of physiologic decline
- Influenza and pneumococcal vaccines

Prognosis is very variable. The condition usually slowly progresses to respiratory failure. At 10 years, 55% of patients have impairing dyspnea, 23% are on LTOT, and 10% are housebound. In terms of survival, 70% of patients are alive at 10 years, 33% are alive at 15 years, and 25% are alive at 20 years.

Future developments

Rapamycin may switch off the defect in LAM cells and prevent their proliferation. Studies are ongoing.

Further information

Johnson SR, Tattersfield AE (2000). Clinical experience of LAM in the UK. *Thorax* **55**:1052–1057.

McCormack FX (2008). Lymphangioleiomyomatosis: a clinical update. *Chest* **133**(2):507–516.

Ryu JH, Doerr CH, Fischer SD, Olson EJ, Sahn SA (2003). Chylothorax in LAM. *Chest* **123**(2): 623–627.

Recurrent respiratory papillomatosis

These are essentially warts of the upper respiratory tract, caused by the human papilloma virus (HPV-6 or HPV-11). The virus infects epithelial cells and mucous membranes, similar to that seen in cutaneous and anogenital infection.

The infection is most commonly acquired during ororespiratory exposure from the mother during vaginal delivery, and typically presents in childhood from 6 months onward, with signs and symptoms of upper respiratory tract infection.

It may also present for the first time in adulthood. It is associated with HLA DR3, and with sexual transmission in adults. Recurrent respiratory papillomatosis is rare (2 per 100,000), but oral HPV infection is common.

Clinical course

This is variable.
- May remit spontaneously
- Progressive voice loss and airway obstruction
- Most cases are confined to the larynx, although up to 25% of patients subsequently develop extralaryngeal spread to the bronchial tree.
- 1% of cases have malignant change to squamous cell carcinomas.

Management

- Surgical excision to maintain airway patency
- Laser therapy—but potential problems of thermal injury, stricture formation, and spread of papillomas
- Photodynamic therapy reduces the recurrence rate, using oral or intravenous photosensitizing agent, then laser therapy to destroy photosensitive tissue.
- Microdebrider is more commonly used.
- Medical treatment—interferon, acyclovir, ribovarin, isoretinoin, and methotrexate have all been tried.
  - *Interferon-*α as a daily subcutaneous injection leads to complete remission in 30%–50% of patients, and partial resolution in 30%. One-third of cases recur when treatment is stopped. Adverse reactions are common: flu-like symptoms, deranged LFTs, leucopenia, and alopecia.
  - *Cidofovir* is a nucleoside monophosphate analogue and inhibits viral polymerase. It is given as an intralesional injection. Potential side effects include nephrotoxicity and neutropenia.

Pulmonary arteriovenous malformations (PAVMs): etiology and diagnosis

Etiology

Pulmonary arteriovenous malformations (PAVMs) are abnormal blood vessels replacing normal capillaries, making a direct, low-resistance connection between the pulmonary arterial and systemic venous circulations. They vary in size from tiny clusters of vessels (telangiectasia) to larger, more complex aneurysmal-type sacs. The disorder is rare, affecting 1 in 15,000 to 24,000.

Several genetic susceptibility loci have been identified on chromosomes 9 and 12. One identified mutation is in the endoglin gene. This modulates signaling via the transforming growth factor-β family of growth factors. This gene is also implicated in the development of idiopathic pulmonary arterial hypertension

Subjects with significant PAVMs have low pulmonary vascular resistance, a low mean PAP, and a high cardiac output—due to long-standing adaptive mechanisms to the effects of the shunt, in addition to vascular remodeling effects.

Most patients present post-puberty, as AVMs probably develop at this time. They probably grow throughout life, especially during puberty and in pregnancy. They may rarely regress spontaneously.

Diagnosis

Most patients present with an abnormal **CXR**, classically showing a smooth, rounded intrapulmonary mass, with draining or feeding vessels.

Mild **hypoxemia** occurs. An AVM is a direct communication between the pulmonary artery and pulmonary vein. Blood therefore bypasses the pulmonary capillary bed, with reduced oxygenation, which poorly corrects with supplementary oxygen.

Orthodeoxia is desaturation upon standing due to an increase in blood flow in the dependent lung areas. Seventy percent of PAVMs are basal, hence the desaturation in the upright position.

CT identifies all AVMS, and can determine those suitable for embolization. Contrast is not required.

Patients may present with the complications of a PAVM, particularly bleeding or peripheral abscess formation. The absence of a normal filtering capillary bed means small particles can reach the systemic circulation, leading to sequelae, particularly in the cerebral circulation, of strokes and cerebral abscesses. These abnormal vessels are also at risk of rupture.

Shunt quantification

- In normal individuals the anatomical shunt is <2%–3.5% of the cardiac output (due to post-pulmonary drainage of bronchial veins into the pulmonary veins and drainage into the left atrium).
- *100% oxygen rebreathing study*, a noninvasive method of shunt quantification
- *99mTC perfusion scan*, a tracer study. The size of the shunt can be assessed from the proportion of radiolabeled macroaggregates reaching the systemic circulation, compared to the total number injected.
- *Contrast echocardiogram* to measure the circulatory transit time of injected echocontrast
- *Angiography*

Clinical features

- Asymptomatic (50%)
- Dyspnea
- Hemoptysis (10%), probably due to additional bronchial telangiectasia, which can cause hemorrhage into bronchi or the pleural cavity
- Chest pain (12%); etiology is uncertain
- Clubbing
- Cyanosis
- Orthodeoxia
- Vascular bruits
- Telangiectasia; 80% of PAVM patients have hereditary hemorrhagic telangiectasia (HHT), and their families should be screened because of the risk of stroke (see p. 629)
- May present with acute stroke, with focal neurological signs

PAVMs: management and complications

Management

Embolization is usually done with coils, which generate local thrombin, leading to cessation of blood flow in AVM feeding vessels. This results in a reduction in the right–left shunt and improvement in hypoxemia. The procedure should be done by an expert in a specialist center only. The small risk of neurological sequelae and angina or arrhythmias is reduced with operator experience.

Some 60%–70% of patients are left with a small persisting shunt following treatment and retain a small risk of abscess formation. Patients are therefore given prophylactic antibiotics for dental and surgical procedures.

Surgical resection may be more appropriate than embolization in some cases.

Antiplatelet therapy (rarely) is used in individual cases, if there are ongoing transient ischemic attacks.

Transplantation is not advised as there is no increased survival benefit over medical treatment.

Screening The majority of patients with PAVMs have HHT, and so screening of family members is important.

Follow-up All patients need regular follow-up with shunt assessment post-surgical resection or embolization, as removal of one shunt may unmask or provoke the development of others.

Female patients should be advised to defer pregnancy until completion of formal assessment, because of the risks of growth and rupture of PAVMs in pregnancy (see Complications).

Complications

- PAVM patients never die of respiratory failure in the absence of additional respiratory disease.
- All patients are at risk of stroke and cerebral abscesses.
- Transient ischemic attack or stroke occurs in 25%
- Abscesses occur in 10%, due to paradoxical emboli through the right-to-left shunt, and the absence of a filtering capillary bed.

Pregnancy is associated with an increase in size of AVMs, and new ones may develop, with potentially catastrophic consequences. Careful shunt assessment is therefore needed prior to pregnancy, along with contraceptive advice. Close liaison between the pulmonary consultant and obstetric team is paramount. AVMs may need embolization in the third trimester to allow safe delivery.

Hereditary hemorrhagic telangiectasia

HHT is also referred to as Osler–Weber–Rendu syndrome. Prevalence is 1 in 5000–8000.

Definition

HHT is an autosomal dominant disorder characterized by the development of abnormal, dilated vessels in the systemic circulation, which may bleed, leading to
- Recurrent epistaxis
- Gastrointestinal bleeding
- Iron deficiency anemia
- Other organ involvement, e.g. hepatic (in 30%, commonly asymptomatic), renal, pulmonary, and spinal AVMs

Screening

Careful questioning of family members (does anyone in the family have frequent nose bleeds?) and examination for telangiectasia should reveal those in whom screening should occur.

All those with HHT should be screened for PAVMs, and all of their offspring should be screened post-puberty and pre-pregnancy. There is increasing penetrance with increasing age (62% at age 16, 95% at age 40). Similarly, the detection of PAVMs in a patient should lead to screening for HHT in family members.

There is no consensus regarding the best screening method, but a combination of the following tests may be used:
- CXR
- Supine and erect oximetry (looking for orthodeoxia)
- CT or the chest
- Shunt quantification techniques, e.g., contrast echocardiogram, 100% oxygen rebreathing

Screening may need to be continued throughout life (every 5 to 10 years) and during times of enlargement or development of AVMs—post-puberty and pre-pregnancy.

Management

- Usually involves liaison with ENT and gastroenterological colleagues for symptomatic treatment
- Iron replacement, transfusions
- Asymptomatic hepatic AVMs—no treatment usually required
- Cerebral AVMs (in 15% of HHT patients)—some specialists argue that these should be treated prophylactically, due to the risk of rupture and bleeding (2% per year, often fatal).

Further information

Shovlin CL, Letarte M (1999). Hereditary haemorrhagic telangiectasia and pulmonary arteriovenous malformations: issues in clinical management and review of pathogenic mechanisms. *Thorax* **54**:714–739.

For patients and their relatives: www.hht.orga
Telangiectasia self-help group Web site: www.telangiectasia.co.uk
US self-help group web site: http://www.hht.org/

Primary ciliary dyskinesia (PCD)

PCD is a rare, genetic cause of disease, encountered in adults as a cause of bronchiectasis.

Cilia are found in
- The whole length of the upper respiratory tract
- Brain ventricles
- Fallopian tube or ductus epididymis

They are made up of dynein arms, with outer and inner connecting rings, and beat at 14 beats/second. Many gene defects have been identified in PCD, causing a number of cilial abnormalities.

Abnormal cilia do not beat normally, leading to reduced mucociliary clearance, microbiological colonization (which further inhibits cilial action), chronic infection, and the development of bronchiectasis.

The main aim following diagnosis in childhood is the prevention of chronic respiratory disease and bronchiectasis.

Clinical features
- Autosomal recessive
- May present with neonatal respiratory distress
- Situs inversus (in about 30%, as cilia determine the side of the organs. Random organ siding occurs with cilial dysfunction, hence the situs inversus of Kartagener's syndrome)
- Nasal blockage or rhinitis
- Persistent wet cough in childhood
- Hearing problems or recurrent ear infections
- Clubbing and signs of chest disease are rare in childhood.
- Wheeze in 20%
- Infertility due to low sperm count in men
- In adults the disease usually presents with the clinical signs of bronchiectasis: cough productive of purulent sputum, recurrent chest infections, and intermittent hemoptysis.

Diagnosis
Conduct a cilial biopsy via the nasal route. Cilia are examined by high-speed digital video, where their beat frequency and pattern can be assessed. Neither of these tests are routinely available and referral to a specialized center may be necessary. Most cases of PCD are diagnosed in childhood. There is an increased frequency in the children of consanguineous marriages.

Consider the diagnosis in
- Bronchiectasis
- Situs inversus
- Persistent upper and lower respiratory infection from early childhood
- Infertility—males may present in infertility clinics.

Management

In adults this involves the treatment of secondary bronchiectasis (see p. 376) with

- Antibiotics as necessary
- Physiotherapy
- Vaccinations
- Management of hemoptysis

Flying, diving, and altitude

Lung disease and flying

Air travel poses respiratory issues for several reasons:
- Lower ambient oxygen concentration
- Barotrauma
- Closed environment and disease transmission

Lower ambient oxygen concentrations

Most airline cabins are pressurized to the equivalent of 5000–8000 feet. This results in a decrease in barometric pressure and partial pressure of oxygen. At sea level, atmospheric pressure is 760 mmHg, resulting in a PaO_2 of 98 mmHg. At 8000 feet, barometric pressure decreases to 565 with a resultant PaO_2 of 55 mmHg.

In patients with underlying lung disease hypoxemia may develop or worsen. In these patients the possibility of developing hypoxemia at altitude should be considered. Both the hypoxia inhalation test (HIT) and regression formulas have been used to estimate the risk. The routine use of a sea level O_2 pressure threshold of 68–72 mmHg as safe or unsafe may misclassify many patients.

At sea level, the HIT exposes patients to 15% O_2 (simulating 8000 feet) mixed with 85% nitrogen. Patients breathe through a mouthpiece with nose clips in place for 15–20 minutes and with a 12-lead ECG monitoring for ischemia. The primary end-point consists of the PaO_2. ECG should be employed in selected patients to monitor for ischemia and arrhythmias. In-flight oxygen is typically prescribed if the PaO_2 at a simulated 8000 feet falls below 55 mmHg.

Regression equations can be used as a screening tool to identify patients with borderline PaO_2 estimates for further testing with the HIT. The estimated PaO_2 at 8000 feet is estimated by this formula:

Estimated PaO_2 at 8000 ft = 0.453(PaO_2 at sea level) + 0.386 (FEV_1 percentage of predicted) + 2.440.

The regression approach does not assess susceptibility to the development of symptoms or ECG changes during hypoxia, nor does it predict the response to exercise.

The timing of pre-flight testing should ideally be within 2–14 days of travel. Airlines should be contacted 48–96 hours prior to flight to arrange for in-flight oxygen.

Barotrauma

According to Boyle's Law, the volume of a gas varies inversely with the pressure to which it is subjected. With ascent, as barometric pressure decreases, volume will increase. Ascent to the equivalent of 8000 feet will increase gas in trapped compartments, such as a pneumothorax or bulla, by up to 40%. *A pneumothorax is an absolute contraindication to air travel due to the danger of tension pneumothorax.*

Invasive procedures increase the risk of introducing air into an area that could expand in a pressurized cabin, increasing the risk for barotrauma. Patients should postpone air travel until at least 10–14 days after most surgical procedures.

Closed environment

Active or contagious infectious diseases, such as tuberculosis and pneumonia, are a contraindication to air travel. Significant attention to respiratory viruses such as influenza and SARS has prompted government agencies to develop protocols to control spread of infection should cases be suspected in-flight.

Diving

Diving is associated with several categories of respiratory problems:
- Barotrauma (i.e., ruptured bullae and pneumothorax)
- Decompression sickness
- Worsening of preexisting disorder while at depth (i.e., asthma)
- Breath-hold diving and ascent hypoxia

Barotrauma

Aside from drowning, barotrauma is the most common form of diving-related injury. In the lungs, the decrease in air volume during descent can lead to mucosal edema, vascular engorgement, and hemorrhage if the lung volume decreases below residual volume. Upon ascent, the air volume will expand, and if air cannot escape quickly enough from whatever compartment, rupture may occur. Alveolar rupture can result in pneumomediastinum or pneumothorax, which may lead to tension pneumothorax with expansion of the gas upon ascent.

The most potentially serious complication of barotrauma is that of arterial gas embolism. This can result from any of three mechanisms:
- Passage of gas bubbles into the pulmonary veins and into the systemic circulation
- Development of venous gas emboli, which overwhelm the filtering capacity of the pulmonary capillaries and appear in the systemic circulation
- Development of venous gas emboli that reach the arterial circulation paradoxically via a functional right-to-left shunt, such as a patent foramen ovale

Arterial gas emboli may cause myocardial infarction, stroke or distal ischemia, and activation of inflammatory cascades. Emergency treatment includes administration of 100% oxygen and hydration as well as hyperbaric oxygen as soon as possible.

Decompression sickness (a.k.a. Caisson disease, or "the bends")

During exposure to high pressure, extra nitrogen dissolves into the blood and other tissue fluids. Upon ascent, this nitrogen bubbles off. If the amount coming out of solution is too great, nitrogen bubbles act as emboli and limit blood flow, producing microinfarction and damage to various organs.

Air travel increases the risk of developing decompression sickness. Divers making only one dive per day may travel after 12 hours from the last dive; divers completing multiple dives or requiring decompression stops should wait 48 hours prior to air travel.

Type I decompression sickness presents with musculoskeletal complaints, cutaneous pruritis, localized erythema, and localized edema or lymphadenopathy.

Type II decompression sickness is more severe. Neurological injury may manifest as memory loss, ataxia, visual disturbance, changes in personality or speech, or spinal cord damage. Within the lungs, occlusion of the pulmonary circulation may produce chest pain, wheezing, dyspnea and pharyngeal irritation or even acute right heart failure.

Limited diving times and slow ascents reduce this problem. Severe cases require treatment in hyperbaric chambers as soon as possible. Delay of treatment results in diminished rates of improvement but should never be withheld even after a long delay.

Worsening of preexisting lung disease

Asthma may be provoked by the dry gases breathed from the scuba gear. Cold-, exercise-, or emotion-induced asthma increases the risk. Only well-controlled asthmatics may dive, but not if they have required a therapeutic bronchodilator within the last 48 hours or have had any other chest symptoms. A bronchodilator may be taken prior to the dive. Lung diseases such as cystic fibrosis, COPD, fibrotic lung disease, previous pneumothorax (with no pleurodesis), and lung bullae are considered *absolute contraindications* to diving.

Breath-hold diving

During a breath-hold dive, the increased pressure on the chest elevates the alveolar PO_2 and thus the arterial PO_2, extending the breath-hold time. During the dive, oxygen is consumed and the PaO_2 falls. Thus, on ascent, the PaO_2 falls precipitously with possible loss of consciousness and drowning.

Altitude sickness

Respiratory complications of altitude are related to hypocapnia and hypoxia:
- Acute mountain sickness including high-altitude pulmonary edema and high-altitude cerebral edema
- High-altitude periodic breathing of sleep
- Chronic mountain sickness

Whether high-altitude illness occurs depends on the rate of ascent, level of ascent, sleeping altitude, and individual physiology. Risk factors include a history of altitude sickness, physical exertion, age <50, residence at altitude <3000 feet, rapid ascent, and obesity.

Acute mountain sickness (AMS)

Two forms exist, based on severity of illness.

In the *minor* form, symptoms are due to hyperventilation provoked by hypoxia, including light-headedness or fatigue, numbness or tingling of extremities, nausea, vomiting, and anorexia, and headache. These common symptoms develop over 6–12 hours after arrival, and affect about one-fourth of those traveling to high altitude. Most of the symptoms are due to a respiratory alkalosis and resolve as the kidney retains $[H^+]$ and excretes $[HCO_3^-]$, returning pH toward normal. This scenario tends to be common in those with a higher hypoxic drive.

In the *major* form, symptoms are due to the hypoxia itself, are more serious, can develop rapidly, and tend to occur more in those with a lower hypoxic drive.

High altitude pulmonary edema (HAPE)

HAPE is a potentially fatal form of noncardiogenic pulmonary edema. Hypoxia provokes a nonuniform and exaggerated degree of pulmonary vasoconstriction, raising pulmonary artery pressure (PAP). Fluid leakage into alveoli and capillary damage with pulmonary hemorrhage produce clinically apparent disease. The dominant findings are dyspnea out of proportion to work, cough, cyanosis, blood-tinged frothy sputum, elevated JVP, and crackles on auscultation.

There may be a genetic susceptibility. Associations have been found between HAPE and specific polymorphisms of the endothelial nitric oxide synthase gene, the angiotensin-converting enzyme gene, and the human leukocyte antigens (HLA) DR6 and DQ4. Also, genetic variations in the structure or function of the sodium channels of type II pneumocytes may promote susceptibility.

Patients with recurrent HAPE or HAPE occurring at <8000 feet should have an echocardiogram to rule out a shunt, pulmonary hypertension, mitral stenosis and other conditions that increase pulmonary vascular resistance.

High-altitude cerebral edema (HACE)

HACE is another life-threatening disease likely related to hypoxia-induced increases in cerebral blood flow along with decreased integrity of the blood–brain barrier. The changes in blood flow may cause cerebral edema, retinal hemorrhage, cerebral thrombosis, and petechial hemorrhage. The dominant symptoms are ataxia, confusion, disorientation, hallucinations, behavioral change, severe headache, reduced consciousness level, and papilledema.

Management

Prevention of altitude sickness centers on the rate and degree of ascent. Keep ascent to <1000 feet/day and rest every third day. The minor form of altitude sickness will likely resolve spontaneously over a few days with simple symptomatic treatment, analgesics, and hydration.

Prophylaxis with acetazolamide is effective and is recommended when rapid ascent to altitudes >8000 feet is unavoidable. *Daily acetazolamide beginning 2 days prior to ascent is probably adequate for most individuals or as a treatment after symptoms develop.*

Slow-release theophylline has demonstrated some effectiveness as prophylaxis. Patients who are unable to tolerate any oral intake should descend to lower altitude.

Aspirin given prophylactically is effective in prevention of altitude-related headaches. First-line treatment for AMS includes acetazolamide and dexamethasone (for sulfa-allergic patients). Dexamethasone should be started for more severe AMS.

The management of severe mountain sickness is urgent. Oxygen tension must be increased, either by rapid descent, portable oxygen, or a portable hyperbaric chamber. In HAPE, patients should be kept upright and warm. Nifedipine may be administered to reduce PAP, provided blood pressure remains acceptable. Investigational therapies for HAPE include sildenafil and inhaled nitric oxide.

For HACE, dexamethasone (4–8 mg followed by 4 mg every 6 hours) can be given, although no studies have been performed to demonstrate effectiveness. Improvement is usually rapid once oxygen tension is raised.

Medications shown to prevent HAPE include prophylactic nifedipine, tadalafil, dexamethasone and high-dose inhaled salmeterol.

High-altitude periodic breathing of sleep

This is a form of periodic respiration that likely occurs due to an exaggerated carotid receptor stimulation secondary to alkalosis and hypoxia and is often considered a subset of AMS.

Acetazolamide is effective in prevention and treatment and contributes to a lower arterial pH, higher minute ventilation, and higher overnight oxygen saturation. Other possible therapies include temazepam and zolpidem, although further evidence is needed.

Chronic mountain sickness

Also known as Monge's disease, this disorder occurs in the setting of excessive elevated hematocrit secondary to hypoxia and may result in pulmonary hypertension and cardiopulmonary compromise. Chronic cerebral effects may also result from hypoxic injury.

Toxic agents

Drug-induced lung disease: clinical presentations

Introduction

Over 300 drugs are known to damage the respiratory system, from the nose to alveoli. It is not feasible to list or discuss all of them here. A useful listing (plus references) is kept at www.pneumotox.com and can be queried by either drug (or drug type) or clinical or radiological presentation.

Drugs can cause different types of lung disease, including large and small airways disease, a wide spectrum of interstitial lung diseases, pleural and pulmonary vascular diseases, and lymph node and neuromuscular involvement (see Box 47.1). This chapter describes the more common drugs that produce respiratory problems.

Diagnosis

Drug-induced lung disease is almost always a diagnosis of exclusion. The clinician has to suspect it to find it. A complete history of approved and over-the-counter (OTC) medications, supplements, herbs, and illicit substances should be obtained from every patient.

A small number of risk factors have been identified for some drugs. Dose-related toxicity has been demonstrated for amiodarone, bleomycin, nitrosoureas, and radiation therapy. Concomitant administration of certain drugs increases risk of pulmonary toxicity, such as bleomycin and supplemental oxygen. Genetic predisposition to pulmonary drug toxicities is suspected, but requires further research.

Classes of drugs with a propensity to lead to pulmonary toxicity include the following:
- Chemotherapeutic agents, e.g., bleomycin, mitomycin C, methotrexate
- Antibiotics, e.g., nitrofurantoin, amphotericin B
- Anti-inflammatory medications, e.g., acetylsalicylic acid, interferons, leukotriene antagonists
- Analgesics
- Cardiovascular drugs, e.g., amiodarone, beta blockers, ACE inhibitors

Box 47.1 Common presentations of drug-induced lung disease and examples of causative agents

- Interstitial lung disease, pneumonitis, fibrosis
  - Acute hypersensitivity pneumonitis (nitrofurantoin, methotrexate)
  - Interstitial pneumonitis eosinophilia (amiodarone, ACE inhibitors)
  - Organizing pneumonia (amiodarone, bleomycin)
  - Pulmonary fibrosis (bleomycin, amiodarone, nitrofurantoin)
- Airways disease
  - Bronchospasm (beta blockers, contrast media)
  - Obliterative bronchiolitis (busulfan, penicillamine)
  - Cough (ACE inhibitors)
- Pleural changes
  - Pleural effusion or thickening (beta blockers, nitrofurantoin, methotrexate, dopamine agonists)
  - Pneumothorax (bleomycin)
- Vascular changes
  - Thromboembolic disease (phenytoin)
  - Pulmonary hypertension (dexfenfluramine, other appetite suppressants)
  - Vasculitis (nitrofurantoin, L-tryptophan)
- Mediastinal changes
  - Node enlargement (bleomycin, phenytoin)
  - Sclerosing mediastinitis (ergot)
- Pulmonary edema (methotrexate, contrast media)
- Pulmonary hemorrhage (methotrexate, nitrofurantoin, penicillamine, contrast media)

Drug-induced lung disease: examples

Amiodarone

Iodinated benzofuran is used to suppress supra- and ventricular tachycardia. Lung toxicity correlates loosely with total dose and usually occurs after a variable number of months. It is seen in 10% of subjects on >400 mg/day, and is rare at <300 mg/day.

Risk factors
- Daily dose >400 mg
- Increasing age of patient
- Use for more than 2 months
- Preexisting lung disease (although not a contraindication to its use)
- Recent surgical intervention or lung infection.

Diagnosis

Diagnosis is usually one of exclusion, and response to cessation of drug (which can take months). A number of side effects occur, including corneal microdeposits, peripheral neuropathy, liver and thyroid dysfunction, and bluish discoloration of the skin.

The most serious side effects are pulmonary. Infiltrative lung disease occurs in 6% of patients, varying from acute respiratory distress (rare) through to organizing pneumonia (cough, pleuritic pain, fever, dyspnea, asymmetric patchy infiltrates, effusion) and the most indolent, chronic interstitial pneumonitis (cough, insidious dyspnea, weight loss, diffuse and/or focal opacities).

On **CT** the liver, thyroid, and lungs will usually show increased attenuation, indicating a significant amiodarone load. A baseline CXR and baseline pulmonary function tests may be useful.

Lung biopsies

Biopsies are not always required, but if obtained can exclude other diagnoses and provide compatible findings; there is dissent as to how diagnostic they are. The finding of foamy macrophages in the airspaces, filled with amiodarone–phospholipid complexes, is indicative only of amiodarone use. Mechanisms of toxicity are unclear, and there are features to suggest both hypersensitivity and direct toxic damage.

Treatment

Drug withdrawal is essential. Steroids are effective and required in severe disease. The half-life of amiodarone in the tissues is in excess of a month, and response to stopping the drug may be slow. Prognosis is good in most patients.

Azathioprine

Extensively used as an immunosuppressant, this drug and has remarkably little pulmonary toxicity other than via opportunistic lung infection. There are case reports of pneumonitis only.

Bleomycin

This DNA-damaging glycopeptide is used in the treatment of lymphomas, germ cell tumors, and squamous carcinomas (cervix, head, neck, and esophagus). Pulmonary fibrosis occurs in about 10%.

Risk factors
- Age >70
- Cumulative dose of >450 U
- Preexisting lung disease
- Increased FiO_2 (even for some time after drug administration), probably via increased superoxide/free radical formation
- Pulmonary radiation, not just in the radiated field
- Renal failure decreases drug elimination and thus increases toxicity
- Associated use of cyclophosphamide

Symptoms (cough, dyspnea, chest pain, fever) develop 1–6 months after taking bleomycin. There is hypoxia and a restrictive defect. Progressive basal subpleural shadowing is evident, as are small lungs and blunting of costophrenic angles.

Histology shows a dominant subpleural distribution of damage and repair with fibrosis; this appearance is nondiagnostic and common to many drugs and disorders. Toxicity is probably due to DNA damage or oxidative injury, with interindividual variation occurring from differing activity of the enzyme bleomycin hydrolase; only low levels of this enzyme exist in the lung (and skin). A rare acute hypersensitivity form comes on within days of administration.

Treatment
- Bleomycin must be stopped on suspicion of damage, and some clinics use serial lung function tests (DLCO) to detect early disease.
- Steroids are used, but there is little evidence they alter long-term prognosis (in the acute hypersensitivity subgroup there is a clear beneficial effect).
- Use minimum FiO_2 to maintain an adequate SaO_2
- Over 50% of patients may experience a relentless decline in lung function.

Busulfan

This DNA alkylating, myelosuppressive agent is mainly used to treat chronic myeloid leukemia, and prior to bone marrow transplantation. It has a low rate of lung toxicity (4%–10%) due to fibrosis.

Risk factors
- Cumulative doses >500 mg (mostly over 120 days)
- Concurrent administration of other alkylating agents
- Pulmonary radiation

Patients present with cough and progressive SOB, often years after exposure (average about 3.5). CXR reveals a combined alveolar and interstitial process. Pulmonary function shows a reduced DLCO and sometimes a restrictive defect. Diagnosis is usually by exclusion. The place of steroids in treatment is unproven.

Chlorambucil

This DNA alkylating agent is used mainly to treat chronic lymphocytic leukemia. There is a low risk (1%) of pulmonary toxicity, and it is confined to those who have received >2 g. As with busulfan, presentation may be many years later. Presents with cough, dyspnea, weight loss, and basal crackles. CXR shows diffuse basal reticular shadowing. Histology is nonspecific. On suspicion, chlorambucil should be stopped. Use of steroids for treatment is unproven.

Cyclophosphamide

A DNA alkylating agent widely used in combination regimens for hematologic cancers and other solid tumors, this drug is particularly useful as an immunosuppressive agent in certain rheumatologic disorders, vasculitides, and nephropathies. Lung toxicity is rare.

Risk factors
• Pulmonary radiation
• Oxygen therapy
• Concurrent drugs causing pulmonary toxicity, e.g., bleomycin.

Clinical presentation
Clinical presentation is usually within 6 months, with a short duration of fever, cough, and fatigue. CT shows reticular shadowing with ground-glass appearance. Later-onset progressive pulmonary fibrosis can also develop insidiously in those on therapy for many months with progressive SOB and dry cough.

Histology of the more acute type can be similar to any of the acute interstitial pneumonias (e.g., organizing pneumonia, diffuse alveolar damage), whereas the more chronic form is indistinguishable from UIP. Cyclophosphamide is not itself toxic to the lung, but its metabolites are. There appears to be genetic variation to susceptibility, as there is no obvious dose–response relationship.

Cessation of the drug along with steroid therapy is used successfully for the acute form, but the chronic form seems to progress inexorably, in a manner similar to UIP. Lung transplantation is an option.

Gemcitabin

This pyrimidine analogue is used to treat non-small cell lung, breast, pancreas, and ovarian cancer. Three patterns of pulmonary toxicity are reported. Within days or hours, nonspecific and self-limiting dyspnea can occur. Acute hypersensitivity with bronchospasm has also been reported. Profound dyspnea with pulmonary infiltrates, which can progress to respiratory failure and death, has been described. Typically, discontinuation of the drug results in resolution of the adverse event.

Gold

Used in rheumatoid arthritis, a >500 mg cumulative dose can produce pneumonitis (possibly organizing pneumonia, obliterative bronchiolitis) with cough, dyspnea, and basal crackles. Although rare (1%), it is associated with certain HLA types and distinctive histological feature of alveolar septal inflammation. There is good prognosis following drug cessation, and the pneumonitis almost always responds to steroids.

Infliximab

Anti-TNF agents represent a large step forward in the treatment of rheumatoid arthritis and Crohn's disease. However, there is a small but important risk of reactivating TB.

Methotrexate

This folic acid derivative inhibits cell division by blocking dihydrofolate reductase and nucleic acid production. It is mainly used in leukemia and as an immunosuppressive in, e.g., rheumatoid arthritis, psoriasis and sarcoidosis. It commonly (4%–10%) causes a variety of lung pathologies not associated with folic acid deficiency.

Risk factors
- Hypoalbuminemia
- Diabetes
- Rheumatoid or other lung or pleural disease
- Not particularly dose-related; can occur at doses of <20 mg/week
- Daily rather than intermittent (weekly) therapy
- Age >60 years

Presentation is both acute (interstitial pneumonitis, fever, and eosinophilia) and over very long time periods. However, the subacute form (within a year, dyspnea, fever, cough, hypoxia, basal crackles, restrictive defect, and reduced DLCO) is more common. CXR shows bilateral diffuse pulmonary infiltrates or a mixed alveolar pattern, with occasional effusions.

Histology is more useful than for other drug toxicities, showing alveolitis, interstitial pneumonitis, epithelial cell hyperplasia, eosinophilic infiltration, and weak granuloma formation in the more acute hypersensitivity form, and more UIP-like changes in the indolent form. The mechanism of damage is unknown but likely to be multifactorial.

Treatment consists of drug withdrawal and the unproven use of steroids. Anecdotal reports support the use of steroids for the more acute hypersensitivity form. Other methotrexate-related lung diseases include opportunistic lung infection.

Nitrofurantoin

Nitrofurantoin is commonly used for long-term prophylaxis against urinary tract infections (UTIs). Acutely, nitrofurantoin causes a hypersensitivity vasculitis and, much less frequently, chronic interstitial fibrosis. Most patients are women, given their much higher prevalence of chronic UTIs.

The acute form presents abruptly with fever, dyspnea, dry cough, rash, chest pain, hypoxia, crackles, and eosinophilia within a week or two of starting nitrofurantoin, and is dose-independent. CXR shows lower-zone diffuse, patchy infiltrates and sometimes unilateral effusions. Lung biopsy reveals vasculitis, eosinophilia, reactive type II pneumocytes, focal hemorrhage, and some interstitial inflammation.

Treatment consists of drug discontinuation, and improvement begins rapidly. Prognosis is good with or without steroids.

Penicillamine

Used in the treatment of rheumatoid arthritis, penicillamine can lead to the development of SLE, bronchiolitis obliterans, and Goodpasture's syndrome. This disease is dose related but rare, with a subacute onset (after several months) of dyspnea and cough. There is a progressive obstructive pattern without bronchodilator response.

Talc

Talc (magnesium silicate) is commonly used for pleurodesis. Talc particles may be small enough to enter the circulation after intrapleural instillation, being found throughout the body at postmortem. They appear to provoke a systemic reaction with fever, raised inflammatory markers, and hypoxia suggestive of an ARDS-like pathology.

Occasional deaths after talc pleurodesis have been reported. Refined talc with fewer smaller particles seems less toxic. Talc is also used as a filler in many medications, including methadone, propoxyphene, methamphetamines, and others. If crushed, mixed with liquids, and injected by addicts, talc can travel to the lung and lead to a granulomatous reaction (talc granulomatosis) and pulmonary arterial occlusion.

Paraquat poisoning

Definitions

Paraquat and related bipyridyl compounds are widely used as contact herbicides. They kill plants by inhibiting NADP reduction during photosynthesis, which involves the production of superoxide radicals. The toxicity of paraquat in animals is also believed to be due to the production of damaging superoxides.

Most cases of poisoning are deliberate. The incidence of suicide attempts with paraquat is greater outside the United States. Ingestion rather than inhalation is the typical route of exposure in humans, although paraquat is absorbed through the skin and mucous membranes, including the conjunctiva and bronchial mucosa. Treatment should be initiated as soon as possible.

- More than 6 g is always fatal
- Less than 1.5 g is rarely fatal
- Between 1.5 and 6 g, the mortality is 60%–70%
- It is usually fatal if the blood level >0.2 mg/mL at 24 hours.

Clinical features

- Oral and esophageal ulceration shortly after contact, with later formation of a pseudomembrane
- Renal failure (reversible) occurs within a few days, but delayed excretion of paraquat prevents falls in blood levels.
- Pulmonary edema occurs early on, evolving into acute respiratory distress syndrome.
- Death usually occurs within 1 to 2 weeks.
- Long-term pulmonary effects consist of accelerated pulmonary fibrosis with varying degrees of recovery. Clinical features include rapidly progressive dyspnea, hypoxemia, and restriction with decreased DLCO on pulmonary function testing.

Management

- No known antidotes
- Gastric lavage to reduce absorption
- Hemoperfusion (hemodialysis is less effective) to reduce blood levels, although benefit is controversial
- Lowest inspired oxygen tension possible (high concentrations probably increase superoxide formation and, thus, toxicity)
- Supportive measures, which may require intubation and ventilation
- Other treatments (e.g., corticosteroids) are experimental.

Inhalational lung injury

Definition

Inhalation of toxic agents, typically at high doses, is capable of injuring the lungs. The acute damage is common to many toxic agents and includes pneumonitis or pulmonary edema, mucosal damage, sloughing, and airway debris. Chronic respiratory sequelae of an inhalational injury include vocal cord dysfunction (VCD), reactive airways dysfunction syndrome (RADS), bronchitis, bronchiolitis obliterans, and bronchiectasis. Secondary infection is common because of breached defenses.

Mechanism

The following factors play a role in determining toxicity of inhalational agents:
- Water solubility (e.g., ammonia and sulfur dioxide are highly water soluble, ozone and phosgene have low water solubility)
- pH
- Chemical reactivity
- Particle size and physical characteristics (<5 μm to reach lower airway)

In addition, a distinction can be made between primarily irritating substances and asphyxiating substances. *Irritating* substances (e.g., ammonia, chlorine gas) cause symptoms instantly, whereas *asphyxiating* agents lead to tissue hypoxia by displacement of oxygen (e.g., methane, carbon monoxide) or by interference with cellular respiration (e.g., cyanide, hydrogen sulfide).

Management

Following acute exposure, supportive therapy is critical.
- Look for respiratory failure, stridor, or distress; this may occur hours later.
- CXR (poor sensitivity until pulmonary edema develops)
- Patient may require intubation or tracheostomy to bypass edematous and sloughing upper-airway mucosa
- Humidified oxygen,
  - Raise SaO_2 into low to mid-90s (higher levels may contribute to oxidative damage)
  - Raise PaO_2 as high as possible if CO poisoning is suspected.
- Bronchodilators
- Mechanical ventilation (low volume/pressure, permissive hypercapnia)
- Fluid replacement, but not excessive, as it encourages pulmonary edema
- Enteral feeding
- Steroids and prophylactic antibiotics—variable opinions on value
- Nebulized dilute heparin/acetylcysteine—variable opinions on value
- Treat cyanide poisoning if suspected (dicobalt edetate, little evidence)

Examples of toxic agents, listed alphabetically

Aldehydes (acetaldehyde, formaldehyde)
- Colorless gas with odor
- Chemical and plastics industry, used for disinfection
- Highly irritant to mucosal membranes
- Acute damage
  - Pneumonitis or pulmonary edema
- Chronic effects
  - Rhinitis and asthma

Ammonia
- Fertilizer and plastics production, used in many chemical industries
- Highly water soluble, clear, colorless, pungent odor
- Highly irritant to mucosal membranes, thermal and chemical airways burn
- Acute damage
  - Upper airway obstruction from secretions and mucosal edema
  - Pulmonary edema
- Chronic effects
  - VCD, RADS, bronchiolitis, and bronchiectasis are described.

Chlorine
- Extensive use in the chemical industry, bleaching agent, household-cleaning product
- Moderately water soluble, yellow–green acrid gas, dense (heavier than air), pungent odor
- Acute damage
  - Overwhelming toxicity producing rapid hypoxia
  - Diffuse alveolar damage and pulmonary edema
- Chronic effects
  - VCD, RADS, bronchiolitis

Hydrocarbons
- Used as lubricant and cooling agent, mineral spirits, lighter fluid, gasoline
- Route of exposure is ingestion rather than inhalation
- Acute damage
  - Pneumonitis
- Chronic effects
  - Pneumonitis
  - Fibrosis

Hydrofluoric acid
- Used in semiconductor manufacture; production of phosphate fertilizers
- Causes severe local and systemic effects, including mucosal burns
- Can induce hypocalcemia and hypomagnesemia
- Treatment includes use of calcium gluconate

Methyl isocyanate (Bhopal disaster: 3800 dead, 170,000 injured)
- Used in chemical industry, carbamate pesticide production
- Acute damage
  - Pneumonitis and pulmonary edema
- Chronic effects
  - Airways obstruction
  - Bronchiolitis obliterans
  - Pulmonary fibrosis

Nitrogen dioxide
- Exposure in chemical industry (explosives), agricultural silos, welding
- Reddish brown gas, low water solubility, sweet odor, dense (heavier than air)
- Acute effects (several hours after exposure)
  - E.g., silo filler's lung (pneumonitis, pulmonary edema, bronchospasm)
- Later effects
  - Bronchiolitis obliterans

More examples of toxic agents

Ozone
- Exposure through welding, waste treatment, cold storage, food preservation
- Moderate water solubility, bleach-like odor
- Both immediate and late effects of pneumonitis, pulmonary edema
- Can cause de novo or aggravated airways hyperresponsiveness

Phosgene
- Chemical warfare, chemical industry, chlorination, welding
- Poorly water soluble
- Acute damage (12–24 hours after exposure)
  - Pneumonitis and pulmonary edema
  - Produces COHb; breath CO therefore reflects degree of exposure

Smoke
- Complex mixture of substances
- Hypoxia due to agents such as CO, cyanide, other oxidants
- Thermal injury typically to the upper airway
- Irritant injury to entire respiratory tract
- Acute damage
  - Mucosal edema and sloughing with airway blockage, bronchospasm
- Chronic effects
  - VCD, RADS, bronchiolitis obliterans, bronchiectasis

Sulfur dioxide

- Used as a fumigant, bleaching agent in the paper industry, component of smog
- Highly water soluble
- Upper airway irritant as it dissolves to form sulfuric acid
- Acute damage
  - Sloughing of airway mucosa
  - Pneumonitis and hemorrhagic pulmonary edema
- Chronic effects
  - De novo or aggravate airways hyperresponsiveness

Welding fumes

- Many agents released
- Specific examples:
  - Cadmium—pneumonitis (12–14 hours after exposure)
  - Zinc—metal fume fever
  - Several agents may cause airways hyperreactivity or COPD.
  - Siderosis (welder's lung) nonfibrogenic pneumoconiosis, iron deposits in lung producing small, rounded opacities

Carbon monoxide poisoning

Definition and epidemiology

- Carbon monoxide is a colorless, odorless gas formed during incomplete carbon compound combustion.
- About 3000–6000 deaths per year in the United States are due to CO poisoning.
- Accidental poisonings are more common in the winter, when faulty heating systems are in use.
- Nonaccidental deaths are mainly from inhaling car exhaust fumes.
- Methylene chloride (industrial solvent, paint remover) is converted to CO in the liver, and overexposure may present as CO poisoning.
- Up to one-third of patients die following acute high-level CO exposure and another third may be left with permanent neurological sequelae.
- Chronic low-grade CO exposure may present as nonspecific ill health and may affect thousands of individuals.

Pathophysiology and related conditions

- Carbon monoxide competes avidly with O_2 (250 times greater) to bind with the iron in hemoglobin, making it less available for oxygen carriage.
- The hemoglobin molecule is also distorted by combination with CO that makes it bind more tightly to O_2, shifting the O_2 dissociation curve to the left.
- This further reduces oxygen delivery to the tissues: a 50% carboxyhemoglobin (COHb) level is far more dangerous than a 50% anemia level.
- CO also binds to extravascular molecules such as myoglobin in the heart and some of the cytochrome chain proteins, interfering with energy production; in this respect it is like cyanide.
- Normal levels of COHb can be up to 3%, and up to 15% in heavy smokers.

Clinical features of CO poisoning
Immediate
- Nausea, headache, malaise, weakness, and unsteadiness
- Loss of consciousness, seizures, cardiac abnormalities (ischemia, arrhythmias, pulmonary edema)
- No cyanosis, healthy looking cherry-red color
- Suspect it if several members of a household have these features.

Symptoms based on carboxyhemoglobin levels
- 0%–5%   No symptoms
- 15%–20%   Headache, tinnitus
- 20%–40%   Nausea, weakness, fatigue, disorientation
- 40%–60%   Confusion, respiratory failure, coma
- >60%   Shock, death

Delayed (approximately 1–3 weeks, can be longer)
- Cognitive defects and personality changes
- Focal neurological and movement abnormalities

Investigations

- Pulse oximetry will appear *normal* because COHb's absorption spectra are similar to those of oxyhemoglobin.
- Arterial PaO_2 levels may be *normal.*
- COHb levels can be measured on a co-oximeter.
- Breath CO can be measured with devices used for smoking cessation.
- Routine tests to rule out other diagnoses

Management

- CO is only removed from the body through displacement by O_2; therefore, use high concentrations of oxygen.
- Raise the PaO_2 as high as possible, intubate, and give 100% O_2 if necessary.
- The half-life of COHb breathing air is about 5 hours; when breathing 100% O_2 it is about 1 hour.

Hyperbaric O_2 more rapidly displaces CO and increases dissolved O_2. It reduced the frequency of delayed neurological symptoms from 46% to 25% after significant exposure in one randomized controlled trial, but it needs to be instituted early. Its use is still controversial but may be justified in selected cases (e.g., coma, pregnancy and COHb >15%, cardiac ischemia).

Facilities are not easily available everywhere. For further information consult the Divers Alert Network (www.diversalertnewtwork.org) and Underwater Hyperbaric Medicine Society (www.uhms.org).

Further information

Juurlink DN, Buckley NA, Stanbrook MB, Isbister GK, Bennett M, McGuigan MA (2005). Hyperbaric oxygen for carbon monoxide poisoning. *Cochrane Database Syst Rev* **25**;(1):CD002041.

Weaver LK, Hopkins RO, Chan KJ, et al. (2002). Hyperbaric oxygen for acute carbon monoxide poisoning. *N Engl J Med* **347**:1057–1067.

Pediatric lung disorders pertinent to adult practice

Chronic lung disease of prematurity and viral wheeze

This chapter concentrates on pulmonary conditions that occur in childhood and are becoming increasingly relevant to adult practice.

Chronic lung disease of prematurity (CLD)

CLD is formerly known as bronchopulmonary dysplasia (BPD).

Advances in neonatal medicine have led to the improved survival of premature babies with immature lungs and respiratory disease. Babies born at lower gestational ages are surviving into adulthood, due to therapy with antenatal steroids to prevent respiratory distress syndrome (RDS), the use of artificial surfactant to decrease the surface tension in the neonatal alveolus, and improvements in ventilatory techniques. CLD usually occurs in babies who have been mechanically ventilated.

CLD is usually caused by barotrauma from prolonged ventilation, high-pressure ventilation, and/or ventilation with high oxygen concentrations in the immature lung and disruption of fetal lung development.

Presentation

Typical presentation is a premature baby who remains oxygen-dependent after 36 weeks postconceptional age. It is now less frequent in those born at 30+ weeks and weighing >1200 g. Mortality is 25%–30% with severe CLD. Infants may require prolonged home oxygen therapy, up to 1 year or beyond.

Typically these infants will have recurrent reactive airway disease–like symptoms associated with upper and/or lower respiratory viral infections during the first several years of life. Half of these patients will need hospital readmission during their first year, with respiratory infection.

Some may have significant pulmonary sequelae during childhood and adolescence, with chronic hypoxia and pulmonary hypertension, but most of the children will not.

Children may have other disabilities associated with prematurity, such as cerebral palsy or learning difficulties. Among these, some may also have other complicating factors such as gastroesophageal reflux, swallow dyscoordination, and/or aspiration.

Pathology

There is cytokine-mediated scarring and repair.
- *Early inflammatory phase*: Bronchial necrosis, alveolar destruction, capillary permeability, and associated obliterative bronchiolitis
- *Subacute fibroproliferative phase*: Type II pneumocyte hyperplasia, bronchial and bronchial smooth muscle hypertrophy, and interstitial and perialveolar fibrosis
- *Chronic fibroproliferative phase*: Airway remodeling in early year(s). Prior to surfactant use, these changes were more severe. Relative pulmonary vascular and alveolar hypoplasia is common in newer forms of CLD.

PFTs

Functional respiratory abnormalities persist with increased airway resistance and airway hyperresponsiveness. RV and RV/TLC levels are raised, indicative of air trapping. Air trapping improves over 3–4 years as lung growth occurs; however, small-airway abnormalities persist, at least until the age of 10 years.

Chest radiology

CT shows persisting mild to moderate abnormalities, with multifocal areas of reduced lung attenuation and perfusion, bronchial wall thickening, and decreased bronchus–pulmonary artery diameter ratios. These radiological abnormalities correlate with physiological evidence of air trapping.

Adulthood

There are few longitudinal studies beyond childhood, and it is unclear what the significance of CLD of prematurity is for adult lung disease.

Viral wheeze and asthma

This is a controversial area. Wheezing is common in infants and toddlers and is often due to viral respiratory tract infections, causing a viral-induced and/or postviral wheeze. This has been found to be associated with passive cigarette smoke exposure, contact with other children, not being breast-fed, and CLD. This transient early wheezing may be distinct from childhood asthma.

The children are often not atopic and have no family history of atopy. The wheeze has usually resolved by the age of 5–6 years, although children may have persistent airway hyperactivity for many years.

Children with asthma may have a family history of eczema, allergies, and/or asthma, may have concomitant atopic dermatitis, and may develop their symptoms at any age, but commonly before age 5–6 years. Half of them have mild symptoms, which regress by puberty. Those with more severe disease requiring regular inhaled steroids often have disease that persists into adult life.

Congenital abnormalities

Tracheomalacia

Tracheomalacia, or floppy trachea, is commonly associated with esophageal atresia and following repair of tracheoesophageal fistula, vascular ring, etc. It may occur as an isolated defect and/or in association with laryngomalacia. Rarely does it require intubation or tracheostomy.

Congenital lobar emphysema

This is overinflation of a lobe due to localized bronchomalacia or bronchial obstruction. It may cause wheeze or produce chest deformity. The condition often resolves spontaneously.

Diaphragmatic hernia

This is a diaphragmatic defect with intra-abdominal contents present in the chest. This may cause respiratory distress soon after birth and may have been detected during the antenatal period by ultrasound. It may also be completely asymptomatic and found incidentally on CXR. There are two types.

Bochdalek hernia is the congenital absence of posterolateral part of diaphragm, with associated hypoplastic lung secondary to abdominal contents limiting its growth. Treatment is with surgical repair of the diaphragmatic defect, but the survival rate is diminished because of underlying lung hypoplasia.

Morgagni hernia is anteromedial herniation through the foramen of Morgagni, which more commonly is found in adulthood. It may be asymptomatic or cause symptoms of fullness, tightness, or pain in the anterior chest; it does not cause intestinal obstruction. CXR shows a cardiophrenic angle density. Surgical repair is difficult and usually not necessary.

Cystic adenomatoid lung

Excessive overgrowth of bronchioles occurs, with multiple cysts in a section of lung, usually a single (lower) lobe. This commonly affects the left lower lobe. The condition can be diagnosed antenatally, and can present in the same way as congenital lobar emphysema. It may be mistaken for diaphragmatic hernia. Treatment is by resection of the affected lobe.

Pulmonary sequestration/sequestrated segment

In this disorder, a segment of lung parenchyma has no bronchial connection and is therefore unventilated. It may be supplied by an aberrant artery from the aorta and have anomalous pulmonary drainage to the right atrium. The sequestrated segment can be intralobar, sharing pleura with the rest of the lung, or extralobar, separated from the lung by a lining of pleural tissue. It is mostly left-sided; 75% of these disorders are situated between the diaphragm and left lower lobe.

Pulmonary sequestration is associated with other congenital abnormalities in 60% of cases. It can be a chance finding on CXR at any age, when cystic change may be seen in this area. Contrast CT or MRI may aid diagnosis. Surgical resection may be necessary if there is repeated infection in this segment.

Hyperlucent lung syndrome

This syndrome is otherwise known as Swyer–James–MacLeod syndrome. Focal hyperlucency of the lung or lobe, often unilateral, is due to paren-chymal and vascular maldevelopment, following a childhood bronchitis or bronchiolitis.

The syndrome is usually asymptomatic. It is diagnosed on CXR, which shows a hypertranslucent lung, with reduced vascular markings and a small pulmonary artery.

Part III

Supportive care

Noninvasive ventilation

Terminology

Ventilatory support may be invasive (via endotracheal tube or tracheostomy) or noninvasive (via facemask or nasal mask). Noninvasive ventilation (NIV) may be subdivided into *positive* or *negative* pressure ventilation.

Positive pressure ventilators deliver volume or pressure support; many different types are available. Bilevel pressure support ventilators are used extensively, and provide pressure support between selected inspiratory and expiratory positive airway pressures (IPAP and EPAP). They function in several modes, including patient-triggered inspiratory support with provision of backup rate that will cut in if the patient fails to breathe. Noninvasive positive pressure support may be provided by specialized portable ventilators or by standard critical care ventilators.

Negative pressure ventilators assist inspiration by expanding the chest wall; expiration occurs through elastic recoil of the lungs. They include devices such as tank ventilators, chest "shell" ventilators, and full body wraps. Other devices such as the rocking bed and "pneumobelt" displace abdominal contents to aid diaphragmatic contraction. Used extensively in the polio epidemics of the 1950s, they are now only rarely used to manage chronic respiratory failure.

Continuous positive airway pressure (CPAP) supplies constant positive pressure during inspiration and expiration and is therefore not generally considered a form of ventilatory support. It provides a "splint" to open the upper airway and collapsed alveoli and improves V/Q matching. CPAP is used extensively in the community to treat obstructive sleep apnea, but it also has a role in improving oxygenation in selected patients with acute respiratory failure, e.g., patients with cardiogenic pulmonary edema.

Abbreviations

NIV = noninvasive ventilation, also referred to as noninvasive mechanical ventilation (NIMV)
NIPPV = noninvasive positive pressure ventilation
IPAP = inspiratory positive airways pressure
EPAP = expiratory positive airways pressure, also referred to as positive end-expiratory pressure (PEEP)
BPAP = bilevel positive airway pressure (IPAP is greater than EPAP)
CPAP = continuous positive airway pressure.

Further information

Mehta S, Hill NS (2001). Noninvasive ventilation. *Am J Respir Crit Care Med* **163**:540–577.

Indications

NIV may be used in an attempt to avoid invasive ventilation and its complications (e.g., upper airway trauma, ventilator-acquired pneumonia); alternatively, NIV may be considered for treatment of patients deemed unsuitable for intubation. NIV is not an alternative to invasive ventilation in patients who require this definitive treatment.

Clinical scenarios

Acute exacerbation of COPD

- Consider NIV in patients with an acute exacerbation of COPD who have a respiratory acidosis (pH <7.35) despite aggressive medical treatment and controlled supplemental oxygen therapy.
- Benefits include reduced mortality and need for intubation, more rapid improvement in physiological outcomes (respiratory rate, pH), and symptomatic relief from breathlessness when compared with standard medical treatment.
- Invasive ventilation, if deemed appropriate, should be considered in patients with severe respiratory acidosis (pH < 7.25), as this is associated with increased mortality and treatment failure with NIV.

Acute cardiogenic pulmonary edema

- Use of CPAP via facemask is effective and should be considered in patients who fail to improve with medical management alone.
- Bilevel NIV has not been shown to be superior to CPAP. It may have a role in patients who do not respond to CPAP.

Decompensated obstructive sleep apnea

Both NIV and nasal CPAP with supplementary oxygen are effective in the treatment of severe decompensated obstructive sleep apnea, although NIV is generally recommended when a respiratory acidosis is present.

Respiratory failure from neuromuscular weakness

NIV is the treatment of choice for decompensated respiratory failure resulting from neuromuscular weakness or chest wall deformity.

Immunocompromised patients

- Immunocompromised patients who develop acute respiratory failure have an extremely high mortality following endotracheal intubation and ventilation.
- In immunocompromised patients with pulmonary infiltrates, fever, and hypoxemic acute respiratory failure, intermittent NIV results in lower intubation rates and hospital mortality than that with standard treatment.
- CPAP is effective in the treatment of PCP.

Facilitation of weaning in COPD patients

Community-acquired pneumonia

- Use of NIV may result in a reduction in need for intubation compared to standard medical treatment, although no significant differences in hospital mortality or length of hospitalization have been shown.
- CPAP may have a role in improving oxygenation in severe pneumonia.
- In patients who would potentially be candidates for intubation, use of NIV or CPAP should not inappropriately delay invasive ventilation and should only be attempted in an ICU or step-down unit setting.

Other conditions

- There is no evidence to support the use of NIV in patients with acute severe asthma.
- There is no strong evidence to support the use of NIV in exacerbations of bronchiectasis and cystic fibrosis, although NIV may be considered as treatment in patients with severe underlying disease who would not be considered suitable candidates for invasive ventilation.
- Bilevel NIV or CPAP may have a role in improving gas exchange following trauma or surgery.

Contraindications

Relative contraindications to the use of NIV are listed below. They should be considered in the context of individual patients; for example, severe hypoxemia may not be considered a contraindication for NIV in a patient who is unsuitable for invasive ventilation.

Contraindications to NIV

- Cardiac or respiratory arrest
- Impaired consciousness or confusion
- Severe hypoxemia
- Copious respiratory secretions
- Hemodynamic instability
- Facial surgery, trauma, burns, or deformity
- Upper airway obstruction
- Tracheal injury
- Untreated pneumothorax
- Inability to cooperate or to protect the airway
- Vomiting, bowel obstruction, recent upper gastrointestinal tract surgery, esophageal injury

Further information

British Thoracic Society Standards of Care Committee (2002). Guidelines on non-invasive ventilation in acute respiratory failure. *Thorax* **57**:192–211.

Nava S, Carbone G, DiBattista N, et al. (2003). Non-invasive ventilation in cardiogenic pulmonary edema. A multicentre randomized trial. *Am J Respir Crit Care Med* **168**(12):1432–1437.

Plant PK, Owen JL, Elliott MW (2000). Early use of non-invasive ventilation for acute exacerbations of chronic obstructive pulmonary disease on general respiratory wards: a multicentre randomized controlled trial. *Lancet* **355**:1931–1935.

NIV in acute respiratory failure

The decision to start NIV should begin after initial stabilization of the patient, including appropriate supplemental oxygen therapy; a proportion of patients will improve and will not require ventilation. Prior to commencing NIV a decision should be made with the patient and their family regarding suitability for invasive ventilation should NIV fail—document this clearly in the medical notes. *If the patient is a candidate for invasive ventilation, care must be taken to avoid inappropriate delays in intubation through the use of NIV or CPAP.*

Setting up NIV

1. Select an appropriate interface and size for the patient. Masks may be nasal or oronasal (full face). Nasal masks require clear nasal passages and may permit mouth leaks, particularly in the acutely breathless patient, but they are more comfortable. Full-face masks avoid mouth leakage and are generally favored for initial use in acute respiratory failure.

2. Explain the procedure to the patient and what you hope to accomplish with this treatment. Allow the patient to hold the mask to their face prior to attaching the head straps—this may increase confidence and compliance. Mask adjustments are often necessary to minimize air leaks, although some leakage may have to be accepted. Avoid excessive strap tension; one or two fingers should fit under the strap.

3. Set up the ventilator. Typical initial pressures for ventilating a patient with hypercapnic respiratory failure due to an exacerbation of COPD would be EPAP 4 cm H_2O and IPAP 8–12 cm H_2O, with a backup rate of ≈15/minute and inspiratory ratio of 1:3 in spontaneous/timed mode. Increase the IPAP in increments of 2 cm H_2O to a maximum of 20, as tolerated by the patient. Similar settings can be used for patients with hypercapnic respiratory failure resulting from neuromuscular weakness. Consider increasing the EPAP (e.g., to 8 or 10 cm) in obese patients with COPD and OSA or in COPD patients to facilitate triggering when auto-PEEP is present. Increasing EPAP may also be needed to treat hypoxemia. In order to maintain a level of pressure support, you need to increase IPAP when you increase EPAP. Pressure support ventilators can also be set to provide CPAP by equalizing the IPAP and EPAP. CPAP may improve oxygenation in selected patients with cardiogenic pulmonary edema or pneumonia.

4. Supplemental oxygen is provided either by an oxygen blender or through a tube connected to the mask or ventilator circuit and adjusted to maintain an oxygen saturation between 90% and 92%.

5. Patient monitoring should involve assessment of comfort, respiratory rate, synchrony with the ventilator, work of breathing, mask leaks, pulse rate, blood pressure, and oxygen saturations (see Table 49.1).

6. Arterial blood gas analysis should be performed within 1 to 2 hours and again after 4 hours if there has been no improvement. Improvement in acidosis and decline in respiratory rate after 1 and 4 hours of treatment are associated with a better outcome. Repeat the blood gas analysis if the clinical condition changes.

7. Lack of response may be indicated by a worsening acidosis or persistently abnormal arterial blood gases, or by a reduced level of consciousness and clinical deterioration. Consider invasive ventilation, if appropriate. The decision to halt NIV depends on the circumstances of the individual patient.

8. Subsequent management depends on the patient's response. Optimal duration of NIV is unclear, but it is typically administered for up to 3 days in acute respiratory failure. NIV does not need to be continuous, and the patient may have breaks for fluid intake or meals and nebulizers treatments. Nebulizer treatments can be done in-line with the ventilator if using a full-face mask. For patients who are too ill to eat, a small-bore feeding tube may be used. Consider switching to a nasal mask after 24 hours to improve patient comfort. Monitor oxygenation and work of breathing when the patient is off NIV.

Table 49.1 Troubleshooting NIV

Problem	Possible solution
Clinical deterioration or worsening respiratory failure	Ensure optimal medical therapy
	Consider complications, e.g., pneumothorax, aspiration, sputum retention
	Does the patient require intubation, if appropriate?
PCO_2 remains high (persistent respiratory acidosis)	Exclude inappropriately high FiO_2
	Check mask and circuit for leaks
	Check for patient–ventilator asynchrony
	Check expiration valve patency
	Consider increasing IPAP
PO_2 remains low (<60 mmHg)	Consider increasing FiO_2
	Consider increasing EPAP
Irritation or ulceration of nasal bridge	Adjust strap tension
	Try cushion dressing
	Change mask type
Dry nose or mouth	Use a heated humidifier
	Check for leaks
Dry sore eyes	Check mask fit
Nasal congestion	Decongestants

NIV in chronic respiratory failure

Chest wall deformity and neuromuscular weakness (see p. 35)

NIV has a well-established role in the management of chronic respiratory failure due to chest wall deformity or neuromuscular weakness, and has been shown to improve symptoms, gas exchange, and mortality.

Common underlying diagnoses include chest wall deformity and kyphoscoliosis, post-polio syndrome, motor neuron disease, spinal cord injury, neuropathies, myopathies, and muscular dystrophies. The nature of the underlying disease must influence the appropriateness of initiating ventilation: progressive conditions such as motor neuron disease often result in increasing dependence on the ventilator, and the patient and their caregivers should be made aware of this.

NIV is typically administered at home during sleep, but as the patient's condition deteriorates, NIV may be needed periodically during the day. Generally, nocturnal ventilation is sufficient to improve daytime gas exchange. The mechanism for this is unclear; it probably resets the central respiratory drive hypercapnia threshold, although respiratory muscle rest and improved compliance may also play a role. Some patients who require daytime use of the ventilator may use a mouthpiece when mobile in their wheelchair.

Small, portable positive pressure ventilators and nasal masks are used in most cases. Negative pressure or abdominal ventilators may have a role in patients who are intolerant of masks, although their use may be limited by upper airway obstruction.

The decision to introduce overnight NIV is difficult and is based on both symptoms (morning headaches, hypersomnolence, fatigue, poor sleep quality) and evidence of respiratory failure (daytime hypercapnia [$PaCO_2$ >45 mmHg] and/or nocturnal hypoventilation with O_2 saturations <88% on overnight oximetry for ≥5 minutes).

Medicare guidelines allow NIV if the forced vital capacity is <50% or the maximal inspiratory pressure is <60 cmH_2O. Daytime respiratory failure, however, is often a late feature and is typically preceded by hypercapnic hypoventilation during sleep.

A recent study in patients with myopathies demonstrated supine inspiratory vital capacity to be an accurate predictor of respiratory reserve: supine IVC <40% of predicted was significantly associated with hypercapnic hypoventilation, and such patients should be considered for treatment with NIV. Supine IVC <20% was typically associated with daytime respiratory failure, whereas supine IVC >60% indicated a minimal risk of respiratory complications. Other factors include signs of cor pulmonale or multiple hospital admissions with respiratory failure

Patients with excessive secretions may not be suitable for NIV, although face-mask ventilation is possible even in the setting of severe bulbar weakness. A cough assist device may be necessary for these patients.

Regular follow-up of patients on overnight ventilation is important. Ask about symptoms and compliance, and repeat arterial blood gas analysis. Lack of improvement in gas exchange may reflect noncompliance, excessive air leakage, inadequate pressure support, or progression of underlying disease; consider repeating nocturnal oximetry monitoring. Patients with persistent severe hypoxia will benefit from long-term supplementary oxygen.

Obstructive sleep apnea (OSA) (see p. 364)

Overnight NIV may have a role in patients with central hypoventilation, Cheyne–Stokes respiration, obesity hypoventilation, overlap syndromes of OSA with coexisting COPD, and in severe OSA unresponsive to nasal CPAP.

Cystic fibrosis (p. 388)

Overnight NIV may have a useful role as a bridge to transplantation in patients with cystic fibrosis and chronic respiratory failure.

COPD (p. 155)

Use of NIV in the management of chronic, stable COPD is controversial. Trials have shown conflicting results, although possibly some benefit in patients with severe hypercapnia and nocturnal hypoventilation.

Further information

Clinical indications for noninvasive positive pressure ventilation in chronic respiratory failure due to restrictive lung disease, COPD, and nocturnal hypoventilation—a consensus conference report. *Chest* 1999; **116**:521–534.

Efrati O, Moday-Moses D, Barak A, et al. (2004). Long-term non-invasive positive pressure ventilation among cystic fibrosis patients awaiting lung transplantation. *Isr Med Assoc J* **6**:527-530.

Ragette R, Mellies U, Schwake C, Voit C, Teschler C (2002). Patterns and predictors of sleep disordered breathing in primary myopathies. *Thorax* **57**:724–728.

Indications for intensive care unit admission

Intensive care units (ICU) provide the medical team with the ability to monitor a patient's status on a minute-to-minute basis, and often have resources that are either more limited or not available in other areas of the hospital. Patients who are unstable, i.e., have physiologically important changes over very short periods of time, need to be cared for in an ICU. Such physiologic instability is commonly seen with serious and life-threatening conditions.

While many hospitals have "criteria" for ICU admission to assist the clinician with resource utilization, it is ultimately up to the clinicians caring for the patient to determine how stable or unstable a patient is, and whether or not ICU level care is necessary for the care of an individual patient.

ICU beds are limited and valuable resources that must be used wisely. It remains the responsibility of the physician to be familiar with the capabilities of the different units and wards within his or her own hospital so that patients may be admitted to the most appropriate location for their condition.

The capabilities of intermediate care units or step-down units may vary widely among facilities.

Indications for ICU admission

Respiratory failure or impending respiratory failure

Patients may or may not require mechanical ventilation with either intubation or noninvasive positive pressure ventilation (NIPPV) at the time of admission. Blood gas analysis, oxygen saturation, respiratory rate, and clinical assessment of the work of breathing, or "respiratory fatigue," are instrumental in determining impending respiratory failure. The term *respiratory failure* encompasses all of the following:

• Ventilatory failure, e.g., COPD exacerbation
• Hypoxemic respiratory failure, e.g., ARDS or severe pneumonia
• Inability to protect or maintain airway, e.g., trauma or overdose

Shock and hemodynamic instability

Shock is defined as end-organ hypoperfusion (inadequate blood flow to meet tissue oxygen demand) and is generally associated with hypotension. Manifestations of end-organ hypoperfusion may include altered mental status, oliguria, respiratory failure, and lactic acidosis.

The restoring of adequate tissue perfusion often requires aggressive, minute-to-minute titration of hemodynamic support, regardless of the underlying etiology. Etiologies of shock may include septic shock and other causes of distributive shock, cardiogenic shock, hypovolemic shock, and obstructive shock.

Life-threatening hemorrhage

• Massive hemoptysis
• Obstetrical patients with massive post- or peripartum hemorrhage
• Gastrointestinal bleeding with "BLEED" criteria (actively **B**leeding, **L**ow blood pressure, **E**levated INR, **E**rratic mentation, and other comorbidities or **D**isorders)

Cardiac arrhythmia and myocardial infarction

Patients at high risk for a lethal arrhythmia, such as those with ventricular arrhythmias or ST-segment elevation myocardial infarctions, will commonly be admitted to either an ICU or CCU (coronary care unit) for close monitoring.

Acute neurologic failure

This includes all patients whose clinical condition requires very frequent neurological checks (i.e., every hour) or intracranial pressure monitoring, patients in severe alcohol withdrawal, patients with status epilepticus, and patients who are unable to protect their airways.

Severe metabolic derangements

This includes those patients whose metabolic, hepatic, or endocrinological disturbance is so severe that they require ICU-level monitoring, such as every-hour laboratories or vital signs. Such disorders may include fulminant hepatic failure, severe diabetic ketoacidosis, and severe hyponatremia.

Major surgical procedures

This category encompasses major surgical procedures that require ongoing hemodynamic monitoring, ventilatory support, or extensive nursing care, such as coronary artery bypass grafting (CABG) or abdominal aortic aneurysm (AAA) repair.

Miscellaneous

The clinical situation, not the diagnosis, ultimately determines the need for ICU-level care. For example, patients receiving thrombolytic therapy for a stroke will often require ICU-level care to monitor for signs and symptoms of a CNS bleed, even though stroke by itself would not fall within the criteria for admission.

ICU resources

Personnel

- Critical care nurses often with 1:1 or 1:2 nurse–patient ratios
- Respiratory therapy (e.g., continuous nebulizer therapies)
- Critical care physicians
- Pharmacy, case managers, nutritionists, etc.

Monitoring

- Continuous or invasive hemodynamic monitoring
- Other invasive monitoring, e.g., intracranial pressure monitor

Therapeutic interventions

- Mechanical ventilation
- Vasopressor or inotropic support
- Renal replacement therapy

Further reading

Kollef MH, O'Brien JD, Zuckerman GR, Shannon W (1997). BLEED: a classification tool to predict outcomes in patients with acute upper and lower gastrointestinal hemorrhage. *Crit Care Med* **25**(7):1125–1132.

Ethical issues

Background and COPD

Most ethical issues faced by doctors arise at the end of a patient's life. This applies particularly to respiratory physicians, who made need to make difficult decisions about the appropriateness of treatment and the prolongation of life in patients with chronic underlying lung disease. In some situations artificial ventilation may prolong the dying process; life has a natural end and the potential to prolong life in the intensive care unit (ICU) can sometimes cause dilemmas.

Doctors have an obligation to respect human life, protect the health of their patients, and put their patients' best interests first. This means offering treatments with benefits that outweigh any risks, and avoiding treatments that carry no net gain to the patient. If a patient wishes to have a treatment that, in the doctor's considered view, is not indicated, the doctor and medical team are under no ethical or legal obligation to provide it (but the patient's right to a second opinion must be respected).

The discussion about resuscitation and formal ventilation is never an easy one. Ideally it should take place with the nursing staff, the patient, and their next of kin, in advance of an emergency situation. In practical terms, this is not always possible. Ideally all decisions regarding resuscitation and the ceiling of treatment (particularly relating to ventilation) should be documented in advance and handed over to the on-call team. Most possible outcomes can be anticipated.

In cases where it has been decided that a treatment is not in the best interests of the patient, there is no ethical distinction between stopping the treatment and not starting it in the first place (though the former may be more difficult to do), and this should not be used as an argument for failing to initiate the treatment in the first place.

Some clinical scenarios are more commonly encountered by the respiratory physician. These are discussed below.

COPD is the fourth most common cause of death in America, and most patients die of respiratory failure during an exacerbation. A commonly encountered clinical situation is one where a patient with COPD is admitted with an exacerbation and is in respiratory failure. Standard treatment does not improve the respiratory acidosis, so noninvasive ventilation (NIV) is commenced. Before starting NIV, a decision must be clearly documented as to whether or not NIV is the ceiling of treatment, especially if the patient has severe or end-stage COPD.

Formal ventilation in the ICU may be appropriate in certain specific situations—for example, in a relatively young patient (i.e., <65 years), a patient with a relatively new diagnosis of COPD for whom the episode is the first or second admission, and a patient having a very obviously potentially reversible cause for the exacerbation, e.g., pneumonia. Sometimes in this situation, a defined time period for intensive care input may be decided, e.g., ventilation for 48 hours (to allow treatments to work and allow time to assess for any improvement), with extubation after that time period if no improvement has been made.

Decisions about formal ventilation and intensive care admission can only be made with knowledge of the patient's usual level of functioning and previous quality of life. The problem in this situation is that quality of life is a very subjective measure. Objective measures of usual functioning, such as measures of daily activity, usual exercise tolerance, and whether home care or assistance with activities of daily living is required, are more useful in guiding the appropriateness of escalating therapy. With particular reference to the patient with COPD, the number of hospital admissions and exacerbations and the need for home oxygen or nebulizers will also be useful. Helpful information may be obtained from the general medical internist if the previous hospital notes are unavailable.

Neither the next-of-kin nor those with enduring power of attorney have the legal right to determine any treatment. The responsibility remains with the doctor and multidisciplinary team, occasionally involving the hospital's ethics committee and sometimes the courts of law.

When there is limited information about the patient and thus uncertainty about the appropriateness of ventilation, it should be started until a clearer assessment can be made. This may be relevant for a patient involved in an accident who presents to the emergency department with little information available. The point about the withdrawal of therapy, should it subsequently be found to be inappropriate, also holds.

There are downsides to invasive ventilation: the risk of pneumothorax is increased in those with end-stage emphysema, and the risk of ventilator-acquired pneumonia increases with time ventilated. Knowledge of the risk of these adverse events helps the medical team to balance the argument and make a decision about whether the risks of ventilation are likely to outweigh its benefits. The issue of limited resources should not influence a decision about formal ventilation or ICU admission.

The average length of intubation of patients with COPD admitted to the ICU is 3.2 days. These patients have a 20%–25% in-hospital mortality, with 50% of patients surviving 1 year after ICU discharge. About 50% will be living independently 1 year after hospital discharge. Clearly, only a very select subgroup of patients is admitted to the ICU, and concerns about prolonged periods of ventilation in this group of patients seem to be unfounded. Patients in whom a clear cause for the exacerbation can be identified (e.g., pneumonia) tend to do better, as there is a treatable cause for the exacerbation and not just progression of the underlying disease.

Lung cancer and neurological disease

Lung cancer

The use of antibiotic treatment for pneumonia in a patient with advanced lung malignancy may be inappropriate in some circumstances. The stage and extent of disease, response to other treatments (e.g., chemotherapy), and the patient's wishes and quality of life are all paramount.

This is another situation in which it might be appropriate to define at the outset the treatments that are appropriate, e.g., 10 days total of intravenous and oral antibiotics. Note that treatments such as antibiotics can lead to improvement in symptoms (e.g., by reducing fever), without necessarily prolonging life, and it may be kinder to continue antibiotics in this situation.

Progressive neurological disease

The decision about noninvasive ventilation in a patient with a progressive neuromuscular disease can be difficult. In this setting, the clinical deterioration can usually be anticipated, and in most situations, discussion should have taken place early on (unless the patient presents in respiratory failure, for example, with pneumonia, and subsequent ventilator weaning is difficult).

Different centers, patients, and their relatives will have differing views as to whether life-prolonging NIV ventilation in the face of progressive neuromuscular disability is warranted. Some centers take the view that if the quality of life and higher mental functioning are good, and the respiratory muscles are affected early on (and other functions and mobility remain good), then NIV is warranted.

Further decisions about withdrawal of treatment with progression of the underlying neurological disease will, of course, still be needed. In motor neuron disease with bulbar palsy, for example, aspiration is a relative contraindication to noninvasive/mask ventilation. Aspiration in these patients is a poor prognostic sign, and often a sign of imminent death.

An advance directive documents the patient's wishes in the event of serious illness. It will usually include a decision about resuscitation and other potential life-prolonging treatments. The patient must understand the implications of his or her decision.

Further information

General Medical Council (2002). Withholding and Withdrawing Life-Prolonging Treatments: Good Practice in Decision-Making. London: General Medical Council.

Tracheostomy

A tracheostomy is most often performed as an adjunct to assisted ventilation. It may be temporary or permanent, depending on the respiratory assistance requirements of the patient. It can be performed as a formal surgical procedure or percutaneously at the bedside.

Tracheostomy in the ICU: indications and advantages

Indications for and advantages of using tracheostomy in the ICU include the following:

- Usually performed after an extended duration of intubation with an endotracheal tube. The usual practice is to convert from endotracheal tube to tracheostomy at day 7 if ventilation is likely to be needed beyond 14 days. Conversion beyond 14 days is considered best practice and certainly by 21 days.
- Improved patient communication over an endotracheal tube (with appropriate cuff deflation and/or tube fenestration)
- Reduction in laryngeal trauma
- Possible reduction in tracheal injury
- Improved nursing care and oral hygiene
- Facilitation of weaning off the ventilator. Importantly, there is no evidence for a reduced incidence of aspiration and pneumonia.

Indications for tracheostomy not in the ICU

Indications for using tracheostomy in patients not in the ICU include the following:

- Severe sleep apnea
- Tracheal or laryngeal stenosis or obstruction
- Acute tracheal or laryngeal trauma
- Neuromuscular disorders requiring respiratory aid
- Need for a secure airway prior to a surgical procedure (i.e., severe facial fractures, craniofacial reconstruction)

Contraindications

No absolute contraindications exist for a tracheostomy. One relative contraindication is a nonemergent tracheostomy in a patient with laryngeal carcinoma. For these patients, a total laryngectomy is the definitive treatment; manipulation of the tumor may lead to an increased risk of stomal recurrence. Abnormal neck or tracheal anatomy may be a relative contraindication to performing a percutaneous tracheostomy.

Percutaneous versus surgical tracheostomy

According to a review of the literature, there are few large studies comparing the two techniques to clearly determine a superior method. However, current studies suggest comparable outcomes in terms of success, cost-effectiveness and complication rates.

One main difference between the techniques is the personnel required to perform the procedure. The standard surgical approach requires a surgeon, while the percutaneous method may be performed by either a surgeon or a critical care physician.

Postoperative care

Fresh tracheostomy precautions, including avoidance of cutting the tracheal tie or stay sutures, should be maintained until the tracheal tract matures. This will prevent accidental dislodgement of the tracheostomy tube and loss of airway. Humidification of the inspired gas is always required to prevent the buildup of thick viscous mucus. Humidification can only be withdrawn in long-term tracheostomy patients after several weeks or months.

Complications

Early complications include mucous plugging, pneumothorax, tracheal stoma bleeding, subcutaneous emphysema, tracheitis, stomal infection, tracheobronchial injury, and tracheostomy tube displacement. Delayed complications include scarring, granulation tissue formation, tracheal stenosis, tracheomalacia, inability to decannulate, bleeding from a tracheo-innominate artery fistula, and tracheoesophageal fistula (particularly if a nasogastric or orogastric tube is in place).

Postoperative chest radiographs are not required after routine tracheostomies. They should be obtained after emergent or difficult procedures, or in patients with signs and symptoms of pneumothorax.

Decannulation

Tracheostomy may still be required to administer intermittent ventilation, reduce ventilatory dead space, aid respiratory secretion clearance, limit aspiration (when cuffed), and bypass any upper airway obstruction. This is weighed against the consequences of a tracheostomy: there is an increased tendency to aspirate when swallowing (because of a reduced ability to protect the laryngeal airway by inhibiting laryngeal elevation), reduced ability to talk, and increased infection brought about from a foreign body in the trachea.

Thus, decannulation should be considered with the following conditions or when there is

- Adequate clearance of secretions, i.e., good cough and thin secretions
- No upper airway obstruction
- No significant aspiration, although a small amount is not an absolute contraindication
- No need to continue ventilation for maintenance of gas exchange
- Possible conversion to noninvasive ventilation

The ability to cope adequately without the tracheostomy can be intermittently tested by capping the tube with the cuff fully deflated, preferably with a fenestrated tube. When considering decannulation it is important that the patient be able to tolerate a plugged tracheostomy overnight without desaturation.

Once a tube has been removed, the stoma can close very quickly and make reinsertion difficult. If necessary for a difficult tracheostomy tube change, introduce a guidewire over which the old tube can be removed and the new one inserted.

The final decision to decannulate is often delayed unnecessarily.

Available tube options

Tracheostomy tubes can be cuffed or uncuffed. If mechanical ventilation is not necessary and aspiration is not a problem, a cuff is not required. Sometimes patients can be adequately ventilated even with the cuff down or no cuff at all; this is usually the case in patients with normal lungs in whom compliance is good and inflation pressures therefore low.

Tracheostomy tubes can be either single or double lumen (with an inner and outer tube). Double-lumen tubes allow better cleaning and patency of the lumen, but the diameter of the lumen is of course less for a similar-sized external diameter.

Extra-long tracheostomy tubes can be used in obese patients with large necks. Adjustable-length tubes are also available in which the length can be adjusted at the tracheostomy site. These tubes should be considered in patients in whom the end of the tracheostomy tube needs to lie closer to the carina (i.e., in obstructive lesions of the trachea or tracheomalacia).

Tracheostomy tubes can be fenestrated to allow partial exhalation via the larynx to aid talking. The fenestration can be closed off with a non-fenestrated inner tube should intermittent mechanical ventilation still be required. A Passy–Muir valve is a one-way valve that attaches to the tracheostomy tube and allows inspiration through the tracheostomy tube but not expiration. This valve allows patients to speak and inspire with the valve cap in place.

Inhalers and nebulizers

Background

Inhalers

There are many different inhaler devices that deliver drugs directly to the airways. Patients should receive advice on techniques for the use of their inhaler. Inhaler technique should be checked regularly and, if patients cannot manage a particular device, they should be switched to another one.

- The percentage of a drug delivered to the airway varies with each device (15%–60% according to the manufacturers), and depends on good technique.
- Spacer devices improve this delivery and are particularly useful for the elderly, children, and those who find it difficult to coordinate inhaler administration with breathing.
- Try to use the same inhaler device for all the drug classes used by a patient.
- Advise the patient how to recognize when a device is empty; some have dose counters on them. For devices without a dose counter, it is best to put a piece of tape with a start date on it and, if the device is used regularly, put a stop date. For a metered dose inhaler (MDI) used as needed, have the patient put a piece of tape on the device and put a tick mark for every 2 puffs taken.
- Titrate inhaler doses with clinical response.

Nebulizers

Nebulizers are sometimes used by patients who cannot use an MDI or a dry powder inhaler (DPI) correctly. It may also be used during acute respiratory illnesses, because of disease severity, or in young children. Patients who are being considered for nebulizer therapy should be seen by a respiratory therapist or nurse to learn how to use the nebulizer correctly. If antibiotics are being nebulized, a different nebulizer and compressor may be needed.

How to use

Open the nebule containing the drug solution and squirt the solution into the nebulizer chamber. Albuterol and ipratropium bromide can be taken together and are available as a Duoneb, but nebulized budesonide or antibiotics should be used separately with a dedicated nebulizer. When ipratropium bromide is being used, it should be delivered via a mouthpiece and not a mask, to avoid eye contact.

Reattach the nebulizer chamber to the compressor. Switch the compressor on and make sure the nebulizer is misting. Position the mouthpiece between the teeth and lips. Breathe slowly in and out. Continue until all the solution is gone.

Depending on the type of nebulizer and compressor, this may take 10–15 minutes. Switch off the machine. Clean the nebulizer chamber with soap and water after each use and allow to air dry.

Every other day, soak the nebulizer in a vinegar solution of 1 part vinegar and 3 parts water for 1 hour, rinse, and air dry. Prior to storing a nebulizer, make sure it is thoroughly dry; this can be done by reattaching the nebulizer to the compressor and turning the compressor on.

If the patient requires oxygen, it can still be used during nebulization by using the oxygen tubing from the oxygen source attached directly to the nebulizer chamber to drive the nebulization. For patients who have repeated infections, review proper cleaning of the nebulizer with them and switch to another device, if possible.

Compressors should be serviced annually. Follow the manufacturer's recommendations for cleaning and care of the machine.

Different inhaler types and instructions for their use

See Table 53.1 and Table 53.2.

Table 53.1 Different inhaler types

Generic name of drug (with product names)	Mechanism of action	Device type
Albuterol (Ventolin HFA®, Proventil HFA®, ProAir HFA®) Levalbuterol (Xopenex) Terbutaline (Bricanyl®)	Short-acting β₂ agonist Duration 4–6 hours	MDI
Salmeterol (Serevent®)s Formoterol (Foradil®)	Long-acting β₂ agonist Duration 12 hours	Diskus (DPI) Aerolizer (DPI)
Ipratropium bromide (Atrovent®) Ipratropium and albuterol (Combivent®)	Short-acting anticholinergic Duration 3–6 hours	MDI MDI
Tiotropium (Spiriva®)	Long-acting anticholinergic Duration 36 hours	Handihaler® (DPI)
Beclomethasone dipropionate (Qvar®)	Corticosteroid	MDI
Budesonide (Pulmicort®)		MDI Turbohaler MDI
Fluticasone propionate (Flovent®)		MDI
Mometasone furoate (Asmanex®)		Twisthaler (DPI)
Salmeterol and fluticasone (Advair®) Formoterol and budesonide (Symbicort®)	Combination steroid and bronchodilator	DPI, MDI MDI
Sodium cromoglycate (Intal®) Nedocromil sodium (Tilade®)	Stabilize mast cells	MDI MDI

Table 53.2 Instructions for use of different inhaler types

Type of device	Instructions for use
Pressurized aerosol metered dose inhaler (MDI) Aerosol	Remove cap and shake the inhaler well. Hold the inhaler upright with your thumb on the base below the mouthpiece and first finger on the metal canister. Then hold the mouthpiece about 1.5–2 inches in front of your mouth. Tilt your head back slightly and open your mouth wide. Breath out gently.
	Press the inhaler and at the same time begin a slow, deep breath. Continue breathing slowly and deeply over 3–5 seconds. Hold your breath for up to 10 seconds if possible. Resume normal breathing and repeat these steps if more than one puff is ordered. Use with the spacer device to improve drug delivery. Clean the plastic case every week.
Spacer (holding chambers) Aero Chamber® InspirEase® Vortex™	Ensure that the spacer is compatible with your inhaler. Remove cap of the inhaler and shake it. Insert it into the end of the spacer device. Place the other end of the spacer in your mouth. Press the inhaler canister once to release one dose of the drug.
	Take one slow (over 3–5 seconds), deep breath in and hold. Repeat as indicated. The valve should not whistle. Clean the spacer at least once a month with mild detergent, rinse, and air dry. Replace it after 6–12 months.
Breath-actuated devices Autohaler®	Prime the device. Remove the cap and lift the red lever. Insert the device into your mouth. Inhale slowly and deeply. Continue inhaling when the device clicks. You're your breath for up to 10 seconds if possible. Slowly breathe out. To take a second inhaled dose, lower the red lever and lift again, and repeat the above sequence.

Table 53.2 (*Cont.*)

Type of device	Instructions for use
Dry powder devices (DPI) Turbohaler®	Prime the device. Remove cap; twist base as far as possible until the click is heard and then twist back again. Repeat this step the first time the device is used. To take a treatment, remove the cap, hold device with the mouthpiece upright, and twist the bottom all the way to the right and back to the left. This loads the medication. Hold the Turbohaler away from your mouth and gently breathe out. Place the Turbohaler in your mouth and seal your lips around it. Inhale rapidly and deeply and hold your breath for up to 10 seconds, if able. If more than one puff is ordered, repeat these steps.
Twisthaler®	Remove cap by twisting;—the dose is then ready. To use the device, hold it level, exhale fully, place the mouthpiece into your mouth between your teeth and inhale steadily. Hold your breath and remove the inhaler. For a second dose, repeat these actions.

Table 53.2 (*Cont.*)

Type of device	Instructions for use
Handihaler®	Flip lid and white mouthpiece open and insert the capsule. Close the mouthpiece back down until it clicks. Pierce capsule by pressing the green button at the side. Take a few breaths in and out and exhale normally. Place the mouthpiece you're your mouth and breathe in slowly and deeply but at a rate sufficient enough to hear the capsule vibrate. Remove inhaler from your mouth and hold your breath for 10 seconds if possible. Slowly breathe out. Repeat if necessary to ensure that all powder from the capsule is gone.
Aerolizer®	Take lid off the Aerolizer; twist top of the Aerolizer to open it. Place capsule in the hole in the center of the Aerolizer. Twist to close the top of the Aerolizer. Hold Aerolizer with the mouthpiece up. Press buttons on the sides of the Aerolizer once firmly. This will pierce the capsule. Hold the Aerolizer away from your mouth and gently breathe out. Place mouthpiece in your mouth and inhale rapidly and deeply to hear the capsule vibrate. Hold your breath for up to 10 seconds if you are able. Then breath out slowly. You may repeat another breath with the capsule to make sure all the powder is gone. Open the top of the Aerolizer and throw away the used capsule.
Diskus®	Hold the device level, place your thumb of the other hand on the thumb grip and pull it back until it clicks. The mouthpiece is now ready to use. Push the lever back until it clicks; the medication is now loaded. Exhale normally, place the mouth-piece between your lips and inhale quickly and deeply. Hold your breath for up to 10 seconds and then exhale normally. You may want to wipe the mouthpiece with a clean tissue and then close it.

Immunosuppressive therapy

Introduction

Immunosuppressive drugs are used mainly in the management of asthma, chronic obstructive pulmonary disease, sarcoidosis and other interstitial lung disease, vasculitis and other pulmonary manifestations of rheumatic disease. Lung cancer and lung transplantation indications will not be addressed in this chapter.

In general, with the exception of lower-dose glucocorticoids, these agents should only be used under the supervision of a physician experienced with prescribing and monitoring immunosuppressive therapy and in conjunction with established protocols (see also Box 54.1). The protocols provided here are examples of many potential approaches.

Box 54.1 General advice for patients on immunosuppressive therapy

- Expect an increased risk of infections and increased likelihood of severe infections
- Expect atypical presentation of infections
- Avoid live vaccines such as measles, mumps, rubella, BCG, yellow fever, oral typhoid, oral polio
- If patient has never had varicella zoster:
  - Avoid contacts with chicken pox or shingles
  - Consider passive immunization
  - Provide immunoglobulin therapy if exposed
  - Hospital treatment with close monitoring is needed if chicken pox develops
- Avoid measles exposure. Provide prophylaxis with immunoglobulin if exposed
- Be aware of drug–drug interactions

Glucocorticoids

Mechanism of action

- Suppresses proinflammatory mediator production (e.g., tumor necrosis factor α [TNF-α], interleukin [IL]-1, IL-12, interferon-γ, prostaglandins, leukotrienes)
- Increases apoptosis of immature and activated T lymphocytes
- Suppresses immune/inflammatory effector cell activation and differentiation (macrophages, T cells, mast cells, natural killer cells, and immature B cells)
- Inhibits macrophage antigen presentation to lymphocytes
- Suppresses neutrophil, eosinophil, and monocyte migration
- Depresses endothelial cell functions including expression of adhesion molecules involved in inflammatory cell recruitment to inflammatory sites
- Decreases fibroblast proliferation, DNA, and collagen synthesis
- Decreases fibroblast production of phospholipase A_2, cyclooxygenase-2, prostaglandins, and metalloproteinases

Pulmonary uses

- Obstructive lung disease
  - Asthma
  - Chronic obstructive pulmonary disease
  - Bronchiectasis
  - Allergic bronchopulmonary aspergillosis
  - Bronchiolitis obliterans
- Interstitial lung disease
  - Connective tissue diseases
  - Hypersensitivity pneumonitis
  - Sarcoidosis
  - Cryptogenic organizing pneumonia
  - Eosinophilic pneumonia
- Vasculitis
- Acute respiratory distress syndrome
- Radiation pneumonitis
- Pleural disease
  - Post–cardiac injury syndrome
  - Radiation pleuritis
  - Connective tissue diseases
- Respiratory muscle weakness
  - Myasthenia gravis
  - Myositis
- Infections (must also treat with appropriate antimicrobial therapy)
  - *Pneumocystis (carinii) jiroveci*
  - *Mycobacterium tuberculosis*
    - Pleurisy
    - Respiratory failure

Commonly prescribed doses (see Table 54.1)

- 5 mg to 1 mg/kg prednisone equivalent, vary dose according to patient response
  - **Low dose:** ≤7.5 mg prednisone equivalent per day
  - **Medium dose:** >7.5 mg, but ≤30 mg prednisone equivalent per day
  - **High dose:** >30 mg, but ≤100 mg prednisone equivalent per day
  - **Very high dose:** >100 mg prednisone equivalent per day
- Induction with pulse dose glucocorticoids may be indicated in life-threatening disease (i.e., vasculitis).
  - **Pulse dose:** >250 mg prednisone equivalent for 1 or a few days
- Twice-daily dosing has a greater immunosuppressive effect than consolidation to once-daily dosing.
- Every-other-day dosing minimizes long-term side effects and hypothalamic–pituitary–adrenal (HPA) axis suppression, but may not adequately suppress inflammation.
- Glucocorticoids have good bioavailability so oral therapy is usually effective.

Table 54.1 Dose equivalents of glucocorticoids

Corticosteroid	Equivalent dose (mg)	Relative anti-inflammatory potency	Relative mineralocorticoid potency	Biologic half-life (hours)
Betamethasone	0.6–0.75	20–30	0	36–54
Cortisone	25	0.8	2	8–12
Dexamethasone	0.75	20–30	0	36–54
Fludrocortisone	—	10	125	18–36
Hydrocortisone	20	1	2	8–12
Methylprednisolone	4	5	0	18–36
Prednisolone	5	4	1	18–36
Prednisone	5	4	1	18–36
Triamcinolone	4	5	0	12–36

Dose adjustments
- Renal impairment: none required
- Hepatic impairment: none required

Drug–drug interactions
- Enhancement of the rate of metabolism of some glucocorticoids has been noted with concurrent administration of phenobarbital, phenytoin, and rifampin, by inducing the cytochrome p450 system.
- Giving aspirin and glucocorticoids concurrently decreases salicylate levels by causing an increased rate of salicylate metabolism. A reduction in glucocorticoid dosage in such patients may result in increased plasma salicylate levels with symptoms of salicylate toxicity.
- Glucocorticoids may make control of diabetes with insulin or oral hypoglycemic drugs more difficult.
- Glucocorticoids may decrease vaccine efficacy.

Corticosteroids and osteoporosis
- All corticosteroids inhibit bone formation and promote the development of osteoporosis (see Box 54.2). Their use may result in vertebral compression fractures.
  - The forced vital capacity may be decreased by as much as 9% with one thoracic vertebral compression fracture.
- The likelihood of developing osteoporosis is associated with the maximum dose and cumulative duration of therapy, but should be anticipated with any extended period regardless of the dose.

Box 54.2 Prevention and treatment of glucocorticoid-induced osteoporosis

On initiation of therapy with glucocorticoid (prednisone equivalent of 5 mg/day) with plans for treatment duration of 3 months

- Modify lifestyle risk factors for osteoporosis
- Smoking cessation or avoidance
- Reduction of alcohol consumption if excessive
- Instruct patient in weight-bearing physical exercise
- Initiate calcium supplementation (1500 mg elemental calcium/day)
- Initiate supplementation with vitamin D (400–800 IU/day)
- Prescribe bisphosphonate (use with caution in premenopausal women)

Already receiving long-term glucocorticoid therapy (prednisone equivalent of 5 mg/day)

- Modify lifestyle risk factors for osteoporosis
- Smoking cessation or avoidance
- Reduction of alcohol consumption if excessive
- Instruct patient in weight-bearing physical exercise
- Initiate calcium supplementation (1500 mg elemental calcium/day)
- Initiate supplementation with vitamin D (400–800 IU/day)
- Prescribe treatment to replace gonadal sex hormones if deficient or otherwise clinically indicated
- Measure bone mineral density (BMD) at lumbar spine and/or hip
- If BMD is not normal (i.e., T-score below −1), then
  - Prescribe bisphosphonate (use with caution in premenopausal women)
  - Consider calcitonin or rPHT as second-line agent if patient has contraindication to or does not tolerate bisphosphonate therapy
- If BMD is normal, follow up and repeat BMD measurement either annually or biannually

From: Recommendations for the prevention and treatment of glucocorticoid-induced osteoporosis: 2001 update. American College of Rheumatology Ad Hoc Committee on Glucocorticoid-Induced Osteoporosis. *Arthritis Rheum* 2001; **44**:1496–1503.

Corticosteroids and adrenal insufficiency

Administration of glucocorticoids suppresses the endogenous HPA axis function and may produce secondary adrenal deficiency.

- May occur with as little as 5 days of prednisone treatment at 20–30 mg/day
- May take up to 12 months for HPA axis function to return to normal
- Consider "stress-dose steroids" (hydrocortisone 50–100 mg IV q6–8 hours) to prevent acute adrenal insufficiency during general anesthesia, surgery, trauma, or an acute infectious disease

Corticosteroids and increased risk of infection

Prednisone dosages >20 mg/day lead to a progressive increase in infection risk after 14 days of treatment.

- Facultative intracellular microbes such as mycobacteria, *Pneumocystis (carinii) jiroveci*, and fungi
- Consider pneumocystis prophylaxis

High-dose corticosteroids can mask the symptoms of infectious diseases such as abscesses and bowel perforation.

Other side effects

These include hypertension, negative balance of calcium and secondary hyperparathyroidism, negative balance of nitrogen, truncal obesity, impaired wound healing, thinning of skin and hair, acne, suppression of growth in children, hyperglycemia, hyperlipoproteinemia and atherosclerosis, sodium retention, hypokalemia, neutrophilia, monocytopenia, lymphopenia, suppression of delayed-type hypersensitivity reactions, myopathy, avascular necrosis, alterations in mood, psychosis, insomnia, increased appetite, posterior subcapsular cataracts, metabolic alkalosis, peptic ulcer disease, "silent" intestinal perforation, increased intraocular pressure and glaucoma, pseudotumor cerebri, congestive heart failure, hirsutism, hepatomegaly, and pancreatitis.

Sudden death with rapid administration of high-dose, pulse therapy has been reported. Consider telemetry.

Pregnancy and lactation

- Pregnancy category C (all steroids)
- Breast-feeding is probably safe.
  - Unknown for fludrocortisone, betamethasone, triamcinolone

Monitoring

- Bone density examination yearly
- Cardiovascular risk factor assessment, including assessment for and treatment of hypercholesterolemia
- Proximal muscle strength
- Blood pressure
- Electrolyte panel
- Mental status
- Ophthalmic exam with prolonged therapy
- HPA axis suppression tests during prolonged therapy
- Weight

Patient recommendations and instructions

- Take with food
- Take in the morning, unless directed differently
- Do not stop abruptly: dosage must be tapered or reduced gradually
- Carry a steroid treatment card or wear a treatment bracelet

Azathioprine

Mechanism of action
- Inhibits T-lymphocytes
- Suppresses delayed hypersensitivity and cellular toxicity
- Antagonizes purine metabolism, resulting in inhibition of mitosis and synthesis of DNA, RNA, and proteins and interferes with cellular metabolism

Pulmonary uses
- Interstitial lung disease secondary to connective tissue diseases
  - Rheumatoid arthritis
  - Polymyositis/dermatomyositis
  - Scleroderma
  - Sjögren's syndrome
  - Lupus pneumonitis
- Idiopathic interstitial lung diseases
  - Idiopathic pulmonary fibrosis (IPF)
  - Cryptogenic organizing pneumonia (COP)
- Sarcoidosis
- Interstitial lung disease secondary to inflammatory bowel disease
- ANCA-associated vasculitis (microscopic polyangiitis, Wegener's granulomatosis)
  - Maintenance therapy
- Churg–Strauss vasculitis
- Idiopathic pulmonary hemosiderosis

Commonly prescribed doses
- Titrate up to 2–3 mg/kg/day orally

Dose adjustments
- Renal impairment
  - Creatinine clearance 10–50 mL/min: 75% of normal dose
  - Creatinine clearance <10 mL/min: 50% of normal dose
  - Dialysis: a maintenance dose of 0.25 mg/kg should be given following hemodialysis
- Hepatic impairment: caution advised

Contraindications
- History of treatment with alkylating agents may increase risk of neoplasia
- Hypersensitivity to azathioprine
- Pregnancy

Drug–drug interactions
- Allopurinol: decrease dose of azathioprine and allopurinol by 50%–75%
- Cyclophosphamide
- Neuromuscular blockers

Black box warning
- Chronic immunosuppression with azathioprine may increase neoplasia risk
- Mutagenic potential to both men and women
- Possible hematologic toxicity

Pulmonary side effects
- Subacute cellular interstitial pneumonitis
- Alveolar hemorrhage
- Bronchospasm ± laryngeal edema and anaphylactic shock
- Vasculitis

Other side effects
- **Serious**: leukopenia, thrombocytopenia, anemia, myelosuppression, immunosuppression, infection, gastrointestinal hypersensitivity reaction, pancreatitis, hepatotoxicity, hepatic veno-occlusive disease, lymphoma, malignancy
- **Common**: leukopenia, thrombocytopenia, anemia, infection, nausea, vomiting, anorexia, diarrhea, elevated liver transaminases, malaise, myalgia, fever, rash, malignancy

Pregnancy and lactation
- Pregnancy category D
- Avoid breast-feeding

Monitoring
- Consider thiopurine methyltransferase (TPMT) genotyping and phenotyping before initiation of therapy
  - Exercise caution and use lower doses in patients heterozygous for TPMT deficiency
  - Avoid in patients homozygous for TPMT deficiency
- Consider pregnancy test <1 week prior to beginning therapy in women of childbearing potential
- Creatinine, CBC, and liver tests at baseline
- CBC weekly × 4 weeks, then biweekly × 4, then monthly
- Liver function biweekly × 2, then monthly

Patient recommendations and instructions
- Take with food
- Use an effective form of birth control throughout treatment course and for at least 2 months after it is stopped

Hydroxychloroquine

Mechanism of action
- Antimalarial
- Unknown immunosuppressant mechanism

Pulmonary uses
- Sarcoidosis
- Idiopathic pulmonary hemosiderosis
- Rheumatoid arthritis
- Systemic lupus erythematosus (SLE)

Commonly prescribed doses
- Hydroxychloroquine: 200–400 mg once daily (or in divided dose twice daily)

Dose adjustments
- Renal impairment: not defined
- Hepatic impairment: caution advised

Contraindications
- Hypersensitivity to drug
- Porphyria
- Retinal and visual field changes

Drug–drug interactions
- Methotrexate: reduced plasma concentrations when administered with hydroxychloroquine
- Digoxin: increased plasma digoxin level
- Beta-blockers: increased bioavailability by inhibiting the cytochrome p450 system

Pulmonary side effects
There are none.

Other side effects
- **Serious:** torsades de pointes, agranulocytosis, thrombocytopenia, aplastic anemia, seizures, exfoliative dermatitis, visual changes, ototoxicity
- **Common:** dizziness, ataxia, headache, abdominal pain, nausea and vomiting, diarrhea, pruritus, weight loss, hair bleaching

Pregnancy and lactation
- Pregnancy category C
- Breast-feeding is probably safe.

Monitoring
- Eye examination at baseline and every 6–12 months
- Liver function testing at baseline and every 6 months
- CBC at baseline and every 6 months

Patient recommendations and instructions
- Take with food or milk

Methotrexate

Mechanism of action
- Reversible inhibition of dihydrofolate reductase resulting in interference with DNA synthesis and repair and cellular replication

Pulmonary uses
- Sarcoidosis
- Pulmonary vasculitis
- Steroid-resistant asthma
- Interstitial lung disease secondary to connective tissue diseases
  - Rheumatoid arthritis
  - Polymyositis/dermatomyositis

Commonly prescribed doses
- 7.5–25 mg orally or subcutaneous weekly
- Administer with folic acid 1–5 mg daily

Dose adjustments
- Renal dosing
  - Creatinine clearance 60–80 mL/hr: decrease dose by 25%
  - Creatinine clearance 50–60 mL/hr: decrease dose by 33%
  - Creatinine clearance 10–50 mL/hr: decrease dose by 50%–70%
  - Creatinine clearance <10 mL/hr: avoid use
  - Hemodialysis: give 50% of dose
- Liver failure: avoid use

Contraindications
- Pregnancy
- Breast-feeding
- Known hypersensitivity to methotrexate
- Alcoholism, alcoholic liver disease, or other chronic liver disease
- Preexisting blood dyscrasias or laboratory evidence of immunodeficiency syndromes

Drug–drug interactions
- Trimethoprim: increased risk of toxicities
- Hydroxychloroquine, chloroquine: decreased levels of methotrexate

Black box warning
- Should be used only by physicians experienced with antimetabolite therapy
- Methotrexate has been reported to cause fetal death and/or congenital abnormalities.
- Methotrexate elimination is reduced in patients with impaired renal function, ascites, or pleural effusion. Such patients require careful monitoring for toxicity.
- Unexpectedly severe bone marrow suppression, aplastic anemia, and gastrointestinal toxicity have been reported with concomitant administration of methotrexate along with some nonsteroidal anti-inflammatory drugs.

- Methotrexate can cause hepatotoxicity, fibrosis, and cirrhosis, but generally only after prolonged use.
- Methotrexate-induced lung disease, including acute or chronic interstitial pneumonitis, may occur at any time during therapy and has been reported at oral doses as low as 7.5 mg/week.
- Diarrhea and ulcerative stomatitis require interruption of therapy. Otherwise, hemorrhagic enteritis and death from intestinal perforation may occur.
- Malignant lymphomas, which may regress following withdrawal of methotrexate, may occur in patients receiving low-dose methotrexate.
- Methotrexate may induce "tumor lysis syndrome" in patients with rapidly growing tumors.
- Severe, occasionally fatal skin reactions have been reported following single or multiple doses of methotrexate.
- Potentially fatal opportunistic infections, especially *Pneumocystis jiroveci*
  - Consider pneumocystis prophylaxis

Pulmonary side effects
- Acute hypersensitivity pneumonitis and respiratory failure
- Subacute cellular interstitial pneumonitis
- Pulmonary infiltrates and eosinophilia
- Pulmonary fibrosis
- Diffuse alveolar damage
- Acute pulmonary edema ± ARDS
- Alveolar hemorrhage
- Bronchospasm ± laryngeal edema and anaphylactic shock
- Pleural effusion
- Chest pain
- Opportunistic infections
  - Consider pneumocystis prophylaxis

Other side effects
- **Serious**: ulcerative stomatitis, diarrhea, thrombocytopenia, leucopenia, anemia, aplastic anemia, agranulocytosis, lymphoproliferative disorders, hepatotoxcity, cirrhosis, hepatic fibrosis, nephrotoxicity, immunosuppression, opportunistic infection, leukoencepthalopathy, stroke-like illness, seizures, neurotoxicity, arachnoiditis, subacute myelopathy, Stevens–Johnson syndrome, exfoliative dermatitis, erythema multiforme, toxic epidermal necrolysis, radiation recall reactions, anaphylaxis
- **Common**: liver function elevation, nausea and vomiting, stomatitis, malaise, fatigue, abdominal discomfort, chills, fever, dizziness, diarrhea, anemia, thrombocytopenia, leukopenia, rash, pruritus, alopecia, photosensitivity

Pregnancy and lactation
- Pregnancy category X
- Breast-feeding is unsafe.

Monitoring

Baseline evaluation

- Consider pregnancy test <1 week prior to beginning therapy in women of childbearing potential
- Complete blood count
- Hepatitis B surface antigen, hepatitis C antibody
- Liver function tests
- With a history of excessive alcohol consumption, persistent elevation of transaminases, or evidence of hepatitis B or C infection consider pretreatment liver biopsy
- Monitor creatinine at 3- to 6-month intervals
- Monitor CBC, AST, ALT, and albumin at 4- to 8-week intervals

During therapy, in the setting of cytopenia or elevation of AST and/or ALT twice the upper limit of normal

- Hold methotrexate, resume at lower dose once laboratory abnormality resolves

During therapy, perform liver biopsy before continuing treatment if

- 5 of 9 or 6 of 12 AST determinations in a 1-year time frame are abnormal
- Albumin decreases below normal range

Patient recommendations and instructions

- Females must use a reliable form of contraception before, during, and after treatment for at least two menstrual periods post-therapy.
- Maintain adequate hydration.
- Take all tablets on the same day at the same time, unless directed differently by your doctor.
- Alcohol significantly increases the risk for liver damage while taking methotrexate, so alcohol intake should be eliminated or minimized to no more than two drinks per month.

Further reading

Kremer JM, Alarcón GS, Lightfoot RH Jr, et al. (1994). Methotrexate for rheumatoid arthritis. Suggested guidelines for monitoring liver toxicity. American College of Rheumatology. *Arthritis Rheum* 37:316–328.

Cyclophosphamide

Mechanism of action
- Alkylating agent of the nitrogen mustard type; alkylates and cross-links DNA

Pulmonary uses
- Vasculitis
  - ANCA-associated vasculitis (microscopic polyangiitis, Wegener's granulomatosis)
  - Behçet disease
  - Churg–Strauss syndrome
- Interstitial lung disease secondary to connective tissue disease
  - Systemic sclerosis (scleroderma)
  - Polymyositis/dermatomyositis
  - Rheumatoid arthritis
  - Sjögren's syndrome
  - Mixed connective tissue disease
- Alveolar hemorrhage secondary to systemic lupus erythematosus
- Idiopathic interstitial lung disease
  - Idiopathic pulmonary fibrosis (IPF)
  - Nonspecific interstitial pneumonia (NSIP)
  - Desquamative interstitial pneumonia (DIP)
  - Lymphocytic interstitial pneumonia (LIP)
  - Cryptogenic organizing pneumonia (COP)
- Sarcoidosis
- Castleman disease

Commonly prescribed doses
- Titrate up to 1.5–2.0 mg/kg orally, once daily
- 750 mg/m^2 intravenously, monthly
  - Intravenous therapy may have fewer adverse effects
  - Prehydrate and consider giving MESNA, which chelates with the urotoxic cyclophosphamide metabolite, acrolein

Dose adjustments
- Renal impairment
  - Creatinine clearance <10 mL/hr: decrease dose by 25%
  - Hemodialysis: give 50% usual dose
- Hepatic impairment: avoid use
- Avoid in leukopenia

Contraindications
- Hypersensitivity to cyclophosphamide products
- Severely depressed bone marrow function

Drug–drug interactions
- Co-administration of cimetidine with cyclophosphamide results in increased exposure to alkylating metabolites and increased bone marrow toxicity.
- Allopurinol increases the half-life of cyclophosphamide and the frequency of leukopenia.

Pulmonary side effects
- Organizing pneumonia ± bronchiolitis obliterans
- Pulmonary fibrosis
- Diffuse alveolar damage
- Acute pulmonary edema
- Bronchospasm ± laryngeal edema and anaphylactic shock
- Pleural effusion
- Opportunistic infections
  - Consider *pneumocystis* prophylaxis

Other side effects
- **Serious**: secondary malignancy (urinary bladder, myeloproliferative, lymphoproliferative), sterility, hemorrhagic cystitis, urinary bladder fibrosis, congestive heart failure, hemorrhagic myocarditis, immunosuppression, infection, anaphylaxis, Stevens–Johnson syndrome, toxic epidermal necrolysis, anemia, leukopenia, thrombocytopenia, SIADH
- **Common**: alopecia, sterility, amenorrhea, nausea, vomiting, anorexia, diarrhea, stomatitis, hemorrhagic cystitis, anemia, leukopenia, thrombocytopenia, rash, headache

Pregnancy and lactation
- Pregnancy category D
- Breast-feeding is unsafe.

Monitoring
- Consider pregnancy test <1 week prior to beginning therapy in women of childbearing potential
- Creatinine, CBC, and liver tests at baseline
- CBC with differential every 2 weeks until blood counts have been stable for 6–8 weeks, then every 4 weeks
- Urinalysis monthly while on therapy; yearly once therapy has been discontinued
- Urine cytologic evaluation: yearly

Patient recommendations and instructions
- Consider banking sperm or ova before treatment.
- Use effective birth control to prevent pregnancy (both men and women) before, during, and 6 months after therapy.
- Take medication with breakfast.
- Drink lots of fluids throughout the day.
- Empty the bladder frequently and before bedtime.

Mycophenolate mofetil

Mechanism of action
- Suppresses antibody formation by B-lymphocytes
- Inhibits proliferative responses of T- and B- lymphocytes
- Inhibits recruitment of leukocytes into sites of inflammation

Pulmonary uses
- Interstitial lung disease secondary to connective tissue disease
  - Systemic sclerosis (scleroderma)
- ANCA-associated vasculitis
- Alveolar hemorrhage secondary to systemic lupus erythematosus
- Interstitial lung disease secondary to inflammatory bowel disease

Commonly prescribed doses
- Titrate up to 1–1.5 g twice daily

Dose adjustments
- Renal impairment
  - Creatinine clearance <25 mL/min/1.73 m^2: max 1 g twice daily
- Hepatic impairment: no adjustment

Contraindications
- Hypersensitivity to mycophenolate mofetil/mycophenolic acid
- Hypersensitivity to polysorbate 80 (IV formulation)

Drug–drug interactions
- Cycloporine: increases mycophenolate mofetil concentrations
- Diflunisal: increases mycophenolate mofetil concentrations
- Mefenamic acid and its congeners: increases mycophenolate mofetil concentrations
- Iron: decreases area under the curve of mycophenolate mofetil by 90%

Black box warning
- Increased susceptibility to infection
- Possible development of lymphoma

Pulmonary side effects
- Pulmonary fibrosis
- Acute permeability edema with or without ARDS
- Cough

Other side effects
- **Serious**: thrombocytopenia, leukopenia, neutropenia, immunosuppression, susceptibility to infection, sepsis, lymphoma, lymphoproliferative disorders, malignancy, gastrointestinal bleeding, gastrointestinal perforation, gastrointestinal ulceration
- **Common**: hypertension, infection, diarrhea, peripheral edema, anemia, abdominal pain, constipation, leukopenia, fever, headache, nausea and vomiting, dyspepsia, hypotension (rapid IV), dyspnea, cough, hypercholesterolemia, hypokalemia, tremor, acne, insomnia

Pregnancy/lactation
- Pregnancy category C
- Avoid breast-feeding

Monitoring
- Consider pregnancy test <1 week prior to beginning therapy in women of childbearing potential
- Creatinine, CBC, and liver tests at baseline
- CBC weekly × 1 month, then biweekly × 2 month, then monthly
- Liver tests monthly

Patient recommendations and instructions
- If the woman is of childbearing potential she should use **two** reliable forms of contraception before, during, and 6 weeks after discontinuation of therapy.
- Take with food

Infliximab

Mechanism of action
- Chimeric human–murine immunoglobulin monoclonal antibody that binds specifically to TNF-α, a proinflammatory cytokine

Pulmonary uses
- Sarcoidosis
- Steroid-refractory asthma
- Interstitial lung disease
  - Rheumatoid arthritis
  - Crohn's disease
- Vasculitis

Commonly prescribed doses
- 3–10 mg/kg intravenously at weeks 0, 2, and 6, then every 4–8 weeks

Dose adjustments
- Renal impairment: none
- Hepatic impairment: none

Contraindications
- Heart failure, moderate to severe
- Hypersensitivity to infliximab

Drug–drug interactions
- Abatacept
- Anakinra

Black box warning
- Increased risk of infections, including progression to serious infections leading to hospitalization or death. These infections have included bacterial sepsis, tuberculosis, and invasive fungal and other opportunistic infections.
- Tuberculosis (frequently disseminated or extrapulmonary at clinical presentation) has been observed in patients receiving infliximab
  - Test for latent tuberculosis
- Rare post-marketing cases of hepatosplenic T-cell lymphoma have been reported in adolescent and young adult patients.

Pulmonary side effects
- Acute hypersensitivity pneumonitis and respiratory failure
- Subacute cellular interstitial pneumonitis
- Pulmonary infiltrates and eosinophilia
- Pulmonary fibrosis
- Bronchospasm ± laryngeal edema and anaphylactic shock
- Eosinophilic pleural effusion
- Pleural or pericardial thickening or effusion, and positive antinuclear or antihistone antibodies (drug-induced lupus)
- Vasculitis
- Opportunistic infections

Other side effects

- **Serious**: acute coronary syndrome, congestive heart failure, leukopenia, neutropenia, pancytopenia, thrombocytopenia, hepatotoxicity, drug-induced lupus, immune hypersensitivity reaction, hepatosplenic T-cell lymphoma, demyelinating disease of the central nervous system, tuberculosis, histoplasmosis, mycosis, sepsis, hepatitis B reactivation, serum sickness, anaphylaxis, rash, malignancy, skin carcinoma, optic neuritis, seizures, multiple sclerosis, vasculitis
- **Common**: fever, chills, myalgias, back pain, arthralgia, dizziness, nausea, urticaria, pruritus, rash, URI, elevated liver transaminases, dyspnea, facial or hand edema, hypotension, hypertension, chest pain, abdominal pain, fatigue, headache

Pregnancy and lactation

- Pregnancy category B
- Breast-feeding: safety is unknown

Monitoring

- Check PPD at baseline
- Signs and symptoms of active tuberculosis infection
- Vital signs during infusion
- Cardiac monitoring in patients with congestive heart failure
- CBC, blood chemistry, liver function tests at baseline and every 3–6 months

Rituximab

Mechanism of action

Rituximab binds to the antigen CD20, located on pre-B and mature B-lymphocytes, resulting in mediation of B-cell lysis.

Pulmonary uses

- ANCA-associated vasculitis (Wegener's granulomatosis, microscopic polyangiitis)
- Sjögren's syndrome
- Rheumatoid arthritis
- Systemic lupus erythematosis
- Lymphocytic interstitial pneumonia
- Pulmonary lymphoma
- Lymphomatoid granulomatosis
- Post-transplant lymphoproliferative disorder

Commonly prescribed doses

- 1000 mg intravenously followed by a second 1000 mg IV dose 2 weeks later
- 375 mg/m^2 intravenously once weekly for 4 doses

Dose adjustments

- **Non-IgE-mediated hypersensitivity reaction**: slow or stop infusion; may resume at 50% reduction in infusion rate when symptoms have resolved
- **Renal impairment**: not defined
- **Hepatic impairment**: not defined

Drug–drug interactions

Concomitant use of biologic agents and other immunosuppressant agents other than methotrexate may place patients at risk of severe infection.

Black box warnings

- Fatal infusion reactions: deaths within 24 hours have been reported
- Severe mucocutaneous reactions
- Progressive multifocal leukoencephalopathy

Pulmonary side effects

- Acute hypersensitivity pneumonitis and respiratory failure
- Subacute cellular interstitial pneumonitis
- Desquamative interstitial pneumonia
- Pulmonary fibrosis
- Alveolar hemorrhage
- Bronchospasm

Other side effects

- **Serious**: infusion reactions, hypotension, angioedema, myocardial infarction, ventricular arrhythmia, cardiogenic shock, anaphylaxis, hypersensitivity reaction, tumor lysis syndrome, renal failure, Steven's–Johnson syndrome, toxic epidermal necrolysis, pemphigus, lichenoid dermatitis, vesiculobullous rash, GI obstruction and perforation, hepatitis B reactivation, fulminant hepatitis, lymphopenia, neutropenia, anemia, thrombocytopenia, sepsis, severe viral infection, progressive multifocal leukoencephalopathy
- **Common**: infusion reaction, fever and chills, nausea, asthenia, headache, angioedema, leukopenia, pruritus, rash, hypotension, rhinitis, bronchospasm, thrombocytopenia, urticaria, vomiting, myalgia and arthralgia, dizziness, abdominal pain, throat pain, hypertension, infection, hyperglycemia

Pregnancy and lactation

- Pregnancy category C
- Avoid breast-feeding

Monitoring

- Hepatitis B surface antigen at baseline if high risk
- Consider pregnancy test <1 week prior to beginning therapy in women of childbearing potential
- CBC before infusion
- Telemetry during infusion

Cyclosporine

Mechanism of action
- Inhibits the activation of T cells
- Inhibits secretion of IL-2
- Calcineurin inhibitor

Pulmonary uses
- Asthma
- Interstitial lung disease secondary to polymyositis/dermatomyositis

Commonly prescribed doses
- The modified and non-modified forms of cyclosporine are not interchangeable.
- Non-modified: titrate up to 2–10 mg/kg/day orally
- Modified: titrate up to 2.5–10 mg/kg/day orally

Dose adjustments
- Renal impairment
  - If serum creatinine rises >30% above baseline on at least 2 occasions, 1 week apart, daily dose should be reduced in decrements of 0.5–0.75 mg/kg/day
  - If creatinine returns to baseline, cyclosporine therapy can continue
  - If serum creatinine remains >30% above baseline, discontinue cyclosporine for 1 month and resume cyclosporine therapy if serum creatinine returns to ≤15% above baseline value.
- **Hepatic impairment**: caution advised
- **Cystic fibrosis** patients may require twice the dose of cyclosporine given to other patients.

Contraindications
- Hypersensitivity to drug
- Hypersensitivity to castor oil derivatives

Drug–drug interactions
- Diltiazem
- Rifampin
- Ketoconazole
- Mycophenolate mofetil concentrations are increased by cyclosporine.
- *Numerous other drug–drug interactions* are associated with the cytochrome p450 system.

Black box warnings
- Should only be used by physicians experienced in immunosuppressive therapy
- Doses should be kept low when used with other immunosuppressants because of the increased risk of infection and lymphoma.
- Modified and non-modified forms of cyclosporine are not bioequivalent.
- Monitor drug levels regularly.

Pulmonary side effects

- Subacute cellular interstitial pneumonitis
- Lipoid pneumonia
- Acute pulmonary edema
- Acute permeability edema ± ARDS
- Alveolar hemorrhage
- Pulmonary hypertension

Other side effects

- **Serious**: hypertension, infection susceptibility, hyperkalemia, nephrotoxicity, hepatotoxicity, glomerular capillary thrombosis, diabetes mellitus, leukopenia, thrombocytopenia, hemolytic anemia, malignancy, seizures, encephalopathy, neurotoxicity, intracranial hypertension, optic disc edema, allergic reactions or anaphylaxis, depression, myocardial infarction, pancreatitis, gastrointestinal hemorrhage
- **Common**: elevated BUN and creatinine, hypertension, hirsutism, infection, tremor, gum hyperplasia, acne, diarrhea, paresthesias, nausea and vomiting, leg cramps, headache, liver dysfunction, abdominal pain, sinusitis, hypomagnesemia, hyperglycemia, hyperkalemia, hyperuricemia and gout, dyslipidemia

Pregnancy and lactation

- Pregnancy category C
- Avoid breast-feeding

Monitoring

- Consider pregnancy test <1 week prior to beginning therapy in women of childbearing potential
- Baseline CBC, BUN, creatinine, and liver tests
- BUN, creatinine every 2 weeks until target dose is reached, and continued for 3 months and then monthly
- Liver function tests frequently
- Serum cyclosporine levels
- Blood pressure at baseline and every 2 weeks until target dose is reached, then continued for 3 months and then monthly

Patient recommendations and instructions

- Avoid sun exposure to decrease risk of skin malignancies.
- Do not eat grapefruit or drink grapefruit juice while taking this drug.
- Consult with a health-care professional prior to new drug use, including over-the-counter and herbal drugs.
- Brush and floss your teeth regularly.

Sirolimus

Mechanism of action
- Inhibition of IL-2-, IL-4-, and IL-15-stimulated T-lymphocyte activation and proliferation
- Inhibitor of ribosomal protein S6 kinase 1, which leads to abnormal cell proliferation
- Inhibitor of antibody production through formation of an immunosuppressive complex with FK binding protein-12

Pulmonary uses
- Lymphangioleiomyomatosis (LAM) (under study)

Commonly prescribed doses
- Loading: 6–15 mg orally × 1
- Maintenance: 2–5 mg daily

Dosage adjustments
- **Renal impairment**: no adjustment, caution advised
- **Hepatic impairment**
  - Decrease maintenance dose by 33%
  - It is not necessary to reduce the loading dose
- **<40 kg**
  - Adjust dose to 1 mg/m^2/day
  - The loading dose should be 3 mg/m^2

Contraindications
Hypersensitivity to sirolimus

Drug–drug interactions
- Carbamazepime
- Cyclosporine
- Diltiazem
- Phenobarbital
- Phenytoin
- Rifabutin
- Rifampin
- Tacrolimus
- Verapamil
- Voriconazole and other azoles

Pulmonary side effects
- Deep venous thrombosis with pulmonary embolism in 3%–20%
- Subacute cellular interstitial pneumonitis
- Desquamative interstitial pneumonia
- Diffuse alveolar damage
- Granulomatous interstitial lung disease
- Alveolar hemorrhage
- Consider *pneumocystis* prophylaxis

Other side effects

- **Serious**: anaphylaxis, angioedema, exfoliative dermatitis, vasculitis, immunosuppression, infection, lymphoma, malignancy, lymphocele, thrombocytopenia, hemolytic uremic syndrome, leukopenia, hypokalemia, thrombotic microangiopathy, interstitial lung disease
- **Common**: peripheral edema, hypertension, hypercholesterolemia, hypertriglyceridemia, asthenia, elevated BUN and creatinine, proteinuria, diarrhea, nausea, vomiting, abdominal pain, constipation, dyspepsia, headache, tremor, arthralgia, fever, pain, anemia, hypophosphatemia, hypokalemia, leukopenia, thrombocytopenia, acne, rash, insomnia, weight gain

Pregnancy and lactation

- Pregnancy category C
- Avoid breast-feeding

Monitoring

- Consider pregnancy test <1 week prior to beginning therapy in women of childbearing potential
- Renal function
- CBC with differential
- Lipid panel
- Pulmonary function
- Blood pressure
- Electrolytes
- Whole-blood sirolimus levels in patients likely to have altered drug metabolism

Patient recommendations and instructions

- Take with or without food consistently
- Solution: take with 2 ounces of water or orange juice ONLY, stir vigorously, and drink immediately after mixing; refill container with 4 ounces of orange juice or water, stir vigorously, and drink at once
- Avoid pregnancy. A woman of childbearing potential should use effective contraception before, during, and 12 weeks after treatment has been discontinued.

Long-term oxygen therapy

Effects of long-term oxygen therapy

Two landmark trials of long-term oxygen therapy (LTOT) were published in the 1980s: the British Medical Research Council (MRC) Working Party trial, and the North American Nocturnal Oxygen Therapy Trial (NOTT).

The *MRC trial* compared a group of COPD patients receiving oxygen for 15 hours per day with a control group receiving no oxygen. Eighty-seven patients were enrolled with a mean age of 58 years, FEV_1 of 0.7 L, and pulmonary artery pressure of 34 mmHg. Mean arterial gas pressures at entry were PaO_2 of 51 mmHg and $PaCO_2$ of 55 mmHg. Over 5 years, there was an improvement in mortality in the group receiving oxygen therapy, although mortality for male patients did not improve until 500 days after commencement of treatment.

The *NOTT trial* compared continuous daily oxygen (average 17.7 hours a day) with 12-hour overnight oxygen. Two hundred and three COPD patients were enrolled with a mean age of 66 years, FEV_1 of 0.7 L, and pulmonary artery pressure of 33 mmHg. Mean arterial gas pressures at entry were PaO_2 of 51 mmHg and $PaCO_2$ of 43.5 mmHg. There was significant improvement in mortality for the group with continuous oxygen treatment at 24 months, but not at 12 months.

Supplemental oxygen can also reduce cardiac work and improve pulmonary hemodynamics. In the NOTT study, continuous oxygen therapy significantly improved pulmonary vascular resistance, pulmonary artery pressure, and stroke volume index. Other studies have confirmed improvement in pulmonary artery pressure after supplemental oxygen therapy. Attempts to correlate pulmonary hemodynamic responses to oxygen with long-term survival have been unsuccessful; the reason for improved survival with LTOT remains unclear.

In many COPD patients, exercise is limited by ventilatory instead of circulatory factors. Supplemental oxygen increases walking distance and improves exercise endurance in COPD patients. In patients with hypoxemia or oxygen desaturation with exercise, supplemental oxygen increases oxygen delivery and utilization during exercise. Supplemental oxygen also reduces ventilatory muscle fatigue and sensation of dyspnea.

In addition to patients with COPD, individuals with interstitial lung disease, neuromuscular or skeletal disorders, cystic fibrosis, pulmonary hypertension, or congestive heart failure may benefit from LTOT. However, survival benefit has only been demonstrated in patients with COPD. LTOT can also be used to relieve dyspnea in patients with lung malignancy or in the terminally ill.

Benefits of LTOT

- Decreased work of breathing via reduction in minute ventilation and respiratory rate
- Improved neuropsychological performance (i.e., alertness, motor speed, hand grip)
- Improved sleep quality via reduction in hypoxia-associated brain arousals during sleep
- Reduction in secondary polycythemia

- Reduced cardiac arrhythmias and possible reduced risk of nocturnal sudden death
- Reduced sympathetic outflow with increased sodium and water excretion, leading to improved renal function

Indications for LTOT

- Hypoxemia at rest: PaO_2 <56 mmHg or SaO_2 <89%
- Cor pulmonale: PaO_2 56–59 mmHg or SaO_2 89% in patients with dependent edema suggesting congestive heart failure, P pulmonale on ECG defined as P wave >2.5 mm in lead II, or polycythemia with Hct >55%
- Nocturnal hypoxemia: PaO_2 <56 mmHg or SaO_2 <89% with associated complications (e.g., pulmonary hypertension, daytime somnolence, cardiac arrhythmias)
- Sleep apnea with nocturnal desaturation: oxygen desaturation not corrected by CPAP or bilevel positive airway pressure
- Oxygen desaturation with exercise: PaO_2 <56 mmHg or SaO_2 <89% with low level of exertion

Adverse effects of LTOT

Adverse effects of oxygen therapy are rare, and progressive carbon dioxide retention is unlikely in stable patients. When carbon dioxide retention does occur, ventilation–perfusion mismatch is the most likely cause.

Although oxygen is not explosive, it markedly enhances combustion. Physicians must therefore caution their patients to not permit smoking, open flames, or spark-producing devices in close proximity to oxygen use.

Nasal cannula use may lead to nasal drying, irritation, or bleeding. These symptoms often respond to humidification or topical measures.

Oxygen supply systems

Three types of stationary sources exist for home supplemental oxygen. Portable oxygen systems are available for ambulatory patients. Unless physicians prescribe a specific oxygen system, vendors will typically provide the least expensive system.

Oxygen concentrators

These are electrically powered and use molecular sieve beds to filter and concentrate oxygen molecules from ambient air. They are the most cost-effective supply system. Flow rates of 3–6 L/min can be obtained with stationary units. However, FiO_2 delivered decreases as flow increases.

Patients should have a compressed gas cylinder for backup in case of power or concentrator failure. Portable concentrators that weigh less than 10 pounds and last up to 8 hours are also available. Flow rates of 1 L/min can be obtained with portable units, but when combined with an oxygen-conserving system, flow equivalence up to 6 L/min can be achieved.

Compressed gas cylinders

These are useful when high flow rates are needed or when the electrical source is unreliable. Stationary cylinders can provide oxygen for nearly 2.5 days at a flow of 2 L/min, and flows up to 15 L/min can be attained. Portable cylinders are also available. However, compressed gas cylinders are bulky and require frequent refills.

Liquid oxygen reservoirs

These last 2–4 weeks at 2 L/min and can be used to refill portable units. Portable liquid oxygen is the only practical ambulatory system for patients who have high continuous liter flow requirements. A container of liquid oxygen will last four times longer than a container of compressed gas of comparable weight. Although more portable and easier to fill, liquid oxygen is more expensive than compressed gas and evaporates when not in use.

Oxygen delivery devices

- Standard *nasal cannulae* are simple and inexpensive. At a flow rate of 6 L/min, maximum delivered FiO_2 is about 0.45.
- A *demand device* detects the initiation of ventilation and delivers a pulse of oxygen during early inspiration. There is no oxygen flow during expiration, reducing oxygen waste. Oxygen-saving estimates range from 50% to 86%.
- A *conserving device* traps an initial portion of expired gas, which comes from the anatomic dead space and contains almost pure oxygen. The conserver also receives continuous oxygen from a supply system, resulting in higher FiO_2 delivery. Increased FiO_2 allows a reduction in total flow.
- A *transtracheal oxygen catheter* delivers oxygen directly through a catheter inserted into the cervical trachea. It has been shown to improve patient adherence and exercise tolerance, and reduce work of breathing and number of hospitalizations. It is expensive, requires placement by an experienced physician, and is associated with risk of local infection and tracheal obstruction from mucus plugs. Patient acceptance can also be a challenge.

Further reading

Noctorunal Oxygen Therapy Trial Group (1980). Continuous or nocturnal oxygen therapy in hypoxemic chronic obstructive lung disease—a clinical trial. *Ann Intern Med* **93**:391–398.

Report of the Medical Research Council Working Party. Long-term domiciliary oxygen therapy in chronic hypoxic cor pulmonale complicating chronic bronchitis and emphysema. *Lancet* 1981; **1**(8222):681–686.

Pulmonary rehabilitation

Definition

Pulmonary rehabilitation is an evidence-based, multidisciplinary, comprehensive intervention for patients with chronic respiratory diseases who are symptomatic and often have decreased daily life activities. Integrated into the individualized treatment of the patient, pulmonary rehabilitation is designed to reduce symptoms, optimize functional status, increase participation of the patient in their care, and reduce health-care costs by stabilizing or reversing manifestations of the disease. It is most commonly employed in patients with COPD.

Aims and evidence

Pulmonary rehabilitation is individually tailored for each patient. It is not available in every center, although it is probably the most cost-effective intervention for COPD.

Aims of rehabilitation
- To reduce functional disability and handicap in people with chronic lung disease
- To improve quality of life and restore independence
- To diminish the health-care burden of disease

Summary of evidence
Numerous randomized clinical trials and meta-analyses evaluating a variety of different style programs have confirmed the benefits of rehabilitation (see Box 56.1), with improvements in functional capacity.
- Patients with COPD who have completed rehabilitation courses perform better than controls on walking tests and have less subjective dyspnea.
- Several uncontrolled studies suggest that pulmonary rehabilitation decreases total hospital stay and recurrent hospitalization rates in patients with COPD.
- Rehabilitation programs that include lower-extremity training are better, when compared to controls, than those using just respiratory muscle training.
- Short-term programs achieve similar overall outcome benefits across the spectrum of patient disabilities. A minimum program length of 6 weeks is recommended.
- Decline in exercise tolerance and health status tends to occur between 6 and 12 months after completion of a course. Whether sustained improvement occurs with ongoing rehabilitation sessions has yet to be evaluated.
- There is no clear mortality benefit from pulmonary rehabilitation.

Patient selection

Candidates

- Anyone with chronic lung disease causing functional impairment
- The majority of candidates will have COPD, but may have cystic fibrosis, asthma, pulmonary fibrosis, or bronchiectasis.
- Any stage of a lung disease, when symptoms are affecting a patient's activity. Ideally, optimum medical treatment should already be in place.
- Well-motivated patients seem to benefit most.
- Patients with poor lower-limb mobility may benefit from upper-limb exercise.
- Oxygen therapy is not a contraindication to rehabilitation.
- Stable ischemic heart disease is not a contraindication to rehabilitation.

Candidates in whom rehabilitation may not be indicated

- Those with unstable ischemic heart disease, severe valvular heart disease, cognitive impairment, difficulties with ambulation
- Poorly motivated people with geographic or transport problems making attendance difficult tend to do less well.

Box 56.1 Benefits of pulmonary rehabilitation in COPD

- Improves exercise capacity
- Reduces perceived intensity of breathlessness
- Improves health-related quality of life
- Reduces the number of hospitalizations and days in the hospital
- Reduces anxiety and depression associated with COPD
- Strength and endurance training of the upper limbs improves arm function
- Benefits extend beyond the immediate period of training
- Improves survival

Program

Programs are usually run on an outpatient basis, but can be done in the community, the home, or in an inpatient facility. They are run by a multi-professional team consisting of a physician, physiotherapist, occupational therapist, dietician, nurse, pharmacist, social worker, respiratory therapist, and psychologist. A minimum program length of 6 weeks is recommended. Programs should be regularly audited to ensure that patient-related outcomes are being achieved.

- **Physical training** is the main component of the program, with aerobic exercise such as walking and cycling 2–3 times per week, starting with supervised sessions and progressing until the patient is independent and will continue life-long exercise. Training may include upper limb strength exercise with weights. Individually prescribed exercise programs are designed for each patient to work toward high intensity. Physiological benefit increases with training intensity. Oxygen supplementation may be required if significant desaturation occurs during exercise.
- **Disease education**
- **Psychological and social intervention** with advice on anxiety and depression, smoking cessation, plus physiotherapy and occupational therapy input
- **Nutritional education** to optimize body weight and muscle mass

Pre-rehabilitation assessment
- Optimize medical treatment
- Oxygen saturation on exercise
- A cardiac stress test such as thallium stress test may be warranted, especially if a history of cardiac disease is present, to rule out unstable ischemic heart disease.

Outcome assessment measures
- Six-minute walk test (6MWT) to assess ability and progress (see Box 56.2)
- **Health status**
  - Disease-specific questionnaires
    Chronic Respiratory Questionnaire (CRQ)
    St. George's Respiratory Questionnaire
  - Generic questionnaires
    Short Form-36 (SF-36)
    Hospital Anxiety and Depression scores (HADS) are measured, but are insensitive to change during pulmonary rehabilitation.
- The Pulmonary Function Status–Dyspnea Questionnaire (PFS-DQ) may be used to measure performance and satisfaction related to activities of daily living.

Box 56.2 Six-minute walk test (6MWT)

This test measures the maximal distance that a patient can walk on a flat surface in a period of 6 minutes. The patients determine their pace and intensity of exercise. They are allowed to rest if they need to. Results may vary according to mood and encouragement. Encouragement phrases should be standardized.

Further information

Lacasse Y, Brosseau L, Milne S, et al. (2002). Pulmonary rehabilitation for COPD. *Cochrane Database Syst Rev* **3**:CD003793.

Nici L, Donner C, Wouters E, et al. (2006). American Thoracic Society/European Respiratory Society statement on pulmonary rehabilitation. *Am J Respir Crit Care* **173**: 1390–1413.

Ries AL, Bauldoff GS, Carlin BW, et al. (2007). Pulmonary rehabilitation: Joint ACCP/AACVPR Evidence-Based Clinical Practice Guidelines. *Chest* **131**(5 Suppl.):4S–42S.

Salman GF, Mosier MC, Beasley BW, Calkins DR (2003). Rehabilitation for patients with COPD: meta-analysis of RCTs. *J Gen Intern Med* **18**(3):213–221.

Smoking cessation

Aims and nicotine replacement therapy

Nearly 438,000 deaths per year in the United States are attributable to smoking, a major cause of chronic obstructive pulmonary disease, stroke, coronary heart disease, and numerous forms of cancers. Medical costs due to smoking are estimated to be nearly $75 billion per year. More deaths are attributed to smoking than to human immunodeficiency virus (HIV), illegal drug use, alcohol use, motor vehicle injuries, suicides, and murders combined.

- 23.9% of men and 18.1% of women in the United States smoke.
- 82% of smokers start as teenagers.
- The incidence of smoking is increasing in developing countries.
- Smoking is also associated with bladder, esophageal, cervical, and renal cancers, as well as cardiovascular and cerebrovascular disease.
- Nicotine exerts its effects on the CNS and is very addictive.
- 70% of smokers want to quit.
- Most smokers require 3–8 quit attempts to stop smoking.

Aims of smoking cessation interventions

In order to achieve the goal of sustained abstinence, the aim is to reduce short-term cravings for nicotine (nicotine and non-nicotine replacement therapy) and, in the long term, modify behavior (through counseling, telephonic or group support [buddy systems]). Research shows that the more a smoker is committed to stop, the more likely they are to quit successfully.

As a health professional it is important to address smoking cessation at all opportunities. Health professionals can trigger quit attempts by giving brief advice to all smokers. When physicians routinely inquire about tobacco use and advise patients to quit, smoking cessation rates increase by 30%. People are especially receptive to smoking cessation messages during times of concern for their own or their family's health.

The "5As" model is a useful guide to approaching the topic:

- **Ask** how much a person smokes, and document pack-years.
- **Advise** on risks of continued smoking and benefits of quitting, and suggest treatments available.
- **Assess** motivation to change.
- **Assist** by referring patient to a counselor and providing nicotine replacement therapy (NRT) if the patient is ready to quit soon, or enhance motivation to quit in the future.
- **Arrange** follow-up to ask about the outcome of prior efforts.

Some hospitals or primary care clinics have smoking cessation counselors on site. The best results for quit rates are achieved by combining counseling with NRT, bupropion, or varenicline tartrate with regular support and follow-up. These can improve quit rates to nearly 30%.

The Tobacco Use and Dependence Clinical Guideline Panel has issued clinical guidelines on the use of NRT and bupropion for smoking cessation.

Nicotine replacement therapy (NRT)

NRT assists in minimizing short- and medium-term nicotine withdrawal symptoms by replacing nicotine. NRT should not be used while the person is still smoking, as it is possible to overdose on nicotine (symptoms include agitation, confusion, restlessness, palpitations, hypertension, dilated pupils, SOB, abdominal cramps, nausea, vomiting). NRT can be bought over the counter or it can be prescribed. It is cheaper than cigarettes!

Contraindications to NRT include recent congestive heart failure, unstable angina, pulmonary disease, severe or chronic skin allergies (patch), pregnancy, breast-feeding mothers, and children under age 18, but it can be used under clinical supervision.

Patches

This craving-controller treatment releases small amounts of nicotine via a transdermal patch (7 mg, 14 mg, 21 mg) to minimize withdrawal symptoms. A 21 mg dose patch should be used in individuals smoking 20+ cigarettes per day. It is convenient and can be worn continuously throughout the day, but is often removed at night because of the vivid nature of dreams associated with its use. Patches can produce localized irritation at the patch site, so suggest use of hydrocortisone cream.

Patches should be used for 6–8 weeks at the higher dose and then weaned to a lower dose for 2–4 weeks. They are available over the counter.

Chewing gum

Different strengths of gum (2 mg, 4 mg) release nicotine as the gum is chewed. It relieves cravings as they occur. When the mouth tingles and has a peppery taste, the smoker should stop chewing and "park" the gum inside the cheek. Nicotine is then absorbed through the lining of the mouth. Chewing the gum continuously can produce nausea.

Nicotine needs to be absorbed through the mouth and not swallowed in saliva, so it is best not to drink while chewing the gum. The physical act of chewing can relieve craving. It can taste unpleasant and patients may need to use several packs of gum a day.

Individuals smoking 20+ cigarettes per day should use high-dose gum. They should use it for 3 months and then reduce the strength and amount of gum. It is available over the counter.

Lozenges

Different strengths of lozenges (2 mg, 4 mg) release nicotine as the lozenge dissolves in the mouth. Lozenges relieve cravings as they occur. The lozenges do not interfere with dental work, there is no special chewing procedure, and they are reported to have a more pleasurable taste. Nicotine is absorbed through the mouth lining.

Lozenges should not be chewed or swallowed, to avoid nausea and upset stomach. It is best not to drink or eat 15 minutes prior to their use. If individuals smoke within the first 30 minutes of waking they should use a higher dose of lozenge.

Smokers should use them for 3 months then reduce the strength and amount of lozenges used. Lozenges are available over the counter.

Inhaler

This is a cigarette-style device that gives small amounts of nicotine when used. It is useful as a quick reliever for people who are habitual or ritualistic and want the hand-to-mouth routine.

Inhalers are expensive. Nicotine is absorbed through the lining of the mouth, not via the lungs. Smokers should use them for 2 months and then gradually reduce their use. Inhalers are available by prescription.

Nasal spray

Nasal spray also provides rapid relief of craving. It provides faster absorption than that with other forms of NRT, so it has higher efficacy rates. It may cause local irritation.

Nasal spray is associated with a low compliance rate. Smokers should use it for 2 months then reduce usage. The spray is available by prescription.

Non-nicotine replacement therapy

Medication in combination with behavioral treatment has been found to nearly triple smoking cessation rates. Studies suggest that varenicline is superior to bupropion in both short- and long-term abstinence rates.

Bupropion (Zyban) is an antidepressant found to reduce the desire to smoke. It weakly inhibits dopamine, serotonin, and norepinephrine reuptake in the CNS. It counteracts nicotine withdrawal symptoms by increasing these levels in the brain. It is suitable for people who smoke 10+ cigarettes a day. It is metabolized by the liver and has a 20-hour half-life.

Smokers start taking bupropion 2 weeks before their intended quit day. They continue taking it for 7–9 weeks after that date. It is thought to lessen weight gain associated with smoking cessation.

Bupropion is contraindicated in patients with epilepsy, seizure disorder, or bulimia, those who are discontinuing benzodiazepine or are pregnant, and those taking monoamine oxidase inhibitors. Reduce the dose if the patient is elderly or has hepatic or renal impairment.

Adverse effects include dry mouth, hypersensitivity, insomnia, and seizures (1 in 1000 users) and death. Bupropion is by prescription only.

Varenicline tartrate (Chantix) is the first approved nicotinic receptor partial agonist that produces low to moderate levels of dopamine, mimicking nicotine's effects. It also acts as an antagonist, blocking the binding of nicotine and thus minimizing the rewarding effects of smoking. It has been found to reduce cravings, withdrawal symptoms, and the pleasurable effects of nicotine in tobacco products. It is suitable for people smoking 10+ cigarettes per day. It is minimally metabolized, unlike nicotine, and has a 24-hour half-life.

Smokers start varenicline 1 week before their intended quit day. They continue taking it for 12 weeks, with an additional 12-week course to increase the likelihood of long-term abstinence. It is well tolerated by most people.

There are no reported contraindications, and no adjustments for mild or moderate renal impairment. Reduce the dose if there is severe renal impairment. Recognized averse effects include nausea, insomnia, abnormal dreams, headache, constipation, flatulence, and vomiting. Vareniciline should be used during pregnancy only if the anticipated benefits outweigh the risks to the fetus. It is available by prescription only.

Hypnosis aims to improve willpower in the subconscious state with therapeutic suggestion. There is anecdotal success, but a Cochrane review of trials showed no greater abstinence rate with hypnosis than with any other treatment or with placebo treatment.

Acupuncture and acupressure have no evidence showing benefit of their use over that of placebo acupuncture.

Future developments

Clinic- and hospital-based smoking cessation services have increased and been improved, with links to community-based services, e.g., telephonic and Web-based quit programs.

In the field of nicotine immunotherapy, laboratory-based models are being used to create a nicotine vaccine (NicVAX) that would prevent abstinent smokers from restarting. The vaccine would induce specific nicotine antibodies to prevent inhaled nicotine from binding to nicotine receptors and causing neurological stimulation.

Further information

A clinical practice guideline for treating tobacco use and dependence: A US Public Health Service report. The Tobacco Use and Dependence Clinical Practice Guideline Panel, Staff, and Consortium Representatives. *JAMA* 2000: **283**: 3244–3254.

Centers for Disease Control and Prevention (2002). Annual smoking-attributable mortality, Years of potential life lost, and productivity losses—United States, 1995–1999. *MMWR Morb Mortal Wkly Rep* [serial online] **51**(14):300–303. Available from: http://www.cdc.gov/mmwr/preview/mmwrhtml/mm5114a2.htm.

Fiore MC, Bailey WC, Cohen SJ, et al. (2000). *Treating Tobacco Use and Dependence. Quick Reference Guide for Clinicians.* Rockville, MD: US Department of Health and Human Services. Public Health Service. Available from: http://www.surgeongeneral.gov/tobacco/tobaqrg.htm.

U.S. Department of Health and Human Services (2004). *The Health Consequences of Smoking: A Report of the Surgeon General.* U.S. Department of Health and Human Services, Centers for Disease Control and Prevention, National Center for Chronic Disease Prevention and Health Promotion, Office on Smoking and Health. Available from: http://www.cdc.gov/tobacco/data_statistics/sgr/sgr_2004/index.htm.

Chapter 58

Palliative care of the chest patient

Pain and dyspnea

Palliative care is defined as the management of patients whose disease is not responsive to curative treatment. Its aim is to provide the best possible quality of life for patients, their careers, and families. It includes controlling pain and other physical symptoms, as well as addressing psychological, social, and spiritual problems.

Within chest medicine, palliative care is most commonly considered for patients with lung cancer and mesothelioma; many other patients with progressive, end-stage respiratory disease (such as COPD, CF, and IPF) also benefit from specific palliative interventions.

- Involve the specialist palliative care team early.
- Recognize that delirium, dyspnea, and decreased mobility often herald the terminal phase of cancer.

Pain

- Aim to determine cause, type, and site.
- Start with simple analgesia and increase according to pain severity, moving from nonopioid analgesia through weak opioids to strong opioids.
- Prescribe analgesia as needed for breakthrough pain.
- Anti-inflammatory drug can be effective for bone pain.
- Treat drug side effects, e.g., constipation, nausea. Consider prophylactic laxatives with chronic morphine use.
- Consider radiotherapy for localized chest wall pain related to cancer.
- Pain from bony metastases may be treated with bisphosphonates.
- Neuropathic pain can be treated with specific antidepressants (e.g., amitriptyline) or anticonvulsants (e.g., carbamazepine or sodium valproate).
- Consider referral to a pain clinic for additional intervention, including nerve blocks, transcutaneous electrical nerve stimulation (TENS), or complementary therapies.

Dyspnea

- Consider possible causes; dyspnea may be due to the underlying lung disease, or due to an additional pathology (see Box 58.1).
- Dyspnea is made worse by anxiety and panic.
- Lung cancer and pulmonary metastases are associated with the sensation of shortness of breath, often due to stimulation of receptors by malignant infiltration or lymphangitic carcinomatosis.
- Optimize treatment of any underlying lung disease with bronchodilators and steroids, if appropriate.
- Treat concurrent chest infections.
- Opioids can be used to relieve the sensation of dyspnea; monitor efficacy and adverse effects closely.
- Intermittent oxygen use may occasionally help relieve symptoms.
- Consider an airway stent in a patient with lung cancer who has dyspnea due to bronchial obstruction or compression with tumor.

Box 58.1 Causes of breathlessness in patients with lung cancer

- Pneumonia
- Underlying chronic lung disease (e.g., COPD, IPF)
- Lobar collapse
- Pleural effusion
- Superior vena cava obstruction
- Upper airway obstruction
- Pulmonary emboli
- Lymphangitic carcinomatosis
- Pericardial effusion
- Anemia
- Depression
- Anxiety and panic

Other symptoms

Anxiety

- Leads to dyspnea, which in turn worsens anxiety
- Benzodiazepines may be tried for respiratory panic; monitor efficacy and adverse effects closely.
- Relaxation exercises and diaphragmatic breathing training may benefit some patients.
- Consider psychiatric consultation to help manage anxiety.

Cough

- Cough suppressants, including opioid agents as codeine, may be tried.
- Nebulized saline may help expectoration.
- Nebulized local anesthetic may be considered for persistent coughing (avoid use in asthmatics, as it may cause bronchospasm).

Pleural effusion

- Drain if symptomatic and consider pleurodesis early if recurrent
- Consider an in-dwelling tunneled catheter to drain fluid if effusion is symptomatic and pleurodesis has failed because of a trapped lung.

Poor appetite

- Common symptom and may be primary due to cachexia–anorexia syndrome, or secondary, due to mouth problems such as candidiasis, nausea, hypocalcemia, drugs, or depression
- Cachexia leads to decreased respiratory muscle strength and increased shortness of breath.
- Consider nutritional supplements and a dietitian consult.

Brain metastases

- Steroids (e.g., dexamethasone) may relieve cerebral edema associated with brain metastases.
- Radiotherapy should also be considered.

Part IV

Practical procedures

Airway management

Patients in emergency or critical care situations may require ventilation support and tracheal intubation. Hypoxic patients who have adequate spontaneous ventilation may only require a higher percentage of inspired oxygen. Patients with impending respiratory failure and in need of positive pressure ventilation will require intubation.

Intubation is also recommended for patients with impaired consciousness and at risk for aspiration, and burned patients in whom swelling of the airway may occur. Close attention should be given to supporting the patient's spontaneous respiratory efforts until everything has been prepared for definitive airway management.

Mask airway

Ventilation using a bag-mask breathing system is a first-line method for assisting a patient's spontaneous ventilation or resuscitating an apneic patient. One person can perform this technique, although a two-person technique may be required for treating those patients who are obese or bearded or have decreased lung compliance.

With a two-person technique, one provider uses two hands to seal the mask on the patient's face while also subluxing the mandible anteriorly (vertical jaw thrust in the supine patient) to open the airway. The second provider squeezes the bag.

Simple airway adjuncts

Oral and nasal airways can be used to overcome backward tongue displacement in an unconscious patient.

Oropharyngeal airway

A curved plastic device with a flanged end is inserted into the mouth. Estimate size by holding the airway at the side of the patient's face and estimating the required length from the mouth to the angle of the jaw. Insert the airway concave side up and then rotate it 180°, or place it in the correct orientation directly over a tongue depressor. Make sure that the distal tip of the airway rests behind the base of the tongue.

In awake or semiconscious patients oral airways may cause coughing, vomiting, or laryngospasm.

Nasopharyngeal airway

For a nasal airway a soft plastic tube with a flange at one end and a beveled tip at the other is used. Nasal airways are better tolerated than oral airways in the semiconscious patient, but may cause nasal trauma and bleeding. They should not be used in patients with some basilar skull fractures, and used only cautiously in those with coagulopathies or nasal deformities.

If time permits before insertion, prepare the nasal passage by applying a topical anesthetic and a vasoconstrictor to reduce discomfort and bleeding. Lubricate nasal airways with a water-soluble lubricant and gently insert the beveled end in a straight-back direction until the flange rests against the nasal opening. Do not apply excessive force. If obstruction is encountered, remove the airway and insert in the other nostril or try a smaller size.

As a general rule, use a nasal airway similar in size to the patient's little finger. Typical adult sizes range from 32 to 36 Fr.

Laryngeal mask airway (LMA)

In the critical care setting, an LMA is most appropriately used to maintain airway patency in a spontaneously ventilating patient, and as a rescue airway in the event of a failed intubation. Positive pressure ventilation can be performed through an LMA unless the patient has high airway resistance or decreased lung compliance. An LMA consists of a wide-bore tube with an inflatable cuff (mask) at one end.

To insert the LMA (see Fig. 59.1, Fig. 59.2, Fig. 59.3, and Fig. 59.4), the mask should be deflated into a "spoon shape" and its posterior surface lubricated with a water-soluble lubricant. The LMA is held with the index finger at the junction of the mask and the tube. The distal tip of the mask is pressed flat against the hard palate. Maintaining constant outward pressure, the index finger traces the palate, advancing the mask behind the tongue and into the hypopharynx until resistance is felt. Inflate the mask with just enough air to obtain a seal. Secure the tube with tape.

Assess breath sounds by auscultation and listen for a leak around the mask. If a large leak is present at <20 cm H_2O inspiratory pressure, remove and replace the same LMA or change sizes.

A size 4 LMA is used in most women and a size 5 in most men. A size 3 is appropriate for small adults and children over 30 kg.

Endotracheal intubation

Placement of an endotracheal tube (ETT) is the definitive method for maintaining airway patency and preventing aspiration of gastric contents. A standard ETT is beveled at one end with an inflatable cuff and has a removable connector (15 mm) at the other end.

Intubation

Tracheal intubation requires specialized training.

- The patient lies supine, with the neck flexed and head extended ("sniffing position"). The occiput should be elevated by pads or folded blankets.
- If possible, the patient should receive 100% oxygen through a snug-fitting facemask for several minutes prior to intubation.
- Anesthetic induction agents and muscle relaxants may be used to facilitate the ease of intubation; however, in patients *in extremis* the advantage of their use must be weighed against the risk of converting "poor ventilation" into a "cannot-ventilate" situation.
- The laryngoscope is held in the operator's left hand while the patient's mouth is opened with the operator's right hand. A curved laryngoscope blade (MacIntosh) is inserted into the right side of the patient's mouth and the tongue is swept to the left. The tip of the blade is advanced along the surface of the tongue into the space between the epiglottis and the base of the tongue (vallecula). With a gentle forward and upward motion in the direction of the laryngoscope handle, the tongue and soft tissue are lifted and the glottic opening is exposed. If the vocal cords are not immediately seen, visualization may be facilitated by external cephalad pressure on the larynx by either the operator's right hand or by an assistant.
- Suction should always be available and may be necessary to clear secretions from the posterior pharynx.

- The ETT is introduced from the right side of the patient's mouth and advanced through the cords until the cuff just disappears.
- Withdraw the laryngoscope and inflate the cuff.
- If the larynx is anterior and only the posterior structures of the glottis are seen (e.g., arytenoids), then a flexible stylet may be passed into the trachea and an ETT guided over it.
- Confirm appropriate ETT position by watching the chest rise symmetrically, auscultating for breath sounds bilaterally and checking for end tidal CO_2. Five breaths showing CO_2 confirms tracheal intubation. If the chest rises asymmetrically or breath sounds are heard unilaterally, usually a main-stem intubation has occurred. Deflate the cuff and slowly withdraw the ETT until bilateral breath sounds are present.
- Secure the ETT with either tape or specialized tube holders. If tape is used, it should wrap tightly around the ETT and encircle the patient's neck.
- Attach the ETT to a self-inflating bag or a ventilator to administer oxygen and begin ventilation.
- Obtain a CXR to confirm correct tube position 2–3 cm above the carina.
- A 7.0 mm I.D. ETT is used for most women. An 8.0 mm I.D. ETT is used for most men.

Special considerations
Certain situations demand advanced training beyond the basic intubation skills. These situations include but are not limited to the following: patients with cervical fractures, increased intracranial pressure, morbid obesity, airway anatomy distorted by tumor or surgery, and patients with a history of difficult intubation. For these patients, seek out help from an experienced anesthesiologist or other airway expert.

Alternative techniques
There are now a large variety of alternative devices for supraglottic ventilation and tracheal intubation. Well-established alternative techniques for intubation include the use of the flexible fiber-optic bronchoscopy and the LMA-Fastrach. Newer fiber-optic laryngoscopes and lighted stylets are also rapidly gaining popularity.

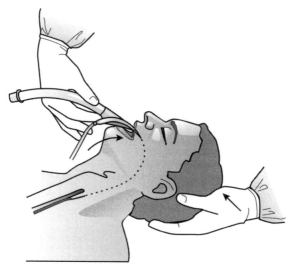

Figure 59.1 With the head extended and the neck flexed, carefully flatten the LMA™Airway tip against the hard palate (courtesy of LMA North America, Inc.).

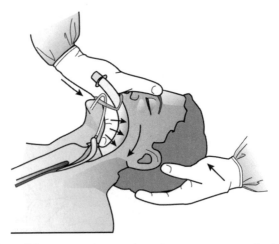

Figure 59.2 Use the index finger to push cranially, maintaining pressure on the tube with the finger. Note position of the wrist. Advance the mask until definite resistance is felt at the base of the hypopharynx (courtesy of LMA North America, Inc.).

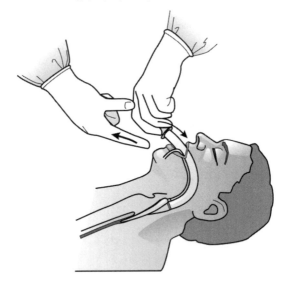

Figure 59.3 Gently maintain cranial pressure with the nondominant hand while removing the index finger (courtesy of LMA North America, Inc.).

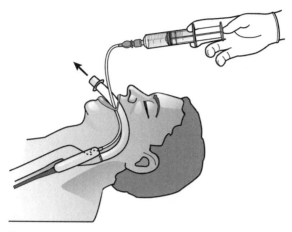

Figure 59.4 Without holding the tube, inflate the cuff with just enough air to obtain a seal (to a pressure of approximately 60 cm H_2O). Never overinflate the cuff (courtesy of LMA North America, Inc.).

Further information

Hagberg CA (Ed.) (2007). *Benumof's Airway Management*, 2nd ed. Philadelphia: Mosby Elsevier.

Ortega R, Mehio AK, Woo A, Hafez DH: Positive-pressure ventilation with a face mask and a bag-valve device. *N Engl J Med* Web site: Videos in Clinical Medicine357:e4. Available at: http://content.nejm.org/cgi/content/short/357/4/e4

Rosenblatt WH (2006). Airway management. In Barash PG, Cullen BF, Stoelting RK (Eds.). *Clinical Anesthesia*, 5th ed. Philadelphia: Lippincott Williams & Wilkins, pp. 595–642.

Cricothyroidotomy

In some situations of facial or laryngeal trauma or pathology, ventilation and tracheal intubation of a patient is impossible. It may be necessary to create an immediate surgical airway below the level of obstruction. All physicians involved with airway management should be familiar with the various methods of establishing an invasive transtracheal airway. Call for help from a surgeon, emergency physician, or anesthesiologist early!

Percutaneous transtracheal jet ventilation (TTJV)

- TTJV is a simple and rapid form of needle cricothyroidotomy reserved for situations in which mask ventilation and intubation are not possible (see Fig. 60.1).
- Position the patient supine with the neck extended.
- Identify the cricothyroid membrane: a soft triangular area above the cricoid ring and below the thyroid cartilage.
- Prep the skin with antiseptic and inject local anesthesia (1% xylocaine) over the membrane as time permits.
- Stabilize the larynx and stretch the skin taut overlying the membrane.
- Using a large-bore angiocatheter (16G or larger) attached to a 5 mL syringe, puncture the membrane and enter the trachea. The angio-catheter should initially be advanced perpendicular to the skin with constant aspiration on the syringe. Aspiration of free air confirms that the angiocatheter has entered the trachea. Be careful not to penetrate the posterior wall of the trachea.
- Once in the trachea, redirect the angiocatheter 45° caudally and advance only the catheter fully into the trachea. Remove the needle and aspirate again from the catheter to confirm that it remains in the trachea.
- Hold the catheter securely and attach an oxygen source.
- Ideally, a handheld jet ventilator is available, which can be Luer-locked onto the transtracheal catheter. Jet ventilators have a hand-controlled valve and can be adjusted to deliver 100% oxygen in short bursts (1–1.5 seconds) at approximately 25–30 psi. With each breath adminis-tered, observe for an adequate chest rise, then release the valve and allow the patient to exhale passively through the upper airway. If the patient has total upper airway obstruction, a second transtracheal catheter may be needed to permit exhalation.
- If a jet ventilator is unavailable, a low-pressure system may be quickly constructed. First remove the plunger from a 10 mL syringe and attach the empty barrel to the transtracheal catheter. Then insert a cuffed tracheal tube (7.0 mm ID) into the barrel and inflate the cuff to create a seal. Connect a self-inflating bag to an oxygen source and attach it to the tracheal tube. Proceed to ventilate. Although a low-pressure system will provide only marginal ventilation, it can help to maintain oxygenation of the patient until a definitive airway is established.
- It is imperative to maintain control of the transtracheal catheter at all times, since TTJV can cause severe barotrauma.

Surgical cricothyroidotomy

- Performing a surgical cricothyroidotomy requires specialized training and should be performed with the help of a surgeon.
- The patient is positioned and prepped as for TTJV.
- With a scalpel, make a vertical skin incision over the cricothyroid membrane.
- Using a curved hemostat, blunt dissect to the membrane surface.
- Maintaining firm traction on the laryngeal soft tissue with one hand, use the point of the hemostat to puncture the membrane and enter the trachea.
- Once in the trachea, spread the hemostat to create a hole in the membrane.
- While keeping the hemostat spread open and maintaining constant control of the trachea, insert a small tracheal tube through the hole. Be careful not to pass the carina with the tip of the tube (main-stem intubation).
- Secure the tube and attach an oxygen source.
- Several commercial kits for percutaneous cricothyroidotomy are available and greatly simplify the process of obtaining a surgical airway.

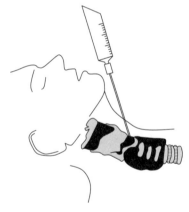

Figure 60.1 Diagram of needle cricothyroidotomy

Further information

Hagberg CA (Ed.) (2007). *Benumof's Airway Management*. 2nd ed. Philadelphia: Mosby Elsevier.

Rosenblatt WH (2006). Airway management. In Barash PG, Cullen BF, Stoelting RK (Eds.). *Clinical Anesthesia*, 5th ed. Philadelphia: Lippincott Williams & Wilkins, pp. 595–642.

Wong EK, Bradick JP (2000). Surgical approaches to airway management for anesthesia practitioners. In Hagberg CA (Ed.). *Handbook of Difficult Airway Management*. Philadelphia: Churchill Livingsone, pp. 185–218.

Bronchoscopy

Bronchoscopy is the procedure of passing a telescope or camera into the central airways to inspect the large and medium-sized airways. It may be performed with a flexible scope, usually by the transnasal technique using local anesthesia and sedation (usually lidocaine for local anesthesia and a combination of a benzodiazepine and an opioid for sedation), or under general anesthesia with a rigid scope. Airways can be visually inspected, samples taken and collected, and therapeutic procedures performed.

Virtual bronchoscopy is a noninvasive procedure used to visualize areas inaccessible to the flexible bronchoscope. It is used to evaluate bronchial obstruction caused by both endoluminal pathology (tumor, mucous, foreign bodies) and external compression, and can be helpful in the preoperative planning of stent placement. This chapter focuses on flexible fiber-optic bronchoscopy.

Indications for bronchoscopy (see Table 61.1)

Suspected lung cancer

A radiographic mass or nodule <4 cm from the origin of the nearest lobar bronchus is likely to be accessible for biopsy by bronchoscopy. Fluoroscopic guidance can expand the range of bronchoscopic biopsy access to the pleural surface.

Autofluorescence bronchoscopy uses inherent tissue properties to identify preinvasive lesions of the central airways. Endobronchial ultrasound can accurately define airway invasion versus compression from tumors, guide transbronchial needle aspiration of hilar and mediastinal lymph nodes, and predict on the basis of ultrasound morphology whether peripheral nodules are benign or malignant.

Suspected pulmonary infection

In a patient who is unable to produce sputum, bronchoscopy allows access to pulmonary secretions. In immunocompromised patients with fever, cough, hypoxemia, or CXR changes, bronchoscopic evaluation may identify infectious organisms not found through sputum analysis.

In neutropenic patients, gram-negative bacterial infections predominate, but fungal infections are common if neutropenia persists. In impaired cellular immunity, viral infections predominate. *Streptococcus pneumoniae* and *hemophilus influenzae* are the primary bacterial infections in patients with impaired humoral immunity.

In HIV-infected patients, fiber-optic bronchoscopy is useful in evaluating for *Pneumocystis jurobeci* (formerly *carinii*), endobronchial Kaposi sarcoma, or suspected cancer.

Suspected interstitial lung disease

An endobronchial or transbronchial lung biopsy may provide an adequate sample for diagnostic purposes in interstitial lung diseases (ILD) such as sarcoidosis. Biopsies adequate for tissue diagnosis in ILD are more often obtained by surgical lung biopsies (either thorascopic or open).

Fiber-optic bronchoscopy with biopsy can diagnose rejection in lung transplant recipients.

Foreign body removal

If an object is within the larger airways and visible, the foreign body may be removed using biopsy forceps, balloon catheters, or wire basket or loop snares. Fluoroscopy may assist in the distal clearance of the object.

Additional therapeutic indications include diathermy, laser (Yag or argon) resection or coagulation, cryotherapy, endobronchial brachytherapy, stenting, fibrin adhesives, balloon dilation, and lung volume reduction. Bronchoscopy is used in difficult intubations such as cervical spine disease or a failed conventional intubation.

Relative contraindications (see Table 61.2)

If a patient is hypoxemic, the risk of significant hypoxemia or hypoxia during bronchoscopy is increased. Continuous positive airway pressure (CPAP) in hypoxemic patients undergoing bronchoscopy may allow maintenance of normoxia.

Risks associated with fiber optic bronchoscopy (see Table 61.3)

Flexible bronchoscopy is a safe procedure, with reported mortality rates in large series of 0.01%–0.04% and major complications of 0.08%–0.12%. Complications include respiratory depression, arrhythmias, cardiorespiratory arrest, vasovagal episodes, fever, nausea and vomiting, laryngospasm, airway obstruction, pneumonia, pneumothorax, and hemorrhage.

Bleeding occurs in approximately 0.7% of patients due to mechanical trauma from the bronchoscope or suctioning brushing, and is more common with transbronchial biopsy (1.6%–4.4%). Patients with malignancy, immunocompromise, or uremia have an increased risk of bleeding.

If bleeding does not stop spontaneously, the bronchoscope should be wedged to tamponade the bleeding in the appropriate segmental bronchus. Use minimal suction to allow clot formation. Administer 1 mL aliquots of 1:20,000 adrenaline solutions via the bronchoscope as near as possible to the bleeding point until it stops. Iced saline may also be useful.

If massive bleeding occurs, the patient should be turned onto the side of the bleeding to protect the other lung. Intubation and assisted ventilation may be necessary.

Table 61.1 Indications for flexible and rigid bronchoscopy

Common indications for flexible bronchoscopy

- Cough (persistent, unexplained)
- Hemoptysis
- Wheeze (localized)
- Abnormal chest radiograph
- Atelectasis (persistent)
- Mediastinal or hilar mass
- Parenchymal mass or nodule
- Determine etiology of pneumonia
- Recurrent or nonresolving
- Nosocomial
- Immunocompromised host
- Foreign body in airway
- Evaluation for rejection in lung transplantation

Common indications for rigid bronchoscopy

- Massive hemoptysis
- Foreign-body removal
- Placement of airway stent
- Laser or photodynamic therapy

Table 61.2 Contraindications for bronchoscopy

Relative contraindications for bronchoscopy

- Inability to cooperate with the procedure
- Refractory hypoxemia
- Uncontrolled arrhythmia
- Recent myocardial infarction or unstable angina
- Uncorrected blood-clotting abnormalities (particularly platelet counts <50,000/mm^3)
- Severe uremia and liver disease
- Pulmonary hypertension

Table 61.3 Complications of bronchoscopy

Common complications of bronchoscopy

Medication- or anesthesia-related

- Respiratory depression
- Hypotension
- Arrhythmias
- Agitation (paradoxical)
- Nausea and vomiting
- Laryngospasm or bronchospasm
- Seizures

Procedure-related

- Hypoxemia
- Arrhythmias
- Fever
- Epistaxis (with nasal approach)
- Laryngeal spasm, edema, injury
- Bacteremia
- Pneumonia
- Bleeding
- Pneumothorax

Thoracentesis

Thoracentesis ("pleural tap," or pleural fluid aspiration) may be diagnostic or therapeutic.

Diagnostic thoracentesis

Indication: undiagnosed pleural effusion
Contraindications: There are no absolute contraindications to pleural aspiration, although care should be taken if the patient is anticoagulated.

Technique
1. Explain the procedure to the patient.
2. Take time with the nursing and technical staff for proper identification of the patient and site of the procedure.
3. Position the patient sitting forward, leaning on a pillow over a table with their arms folded in front of them.
4. Double-check the correct side from chest examination and CXR.
5. Choose the aspiration site using ultrasonography. Use a posterior or lateral approach (although avoid very posterior approaches close to the spine, as the intercostal artery drops medially to lie in the mid-intercostal space).
6. Use sterile skin preparation and aseptic technique.
7. Infiltrate the skin, intercostal muscle, and parietal pleura with 10 mL 1% lidocaine. Aim just above the upper border of the appropriate rib, avoiding the neurovascular bundle that runs below each rib. The parietal pleura is extremely sensitive; use the full 10 mL lidocaine.
8. Aspirate pleural fluid with a 21G needle and 50 mL syringe.
9. Following diagnostic tap:
   - Note pleural fluid *appearance*
   - Send sample in a sterile container to biochemistry for measurement of *protein* and LDH
   - Send fresh 20 mL sample in a sterile container to cytology for examination for malignant cells and differential cell count. A 3.8% sodium citrate tube may help preserve cells in cytology samples.
   - Send samples in a sterile container and blood culture bottles to *microbiology* for Gram stain and microscopy, culture, and AFB stain and culture.
   - Process nonpurulent, heparinized samples in arterial blood gas analyzer for *pH* (consult biochemistry laboratory for local policy of pH analysis beforehand; never put purulent samples in the arterial blood analyzer).
   - Consider measurement of cholesterol and triglycerides, hematocrit, glucose (with paired blood sample), and amylase, depending on the clinical circumstances.
10. There is no need for a routine CXR following aspiration.

Complications of thoracentesis include pneumothorax, cough, bleeding, empyema, spleen or liver puncture, and malignant seeding down the aspiration site (particularly in mesothelioma).

Therapeutic thoracentesis

Indication: symptomatic relief of breathlessness due to a pleural effusion, most commonly due to malignancy

Technique

In many cases, this can be performed as an outpatient procedure.

1. The initial procedure is identical to that of diagnostic thoracentesis (steps 1–8). It is important to verify that the insertion site is correct by first aspirating pleural fluid with a 21G needle. If you are unable to aspirate fluid, abort the procedure and obtain a chest ultrasound to check the presence and location of fluid.
2. Carefully advance a large-bore IV cannula along the anesthetized track.
3. Remove the inner needle and attach the cannula to a three-way tap.
4. Aspirate fluid from the chest with a 50 mL syringe via the three-way tap, and flush the fluid into a bag through extension tubing. Drain fluid in one sitting. Stop the procedure if resistance is felt, or the patient experiences chest pain (usually anterior), discomfort, or severe coughing, suggesting an unexpandable lung. Mild cough is common when large amounts of fluid are removed.
5. Apply dressing to the aspiration site.
6. Obtain repeat CXR to document the extent of improvement in effusion size and to exclude pneumothorax or unexpandable lung.

Aspiration
of pneumothorax

Indications

Primary spontaneous pneumothorax

Consider aspiration if the patient is breathless and/or pneumothorax is large (rim of air >2 cm on CXR).

Secondary spontaneous pneumothorax

Consider aspiration if the patient is <50 years of age, with small pneumothorax (rim of air <2 cm on CXR) and minimal breathlessness.

Technique

Refer to pp. 322–3 for treatment algorithms.

Discuss procedure with the patient and obtain written consent (unless this is an emergency situation).

1. Take time with the nursing and technical staff for proper identification of the patient and site of procedure.
2. Insert an IV cannula.
3. Position the patient sitting upright, supported on pillows.
4. Double-check the correct side from chest examination and CXR.
5. Choose the aspiration site: the second intercostal space in a mid-clavicular line on the side of the pneumothorax.
6. Infiltrate the skin, intercostal muscle, and parietal pleura with 10 mL 1% lidocaine. Aim just above the upper border of the appropriate rib, avoiding the neurovascular bundle that runs below each rib. Parietal pleura is extremely sensitive; use the full 10 mL lidocaine.
7. Perform sterile skin preparation. Wear sterile gloves and gown.
8. While waiting for an M 12/17 anesthetic to work, connect a 50 mL syringe to a three-way tap, with the tap turned off to the patient.
9. Confirm presence of pneumothorax by aspirating air with a 21G needle.
10. Insert a 16G cannula over the upper border of the rib. Remove the inner needle, and quickly connect cannula to a three-way tap and 50 mL syringe.
11. Aspirate 50 mL air with the syringe, turn tap, and expel air into the atmosphere. Repeat until resistance is felt, or 2.5 L air is aspirated (aspiration of >2.5 L suggests a large air leak, and aspiration is likely to fail). Halt the procedure if it is painful or if the patient is coughing excessively.
12. Remove cannula. Cover the insertion site with a dressing.
13. Repeat CXR. Ideal timing of the CXR following aspiration is unknown. It may be advisable to wait several hours before performing the CXR, to detect slow air leaks.
14. Aspiration is successful if the lung is fully re-expanded on CXR.
15. If initial aspiration of a primary pneumothorax fails, repeat aspiration should be considered (unless ≥2.5 L has already been aspirated). At least one-third of patients will respond to a second aspiration.

Abrams pleural biopsy

Indications
- Diagnosis of tuberculous pleural effusion
- Diagnosis of malignant pleural disease in many centers, although a recent randomized, controlled trial has shown that CT-guided cutting-needle biopsy has a greater sensitivity (87% sensitivity in the CT-guided biopsy group vs. 47% in the Abrams group)

Technique
An assistant is required. Discuss procedure with the patient and obtain written consent.

1. Take time with the nursing and technical staff for proper identification of the patient and site of procedure.
2. Insert an IV cannula.
3. Position the patient sitting forward, leaning on a pillow over a table with their arms folded in front of them.
4. Double-check the correct side from chest examination and CXR.
5. Choose the biopsy site using ultrasonography. Use a posterior or lateral approach (although avoid very posterior approaches close to the spine, as the intercostal artery drops medially to lie in the mid-intercostal space).
6. Perform sterile skin preparation. Wear sterile gloves and gown.
7. Infiltrate the skin, intercostal muscle, and parietal pleura with 10 mL 1% lidocaine. Aim just above the upper border of the appropriate rib, while avoiding the neurovascular bundle that runs below each rib. Anesthetize the area behind the rib below the insertion point.
8. While waiting for anesthetic to work, assemble the Abrams reverse-bevel biopsy needle. The needle consists of an outer sheath with a triangular opening (biopsy port) that can be opened or closed by rotating an inner sheath.
9. Verify that the insertion site is correct by aspirating pleural fluid with a 21G needle. If you are unable to aspirate fluid, do not proceed.
10. Make a small (5 mm) skin incision; dissect the intercostal muscles with blunt forceps.
11. Insert the biopsy needle gently with the biopsy port closed. Do not apply force; the needle should slip into the pleural space without resistance. When in the pleural cavity, fluid can be withdrawn by attaching a syringe to the needle and opening the biopsy port.
12. To take a biopsy, attach a syringe to the needle. Open the biopsy port and angle it downward and then pull the biopsy port firmly against the parietal pleura on the rib beneath the entry point (6 o'clock position relative to entry point). Close the biopsy port, thereby pulling a sample of parietal pleura into the needle.
13. Remove the biopsy needle, open the biopsy port, and remove the biopsy sample.
14. Repeat the procedure 4–6 times in positions 4–8 o'clock, always sampling below the insertion point (to avoid the neurovascular bundle beneath the rib above).
15. Send biopsy samples in saline for analysis for tuberculosis and in formalin if malignancy is suspected.

16. Apply dressing to the biopsy site. It may require a single stitch.
17. Obtain a CXR to exclude pneumothorax.

Complications

These include pain, pneumothorax, hemothorax, and empyema. Hemorrhage from trauma to an intercostal artery may necessitate emergency thoracotomy. Fatalities are well documented but are extremely rare.

Further information

Maskell NA, et al. (2003). Standard pleural biopsy versus CT-guided cutting-needle biopsy for diagnosis of malignant disease in pleural effusions: a randomised controlled trial. *Lancet* **361**:1326–1331.

Chest drains

Indications, drain types, and complications

Different types of tubes and catheters are used to remove air or fluid from the pleural cavity (see Box 65.1). The fluid can be blood, pus, or pleural effusion. Chest drainage allows re-expansion of the underlying lung and prevents entry of air or drained fluid back into the chest. A chest drainage system has three components:

1. An unobstructed chest drain
2. A collecting container below chest level
3. A one-way mechanism such as a water seal or Heimlich valve.

Chest drain insertion is an invasive procedure that can be associated with both morbidity and mortality (see Box 65.2 for complications). Ultrasound guidance should be used for small or loculated effusions. Occasionally, pre-procedure CT of the chest can be very useful to ascertain the nature of the pleural space.

Indications
- Pneumothorax
  - Tension pneumothorax (e.g., following needle decompression)
  - Symptomatic pneumothorax with failed aspiration or underlying lung disease.
  - Pneumothorax of any size in a patient receiving mechanical ventilation
- Complicated parapneumonic effusion and empyema
- Malignant pleural effusion for symptomatic relief and/or pleurodesis
- Hemothorax
- Chylothorax
- Penetrating chest trauma (e.g., traumatic hemopneumothorax)
- Trapped lung
- Bronchopleural fistula

Contraindications
- No absolute contraindication
- Relative contraindications
  - Anticoagulation or bleeding diathesis
  - Complicated pleural space with multiple loculations or previous pleurodesis

Box 65.1 Types of chest drains
- Large-bore chest drains (>24 French)
- Medium-bore chest drains (16–24 French)
- Small-bore chest drains (8–14 French)
  - Pigtail tubes (8–14 French)
  - Pneumothorax tubes (8 French)
- Tunneled pleural catheters (15.5 French)

Selection of the appropriate-size chest tube is determined by the viscosity and accumulation rate of the pleural material to be drained.

For pneumothoraces usually 16–24 Fr chest tubes are sufficient. For small air leaks, an 8–14 Fr catheter can be used, whereas for a large air leak or traumatic pneumothoraces, a 28–40 Fr chest tube should be used for drainage of blood in addition to air.

For malignant pleural effusions a 20–24 Fr chest tube is usually adequate. Small-bore tunnel pleural catheters (15.5 Fr) are now successfully used in long-term outpatient and inpatient management of malignant pleural effusions.

For complicated parapneumonic effusions or empyema usually large-bore (28–36 Fr) chest tubes are needed. In multiloculated effusions with failed evacuation by large-bore tubes, fibrinolytic agents can be instilled into the intrapleural space to break adhesions and facilitate drainage.

For a hemothorax usually large 32–40 Fr chest drains are needed.

Box 65.2 Complications of chest drains

- Empyema (1%–3%)
- Chest drain malpositioning (the most common complication, detected in 26% of patients in one series)
- Pain is very common after drain placement.
- Surgical emphysema (air leaks into subcutaneous tissues) may occur if the tube is blocked or positioned with holes subcutaneously, or with very large air leaks.
- Lung parenchymal perforation (0.2%–0.6%)
- Diaphragmatic perforation (0.4%)
- Other complications
  - Perforation of right ventricle, right atrium, or abdominal organs (spleen, liver, stomach, colon)
  - Cardiogenic shock from chest tube compressing right ventricle
  - Bleeding from intercostal artery injury
  - Infection at chest drain site
  - Re-expansion pulmonary edema
  - Vasovagal reaction

Insertion technique

Steps in chest drain insertion

1. Discuss procedure with the patient and obtain written consent (unless this is an emergency situation). Take a few seconds with the nursing staff and technicians for proper identification of the patient and site of the procedure.
2. If the patient's hemodynamic status permits, consider conscious sedation before beginning the procedure (e.g., midazolam 2 mg IV and Fentanyl 25–50 µm initially and then during the procedure on an as-needed basis).
3. Blood pressure, oximetry, and cardiac monitoring should be performed throughout the procedure.
4. Position the patient supine with the arm of the involved side placed behind the head, or the patient can be positioned sitting forward, leaning over a table.
5. Check the correct side from chest examination and CXR.
6. Choose the insertion site—ideally within a "triangle of safety" that avoids major vessels and muscles (boundaries: anteriorly, anterior axillary line and border of pectoralis major; posteriorly, posterior axillary line; inferiorly, horizontal to level of nipple in men or fifth intercostal space in women). More posterolateral approaches are safe but less comfortable for the patient when lying. Avoid posteromedial approaches close to the spine, as the intercostal artery drops medially to lie in the mid-intercostal space.
7. Prep the area of insertion with 10% povidone-iodine or chlorhexidine and drape with sterile towels. Wear sterile gloves and gown.
8. Infiltrate the skin, intercostal muscle, and parietal pleura with 10 mL 1% lidocaine. Aim just above the upper border of the appropriate rib, avoiding the neurovascular bundle that runs below each rib. The subcutaneous fat lacks pain receptors and does not require anesthetic. The parietal pleura, however, is extremely sensitive; use the full 10 mL lidocaine.
9. Confirm the correct site by aspirating pleural fluid or air. If you are unable to aspirate fluid or air, do not proceed with drain insertion; consider image-guided drainage. Occasionally, in obese patients a longer needle is required.
10. Perform chest drain insertion.

Standard technique

Make a 2 cm skin incision parallel to the intercostal space immediately above the rib to prevent injury to the neurovascular bundle. Using blunt dissection with a Kelly clamp, create a subcutaneous tunnel. With the Kelly clamp in the closed position, push the clamp through the parietal pleura; the clamp is then opened to spread parietal pleura and intercostal muscles. Insert a finger through the tract into the pleural space to confirm proper positioning and lack of adhesions between the lung and the pleural surface. Clamp the chest tube at the proximal end with a Kelly clamp and insert tube through the tract into the pleural space. Aim toward the apex for a pneumothorax, and the lung base for a pleural effusion.

Seldinger technique

Make a 2 cm skin incision parallel to the intercostal space. Insert an introducer into the pleural space with aspiration of air or fluid. Place a guidewire through the introducer needle into the pleural space. Graduated-size dilators are serially passed over the guidewire to dilate a tract for chest tube. Pass the chest tube with its dilator into the pleural space. Remove the guidewire and dilator, leaving the chest tube in place.

Insertion technique for tunneled pleural catheters

Here a modified Seldinger technique is employed. Localize pleural effusion by needle thoracentesis. Pass a flexible wire through the needle into the pleural space. Make a 1.5 cm horizontal incision at this site. Make a second horizontal incision 5 cm inferiorly with a subcutaneous tunnel created between the two horizontal incisions. A trocar guides the pleural catheter through the subcutaneous tunnel. Place a dilator with a peel-away sheath over the guidewire into the pleural space. Remove the dilator and thread the pleural catheter over the sheath into the pleural space. Remove the sheath and close the incision using interrupted non-absorbable sutures.

11. Connect the drain to an underwater seal bottle via a three-way tap and tubing. If the drain is correctly positioned in the pleural space it should swing in time with respiration and drain air or fluid.
12. Stitch and tape the drain in place on the chest wall.
13. Ensure adequate analgesia.
14. Warn the patient not to disconnect the tubing or lift the underwater bottle above the level of the insertion site on the chest; give patient a chest drain information sheet or pamphlet.
15. Obtain CXR to check position. The ideal tube position (apex for pneumothorax, base for effusion) is not necessary for effective drainage, so do not reposition functioning drains on this basis. CT may be useful in confirming drain position in certain circumstances.
16. In patients requiring assisted ventilation, especially those requiring high levels of positive end expiratory pressure (PEEP), it is essential to decrease PEEP during chest tube insertion to avoid the potentially serious complication of lung penetration.

Drain management

General considerations

Patients should be managed on a specialist ward by experienced nursing staff. Chest drain observations should be charted regularly, including swinging, bubbling, and volume of fluid output.

If the drain water level does not swing with respiration the drain is kinked (check underneath dressing, as tube enters the skin), blocked, clamped, or incorrectly positioned (drainage holes are not in the pleural space; check CXR). Occluded drains may sometimes be unblocked by a 30 mL saline flush. Nonfunctioning drains should be removed (risk of introducing infection).

Suction is sometimes used to encourage drainage, although there is a lack of evidence regarding its use. Consider using suction in cases of pneumothorax with persistent air leak or following chemical pleurodesis.

Chest drain removal

- Chest drains should be removed when the indication for placement is no longer present or the drain is nonfunctional.
- Chest drains can be removed if the lung is fully expanded and the fluid output is <200 mL/day in patients with pleural effusions. In patients with pneumothoraces, there should be no air leak during either suction or coughing.
- The chest drain should be removed while the patient either performs a Valsalva maneuver or is breath-holding in expiration. Recent data suggest that discontinuation of chest tubes at the end of inspiration or expiration have similar rates of post-removal pneumothoraces.
- Tie the previously placed mattress suture, if applicable. Apply dressing.
- A CXR should be obtained immediately following chest tube removal to document lung position, and 24 hours later to evaluate for pneumothoraces or reaccumulation of fluid.

Clamping vs. unclamping

Never clamp a bubbling chest drain (because of the risk of tension pneumothorax). Clamping may be considered in two situations:

- To control the rate of drainage of a large pleural effusion. Rapid drainage of large volumes may result in re-expansion pulmonary edema; clamping, e.g., for 1 hour after draining 1 L, may prevent this.
- To avoid inappropriate drain removal in cases of pneumothorax with a slow air leak, when bubbling appears to have ceased. In these situations, clamping of a drain for several hours followed by repeat CXR may detect very slow or intermittent air leaks. This approach is controversial, however, and should only be considered on a specialist ward with experienced nursing staff. If the patient becomes breathless, the drain should be immediately unclamped.

Chemical pleurodesis

Background
The purpose of pleurodesis is to eliminate potential space between the parietal and visceral pleura by creating inflammatory adhesions. Elimination of this space prohibits the accumulation of pleural fluid or air. Pleural inflammation is induced by the sclerosant to create the adhesions.

Indications
- Recurrent symptomatic pleural effusion due to malignant disease
- Recurrent, uncontrollable symptomatic effusions of benign origin: CHF, hepatic hydrothorax, yellow nail syndrome, etc.
- Recurrent pneumothorax

Contraindications and cautions
Failure of lung expansion may be due to trapped lung or bronchial obstruction. If bronchial obstruction is present, endobronchial laser ablation or stent placement may allow re-expansion and successful pleurodesis.

Methods of pleurodesis
- Chemical pleurodesis via tube thoracostomy
- Talc insufflation via pleuroscopy or thoracoscopy

Chemical pleurodesis
Common types of sclerosant include the following:
- Talc
  - 3–5 g, inexpensive
  - 90% success rate reported
- Bleomycin
  - 60 units, expensive
  - Efficacy approximately similar to that of talc
- Silver nitrate
  - May be as effective as talc

Technique
Preparation
1. Obtain informed consent after discussing the procedure, alternative methods, and risks and benefits with the patient.
2. Take time with the nursing and technical staff for proper identification of the patient and the site of procedure.
3. Use an established small-bore (8–14 Fr) chest tube for complete drainage. If daily drainage is >500 cc/day, consider palliative drainage with a tunneled catheter or surgical pleurodesis.
4. Evaluate CXR for complete fluid drainage and full expansion of the lung.

Talc pleurodesis
1. Establish IV access. Monitor blood pressure, pulse, temperature, respiratory rate, and oxygen saturation every 30 minutes for 2 hours, then hourly for an additional 6 hours. Provide oxygen supplementation as needed.

2. Systemic premedication is with opiates for analgesia and benzodiazepines for anxiolysis. Pleurodesis can be extremely painful. Exercise appropriate caution in elderly patients and those with hepatic or renal disease. Use acetaminophen to reduce fever.

3. Provide intrapleural analgesia with 1% lidocaine (max 3 mg/kg) using a sterile technique via chest tube. Clamp the tube and allow 10 minutes for dwell time.

4. Administer 4 g sterile talc suspension (range 3–5 g) in 30–50 cc saline using a sterile technique via chest tube. Ensure complete suspension of talc before administration.

5. Flush the chest tube with saline.

6. Clamp the chest tube for 1 hour. Some physicians use rotational positioning. After 1 hour, unclamp the tube and start drainage with -20 cm/H_2O suction.

7. Continue systemic analgesia, antipyretics, and anxiolytics every 4–6 hours as needed for the next 24–48 hours.

8. The duration of chest tube drainage after sclerosant administration is unclear. A good guideline is reduction of daily drainage <150–200 cc in 24 hours. Removal at 12–72 hours has been reported.

Complications

- *Common*: Fever, pleurisy, mild hypoxemia, diffuse pulmonary infiltrates
- *Uncommon*: Acute lung injury or ARDS, empyema, arrhythmia, hypotension
- In patients with mesothelioma, consider prophylactic radiation of the chest tube insertion site to prevent seeding of the tract.
- Because of long-term concerns regarding potential asbestos contamination, talc is usually reserved for malignant processes. In benign conditions, mechanical abrasion is the method of choice, with chemical pleurodesis used in those with surgical contraindications.

Further reading

Glazer M, Berkman N, Lafair JS, Kramer MR (2000). Successful talc slurry pleurodesis in patients with nonmalignant pleural effusion. *Chest* **117**(5):1404–1409.

Goodman A, Davies CWH (2006). Efficacy of short-term versus long-term chest tube drainage following talc slurry pleurodesis in patients with malignant pleural effusions: a randomised trial. *Lung Cancer* **54**:51–55.

Haddad FJ, Younes RN, Gross JL, Deheinelin D (2004). Pleurodesis in patients with malignant pleural effusions: talc slurry or bleomycin? Results of a prospective randomized trial. *World J Surg* **28**(8):749–754.

Kennedy L, Rusch VW, Strange C, Ginsberg RJ, Sahn SA (1994). Pleurodesis using talc slurry. *Chest* **106**:342–346.

Paschoalini MS, Vargas FS, Marchi E, Pereira JR, Jatene FB, Antonangelo L, et al. (2005). Prospective randomized trial of silver nitrate vs. talc slurry in pleurodesis for symptomatic malignant pleural effusions. *Chest* **128**(2):684–689.

Zimmer PW, Hill M, Casey K, Harvey E, Low DE (1997). Prospective randomized trial of talc slurry vs bleomycin in pleurodesis for symptomatic malignant pleural effusions. *Chest* **112**(2):430–434.

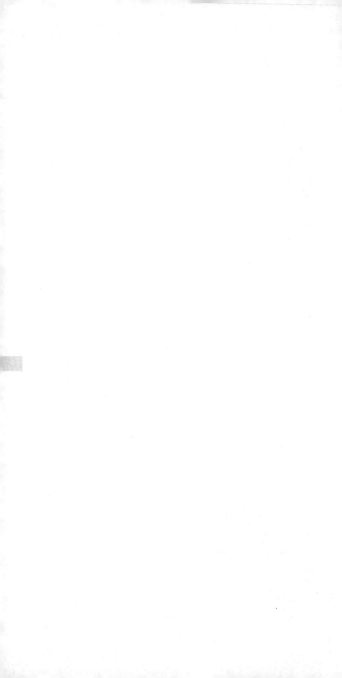

Medical thoracoscopy

Medical thoracoscopy or pleuroscopy, in contrast to video-assisted thoracic surgery (VATS), is performed by chest physicians, using conscious sedation and local anesthetic. The procedure involves examination of the pleural cavity, which includes the chest wall, parietal and visceral pleura, lung, and diaphragm, by means of a pleuroscope and is used for taking a biopsy of the parietal pleura. Chemical pleurodesis can also be performed at the same time.

An adequate pleural space for insertion of the pleuroscope is required to avoid damaging the underlying lung. Patients suitable for thoracoscopy are those who have an underlying pleural effusion or a pneumothorax where the lung is away from the predetermined insertion site.

The procedure can be performed with rigid telescopes or flex-rigid pleuroscopes in an endoscopy suite.

Indications for thoracoscopy
- Undiagnosed exudative pleural effusion where the diagnostic accuracy of medical thoracoscopy is 95%
- Suspected mesothelioma
- Staging of pleural effusion in lung cancer
- Treatment of recurrent pleural effusions with talc poudrage
- Pneumothorax requiring chemical pleurodesis as an alternative in a patient unfit for VATS

Contraindications and cautions
- Obliterated pleural space
- Pleural adhesions, as these may tear underlying lung when pneumothorax is induced
- Bleeding disorder
- Hypoxia <92% on air
- Unstable cardiovascular disease
- Persistent, uncontrollable cough

Risks associated with thoracoscopy
The mortality rate is low (0.09%–0.24%).
- Hemorrhage, which may need diathermy in the pleural space; rare
- Lung laceration; rare
- Air or gas embolism during pneumothorax induction; rare, <0.1%
- Local wound infection
- Empyema
- Fever, ARDS with talc poudrage (see pp. 786–7).

Preparation of patient and consent
- The patient should have written information >24 hours before the procedure. The doctor performing the procedure should obtain written consent.
- Check recent CXR and any CT scans that are available.
- Check CBC, coagulation profile, electrolytes, and renal panel.
- Nothing should be taken by mouth 4 hours pre-procedure.
- Take time with the nursing and technical staff for proper identification of the patient and site of the procedure.

- Insert an IV cannula in the arm on the same side as the thoracoscopy to enable repeated sedative administration during the procedure.
- Premedication is with analgesia, such as a single dose of oral ibuprofen 800 mg, 1–2 hours before the procedure.
- Provide antibiotics, such as cefuroxime 1.5 g IV, for infection prophylaxis.
- Monitor baseline oxygen saturations, pulse, BP, and temperature.

Equipment

- Rigid instruments: stainless steel trocars measuring 5–10 mm, telescopes with different viewing angles (0°, 30°, 50°), 5 mm optical forceps or coagulating tooth forceps for parietal pleural biopsy. A cold (xenon) light source, endoscopic camera to attach to the eyepiece of a telescope, video monitor, and recorder are also required.
- Autoclavable flex-rigid pleuroscope (Olympus LTF 160) fashioned like a bronchoscope with a rigid shaft and flexible tip that allows two-way angulation. A 10 mm disposable trocar, flexible biopsy forceps, and standard accessories that can be inserted through a 2.8 mm working channel of the pleuroscope are also needed. This instrument interfaces well with processors (CV-160, CLV-U40) and light sources (CV-240, EVIS-100 or 140, EVIS EXERA 145 or 160) made by the manufacturer for flexible bronchoscopy or GI endoscopy.

Procedure

- Place the patient in the lateral decubitus position with the affected side (pleural effusion or pneumothorax) up and arm raised above the head.
- Continuously monitor oxygen saturation by pulse oximetry, as well as ECG and BP.
- Administer sedation (midazolam) intravenously and titrate according to patient comfort.
- Administer oxygen (2–4 L/min) via nasal cannula.
- Clean the skin and administer local anesthetic to the selected intercostal space in the same way as for a chest tube.
- Aspiration of fluid or air from the pleural space confirms that it is safe to proceed with pleuroscopy. Make an incision and perform blunt dissection until the pleural space is entered. Then insert the trocar and drain pleural fluid via a suction tube through the trocar or under visualization using the flex-rigid pleuroscope.
- Allow air to enter the pleural space through this port so that the lung does not reinflate, and create a pneumothorax. Insert the telescope with its light source or flex-rigid pleuroscope through the port and inspect the chest cavity. Usually a single puncture is sufficient for pleural space examination and for obtaining biopsy of the parietal pleura. Occasionally, a second port of entry is required for other instruments such as diathermy for control of hemorrhage or lung biopsy with the coagulating forceps.
- Thoracoscopic biopsies are usually large and yield good diagnostic results. If the pleural surfaces have appearances consistent with malignancy, pleurodesis can be performed at the end of the procedure with talc via an insufflator.

Post-thoracoscopy care

- Monitor oxygen saturations, pulse, BP, and temperature.
- The patient will have a chest drain in situ. This should be on free drainage initially, then continuous suction is required when the drain stops bubbling
- Analgesia as required, such as IV fentanyl or Versed, and po Percocet.
- DVT prophylaxis with subcutaneous heparin (increased coagulopathy is observed with talc pleurodesis)
- CXR on the morning after thoracoscopy
- Remove the chest drain when the lung is reinflated on CXR with minimal fluid drainage or absence of bubbling in the chest drain. Trapped lung occurs if the visceral pleura is too thick to allow lung reinflation.
- If mesothelioma is diagnosed, refer patient for radiation to thoracoscopy and chest drain tract sites.

Further information

Lee P, Colt HG (2005). Rigid and semi-rigid pleuroscopy: The future is bright. *Respirology* **10**:418–425.

Lee P, Colt HG (2005). Flex-rigid pleuroscopy: step by step. In *CMP Medica Asia* 2005.

Rodriguez-Panadero F, Janssen JP, Astoul P (2006). Thoracoscopy: general overview and place in the diagnosis and management of pleural effusion. *Eur Respir J* **28**:409–422.

Tassi GF, Davies RJ, Noppen M (2006). Advanced techniques in medical thoracoscopy. *Eur Respir J* **28**:1051–1059.

Some diagnostic tests

Skin-prick tests

These may be useful in identifying specific allergens causing immediate hypersensitivity reactions. They may influence management and guide allergen avoidance. They are also used to help define atopy. Triggers in contact urticaria, atopic eczema, and suspected food allergy may also be identified. The results are available almost immediately (compared to a RAST test for specific IgE), and correlate well with RAST test results. They should be carried out by staff trained to deal with adverse reactions and to read the tests.

The allergens chosen for testing should be identified from the history, and usually include common aeroallergens, e.g., grass, house dust mite (*D. pteronyssinus*), and cat dander.

Practical points

- All antihistamines should be stopped prior to testing; chronic steroid use may influence skin reactivity.
- There is a very small risk of anaphylaxis; adrenaline and resuscitation equipment should be available. Particular care is needed with food and latex testing.
- Put a drop of allergen on the skin (usually the inside forearm).
- A range of allergens are commercially available. Fresh produce should be used for suspected fruit and vegetable hypersensitivity.
- Lance the skin through the allergen drop using a needle (do not draw blood). This should be with a calibrated lancet (1 mm) held vertically, or a hypodermic needle held at a 45° angle to the skin.
- The positive control is usually histamine, and the negative control the dilutent (usually saline).
- Read the test after 15 to 20 minutes
- A positive result is an itchy weal, which should be compared with the controls, as some subjects may react to the skin prick alone (dermatographism).
- A wheal of 3 mm or more larger than the saline control is considered positive (indicating allergen sensitization).
- A positive result does not prove that the clinical symptoms are due to bronchial hyperresponsiveness to the tested allergen, but does raise clinical suspicion. Positive results can occur in those without symptoms, and false negatives do occur.

RAST, or radioallergosorbent blood tests, are more specific but less sensitive and more expensive than skin-prick tests, and they give similar information. There is no risk of anaphylaxis and the patient does not need to stop steroids or antihistamines for the test to be performed.

Technique of induced sputum

- Used to investigate for infection (e.g., TB, PCP) or airway inflammation
- Patients rinse their mouth and clean their teeth to minimize oral contamination. They are given an inhaled bronchodilator (e.g., albuterol) to minimize bronchoconstriction when indicated.
- Nebulized hypertonic (3%, 5%, or 10%) saline is administered via a mouthpiece or a facemask. Afterwards, the patient expectorates sputum into a sterile container.
- If infection is likely, perform the test in a negative pressure room or booth, with appropriate protection of staff and other patients. Do not perform it on the open ward or outpatient department unless in an enclosed booth.
- Send sputum promptly to microbiology for staining and culture, and direct immunofluorescent testing for PCP (if indicated). Sputum for cell counts is mixed with 0.1% dithiothreitol and diluted with saline, then filtered and centrifuged.

Methacholine challenge testing

- This testing is helpful if there is doubt about the diagnosis of airway hyperreactivity or asthma.
- Low concentrations of inhaled methacholine induce clinically significant airway obstruction (bronchospasm) in patients with hyperreactive airways.
- Testing should be performed by experienced personnel, with facilities to deal with acute severe bronchospasm.
- Beginning with very low concentrations, increasing doses of nebulized methacholine are given by inhalation, with the FEV_1 measured after each dose.
- The test is stopped after a 20% fall in FEV_1, or if the highest concentration of methacholine has been given.
- The concentration of drug causing the 20% fall is known as the PC_{20}.
- Airway hyperreactivity is indicated by a PC_{20} of below 8 mg/mL. Normal subjects have a PC_{20} >16 mg/mL.

Appendices

Lung function testing

Flow–volume loop

The flow–volume loop plots inspiratory and expiratory flow against lung volume during a maximal expiratory and maximal inspiratory maneuver (see Fig. App.1.1).

At the beginning of **expiration** after taking a full breath in, the expiratory muscles are at their strongest, the lungs at their biggest, and hence the airways are at their most open (A). The lungs at this point are at total lung capacity (TLC). Because the lungs are at their largest, the radial attachments to the airways, effectively the alveolar–capillary membranes and their connective tissue, are pulling the hardest and supporting the airways against **dynamic compression** during the exhalation maneuver.

This means that the highest flow rates are possible at the beginning of the blow, hence the sudden rise to a **peak expiratory flow rate** in the 100 ms or so of the forced breath out, (B). This is the **peak flow** and is essentially what a peak flow meter measures.

As the lung empties and the lung volume drops, the dilatory pull on the airways from the radial attachments of the surrounding lung tissue reduces (C). Hence the airways narrow and become less supported and are less able to resist dynamic compression. This means that the maximal airflow obtainable, regardless of effort, falls too.

Eventually the expiratory muscles cannot squeeze the chest anymore. Also, increasingly with age, the small airways may actually close off, preventing further emptying (D). The volume at which this begins to happen is called the **closing volume**. The final lung volume at the end of expiration is called the *residual volume* (RV).

As maximal **inspiration** starts, although the inspiratory muscles are at their strongest, the airways are at their smallest. Thus flow rates start low and increase as the airways open up. However, as the airways open up, the inspiratory muscles approach their limit and, accordingly, the flow rates fall again; hence the different, rounded, appearance of the inspiratory limb of the flow–volume curve.

Normally the inspiratory and expiratory flow rates depend on lung volume and are termed "volume-dependent." If there is a **fixed upper airway narrowing**, such as from a fibrous tumor in the trachea, the size of the airway will not vary with lung volumes and flow becomes "volume-independent." Figure App.1.2 shows this.

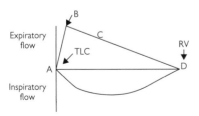

Figure App.1.1 Flow–volume loop: maximal expiratory and inspiratory maneuver.

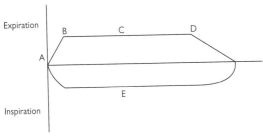

Figure App.1.2 Flow–volume loop: fixed upper airway narrowing.

At A, the rise in flow will initially be normal, but at some point the maximum flow imposed by the upper airway narrowing will cut in (B). From that point onward the flow rate will be fixed at this maximum (C) until the lower recoil and narrowing small airways again determine the maximum flow (D). The flow volume curve has been severely "clipped" with a square-like appearance. The same clipped appearance will be present on the inspiratory limb (E).

   Sometimes, such upper airway restriction may be *variable* rather than fixed and is only present on inspiration (e.g. paralyzed and collapsing vocal chords being sucked in, and then blown open again on expiration).

- Thus a square inspiratory limb, but normal expiratory limb, provides evidence of a mobile, **extrathoracic upper airways obstruction** (see Fig. App.1.3).

Conversely, a mobile intrathoracic upper airway obstruction (e.g., fleshy tumor at the carina, or retrosternal thyroid) may obstruct more during expiration with corresponding lower lung volumes, compared to inspiration when the chest is being expanded.

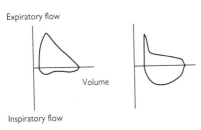

Figure App.1.3 Flow–volume loop: extrathoracic upper airways obstruction.

- Thus a square expiratory limb, but normal inspiratory limb, is evidence of a *variable intrathoracic upper airways obstruction*.

The other, more common causes of airway obstruction are due to narrowing of the lower airways (asthma, COPD). In these conditions the airway caliber (and thus flow rates) still remain dependent on lung volume. Hence the flow rates decrease as the lung volume decreases, but particularly so at low lung volumes. This is because resistance to flow is proportional to the airway radius raised to the power of 4 (r^4) and thus is most significant when airways are already small.

Hence increasing airflow obstruction produces expiratory flow–volume curves like those in Figure App.1.4. This greater effect of small airways narrowing at low lung volumes has led some units to report flow rates at, for example, 25% expired lung volume, or averaged between 25% and 75% of the total expired lung volume.

The airways can be so small that some begin to close off at lower lung volumes (the *closing volume*); hence a full breath out is not possible, producing air trapping and a raised residual volume (RV) (A). Sensitive tests of small airways narrowing have to concentrate on flows at low lung volumes, and peak flow measurements are relatively insensitive.

- Peak flow measurements are most sensitive to upper airway narrowing.

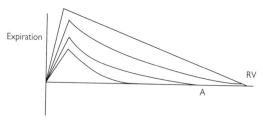

Figure App.1.4 Expiratory flow–volume curve for increasing airflow obstruction.

Spirometry, peak flow measurements, and CO transfer

Spirometry and peak flow measurements

- The ordinary spirometer records **volumes against time** rather than **flows against volume.**
- The two essential measures are **FEV₁** and **VC**.

The *vital capacity (VC)* is the maximum amount of air that can be blown out completely. This will be **reduced** if the lungs or chest wall are **stiff** (preventing a full breath in), the **inspiratory muscles are weak** (preventing a full breath in), or the **airways are narrowed** such that the small airways collapse during expiration (preventing a full breath out). Suboptimal effort will also result in a low VC.

The FEV_1 is the amount (forced expiratory volume) that can be blown out in 1 second. It is less effort-dependent and generally more robust. The ratio of the two values (FEV_1/VC) reveals whether airflow obstruction is present.

A ratio of FEV_1/VC of less than about 70%–75% indicates airflow obstruction, although this varies with age. A more accurate indicator is whether the ratio is within the normal range as defined by the lower limit of normal based on predicted values derived from the National Health and Nutrition Examination Survey (NHANES) III reference equations. These are based on NHANES III data (see end of Appendix 1).

The degree, or severity, of airflow obstruction is gauged by the FEV_1 expressed as a percentage of the predicted value based on the NHANES III reference range.

- Airflow obstruction ratings are as follows:
  - Mild FEV_1 = >70% predicted
  - Moderate FEV_1 = 60%–69% predicted
  - Moderately severe FEV_1 = 50%–59% predicted
  - Severe FEV_1 = 35%–49% predicted
  - Very severe FEV_1 = <35% predicted

It is important to realize that the range of normality is considerable, and it may not be clear if a set of results is simply at the bottom end of normal or is considerably reduced from the patient's normally much higher figures. Serial measurements indicating continuing deterioration may be the first clue.

When airflow obstruction is present, one may further determine whether obstruction is reversible with bronchodilator therapy. This is done by repeating spirometry 15 minutes after inhalation of a short-acting bronchodilator such as albuterol. A bronchodilator response is present if the FEV_1 or FVC increase by at least 12% and 200 mL from baseline values.

A restrictive pattern may occur in any lung disease that results in loss of lung volume (e.g., interstitial lung disease, pleural disease, or chest wall stiffening), as well as in the setting of severe obstruction, neuromuscular weakness, or suboptimal effort. To accurately define restriction (low TLC) one needs to measure lung volumes directly. The FEV_1/VC ratio may actually be raised in interstitial lung disease, as the airways are better supported by the fibrosed radial attachments, which reduces dynamic compression.

The *slope* of the volume–time plot from a spirometer is effectively the *flow rate* at any particular point.

Diffusing capacity (carbon monoxide transfer)

This test is an index of the amount of **gas exchanging surface area** available. A gas mixture containing CO is inhaled, the breath held for 10 seconds, and then exhaled. The amount that has disappeared (by crossing the alveolar–capillary membrane and being taken up by red cells) is calculated. A correction for hemoglobin concentration is required, as the amount of CO transferred will fall as the available hemoglobin is reduced.

The **total amount of CO transferred is the diffusing capacity of the lung for CO (DLCO)**. The total lung volume "reached" by the CO is the amount breathed in, *plus* the amount of air already in the lung at the start of inspiration. This is measured by including an inert gas such as helium in the inhaled gas mixture that is then diluted by the air already in the lung; thus by comparing the concentration of the inspired inert gas with the expired concentration, total lung volume can be calculated. The total lung volume measured in this way is called the *alveolar volume*, VA.

The DLCO is often expressed as a ratio of DLCO to VA, which appears to "correct" the DLCO for the VA. However, this is not accurate, as the DLCO/VA actually reflects the intrinsic ability of the lung to transfer CO. Thus, the DLCO is a global measure of gas transfer that reflects the product of intrinsic diffusing capacity of the lung (DLCO/VA) and the total lung volume available for gas transfer (VA).

- The DLCO and DLCO/VA are *reduced* most in emphysema when alveoli have been destroyed, or in pulmonary vascular disease, which disrupts capillary function directly. They are also reduced in interstitial and fibrotic lung diseases.
- The DLCO is usually *normal* in asthma or chronic bronchitis. In some patients with asthma, the DLCO may be slightly elevated.
- The DLCO and DLCO/VA may be *increased* in the presence of pulmonary hemorrhage, as can occur in SLE, Goodpasture's disease, and pulmonary vasculitis. This is because the free red cells lining the alveoli take up CO directly and "falsely" elevate the figure.

The diffusing capacity test requires more cooperation than simple spiroetry, as well as a minimum inspired volume.

Respiratory muscle function, body plethysmography, and lung volumes

Respiratory muscle function

See Figure App. 1.5 and Table App. 1.1.

Respiratory failure and a small VC may be due to weak respiratory muscles. It is therefore useful to be able to assess inspiratory and expiratory muscle power. There may be global weakness or specific inspiratory, usually diaphragm, weakness.

In the clinic the simplest test is a **lying and standing VC**. If the diaphragm is paralyzed, then on lying down the abdominal contents will push up on the diaphragm and limit inspiration. On standing the abdominal contents drop and aid inspiration.

- A fall in VC of <10% on lying down is probably normal.
- A fall of 10%–20% is suspicious for diaphragm paralysis.
- A fall of >20% is abnormal and suggests significant, usually bilateral, diaphragm paralysis.

In the laboratory there are various ways to test respiratory muscle function. In one approach the patient blows against a *pressure meter* after a maximum inspiration (maximal expiratory pressure [MEP]), and inspires against the meter after a full expiration (maximal inspiratory pressure [MIP]). This is, of course, highly effort-dependent.

More accurate assessments of inspiratory muscle function, particularly the diaphragm, can be obtained using two esophageal balloons placed above and below the diaphragm and connected to pressure transducers. *Transdiaphragmatic pressures* during maximal inspiratory efforts, sniffing, and breathing to TLC all provide reproducible measures of diaphragm function, but depend on good cooperation and effort by the patient.

Body plethysmography

In this procedure the patient sits in a closed cabinet (a "body box") and breaths through a mouthpiece connected to the outside. It has two particular advantages over simpler lung function tests: it can measure the TLC and it provides a measure of airways obstruction (airways resistance), requiring little or no effort by the patient.

The other main method of measuring TLC involves inert gas dilution as described above. However, in the presence of small airways obstruction, the inert gas may not reach all parts of the lung during the 10-second breath hold, and the volume of dilution will therefore be lower than the real TLC. The body plethysmograph relies on the pressure changes that occur when all the air in the chest is alternately compressed and expanded by the patient making breathing efforts against a airway closed by a shutter at the mouth. The pressure changes in the oral cavity are then proportional to the volume of air being compressed and expanded, thus allowing calculation of the volume of air in the chest at the time.

Note that this volume will include any bullae or cysts in the lung. The *difference between the plethysmographic lung volume and the inert gas dilution volume will reflect the volume of these bullae or cytsts* as well as areas not reached by the helium due to increased airways resistance.

Measurement of *airways resistance* with the body box relies on a similar principle. If there were no airways resistance, then breathing in and out would not compress or expand the air in the chest. With increasing resistance, the air in the chest will be compressed during expiration and expanded on inspiration. This results in the generation of pressure with flow, thus allowing calculation of airways resistance during quiet breathing or panting (the latter ensures the vocal chords are fully open and not contributing to the measured resistance).

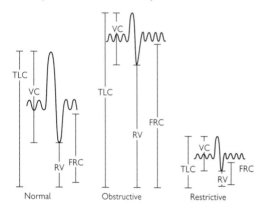

Figure App.1.5 Lung volumes in normal, obstructive, and restrictive lung conditions. TLC, total lung capacity; VC, vital capacity; RV, residual volume; FRC, functional residual capacity; FEV$_1$, forced expiratory volume in 1 second.

Table 1 Typical lung function changes in obstructive and restrictive diseases

Derivative	Obstructive	Restrictive
FEV$_1$ (% predicted)	↓	↓
VC (% predicted)	N or ↓	↓
FEV$_1$/VC ratio	↓	N or ↑ (increased recoil)
TLC (% predicted)	N or ↑	↓
RV (% predicted)	↑	↓
FRC (% predicted)	N or ↑	↓
RV/TLC ratio	↑ (gas trapping)	N

N = normal; ↓ = decreased; ↑ = increased.

Predicted values for FEV$_1$, VC, and peak flow can be determined by reference equations in Hankinson JL, Odencrantz JR, Fedan KB (1999). Spirometric reference values from a sample of the general US population. *Am J Respir Crit Care Med* **159**:179–187.

Blood gases and acid–base balance

Introduction

Normal ranges

Normals ranges are as follows:
- pH 7.35–7.45
- $PaCO_2$ (partial pressure of CO_2) 35–45 mmHg
- HCO_3^- (serum bicarbonate) 22–26 mmol/L

How to take

Arterial blood gases (ABGs) can be drawn from the radial, brachial, femoral, dorsalis pedis, and, rarely, axillary arteries. The radial artery is the most commonly used site because of ease of access and dual radial–ulnar supply to the hand.

The Allen test should be preformed before puncture of the radial artery to evaluate for sufficient dual circulation. The test involves lifting the arm high with a clenched fist and with the radial and ulnar arteries compressed. Then the arm is lowered and pressure on the ulnar artery released. If the circulation is sufficient, the hand should turn pink within 6 seconds. This procedure is repeated with the radial artery. After sterile preparation, the artery can be punctured with a heparinized syringe. If it takes >10 seconds an abnormal circulation is indicated and that side arm should not be used.

The specimen should be analyzed immediately, or within 15 minutes if kept on crushed ice. Always record the date and time of the specimen and the percent of inspired O_2.

Interpretation of arterial blood gases: 1. Hypoxia

Hypoxia

PaO_2 (partial pressure of O_2) is <60 mmHg; however, the normal range changes according to altitude and atmospheric pressure.

Hypoxia can occur in the following conditions:

- V/Q mismatch—the differential includes chronic lung disease (asthma, COPD, alveolar disease, interstitial disease, pulmonary embolism, pulmonary hypertension). Oxygenation improves with 100% oxygen.
- Right-to-left shunt, such as with pneumonia, ARDS, pulmonary AV malformation, and intracardiac shunt. Oxygenation does not improve with 100% oxygen.
- Hypoventilation, such as with narcosis and obesity hypoventilation syndrome
- High altitude, because of a low partial pressure of oxygen
- Low mixed venous oxygen, because of increased oxygen consumption (sepsis), poor oxygen delivery (anemia, methemoglobinemia, CO poisoning), or low cardiac output
- Decreased diffusion can cause hypoxia in end-stage COPD and late-stage fibrosis.

To further understand the cause of hypoxia, an alveolar–arterial (A–a) oxygen tension gradient should be calculated.

The A–a gradient at sea level = $150 - (PaO_2 + 1.25[PaCO_2])$.

The equation for higher altitude = $PAO_2 - PaO_2$

PAO_2 = partial pressure of oxygen in the alveoli

PaO_2 = partial pressure of oxygen in the artery

$PAO_2 = [(P_b - P_{H2O}) \times FiO_2] - [PaCO_2/0.8]$.

FiO_2 = fraction of inspired oxygen (room air $FiO_2 = 0.21$)

P_b = barometric pressure

P_{H2O} = partial pressure of water at 37°C = 47.

Normal A–a is ~5–15. More accurately, normal can be calculated by ≤0.3 × age or (age/4) + 4.

The A–a gradient is normal in hypoxia because of hypoventilation or high altitude, while the other causes result in an increased A–a gradient.

Interpretation of arterial blood gases: 2 Acid–base disorders

Acid–base balance is maintained by the kidneys and lungs via buffering:

$$HCO_3^- + H^+ \leftrightarrow H_2CO_3 \leftrightarrow H_2O + CO_2$$

The bicarbonate is managed by the kidney, and the CO_2 by the lung.

Acidemia occurs when there is an increased production of acid or an increased loss of bicarbonate, which lowers the pH. Conversely, *alkalemia* occurs from excessive bicarbonate accumulation or loss of acid.

Compensation occurs in response to acid–base disorders to lessen the overall change in pH from normal. The respiratory compensation commences immediately and full response occurs in 12–24 hours. Renal compensation is slower and can take 3–5 days.

Complex acid–base disorders can exist depending on the patient's clinical setting. A triple acid–base disorder can occur, but a quadruple acid–base disorder cannot, because a respiratory acidosis and a respiratory alkalosis cannot occur simultaneously.

Steps to ABG interpretation

1. Are the data accurate?
2. What is the primary process—acidemia or alkalemia? Is the disorder metabolic or respiratory?
3. If metabolic acidosis is present, is there an anion gap? Is the respiratory compensation appropriate?
4. If metabolic alkalosis is present, is it saline responsive or unresponsive? Is the respiratory compensation appropriate?
5. If respiratory acidosis or alkalosis is present, is it acute or chronic?
6. What is the anion gap?

Other blood work necessary for ABG interpretation is an electrolyte panel and albumin.

Step 1

- Data inconsistency can occur due to lab error or when evaluating data points from different blood draws.
- To evaluate for accuracy of data, use the Henderson–Hasselbach equation.

- Calculated $[H^+] = 24 \times (PaCO_2/[HCO_3^-])$
- To obtain the expected $[H^+]$ for a given pH, use Table App.2.1 **or** calculate using the rule that with every change in pH by 0.01 units from 7.4, the expected $[H^+]$ inversely changes by 1 mmol/L. If there is a difference between the calculated and the expected $[H^+]$, there is data inaccuracy and the blood draw should be repeated.

Step 2

- Evaluate the pH. Normal pH is 7.35–7.45. Alkalemia is defined as pH >7.45 and acidemia is defined at pH <7.35.
- If the pH indicates acidemia
  - There is a metabolic component if the bicarbonate is <22 mmol/L (proceed to Step 3)
  - There is a respiratory component if the pCO_2 is >45 mmHg (proceed to Step 5)
- If the pH indicates alkalemia
  - There is a metabolic component if the bicarbonate is >26 mmol/L (proceed to Step 4)
  - There is a respiratory component if the $PaCO_2$ is <35 mmHg (proceed to Step 5)
- When there is compensation or in complex disorders, the pH may be normal, therefore the HCO_3^- and $PaCO_2$ should be assessed for abnormalities despite a normal pH.

Step 3

Metabolic acidosis (bicarbonate <22 mmol/L)

Causes are listed in Table App.2.2 and Table App.2.3.

- The anion gap (AG) is a calculation to evaluate the difference between the unmeasured anions and unmeasured cations:

  $[Na^+] - ([Cl^-] + [HCO_3^-])$; normal is 12 ± 2 mEq/L

- Factors that can cause an inaccurately low AG are hypoalbuminemia, hyponatremia, paraproteinemia, and increased potassium, magnesium, calcium, and ammonium. Evaluate the history of the patient and obtain an albumin level. If the albumin is low, estimate a 2.5–3 increase in AG for every 1 g/dL decrease in albumin or calculate the corrected AG:

  AG correct $= AG + 0.25 \times (40 - albumin)$

- Lactate, urine, and serum ketones should be checked with an AG acidosis and the delta and osmolal gap should be calculated:

  Delta gap = (Patient's AG − Normal AG) − (Normal HCO_3^- [Patient's HCO_3^-]) = (Patient's AG − 12) − (24 − Patient's HCO_3^-)

  - Normal delta gap is 0 ± 6.
  - A positive delta gap (especially if >6) indicates an additional acid–base disorder of metabolic alkalosis or respiratory acidosis.
  - A negative delta gap (especially if < −6) indicates an additional non-AG metabolic acidosis or chronic respiratory alkalosis.

  Osmolal gap = measured osmolality − calculated osmolality

  $Osmolal_{calc}$ = 2[Na] + (BUN/2.8) + (glucose/18)

  - Normal osmolal gap is <10 mOsm. Osmolal gap of >10 mOsm suggests ingestion of toxin such as ethylene glycol or methanol.
- If the AG is normal, even with correction for albumin, then the cause is a non-AG metabolic acidosis, which indicates a high Cl and low bicarbonate. Low or negative corrected AG can result from lab error, lithium toxicity, severe hypernatremia, IgG myeloma, hypercalceimia, and hypermagnesemia.
- Calculate the urine AG for non-AG acidosis:

  (Urine Na^+ + Urine K^+) − Urine Cl

  - Normal is −10 to +10.
- Negative urine gap (especially < −10): consider GI loss of bicarbonate
- Positive urine anion gap (especially > −10): consider renal loss of bicarbonate
- To evaluate for appropriate respiratory compensation in metabolic acidosis, calculate the expected:

  $PaCO_2$ = 1.5 × $[HCO_3^-]$ + 8 ± 2 = Winter's equation.

Step 4

Metabolic alkalosis (bicarbonate >26 mmol/L)
A list of causes is listed on Table App.2.4.
- Calculate expected respiratory compensation:

  $PaCO_2$ = (0.7 x HCO_3^-) + 21 ± 1.5

- The maximum respiratory compensation is 50–55 mmHg. If the $PaCO_2$ is higher than 55 mmHg, the respiratory component likely has an underlying respiratory acidosis.
- To evaluate if the cause is saline responsive or saline resistant, check the Urine Cl. Urine Cl <20 mmol/L is saline responsive while Urine Cl >20 mmol/L is saline resistant.

Step 5

Respiratory acidosis ($PaCO_2$ >45 mmHg)
A list of causes is listed on Table App.2.5.

Acute
- Expected increase from normal $[HCO_3^-] = [(PaCO_2 - 40) \times 0.1] \pm 3$
  or for every 10 mmHg increase in $PaCO_2$, an estimated increase in HCO_3^- by 1 mmol/L and a drop in pH by 0.08 units
- Maximum acute metabolic compensation is $[HCO_3^-]$ 30–32 mmol/L

Chronic
- Expected increase from normal $[HCO_3^-] = [(PaCO_2 - 40) \times 0.35] \pm 4$
  or for every 10 mmHg increase in $PaCO_2$, an estimated increase HCO_3^- by 4 mmol/L and a drop in pH by 0.034 units
- Maximum chronic metabolic compensation is $[HCO_3^-]$ 45–50 mmol/L

Respiratory alkalosis ($PaCO_2$ <35 mmHg)
A list of causes is listed on Table App.2.6.

Acute
- Expected decrease from normal $[HCO_3^-] = (40 - PaCO_2) \times 0.2$ **or** for every 10 mmHg decrease in $PaCO_2$, an estimated decrease in HCO_3^- by 2 mmol/L and an increase in pH by 0.08 units

Chronic
- Expected decrease from normal $[HCO_3^-] = (40 - PaCO_2) \times 0.4$ **or** for every 10 mmHg decrease in $PaCO_2$, an estimated decrease in HCO_3^- by 5 mmol/L and an increase in pH by 0.04 units

Step 6

Always calculate an anion gap, regardless of pH and serum bicarbonate. If there is an anion gap, always calculate the delta gap and osmolal gap as discussed above.

Base excess
- Evaluating the base excess (BE) is another form of assessing a patient's acid–base status. The BE is calculated by:

  $$BE = 0.93 \times ([HCO_3^-] + 14.84 \times (pH\ 7.4) - 24.4)$$

  - Normal is −3 to +3 mEq/L
- BE >3 mEq/L indicates a primary metabolic alkalosis or compensation for respiratory acidosis.
- BE < −3 mEq/L indicates a primary metabolic acidosis or compensation for respiratory alkalosis.

Table App.2.1 pH levels with corresponding expected [H+]

pH	[H+]
7.80	16
7.75	18
7.70	20
7.65	22
7.60	25
7.55	28
7.50	32
7.45	35
7.40	40
7.35	45
730	50
7.25	56
7.20	63
7.15	71
7.10	79
7.05	89
7.0	100

Table App.2.2 Causes of anion gap metabolic acidosis

- Lactic acidosis
  - D-lactic acidosis
  - Liver disease
  - Shock, cardiac arrest, sever hypoxia, tissue ischemia
  - Severe exercise
  - Seizure
  - Hereditary (enzyme deficiencies or mitochondrial diseases)
  - Malignancies
  - Renal replacement fluids
  - Rhabdomyolysis
  - Toxins: e.g., toluene (glue sniffing)
  - Medications: metformin, nucleoside reverse transcriptase inhibitors, linezolid, lorazepam, propofol, β_2 agonists, salicylates, HIV medications
- Ketoacidosis
  - Diabetic
  - Alcohol-induced
  - Starvation
- Kidney failure
- Toxin ingestion
  - Ethylene glycol
  - Methanol
  - Salicylates
- Paraldehyde

Table App.2.3 Causes of non-anion gap metabolic acidosis

- GI losses
  - Diarrhea
  - Ostomy (ileal or proximal colon)
  - Ureteral/enteric diversion
- Renal losses
  - Renal tubular acidosis (RTA)
  - Acute tubular necrosis (ATN)
- Chronic tubulointerstitial disease
  - Hypoaldosteronism
- Medications
  - Carbonic anhydrase inhibitor
  - Aldosterone inhibitors
  - Ammonium chloride
  - Total parenteral nutrition (TPN)
  - Large-volume saline—dilutional acidosis
  - Exogenous hydrochloric acid
- Post-hypocapnia

Table App.2.4 Causes of metabolic alkalosis

- GI losses: emesis, nasogastric suctioning, diarrhea with high Cl⁻, e.g., laxative abuse
- Villous adenoma
- Chronic diuretic use
- Refeeding syndrome
- Posthypercapnia
- High-dose carbenicillin
- Increased mineralocorticoid activity
  - Primary hyperaldosteronism
  - Primary hypercortisolism
  - Exogenous steroid
  - Hyperreninemic state
  - Bartter's and Gitelman's syndromes
- Excess licorice injection
- Chronic kidney failure
- Hypokalemia
- Milk-alkali syndrome
- Hypercalcemia
- Massive blood transfusions
- Sweat losses in cystic fibrosis

Table App.2.5 Causes of respiratory acidosis

- Diseases of airway obstruction: bronchospasm, upper airways obstruction, laryngospasm
- Parenchymal abnormalities: pneumonia, pulmonary edema, acute ARDS, obstructive and restrictive diseases, pulmonary hemorrhage
- Abnormal thoracic mechanics: hemothorax, pneumothorax, flail chest, large effusion, abdominal distension
- Neuromuscular diseases: neuropathy, myopathy
- Depression of respiratory centers: medications, toxins, brain injury, obesity hypoventilation, CNS infection
- Mechanical ventilator
- Increased CO_2 production: malignant hyperthermia, hypermetabolism, high-carbohydrate diet
- Metabolic: hypermagnesemia, hypokalemia

Table App.2.6 Causes of respiratory alkalosis

- Pulmonary disease: pulmonary edema, right-to-left cardiac shunt, high-altitude pulmonary edema, pulmonary embolism, acute lung injury, pneumonia
- Mechanical ventilation
- Stimulation of respiratory center: CNS infection, CVA, pregnancy, sepsis, hepatic encephalopathy, anxiety
- Medications: salicylates, SSRI, progesterone
- Hypoxemic drive
- Pain

Cases

1. A 55-year-old female presents with shortness of breath. Lab values are as follows: pH 7.32, $PaCO_2$ 24 mmHg, PaO_2 95 mmHg, Na = 135 mmol/L, K = 4.5 mmol/L, Cl^- = 101 mmol/L, HCO_3^- = 20 mmol/L. What is the acid–base disorder?

Step 1
Calculated $[H^+]$ = 24 × ($PaCO_2/[HCO_3^-]$) = 24 × (24/20) = 29
Expected $[H^+]$ based on Table App. 2.1 is ~47
Therefore, there is an inconsistency in the data.

2. A 32-year-old patient with type 1 diabetes mellitus presents with cough, fever, productive sputum, and nausea and vomiting. Lab values are as follows: pH 7.6, $PaCO_2$ 21 mmHg, PaO_2 60 mmHg, Na = 136 mmol/L, K = 4.6 mmol/L, Cl^- = 80 mmol/L, HCO_3^- = 19 mmol/L. What is the acid–base disorder?

Step 1
Calculated $[H^+]$ = 24 × ($PaCO_2/[HCO_3^-]$) = 24 × (21/19) = 26
Expected $[H^+]$ based on Table App.2.1 is 25
Therefore, the data are consistent.

Step 2
Based on the pH of 7.6, this suggests alkalemia and the source is respiratory, given a low $PaCO_2$ of 21 mmHg.

Step 5
Expected decrease in HCO_3^- from normal for an acute process is
(40 − $PaCO_2$) × 0.2 = 4. Thus the expected HCO_3^- is (22 − 4) = 18.
Expected decrease in HCO_3 from normal for a chronic process is
(40 − $PaCO_2$) × 0.4 = 8. Thus the expected HCO_3^- is (22 − 8) = 14.
Measured HCO_3^- is 19, which suggests an acute respiratory process.

Step 6
The AG is elevated at 37, which indicates an underlying anion gap metabolic acidosis (DKA). The delta gap is elevated at 10, indicating a metabolic alkalosis (emesis) as well.

Thus the patient has acute respiratory alkalosis, anion-gap acidosis, and a metabolic alkalosis.

CT anatomy of the thorax

Mediastinal window

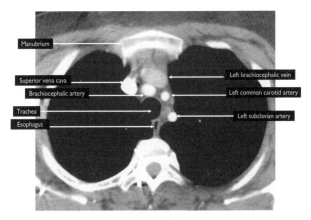

Figure App.3.1 Level of head and neck vessels.

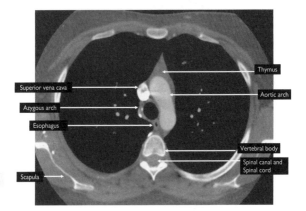

Figure App.3.2 Level of aortic arch.

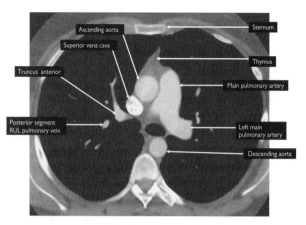

Figure App. 3.3 Level of left main pulmonary artery. RUL, right upper lobe.

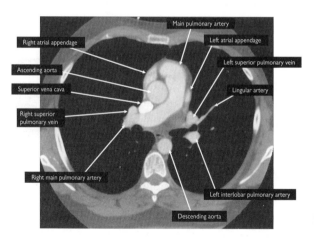

Figure App. 3.4 Level of right main pulmonary artery.

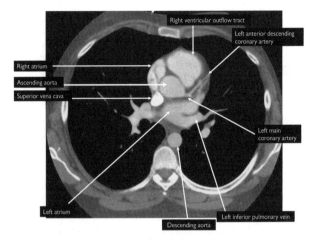

Figure App. 3.5 Level of right ventricular outflow tract.

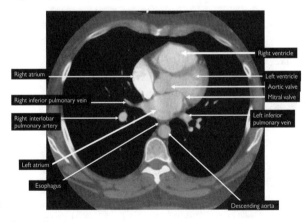

Figure App.3.6 Level of aortic valve.

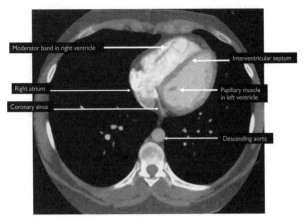

Figure App. 3.7 Level of coronary sinus.

Lung window

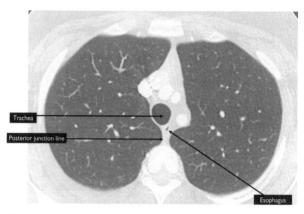

Figure App. 3.8 Level of trachea.

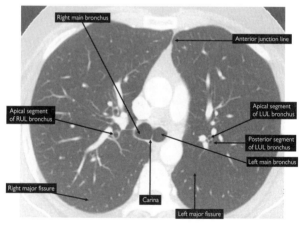

Figure App. 3.9 Level of carina. LUL, left upper lobe; RUL, right upper lobe.

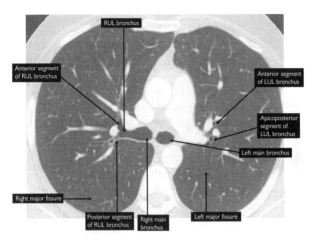

Figure App. 3.10 Level of bifurcation of right upper lobe (RUL) bronchus. LUL, left upper lobe.

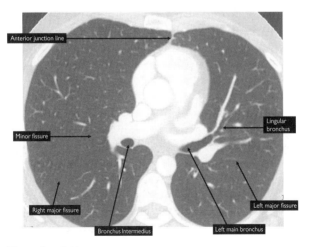

Figure App. 3.11 Level of lingular bronchus.

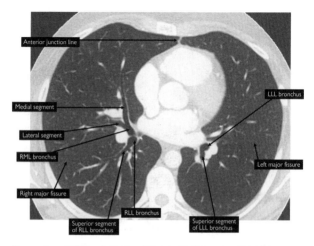

Figure App. 3.12 Level of right middle lobe (RML) bronchus. LLL, left lower lobe; RLL, right lower lobe.

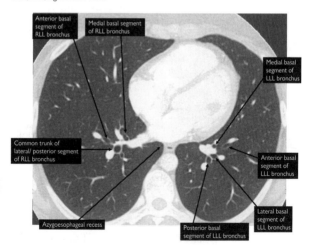

Figure App. 3.13 Level of basal segmental bronchi. LLL, left lower lobe; RLL, right lower lobe.

CT patterns of lung disease

CT patterns of lung disease

Findings	Causes
Air space consolidation: Fluid (pus, blood, or water), secretion, or cells in the alveoli	1. Acute: Pneumonia, pulmonary edema or hemorrhage, ARDS, AIP, aspiration, acute radiation pneumonitis, acute hypersensitivity pneumonitis 2. Chronic: COP, eosinophilic pneumonia, neoplasm (BAC, lymphoma), TB/fungal infection, alveolar proteinosis, lipoid pneumonia
Mosaic attenuation: Sharply demarcated, geographic differences in lung attenuation (darker and lighter regions) as compared to normal	Ground-glass infiltrative disease (abnormal areas of increased attenuation without bronchovascular obscuration): 1. Acute: Pneumonia (atypical, viral, CMV, or *Pneumocystis jiroveci*), pulmonary edema or hemorrhage, ARDS, AIP, acute radiation pneumonitis 2. Chronic: COP, eosinophilic pneumonia, neoplasm (BAC, lymphoma), hypersensitivity pneumonitis (acute and subacute), collagen vascular disease, cellular NSIP, DIP, respiratory bronchiolitis/RB-ILD, alveolar proteinosis, lipoid pneumonia
	Mosaic perfusion (abnormal areas of decreased attenuation due to decreased perfusion): 1. Vascular: • Chronic pulmonary embolism • Pulmonary arterial hypertension from other causes: obstructive sleep apnea, COPD/emphysema, pulmonary venoocclusive disease, high altitude, *Schistosomiasis*, vasculitis (lupus, rheumatoid disease, scleroderma, polymyositis, Churg–Strauss, Wegener's), cardiac shunt (VSD, ASD, PDA, PAPVR), hepatopulmonary syndrome, AIDS 2. Airway disease: infectious bronchiolitis, constrictive bronchiolitis, asthma, cystic fibrosis
Predominantly upper lobe process	Centrilobular emphysema, radiation injury or fibrosis, sarcoidosis, silicosis, berylliosis, talcosis, TB/fungal infection, chronic hypersensitivity pneumonitis, respiratory bronchiolitis/RB-ILD, Langerhans cell histiocytosis, cystic fibrosis, ankylosing spondylitis
Predominantly lower lobe process	UIP, IPF, fibrotic NSIP, asbestosis, collagen vascular disease, drug-induced (amiodarone, methotrexate, cyclophosphamide, bleomycin), neurofibromatosis, lipoid pneumonia
Predominantly peripheral process	UIP, NSIP, COP, eosinophilic pneumonia, pulmonary contusion or trauma, pulmonary infarct
Predominantly central (perihilar) process	Sarcoidosis, silicosis, berylliosis, talcosis, large airway disease (cystic fibrosis)

Thickened interlobular septae or Kerley's lines	Hydrostatic pulmonary edema or hemorrhage, pneumonia (viral or mycoplasmal), lymphangitic carcinomatosis, lymphoma, leukemia, Kaposi's sarcoma, alveolar proteinosis
Crazy-paving pattern: Interlobular septal thickening and superimposed ground-glass opacity	Alveolar proteinosis, pulmonary edema or hemorrhage, pneumonia (atypical, viral, CMV, or *Pneumocystis jiroveci*), cellular NSIP, COP, chronic eosinophilic pneumonia, BAC, subacute hypersensitivity pneumonitis
Nodules: small, discrete, rounded opacities, generally of 2–10 mm in diameter, in the alveoli or interstitium	Metastases, sarcoidosis, pneumoconiosis, hypersensitivity pneumonitis, Langerhans cell histiocytosis, miliary TB, fungal or varicella infection, alveolar microlithiasis, amyloidosis
Perilymphatic nodules: Distributed along the pulmonary lymphatics (peribronchovascular, centrilobular, surrounding the secondary lobules, and along the pleura)	Sarcoidosis, lymphangitic carcinomatosis, lymphoma, Kaposi's sarcoma
Poorly defined centrilobular nodules: Peribronchiolar or periarteriolar inflammation	1. Infectious bronchiolitis (viral or mycoplasmal) 2. Hypersensitivity pneumonitis (no smoking history) 3. Smoking-related disease: respiratory bronchiolitis/RB-ILD, Langerhans cell histiocytosis, DIP 4. Follicular bronchiolitis (collagen vascular disease) 5. Vasculitis
Tree-in-bud pattern: Mucus, pus, or secretion filling the dilated bronchioles	Bronchopneumonia, panbronchiolitis/Asian bronchiolitis, asthma, cystic fibrosis, endobronchial TB or MAI, allergic bronchopulmonary aspergillosis
Cysts: Small air-containing spaces with thin (<5 mm) walls	Paraseptal emphysema, UIP (honeycombing cysts), LAM (female, uniformed cysts), tuberous sclerosis (male), Langerhans cell histiocytosis (different sizes and shapes), *Pneumocystis jiroveci* pneumonia, LIP (collagen vascular disease, HIV), pneumatoceles (prior infection), cystic bronchiectasis
Cavity: A collection of air and/or fluid, with thick (>5 mm) wall	Neoplasm (sarcoma, squamous cell), infection (bacterial, TB, fungal), autoimmune/collagen vascular disease (rheumatoid nodules, Caplan's syndrome, Wegener's), traumatic lung cyst, congenital (CPAM), papillomatosis/HPV

BMI calculator
and height converter

BMI calculator

Height in metres

Weight (kg)	1.36	1.40	1.44	1.48	1.52	1.56	1.60	1.64	1.68	1.72	1.76	1.80	1.84	1.88	1.92	1.96	2.00
125	68	64	60	57	54	51	49	46	44	42	40	39	37	35	34	33	31
123	67	63	59	56	53	51	48	46	44	42	40	38	36	35	33	32	31
121	65	62	58	55	52	50	47	45	43	41	39	37	36	34	33	31	30
119	64	61	57	54	52	49	46	44	42	40	38	37	35	34	32	31	30
117	63	60	56	53	51	48	46	44	41	40	38	36	35	33	32	30	29
115	62	59	55	53	50	47	45	43	41	39	37	35	34	33	31	30	29
113	61	58	54	52	49	46	44	42	40	38	36	35	33	32	31	29	28
111	60	57	54	51	48	46	43	41	39	38	36	34	33	31	30	29	28
109	59	56	53	50	47	45	43	41	39	37	35	34	32	31	30	28	27
107	58	55	52	49	46	44	42	40	38	36	35	33	32	30	29	28	27
105	57	54	51	48	45	43	41	39	37	35	34	32	31	30	28	27	26
103	56	53	50	47	45	42	40	38	36	35	33	32	30	29	28	27	26
101	55	52	49	46	44	42	39	38	36	34	33	31	30	29	27	26	25
99	54	51	48	45	43	41	39	37	35	33	32	31	29	28	27	26	25
97	52	49	47	44	42	40	38	36	34	33	31	30	28	27	26	25	24
95	51	48	46	43	41	39	37	35	34	32	31	29	28	27	26	25	24
93	50	47	45	42	40	38	36	35	33	31	30	29	27	26	25	24	23
91	49	46	44	42	39	37	36	34	32	31	29	28	27	26	25	24	23
89	48	45	43	41	39	37	35	33	32	30	29	27	26	25	24	23	22
87	47	44	42	40	38	36	34	32	31	29	28	27	26	25	24	23	22
85	46	43	41	39	37	35	33	32	30	29	27	26	25	24	23	22	21
83	45	42	40	38	36	34	32	31	29	28	27	26	25	23	23	22	21
81	44	41	39	37	35	33	32	30	29	27	26	25	24	23	22	21	20
79	43	40	38	36	34	32	31	29	28	27	26	25	24	22	21	21	20
77	42	39	37	35	33	32	30	29	27	26	25	24	23	22	21	20	19
75	41	38	36	34	32	31	29	28	27	25	24	23	22	21	20	20	19
73	39	37	35	33	32	30	29	27	26	25	24	23	22	21	20	19	18
71	38	36	34	32	31	29	28	26	25	24	23	22	21	20	19	18	18
69	37	35	33	32	30	28	27	26	24	23	22	21	20	20	18	18	17
67	36	34	32	31	29	28	26	25	24	23	22	21	20	19	18	17	17
65	35	33	31	30	28	27	25	24	23	22	21	20	19	18	18	17	16
63	34	32	30	29	27	26	25	23	22	21	20	19	19	18	17	16	16
61	33	31	29	28	26	25	24	23	22	21	20	19	18	17	17	16	15
59	32	30	28	27	26	24	23	22	21	20	19	18	17	17	16	15	15
57	31	29	27	26	25	23	22	21	20	19	18	18	17	16	15	15	14
55	30	28	27	25	24	23	21	20	19	18	17	16	16	15	14	14	14
53	29	27	26	24	23	22	21	20	19	18	17	16	16	15	14	14	13
51	28	26	25	23	22	21	20	19	18	17	16	16	15	14	14	13	13
49	26	25	24	22	21	20	19	18	17	16	16	15	14	14	13	13	12
47	25	24	23	21	20	19	18	17	16	16	15	15	14	13	13	12	12
45	24	23	22	21	19	18	18	17	16	15	15	14	13	13	12	12	11
43	23	22	21	20	19	18	17	16	15	15	14	13	13	12	12	11	11

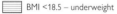

- BMI <18.5 – underweight
- BMI 18.5–24.9 – acceptable weight
- BMI 25–29.9 – overweight
- BMI 30–39.9 – obese
- BMI >= 40 – morbid obesity

Height converter

Height (ft and in)	Height (m)
5'0"	1.52
5'1"	1.55
5'2"	1.58
5'3"	1.60
5'4"	1.63
5'5"	1.65
5'6"	1.68
5'7"	1.70
5'8"	1.73
5'9"	1.75
5'10"	1.78
5'11"	1.80
6'0"	1.83
6'1"	1.85
6'2"	1.88
6'3"	1.90
6'4"	1.93
6'5"	1.96
6'6"	1.98

Index

FEV₁/VC Caucasian <u>MALES</u> courtesy of Vitalograph

Prediction Nomogram

MALES ○↗ BTPS

Height		FVC	FEV₁	Age
(cm)	(inches)	(liter)	(liter)	(years)

```
190 ┬          ┬    ┬         ┬ 20
    ├ 74       │    │         │
    ├ 73       │    │         │
    ├          ┼ 6  │         │
    ├ 72       │    ┼ 5       │
180 ┼ 71       │    │         ┼ 30
    ├ 70       │    │         │
    ├ 69       │    │         │
    ├          ┼ 5  │         │
    ├ 68       │    ┼ 4       │
170 ┼ 67       │    │         ┼ 40
    ├ 66       │    │         │
    ├          ┼    │         │
    ├ 65       │    │         │
    ├ 64       ┼ 4  ┼ 3       │
160 ┼ 63       │    │         ┼ 50
    ├ 62       │    │         │
    ├ 61       │    │         │
    ├          ┼ 3  │         │
    ├ 60       │    ┼ 2       │
150 ┼ 59       │    │         ┼ 60
    ├ 58       │    │         │
    ├ 57       │    │         │
    ├          ┼ 2  │         │
    ├ 56       │    │         │
140 ┴          ┴    ┴         ┴ 70
```